Transfusion Therapy: Clinical Principles and Practice

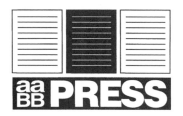

Other related publications available from the AABB:

Transfusion Support in Patients With Sickle Cell Disease
By Wendell F. Rosse, MD; Marilyn J. Telen, MD; and Russell E. Ware, MD, PhD

Cellular Characteristics of Cord Blood and Cord Blood Transplantation
Edited by Hal E. Broxmeyer, PhD

Apheresis: Principles and Practice
Edited by Bruce C. McLeod, MD; Thomas H. Price, MD; and Mary Jo Drew, MD

Cytokines in Transfusion Medicine: A Primer
Edited by Robertson D. Davenport, MD, and Edward L. Snyder, MD

New Directions in Pediatric Hematology
Edited by Steven M. Capon, MD, and Linda A. Chambers, MD

Transfusion Reactions
Edited by Mark A. Popovsky, MD

Introduction to Transfusion Medicine: A Case Study Approach
By Elaine K. Jeter, MD, and Mary Ann Spivey, MHS, MT(ASCP)SBB

To purchase books, please call our sales department at (301)215-6499, fax orders to (301)907-6895, or email orders to sales@aabb.org. View the AABB Publications Catalog and order books on the AABB Website at www.aabb.org. For other book services, including chapter reprints and large quantity sales, ask for the Senior Sales Associate.

Transfusion Therapy: Clinical Principles and Practice

Editor

Paul D. Mintz, MD
University of Virginia Health Sciences Center
Charlottesville, Virginia

AABB Press
Bethesda, Maryland
1999

American Association of Blood Banks
8101 Glenbrook Road
Bethesda, Maryland 20814-2749

ISBN NO. 1-56395-099-5
Printed in the United States

Library of Congress Cataloging-in-Publication Data

Transfusion therapy : clinical principles and practice / editor, Paul D. Mintz.
p. cm.
Includes bibliographical references and index.
ISBN 1-56395-099-5
1. Blood—Transfusion. 2. Blood products—Therapeutic use. 3. Anemia—Treatment.
I. Mintz, Paul D. [DNLM: 1. Blood Transfusion. WB 356 T77405 1998]
RM171.T723 1998 615'.39—dc21
DNLM/DLC
for Library of Congress

98-42095
CIP

Contributors

James P. AuBuchon, MD
Dartmouth-Hitchcock Medical Center
Lebanon, New Hampshire

Linda A. Chambers, MD
The Ohio State University School of Medicine;
and Children's Hospital
Columbus, Ohio

Robertson Davenport, MD
University of Michigan Medical School
University of Michigan Hospitals
Ann Arbor, Michigan

Sunny Dzik, MD
Harvard Medical School
Beth Israel-Deaconess Medical Center
Boston, Massachusetts

Anne Eder, MD, PhD
University of Pennsylvania School of Medicine
Hospital of the University of Pennsylvania
Philadelphia, Pennsylvania

Richard C. Friedberg, MD, PhD
University of Alabama at Birmingham
Birmingham Veterans Affairs Medical Center
Birmingham, Alabama

Lawrence T. Goodnough, MD
Washington University Medical Center
St. Louis, Missouri

Jed Gorlin, MD
University of Minnesota School of Medicine
Memorial Blood Centers of Minnesota
Minneapolis, Minnesota

Jay H. Herman, MD
Temple University School of Medicine
Temple University Hospital
Philadelphia, Pennsylvania

John Humphries, MD
University of Virginia Health Sciences Center
Charlottesville, Virginia

Leigh C. Jefferies, MD
University of Pennsylvania School of Medicine
Hospital of the University of Pennsylvania
Philadelphia, Pennsylvania

Elaine K. Jeter, MD
University of South Carolina School of
Medicine and Providence Hospital
Columbia, South Carolina

Harvey G. Klein, MD
National Institutes of Health
Bethesda, Maryland

Jong-Hoon Lee, MD
Center for Biologics Evaluation and Research
Food and Drug Administration
Rockville, Maryland

Naomi L.C. Luban, MD
George Washington University School of
Medicine
Children's Hospital National Medical Center
Washington, DC

Jeanne Lusher, MD
Wayne State University School of Medicine
Children's Hospital of Michigan
Detroit, Michigan

Jay E. Menitove, MD
University of Missouri-Kansas City School of
Medicine
Kansas University School of Medicine
Community Blood Center of Greater Kansas City
Kansas City, Missouri

John P. Miller, MD, PhD
American Red Cross Blood Services
Cleveland, Ohio

Paul D. Mintz, MD
University of Virginia Health Sciences Center
Charlottesville, Virginia

Glenn Ramsey, MD
Northwestern University Medical School
Northwestern Memorial Hospital
Chicago, Illinois

Bruce I. Sharon, MD
University of Illinois College of Medicine
University of Illinois Hospital
Chicago, Illinois

Richard K. Spence, MD
State University of New York Health Sciences
Center at Brooklyn
Brooklyn, New York

William D. Spotnitz, MD
University of Virginia Health Sciences Center
Charlottesville, Virginia

E. Richard Stiehm, MD
UCLA Children's Hospital
UCLA Medical Center
Los Angeles, California

Ronald G. Strauss, MD
University of Iowa College of Medicine
DeGowin Blood Center
Iowa City, Iowa

Roseanne Welker, PhD
University of Virginia Health Sciences Center
Charlottesville, Virginia

Carolyn F. Whitsett, MD
Emory University School of Medicine
Crawford Long Hospital
Atlanta, Georgia

Table of Contents

Preface

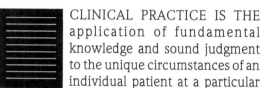CLINICAL PRACTICE IS THE application of fundamental knowledge and sound judgment to the unique circumstances of an individual patient at a particular moment. No set of rules can be written to apply to the constellation of variables that will be present when a physician is confronted with a therapeutic decision. Rather, guidance may be offered to direct practices in typical settings. The intent of this book is to provide assistance to clinicians who need to decide whether to prescribe a blood component transfusion.

The information necessary to define precisely when a transfusion should be given is not available. We do not know myocardial cell mitochondrial pO_2. We do not know the delivery of oxygen to the myocardium or other organs or tissues. Furthermore, we do not know their precise oxygen requirements. We do not know the exact concentration of platelets or each coagulation factor required to prevent bleeding in any particular circumstance. We do not know how to quantify associated benefits of transfusion, such as the contribution to hemostasis of raising a patient's hematocrit. We use surrogate measurements to guide us. For example, almost all guidelines for red blood cell transfusion use hemoglobin concentration as an indication for therapy. Yet, this measurement does not tell us the oxygen delivery or requirement for any organ or tissue or for the patient as a whole. Because of these limitations, a book that offers practical suggestions will be useful for clinicians.

It is not surprising that the editor of a book with 27 authors will encounter informed differences of opinion. I have tried to provide a unified text by addressing specific topics only once and cross-referencing the subjects from other chapters. For example, gamma irradiation of blood components to prevent transfusion-associated graft-vs-host disease in neonates is addressed in the chapter on blood irradiation and not in the pediatric transfusion chapter. Needless to say, a number of discussions among authors occurred to ensure concurrence with the text. Where genuine differences of opinion exist and variations in clinical or laboratory practice are found, these are noted.

This book is intended to fill a niche between the weightier compendia and the handbooks already available. The emphasis of the text is on clinical practices with some pathophysiology included to support recommendations. A pleasant surprise of electronic publishing has been the ability to include in the text and references some reports published only 10 weeks before the book's scheduled publication date.

I thank each of the authors for their capable and diligent work as well as their patience with me. I am particularly grateful for the expert editorial assistance of Laura Henning in the Office of the AABB Press and my indefatiguable and talented secretary, Susan Bywaters, who has mastered the art of gentle patience amidst turbulance.

I hope that physicians will find practical and useful information in this book. The intended audience is clinicians who prescribe blood transfusions; although I hope specialists in transfusion medicine and other health-care professionals will find the text helpful as well. I welcome comments and suggestions from readers.

Paul D. Mintz, MD
Editor
pdm2q@virginia.edu

Note: All drug doses given in this book are intended as guidelines only. Doses should be adjusted according to the clinical status, weight, and age of the patient.

About the Editor

 Paul D. Mintz, MD, is Associate Chair and Professor of Pathology, Professor of Internal Medicine, and Director of the Clinical Laboratories and Blood Bank at the University of Virginia Health Sciences Center in Charlottesville, Virginia. Dr. Mintz received his medical degree from the University of Rochester School of Medicine.

Dr. Mintz is a member of the Board of Directors of the American Association of Blood Banks (AABB) serving as District Director for the Mid-Atlantic region. He has been on many national and regional committees of blood banking organizations including the AABB's Standards Committee as well as its Scientific Section Coordinating Committee. He is a former Chair of both the AABB Transfusion Practices Committee and the Committee on the Circular of Information. Dr. Mintz was the recipient of a Transfusion Medicine Academic Award from the National Heart, Lung, and Blood Institute as well as a grant from the National Blood Foundation. He is a former President of the Mid-Atlantic Association of Blood Banks and is a recipient of the Association's Charles E. Walter Memorial Award.

Dr. Mintz has published numerous journal articles related to blood component collection, preservation, and transfusion. He is a member of the Editorial Board of the *American Journal of Clinical Pathology* and has served as a Contributing Editor for the *Yearbook of Pathology and Laboratory Medicine*. Dr. Mintz previously edited *Transfusion Medicine*, a two-volume edition of *Hematology/Oncology Clinics of North America.*

In: Mintz PD, ed.
Transfusion Therapy: Clinical Principles and Practice
Bethesda, MD: AABB Press, 1999

1

Red Cell Transfusion Therapy in Chronic Anemia

JAY E. MENITOVE, MD

 RED CELL TRANSFUSIONS AUG-
ment oxygen-carrying capacity and are
indicated for patients with abnormally
low hemoglobin concentration/hema-
tocrit measurements whose physiologic compensatory mechanisms are inadequate or at the verge of
becoming inadequate. Currently, a physician's decision to order red cell transfusions rests on clinical
judgment, an interpretation of laboratory test results, and a balancing of transfusion-associated
risks against the benefits derived from increasing
the hemoglobin concentration. In patients with
compensated chronic, normovolemic anemia, appropriate pharmacologic intervention such as iron,
folate, vitamin B_{12}, or erythropoietin administration should precede transfusion. This reflects a concern about transfusion-associated complications
that include infection transmission, alloimmunization, immunohematologic reactions, and allergic
reactions. A transfusion avoidance strategy pre-
sumes that patient monitoring and medical judgment alert physicians to the need for transfusion
before clinical deterioration occurs. For this reason, this chapter begins with a discussion of oxygen
transport and physiologic adaptation mechanisms
in anemic patients, followed by a review of clinical
and experimental observations in these patients. It
concludes with a description of the several contem-
poraneous guidelines addressing red cell transfusion practice.

Jay E. Menitove, MD, Executive Director and Medical Director, Community Blood Center of Greater Kansas City, Clini-cal Professor of Medicine, University of Missouri, Kansas City, Missouri, and Kansas City School of Medicine, and Kan-sas University - School of Medicine, Kansas City, Kansas

Oxygen Transport Physiology

The principal determinants of oxygen transport are hemoglobin concentration and oxygen saturation, cardiac output, oxygen extraction, and organ blood flow. Oxygen delivery to the whole body or to specific organs varies according to the product of blood flow or cardiac output and arterial oxygen content.[1-3] The principal formula and normal ranges related to oxygen transport are provided in Table 1-1. By substituting the equation for arterial oxygen content in the equation for oxygen delivery, it is evident that cardiac output and hemoglobin concentration become the major variables determining tissue oxygen delivery.

Hemoglobin Concentration and Oxygen Saturation

Hemoglobin consists of two alpha and two beta chains that each bind heme groups containing a porphyrin ring and iron atom.[1,4] The binding relationship between hemoglobin and oxygen follows a sigmoid shape, the oxyhemoglobin dissociation curve. The P_{50} defines the oxygen tension at which 50% of hemoglobin-oxygen binding sites are saturated. Normally, this is 26.3 mm Hg, but it varies in response to changes in carbon dioxide tension; pH; 2,3-bisphosphoglycerate concentration; and temperature.

When carbon dioxide binds to hemoglobin, the pH decreases (Bohr effect) and the binding affinity of hemoglobin for oxygen declines, leading to a higher P_{50}. Increasing the pH leads to tighter oxygen binding. Hemoglobin-oxygen affinity varies inversely and the P_{50} increases directly with red cell 2,3-bisphosphoglycerate content. The P_{50} increases during anemia, hypoxia, or alkalosis when glycolysis is stimulated. Fever or other causes of body temperature elevation, such as exercise, decrease the affinity of hemoglobin for oxygen.

Cardiac Output

The major determinants of cardiac output—the measure of blood flow to the body per minute—include stroke volume and heart rate.[1,5-7] Stroke volume relates directly to cardiac filling pressures, arterial pressure and peripheral resistance, and cardiac contractility force. Myocardial oxygen con-

Table 1-1. Oxygen Transport Formulas

Parameter	Formula	Normal Range
Cardiac output (CO)	Stroke volume × Heart rate	4-6 L/min
Arterial oxygen content (CaO_2)	$1.34 \times Hgb \times SaO_2 + (0.003 \times PaO_2)$*†‡	16-22 mL/dL
Mixed venous oxygen content ($C\overline{v}O_2$)	$1.34 \times Hgb \times S\overline{v}O_2 + (0.003 \times P\overline{v}O_2)$*§‖	12-17 mL/dL
Oxygen delivery ($\dot{D}O_2$)	$CO \times CaO_2 \times 10$	500-750 mL/min/m^2
Oxygen consumption ($\dot{V}O_2$)	$CO \times (CaO_2 - C\overline{v}O_2) \times 10$	100-180 mL/min/m^2
Oxygen extraction ratio	$\dot{V}O_2 / \dot{D}O_2$	0.23 - 0.30

*Hgb = hemoglobin concentration in g/dL

†SaO_2 = arterial oxygen saturation

‡PaO_2 = arterial oxygen tension

§$S\overline{v}O_2$ = mixed venous oxygen saturation

‖$P\overline{v}O_2$ = mixed venous oxygen tension

sumption correlates predominantly with contracting myocyte needs and, to a lesser extent, changes in volume. Oxygen delivery to myocardial tissue depends on increasing the coronary blood flow.[8]

Oxygen Extraction

With the exception of the heart, tissue oxygen delivery exceeds resting demand by approximately fourfold.[1,7-9] Assuming a normal cardiac output of 5 L per minute in a patient with a hemoglobin concentration of 15 g/dL, oxygen delivery is approximately 1000 mL per minute. The corresponding oxygen consumption rate ranges from 200 to 300 mL per minute. At a hemoglobin concentration of 10 g/dL, oxygen delivery approximates 680 mL per minute. Oxygen delivery falls to approximately 340 mL per minute when the hemoglobin concentration approaches 5 g/dL if cardiac output remains unchanged. Oxygen consumption remains independent of oxygen delivery above a threshold level but enters a dependent relationship when tissue hypoxia occurs. Available evidence suggests that the critical oxygen delivery rate ranges between 4 and 10 mL per minute per kilogram and may be higher in the presence of disease states that include sepsis and pulmonary dysfunction.

Organ Blood Flow

Arterial tone determines the blood flow to different organs. Changes in autonomic stimulation and vasodilating factors regulate the tone in medium-sized arterial vessels.[1] Responses to such changes correspond to the shunting of blood flow from capillary beds with lesser oxygen requirements to those in which oxygen demand is higher.[2,10-14]

Physiologic Adaptive Mechanisms in Anemia

Cardiac Output

Cardiac output increases in response to normovolemic anemia. Sympathetic nervous stimulation raises the heart rate, and changes in blood viscosity affect stroke volume by augmenting venous return to the heart and decreasing left ventricular afterload.

Increases in heart rate are not observed universally, however.[6,10,15] At rest, patients with chronic anemia have normal heart rates that, during submaximal exercise, increase more than those of patients without anemia.[6,10] During maximal exercise, the heart rate and cardiac output in patients with chronic anemia are lower than those in patients without anemia. Increasing the heart rate decreases diastole and thereby adversely affects myocardial perfusion. While this does not cause myocardial ischemia in most patients, those with coronary artery disease may be at risk.

Normovolemic hemodilution that occurs in chronic anemia results in decreased blood viscosity that is most pronounced in postcapillary venules. This, in turn, enhances venous return or left ventricular preload. In response, cardiac output increases in conjunction with decreased left ventricular afterload, another effect of decreased viscosity. Sympathetic stimulation may act synergistically via beta-adrenergic receptors to increase contractility.[15]

Coronary Artery Blood Flow

Myocardial oxygen extraction approaches 60-75% of oxygen delivered through the coronary circulation,[8,11,12,14,16] significantly exceeding the degree of oxygen removed by other organs. Oxygen delivery to the myocardium increases only through enhanced coronary artery blood flow.[12,17] If the coronary circulation is normal, diminution of hemoglobin concentration to 7g/dL is tolerated. In the presence of coronary stenosis, myocardial ischemia and dysfunction occur at higher hemoglobin levels in most but not all reports.[18-20]

Redistribution of Blood Flow

Studies involving acute hemodilution show alterations in the distribution of blood flow among various organs.[2,10] Cerebral blood flow increases when cardiac output is diverted to the cerebral circulation.[13] Shunting blood from high-flow, low-extraction areas to tissues with high oxygen requirements produces an oxygen reservoir. Such re-routing of blood potentially compensates for a one-third decrease in cardiac output or a 50% increase in oxygen requirements.[2,10] Unfortunately, this redistribution may result in gastrointestinal ischemia and septicemia.[1]

Increased Oxygen Extraction

Normally, peripheral tissues extract approximately one-quarter of the blood's oxygen-carrying capacity. This oxygen extraction of 25% increases threefold during stress.[9] In skeletal muscle during strenuous exercise, oxygen extraction may rise to 80-90% of available oxygen.[2,21,22]

Increased Red Cell 2,3-Bisphosphoglycerate

Oxygen delivery to tissues increases up to 18% as a result of a rightward shift in the oxyhemoglobin dissociation curve following increased production of 2,3-bisphosphoglycerate.[5] Another rightward shift in the dissociation curve follows pH decreases. However, significant changes in pH must occur to alter red cell oxygen affinity. Thus, the Bohr effect has minimal clinical significance.[1]

The principal physiologic adaptive mechanisms in anemia are listed in Table 1-2.

Clinical and Experimental Observations in Anemia

The background information about oxygen transport and physiologic adaptive mechanisms in anemia provides evidence that adequate compensatory mechanisms exist to prevent mortality and morbidity in patients with markedly reduced hemoglobin concentrations. Several randomized clinical trials and a few observational reports provide data for determining the hemoglobin concentration levels at which anemia is tolerated without the need for transfusion. Most of these studies involve patients suffering blood loss during cardiac surgery, hip replacement surgery, or trauma. Others investigate patients in intensive care settings, undergoing pre-

---

Table 1-2. Physiologic Adaptive Mechanisms in Anemia

Increased cardiac output
- Increased heart rate (predominant mechanism)
- Increased stroke volume

Increased coronary artery blood flow
- Impaired in patients with stenotic lesions

Redistribution of blood flow
- Shunting blood flow from high-flow, low-extraction areas to tissues with high oxygen requirements

Increased oxygen extraction
- Oxygen extraction percentage increases from 0.25 to 0.75

Increased red cell 2,3-bisphosphoglycerate
- Rightward shift in oxyhemoglobin dissociation curve increases oxygen off-loading to tissues

operative normovolemic hemodilution, or refusing transfusion because of religious reasons. The principal signs and symptoms of anemia are dyspnea, tachypnea, tachycardia, angina, postural hypotension, syncope, and transient ischemic attacks.

Randomized Studies

In one randomized study involving patients undergoing coronary artery bypass graft surgery,[23] the hematocrit was maintained at 25% in 20 patients and at 32% in another 18 patients. The mean cardiac index was the same in the operating room and on the first postoperative day. No relation occurred between exercise tolerance and hematocrit on the fifth and sixth postoperative days. The group transfused at a hematocrit of 25% received 1.0 unit of blood compared with 2.05 units for the group transfused at a higher level. The hospital length of stay was similar for both groups, and no differences were observed in hemodynamic parameters.

In another study involving patients undergoing coronary artery bypass graft surgery,[24] a group of 13 patients received red cell transfusions if their hemoglobin concentration fell below 12 g/dL. Another 14 patients received red cells when their hemoglobin concentration was below 7 g/dL. The authors reported no differences in morbidity, mortality, or exercise tolerance. However, higher myocardial lactate levels, indicating myocardial ischemia, occurred in the patients who were transfused at the lower hemoglobin level.

Another study among patients suffering acute injury and hemorrhage, randomly assigned 13 patients to receive transfusions when the hematocrit was 40% and 12 patients to receive transfusions when the hematocrit was 30%.[25] Only physiologic measurements were conducted, and no differences in hemodynamic parameters occurred. Oxygen extraction was significantly lower in the high hematocrit group, 22.9% vs 28.5%. Since both values were less than 30%, oxygen delivery was considered adequate. However, oxygen consumption appeared to be more dependent on delivery in the 30% hematocrit group. The patients transfused at a hematocrit of 40% received five more units of red cells than patients in the other group.

Hébert et al[26] studied 69 normovolemic, critically ill patients in intensive care units in a randomized clinical trial. The hemoglobin concentration was maintained between 10 and 12 g/dL (average 10.6 g/dL) in 36 patients and between 7 and 9 g/dL (average 9.0 g/dL) in 33 patients. The group transfused at the lower hemoglobin level received 48% fewer red cells: 2.5 vs 4.8. The 30-day mortality rate was similar in both groups: 25% and 24%, respectively. Organ dysfunction scores were also similar.

The above reports, selected because they represent randomized studies, each contain small numbers of patients. For this reason, additional observational studies containing larger numbers of patients are cited below. Although the study designs are descriptive rather than comparative, inferences can be made about the ability to tolerate reduced hemoglobin levels.

Descriptive Studies

A review of published reports of patients refusing transfusion for religious reasons found few deaths attributed to anemia if the hemoglobin concentration was above 5 g/dL.[27]

In a retrospective cohort study involving 1958 surgical patients who declined blood transfusion for religious reasons, the 30-day mortality rate was 1.3% in patients with a preoperative hemoglobin concentration of 12 g/dL or greater compared with 33.3% in patients with a preoperative hemoglobin concentration of less than 6 g/dL.[19] Anemia accounted for 27.9% of the deaths, and cardiovascular disease accounted for 17.7%. The death rate was 10% among patients with cardiovascular disease, 4.3 times greater than that observed among patients without cardiovascular disease. However, a subsequent study conducted by the same investigators did not confirm the increased risk attributed to cardiovascular disease.[28] This latter study involved consecutive patients undergoing surgery to repair fractured hips and excluded patients who refused transfusion. Among patients whose hemoglobin concentration fell below 8 g/dL, 90.5% received postoperative transfusions compared with 55.6% of those with hemoglobin concentration levels between 8 and 10 g/dL. Patients with hemoglobin levels of 8 g/dL or higher had similar 30- and 90-postoperative-day mortality rates regardless of whether they received a transfusion. Because almost all patients whose hemoglobin was below 8 g/dL received a transfusion, the ability to determine the benefit of such transfusions was negated.

Isovolemic Hemodilution

Another approach to determining the consequences of anemia involves studies in which patients or volunteers are subjected to acute anemia via isovolemic hemodilution. Study subjects undergo phlebotomy with replacement of 5% human serum albumin solutions to retain isovolemia. The process of blood removal followed by volume replacement is continued until the target hemoglobin concentration is achieved. In a report published in 1998, 21 paid volunteers and 11 surgical patients participated in a study in which the hemoglobin concentration was reduced to 5 g/dL.[29] Their systemic vascular resistance index decreased by 58%, their heart rate increased from 58 to 92 beats per minute, their stroke volume index increased from 52 to 62 mL per minute, and their cardiac index increased from 3.05 to 5.71 L per minute. Increased heart rate accounted for 75% of the increased cardiac output; the other 25% was associated with increased stroke volume. Oxygen transport was considered adequate during the 2.4-hour duration of the experiments. The mean oxygen transport was 10.7 mL of oxygen per kilogram per minute when the hemoglobin was 5 g/dL. This suggests that the critical oxygen transport value is less than 10 mL of oxygen per kilogram per minute in normal humans at rest in the supine position when the hemoglobin concentration is 5 g/dL. Unfortunately, this study provides no information about patients with an inability to increase their cardiac output or flow to vital tissues or with an increased oxygen consumption associated with activity or other events.

Other investigators found that patients undergoing coronary artery bypass surgery with preserved ventricular function, ejection fraction greater than 50%, and hemoglobin levels as low as 5.8 g/dL did not experience myocardial ischemia so long as normal hemodynamics were maintained.[18] Animal studies provide evidence of myocardial ischemia at higher hemoglobin levels in the presence of coronary stenosis compared with conditions in which blood flow is not impaired.[11]

Effect of Chronic Anemia on Exercise Tolerance

The effect of chronic anemia on exercise tolerance has been the subject of several studies. Davies et al[30] evaluated African industrial workers with hemoglobin concentrations between 8 g/dL and 10 g/dL, those with hemoglobin levels below 8 g/dL, and normal control subjects with hemoglobin levels greater than 13 g/dL. Anemia was attributed to iron deficiency. When subjects exercised on a stationary bicycle ergometer, maximal aerobic power declined by 34% in the severely anemic group and by 24% in the moderately anemic group compared with the control subjects. During light work, heart rates were not different among the groups, but at higher workloads, the increases in heart rate and cardiac output were greater in anemic subjects.

Woodson[5] repeatedly withdrew 50-100 mL of blood from four normal volunteers until their hemoglobin dropped from an average of 14.8 g/dL to 9.9 g/dL. With the use of a treadmill protocol, the volunteers were studied for 10-14 days after anemia occurred. Maximal oxygen consumption fell in all four subjects by 16% during chronic anemia. Cardiac output at maximal oxygen consumption during established anemia was similar to control measurements and less than the 18-20% increase observed during acute anemia. The increase in cardiac output resulted from a 15-20% increase in heart rate. The percentage of oxygen extraction was greater during established anemia than during acute anemia. A linear relationship was found between hemoglobin concentration and maximal exercise capacity: a 20% decrease in hemoglobin produced a 12% decrement in exercise capacity.

In another study involving experimentally induced chronic anemia,[6] nine healthy subjects underwent repeated phlebotomies to decrease their hemoglobin from 14.6 g/dL to 11.0 g/dL. Following 8-11 weeks in the anemic state, their maximal cardiac output declined to 27.5 L per minute from a control value of 29.5 L per minute. The difference was attributed to a reduction in their maximal heart rate (178 beats per minute compared to 185). During the subjects' submaximal exercise in the anemic state, increased cardiac output occurred as a result of a raised heart rate, not stroke volume, and accounted for approximately 50% of the adaptive response. Increased oxygen extraction by peripheral tissues contributed significantly to the compensatory process; the mixed venous oxygen content was 4.9 mL/dL compared with 8.2 mL/dL. The investigators concluded that long-term anemia is associated with a decrease in heart rate and cardiac output compared with control levels at maximal exercise capacity and that a clear correlation exists between hemoglobin concentration and maximal oxygen uptake.

Hence, different adaptations to anemia occur in acute normovolemic hemodilution and chronic anemia. The extent to which studies involving acute lowering of the hemoglobin concentration can be extrapolated to patients with chronic anemia is uncertain.

The clinical studies discussed above are summarized in Table 1-3.

Quality of Life

An alternative approach to seeking a correlation between hemoglobin concentration and symptoms attributable to anemia involves studies in which exogenous erythropoietin is given to anemic patients and quality-of-life measurements are conducted.

In one observational study,[31] 304 patients with chronic renal failure undergoing hemodialysis received erythropoietin three times per week. The baseline 24% hematocrit increased to 34% in 130

patients. The percentage of patients able to carry on normal activities increased from 26 to 45, the percentage of those very or mostly active increased from 20 to 37, the percentage of those very full of energy increased from 26 to 45, and the percentage of those reporting low or no energy declined from 46 to 23. In another study involving patients with end-stage renal disease,[32] energy and activity levels improved in those patients whose hematocrits increased from less than 30% to 34-35%.

In a double-blind, randomized, placebo-controlled study,[33] 118 patients received placebo or two different erythropoietin doses. The hemoglobin concentration in the placebo group was 7.4 g/dL compared with 10.2 g/dL and 11.7 g/dL in the two groups receiving erythropoietin. Improvement in quality of life or exercise capacity did not differ in the two groups given erythropoietin, but those patients receiving erythropoietin had significantly improved scores for fatigue, physical symptoms, relationships, and depression when compared with the placebo group. The distance walked in the stress test also increased, but there was no improvement in the six-minute walk test.

Among patients with acquired immune deficiency syndrome (AIDS) with baseline hematocrits of 27-28%, those achieving a 3.9% hematocrit increase while treated with erythropoietin had an improvement in quality of life.[34] A double-blind, randomized, placebo-controlled study involving patients with malignancies evaluated the response to erythropoietin or placebo.[35] At baseline, the hematocrit was 29% in both groups. The hematocrit increased at least 6 percentage points in 58% of the erythropoietin-treated patients. Energy levels and ability to perform daily tasks as assessed by questionnaire improved in the erythropoietin treated group, but a statistically significant improvement in overall quality of life was not observed.

These studies show an improvement in subjective and some objective quality-of-life measurements as hemoglobin concentrations in chronically ill patients increase. They imply that a significant variance exists between the minimal hemoglobin level needed to maintain oxygen-carrying capacity and that needed for many daily activities. In light of

Table 1-3. Clinical Studies Involving the Effect of Chronic Anemia on Exercise Tolerance

Diagnosis	Study Design	Conclusion	Reference
Coronary artery bypass graft	Prospective, randomized	No adverse consequences found in patients receiving transfusions - hematocrit 25% vs 32%	Johnson et al, 1992[23]
Coronary artery bypass graft	Prospective, randomized	No difference in morbidity, mortality, or exercise tolerance - hemoglobin 7 vs 12 g/dL	Weisel et al, 1984[24]
Trauma	Prospective, randomized	Adequate tissue oxygenation hematocrit 30% vs 40%	Fortune et al, 1987[25]
Intensive care unit patients	Prospective, randomized	30-day mortality rate and organ dysfunction scores similar - hemoglobin 9.0 vs 10.6 g/dL	Hébert et al, 1995[26]
Jehovah's Witness patients	Retrospective review	Operative mortality increased if hemoglobin <5-6 g/dL	Carson et al, 1996[19] Viele and Weiskopf, 1994[27] Carson et al, 1998[28]
Isovolemic hemodilution	Prospective, observational	Hemoglobin 5 g/dL tolerated in resting, supine volunteers/patients	Weiskopf et al, 1998[29]
Chronic anemia	Prospective, observational	Exercise tolerance decreased for hemoglobin <8 g/dL vs 8-10 g/dL vs >13 g/dL	Davies et al, 1973[30]
Chronic anemia	Prospective, observational	Increased heart rate raises cardiac output; increased oxygen extraction	Woodson, 1984[5]
Chronic anemia	Prospective, observational	Increased heart rate raises cardiac output; increased oxygen extraction	Celsing et al, 1986[6]

the dramatic concern about transfusion-transmitted infections and other adverse consequences of transfusion, it is not surprising that current transfusion recommendations focus on minimal hemoglobin levels achieving acceptable tissue oxygen delivery.

Clinical Guidelines

Guidelines for transfusion advocated by several professional organizations reflect observed data and expert opinion. Of note, these recommendations and algorithms have been made in the absence of blinded, randomized, controlled studies.

In 1988, a National Institutes of Health Consensus Development Conference concluded that the decision to transfuse should include consideration of the duration of anemia and the presence of existing conditions that affect oxygen delivery, such as impaired pulmonary function, inadequate cardiac output, myocardial ischemia, or cerebrovascular or peripheral circulatory disease.[36] The conference panel noted that some patients with chronic anemia tolerate hemoglobin concentrations of less than 7 g/dL.

In 1992, the American College of Physicians published clinical guidelines addressing elective red cell transfusions.[37,38] These guidelines advise weighing the benefits of transfusion against the risks while considering the natural history of the patient's illness and the patient's expected survival. They contain a cautionary note to determine treatable causes of anemia and administer iron, folate, vitamin B_{12}, or erythropoietin, if appropriate. In the absence of signs or symptoms of anemia (syncope, dyspnea, tachypnea, tachycardia, angina, postural hypotension, or transient ischemic attack), transfusion should be avoided regardless of hemoglobin level. If symptoms occur, transfusions should be administered on a case-by-case basis. The guidelines also state that, in general, normovolemic anemia in which the hemoglobin concentration is 7-10 g/dL can be well tolerated in asymptomatic patients. Criticism of these guidelines has focused on a need to prevent symptoms rather than waiting for them to occur and selecting a strategy that minimizes the complexity of the decision-making process for prescribing transfusions.[39]

Practice guidelines issued by the American Society of Anesthesiologists[40] reference reports showing that oxygen delivery is adequate in most individuals at hemoglobin concentrations as low as 7 g/dL, that the heart does not begin to produce lactic acid until the hematocrit drops to 15-20%, and that heart failure usually does not begin until the hematocrit falls below 10%.[40] These guidelines note that chronic anemia is tolerated better than acute anemia. They conclude that red cell transfusion is rarely indicated when the hemoglobin concentration is greater than 10 g/dL and is almost always needed when the hemoglobin concentration is less than 6 g/dL.

The Canadian Expert Working Group issued guidelines for transfusion in 1997.[41,42] These guidelines reiterate the belief that otherwise healthy people at rest have few signs or symptoms of anemia when the hemoglobin concentration is greater than 7-8 g/dL. They note that dyspnea with exertion occurs at this hemoglobin level, that weakness occurs at a hemoglobin of 6 g/dL, that dyspnea at rest occurs at a hemoglobin of 3 g/dL, and that congestive heart failure often occurs when the hemoglobin concentration is 2-2.5 g/dL. When transfusion is given to treat chronic anemia, these guidelines suggest that the goal should be to avert inadequate tissue oxygenation or heart failure. Considerations for devising strategies for ongoing transfusion needs include an assessment of symptoms caused or aggravated by anemia, a determination of whether these signs or symptoms are alleviated by transfusion, the minimal hemoglobin level at which patients function satisfactorily, and an evaluation of the risk:benefit ratio that includes consideration of lifestyle factors, coexistence of other medical disorders, the likely duration of anemia, and the patient's prognosis.

Practice guidelines developed by the College of American Pathologists[43] indicate that red cell transfusions should be given to patients with chronic anemia to minimize symptoms and the risks of anemia. The guidelines indicate that these symptoms and risks occur at hemoglobin concentrations of 5-8 g/dL.

The University Health System Consortium[44] surveyed member institutions and reported in 1997 that 59% of their members used a hemoglobin of 8 g/dL or a hematocrit of 24% as the level for red cell transfusion in patients with chronic anemia, 25% used a hemoglobin of 7 g/dL or a hematocrit of 21%, and 16% used a hemoglobin of 9 g/dL and a hematocrit of 27%. Factors other than hemoglobin or hematocrit values, such as age, sex, rapidity of onset of anemia, physiologic adaptations, cardiopulmonary function, history of ischemic comorbidities, and signs and symptoms of anemia, made up the major criteria for considering the need for transfusion. Only 11% of consortium members used hemoglobin or hematocrit values alone as a justification for transfusion.

From a practical point of view, a reasonable strategy for patients requiring repetitive transfusions involves minimizing the inconvenience associated with repeat visits for red cell infusions. Most patients achieve a 1 g/dL hemoglobin or 3% hematocrit increase per unit given. In the absence of hemolysis, the hemoglobin and hematocrit values decline by a similar amount per week. Thus, an infusion of two units of red cells would provide a biweekly dose of red cells for patients totally lacking erythropoiesis.

The clinical guidelines discussed above are listed in Table 1-4.

Conclusion

Multiple physiologic mechanisms exist to compensate for the decrease in oxygen-carrying capacity associated with anemia. In patients without pulmonary, cardiac, coronary, cerebrovascular, or peripheral vascular disease, it appears that hemoglobin concentrations of approximately 8 g/dL (range= 7-9 g/dL) are tolerated albeit with diminished activity capacity. In patients with impairment of the

above-cited critical organs or tissues, higher hemoglobin concentrations may be necessary. The goal is to avoid complications associated with anemia while balancing the risks attributed to transfusion. To do this, clinicians must consider the patient's age, physiologic adaptations to anemia, cardiopulmonary function, ischemic comorbidities, prognosis, and hemoglobin/hematocrit values. When required, transfusion should be given on a unit-by-unit and a case-by-case basis. The expected outcome is ongoing avoidance of the significant signs and symptoms of anemia.

References

1. Hébert PC, Hu LQ, Biro GP. Review of physiologic mechanisms in response to anemia. Can Med Assoc J 1997;156:S27-40.
2. Finch CA, Lenfant C. Oxygen transport in man. N Engl J Med 1972;286:407-15.
3. Greenburg AG. A physiologic basis for red blood cell transfusion decisions. Am J Surg 1995;170:44S-8S.
4. Hsia C. Respiratory function of hemoglobin. N Engl J Med 1998;338:239-47.
5. Woodson RD. Hemoglobin concentration and exercise capacity. Am Rev Respir Dis 1984; 129:S72-5.
6. Celsing F, Nyström J, Pihlststedt P, et al. Effect of long-term anemia and retransfusion on central circulation during exercise. J Appl Physiol 1986;61:1358-62.
7. Levine E, Rosen A, Sehgal L, et al. Physiologic effects of acute anemia: Implications for a reduced transfusion trigger. Transfusion 1990; 30:11-4.
8. Messer JV, Neill WA. The oxygen of the human heart. Am J Cardiol 1962;9:384-94.
9. Wilkerson DK, Rosen AL, Gould SA, et al. Whole body oxygen extraction ratio as an indicator of cardiac status in anemia. Curr Surg 1988;45:214-7.
10. Woodson RD, Wills RE, Lenfant C. Effect of acute and established anemia on O_2 transport at rest, submaximal and maximal work. J Appl Physiol 1978;44:36-43.

Table 1-4. Clinical Guidelines for Transfusion in Patients With Chronic Anemia

Factors to consider
  Natural history of patient's illness
  Expected survival
  Rapidity of onset of anemia
  Physiologic adaptations
  Cardiopulmonary function
  History of ischemic comorbidities
  Signs and symptoms of anemia
  Hemoglobin/hematocrit values
Decision basis
  Case-by-case
  Unit-by-unit
Hemoglobin/hematocrit trigger
  8 g/dL/24% (range: 7g/dL/21% to
  9 g/dL/27%)

11. Case RB, Berlung E, Sarnoff SJ. Ventricular function. Am J Med 1955;18:397-405.
12. Jan KM, Chien S. Effect of hematocrit variations on coronary hemodynamics and oxygen utilization. Am J Physiol 1977;233:H106-13.
13. Tu YK, Liu HM. Effects of isovolemia on hemodynamics, cerebral perfusion, and cerebral vascular reactivity. Stroke 1996;27:441-5.
14. Jan KM, Heldman J, Chien S. Coronary hemodynamics and oxygen utilization after hematocrit variations in hemorrhage. Am J Physiol 1980;239:H326-32.
15. Spahn DR, Leone BJ, Reves JG, Pasch T. Cardiovascular and coronary physiology of acute isovolemic hemodilution: A review of non-oxygen-carrying and oxygen-carrying solutions. Anesth Analg 1994;78:1000-21.
16. Crystal GJ, Rooney MW, Salem MR. Myocardial blood flow and oxygen consumption during isovolemic hemodilution alone and in combination with adenosine-induced controlled hypotension. Anesth Analg 1988;67:539-47.
17. Spahn DR, Smith LR, Veronee CD, et al. Acute isovolemic hemodilution and blood transfusion. J Thorac Cardiovasc Surg 1993;105:694-704.
18. Doak GJ, Hall RI. Does hemoglobin concentration affect perioperative myocardial lactate flux in patients undergoing coronary artery bypass surgery? Anesth Analg 1995;80:910-6.
19. Carson JL, Duff A, Poses RM, et al. Effect of anemia and cardiovascular disease on surgical mortality and morbidity. Lancet 1996;348:1055-9.
20. Levy PS, Chavez RP, Crystal GJ, et al. Oxygen extraction ratio: A valid indicator of transfusion need in limited coronary vascular reserve? J Trauma 1992;32:769-74.
21. Viteri FE, Torún B. Anemia and physical work capacity. Clin Haematol 1974;3:609-25.
22. Schumacker PT, Samsel RW. Oxygen delivery and uptake by peripheral tissues: Physiology and pathophysiology. Crit Care Clin 1989;5:255-69.
23. Johnson RG, Thurer RL, Kruskall MS, et al. Comparison of two transfusion strategies after elective operations for myocardial revascularization. J Thorac Cardiovasc Surg 1992;104:307-14.
24. Weisel RD, Charlesworth DC, Mickleborough LL, et al. Limitations on blood conservation. J Thorac Cardiovasc Surg 1984;88:26-38.
25. Fortune JB, Feustel PJ, Saifi J, et al. Influence of hematocrit on cardiopulmonary function after acute hemorrhage. J Trauma 1987;27:243-9.
26. Hébert PC, Wells G, Marshall J, et al. Transfusion requirements in critical care. JAMA 1995;273:1439-44.
27. Viele MK, Weiskopf RB. What can we learn about the need for transfusion from patients who refuse blood? The experience with Jehovah's Witnesses. Transfusion 1994;34:396-401.
28. Carson JL, Duff A, Berlin JA, et al. Perioperative blood transfusion and postoperative mortality. JAMA 1998;279:199-205.
29. Weiskopf RB, Viele MK, Feiner J, et al. Human cardiovascular and metabolic response to acute, severe isovolemic anemia. JAMA 1998;279:217-21.
30. Davies CTM, Chukweumeka AC, Van Haaren JPM. Iron-deficiency anemia: Its effect on maximum aerobic power and responses to exercise in African males aged 17-40 years. Clin Sci 1973;44:555-62.
31. Eschbach JW, Abdulhadi MH, Browne JK, et al. Recombinant human erythropoietin in anemic patients with end-stage renal disease. Ann Intern Med 1989;111:992-1000.
32. Evans RW, Rader B, Manninen DL. The quality of life of hemodialysis recipients treated with recombinant human erythropoietin. Cooperative Multicenter EPO Clinical Trial Group. JAMA 1990;263:825-30.
33. Canadian Erythropoietin Study Group. Association between recombinant human erythropoietin and quality of life and exercise capac-

ity of patients receiving haemodialysis. Br Med J 1990;300:573-8.

34. Henry DH, Beall GN, Benson CA, et al. Recombinant human erythropoietin in the treatment of anemia associated with human immunodeficiency virus (HIV) infection and zidovudine therapy. Ann Intern Med 1992; 117:739-48.

35. Case DC, Bukowski RM, Carey RW, et al. Recombinant human erythropoietin therapy for anemic cancer patients on combination chemotherapy. J Natl Cancer Inst 1993;85:801-6.

36. Office of Medical Applications of Research, National Institutes of Health. Preoperative red blood cell transfusion. JAMA 1988;260: 2700-3.

37. Audet AM, Goodnough LT. Practice strategies for elective red blood cell transfusion. Ann Intern Med 1992;116:403-6.

38. Welch HG, Meehan KR, Goodnough LT. Prudent strategies for elective red blood cell transfusion. Ann Intern Med 1992;116:393-402.

39. Sherrard DJ. Perioperative indications for red blood cell transfusion—Has the pendulum swung too far? Mayo Clin Proc 1993;68: 512-3.

40. American Society of Anesthesiologists Task Force on Blood Component Therapy. Practice guidelines for blood component therapy. Anesthesiology 1996;84:732-47.

41. Expert Working Group. Guidelines for red blood cell and plasma transfusion for adults and children. Can Med Assoc J 1997;156:S1-24.

42. Hébert PC, Schweitzer I, Calder L, et al. Review of the clinical practice literature on allogeneic red blood cell transfusion. Can Med Assoc J 1997;156:S9-26.

43. Simon TJ, Alverson DC, AuBuchon J, et al. Practice parameter for the use of red blood cells. Arch Pathol Lab Med 1998;122:130-8.

44. Cummings JP. Technology assessment: Red cell transfusion guidelines. Oakbrook, IL: UHC Services Corporation, 1997.

In: Mintz PD, ed.
Transfusion Therapy: Clinical Principles and Practice
Bethesda, MD: AABB Press, 1999

2

Transfusion Therapy in Congenital Hemolytic Anemias

BRUCE I. SHARON, MD

 THE CONGENITAL HEMOLYTIC anemias are composed of a heterogeneous group of intrinsic red cell abnormalities, including hemoglobin disorders (hemoglobinopathies and thalassemia syndromes), red cell enzyme deficiencies, and abnormalities of the red cell membrane and cytoskeleton. In patients with these conditions, transfusion of red blood cells may be necessary to treat the paramount abnormality—that is, anemia, and its associated decrease in oxygen-carrying-capacity. Transfusion also may be indicated to alleviate a variety of secondary pathophysiologic consequences that are unique to each disorder. The hemoglobin disorders are the most prevalent, and most of this chapter is devoted to them. In particular, the role of RBC transfusion in the management of sickle cell disease (SCD) engenders the greatest controversy,

and this entity is discussed in greatest detail. Much like democracy, transfusion therapy for congenital hemolytic anemia is highly flawed but often superior to any alternative currently available.

Hemoglobinopathies and Thalassemias

The most prevalent hemoglobin disorders are caused by DNA base substitutions that lead to either synthesis of hemoglobin with abnormal structure (eg, SCD), or quantitatively diminished production of hemoglobin (ie, the thalassemias). A few uncommon hemoglobinopathies are characterized by both quantitative and qualitative abnormalities, including hemoglobin E (a β-globin abnormality) and hemoglobin Constant Spring (an α-globin abnormality).

Bruce I. Sharon, MD, Associate Professor of Clinical Pediatrics, University of Illinois at Chicago, Chicago, Illinois

Sickle Cell Disease

In North America, approximately 10% of Blacks have sickle cell trait (ie, are heterozygous for the sickle gene: HbAS). Other hemoglobin disorders are also prevalent within the same population, and the coinheritance of these abnormalities together with the sickle gene is responsible for the genesis of *sickle cell syndromes* (see below). For example, coinheritance (compound heterozygosity) of hemoglobin C(HbC), a β-globin mutation that originated in West Africa, together with the sickle cell (HbS) gene, produces HbSC disease, a typically milder sickle syndrome. In the United States, the gene frequency of β^c is approximately one-third to one-fourth that of β^s. Genes for β-thalassemia and α-thalassemia are also found in African populations, and may also be inherited together with the sickle gene.

Pathophysiology

The molecular basis for the pathophysiology of SCD has been well described, but increasing attention has been devoted recently to secondary, and perhaps even independent, phenomena that occur at higher levels of complexity, including the red cell, vascular wall, and tissue. Recent reviews on the pathophysiology of SCD[1,2] provide further details to complement the summary here.

The crucial first step in the sickling process is sickle hemoglobin polymer formation. In this biphasic process, nucleation occurs first and transpires over a relatively slow interval, the *delay time*. This interval, which represents the time required to achieve a critical minimum nucleus of gelation, is critically dependent on the intraerythrocytic deoxy-HbS concentration. As the concentration of deoxy-HbS rises, the delay time decreases exponentially, approximately on the order of the 15-30th magnitude.[3] Once a critical minimum nucleus of gelation has been established, consisting of approximately 30 tetramers of deoxy-HbS, sickle polymer formation proceeds swiftly through the second phase.[1]

The generation of sickle polymers is reflected at the cellular level by the transformation of normal, biconcave erythrocytes into rigid, highly viscous cells with the distinctive sickle shape. Ordinarily, the sickling process is reversed during the (re-)oxygenation phase, but, after repeated cycles (of deoxygenation/oxygenation), these cells may become irreversibly sickled cells. Such cells maintain their sickle shape even in the absence of HbS polymer formation, probably as a result of incremental membrane damage. They are much more rigid than their normal counterparts and have a distinctly shorter life span, thus contributing to the hemolytic anemia that is a hallmark of this disease. Oddly, there is no appreciable correlation between the percentage of circulating irreversibly sickled cells in an individual and the severity of disease experienced.

Sickle erythrocytes have a heterogeneous distribution of densities. The most dense have an elevated mean corpuscular hemoglobin concentration and are therefore the most prone to undergo sickle polymer formation. The population of dense sickle cells substantially overlaps with the population of irreversibly sickled cells, but not completely.

As sickle polymer formation progresses, increasing numbers of cells assume the sickle shape, and the viscosity of the circulating blood rises sharply. Transit through the microcirculation is impaired, and greater numbers of sickle cells fail to traverse the microcirculation in less than the delay time. In a manner analogous to HbS polymer formation, there appears to be a threshold number of sickled cells with impeded flow, beyond which vascular obstruction is likely to occur.[4] Once this threshold is reached, a self-propagating process ensues in which sluggishly moving red cells lose additional oxygen to adjacent tissues. Further sickling follows, ultimately causing ever larger areas of vascular obstruction.

Various membrane abnormalities have been described in sickle red cells,[2,5] and they may contribute to the vaso-occlusive process. Important findings include abnormally increased cation permeability, which is triggered by polymerization of HbS and is the likely cause of free water efflux, causing intracellular dehydration[2]; membrane deposits of heme and nonheme iron; membrane protein defects, including abnormal interaction with HbS; and abnormalities of the lipid bilayer.

Oxidative injury is the primary cause of membrane damage in sickle red cells, and other intracellular constituents are targets as well.[6] Oxidant damage in these cells stems from both excessive production of toxic oxidants and impaired function of the cells' antioxidant systems. In-vitro data show that sickle erythrocytes produce twice the normal amount of superoxide. Sickle erythrocyte membranes are particularly susceptible to oxidant injury because they cannot isolate cellular iron properly, which, with its propensity to promote lipid peroxidation, is normally segregated from cell membranes. Sickle erythrocytes are poorly deformable even in the oxygenated state because of increased cytoplasmic viscosity and increased membrane stiffness.[5]

Other membrane-associated abnormalities also appear to contribute to the vaso-occlusive process.[5] Sickle erythrocytes are abnormally adherent to vascular endothelium, perhaps even 100-fold more than normal erythrocytes. This effect appears to be most evident in postcapillary venules and is possibly mediated by high-molecular-weight von Willebrand factor multimers. The increased adherence of sickle erythrocytes to the vascular endothelium may be an important trigger of the vaso-occlusive process. The vascular endothelium also produces a variety of vasoactive relaxants, including prostacyclins, and constrictors, such as endothelin, which may play a role in promoting or inhibiting sickle cell vaso-occlusion.

One of the most significant and perplexing features of SCD is the diversity of clinical expression. In addition to the variability that can be explained by compound heterozygous conditions (ie, the sickle cell syndromes), other distinct, inherited conditions, as well as seemingly ill-defined factors, appear to play a role in governing the clinical course. For example, coinheritance of α-thalassemia appears to ameliorate certain complications, including hemolytic anemia, leg ulcer, and possibly even premature death, but it may exacer-

bate others, including aseptic necrosis of the hip and retinopathy. The presence of high percentages of fetal hemoglobin (HbF) also appears to exert a beneficial effect on the clinical course.[7,8] This finding is expected on the basis of the ability of HbF to inhibit sickle hemoglobin polymerization.

The genetic background upon which the sickle mutation is found, as defined by the DNA haplotype in the β-globin region, has also been linked to disease expression. Three major DNA haplotypes for the African β[S]-globin gene have been identified, originating in the Central African Republic (CAR), Benin (Ben), and Senegal (Sen).[9] Increased disease severity has been linked to the CAR haplotype, whereas patients with the Sen haplotype appear to experience milder disease. For example, the presence of at least one CAR haplotype in an individual increases the relative risks of stroke to 2.01 and of kidney disease to 5.00, compared with individuals who lack that haplotype. Patients who are heterozygous for the CAR and Ben haplotypes (CAR/Ben) are twice as likely as Ben/Ben patients, and three times as likely as Sen/Ben patients, to experience major soft-tissue organ damage.[10] These clinical features are perhaps explained in part by the finding of the greatest HbF production in Sen patients, compared with the least HbF production in CAR patients.[11] However, even patients with the same haplotype status have substantial heterogeneity of HbF production and clinical expression, and patients with different haplotype combinations have considerable overlap in their HbF levels. Thus, neither haplotype status nor HbF production is sufficient to explain the spectrum of clinical disease seen in patients with SCD. It is therefore apparent that the clinical expression of disease in sickle cell patients is modulated by inherited factors related to the β-globin gene (eg, compound heterozygosity), regions nearby the β-globin gene (DNA haplotypes, HbF production), inherited factors unlinked to the β-globin gene (α-thalassemia), and epistatic phenomena that have no clearly recognizable inheritance pattern (adherence to vascular endothelium).

Basis for Anemia

The leading cause of anemia in patients with SCD is increased destruction of circulating erythrocytes. These misshapen, poorly deformable cells sustain progressive membrane damage, intensified by oxidant injury. Sickle erythrocytes typically survive only approximately 5-20 days. To compensate, red cell production is increased by up to six or more times above normal, but full correction of the hemoglobin concentration is not achieved. Polymerized deoxy-HbS intrinsically has a low oxygen affinity (rightward shift of the oxygen-hemoglobin binding curve) and is subject to an exaggerated Bohr effect; in addition, sickle (SS) cells have higher than normal levels of 2,3-diphosphoglycerate (2,3-DPG), which also contributes to lowering of the affinity to oxygen.[2] The decrease in oxygen affinity, and therefore the relatively increased delivery of oxygen to tissues, attenuates the drive for erythropoiesis. In addition, a variety of sickle cell complications, including acute splenic sequestration crisis and aplastic crisis, can exacerbate the anemia, and other conditions common in sickle cell patients—for example, fever or infection, immune-mediated hemolysis, glucose-6-phosphate dehydrogenase (G6PD) deficiency, and folic acid deficiency—can contribute further to the anemia.

Sickle Cell Syndromes

A variety of other α- and β-globin mutations are prevalent within the African sickle cell population, and, when coinherited together with the sickle mutation, they modify its clinical expression. SCD is therefore a heterogenous group of disorders. In any particular syndrome, the tendency toward sickling depends upon the intracellular concentration of HbS and the proclivity of the nonsickle hemoglobins to influence the polymerization process. For example, HbA and HbC are permissive toward, and even mildly promote, sickle polymer formation, whereas HbF distinctly inhibits this process. Compared with patients who are compound heterozygotes for Hbs A and S (sickle trait), individuals

with HbSC disease have a higher intracellular concentration of HbS, thereby explaining the greater clinical impact of the latter condition. As would be predicted from these considerations, the anticipated and observed ranking of disease severity is as follows: HbSS, HbS/β°-thalassemia, HbSC, HbS/β⁺-thalassemia, HbS/HPFH (hereditary persistence of fetal hemoglobin), and HbAS.

General Guidelines for Transfusion Therapy

There are two fundamental indications for the transfusion of red cells in SCD: anemia and vaso-occlusion. (The latter indication is unique to this disorder.) Depending on the severity and relative contribution of each of these complications, the threshold, method, and endpoint for transfusion therapy differ markedly. The general approach to transfusion therapy is reviewed first, and specific guidelines for transfusion are reviewed for each of the various sickle cell complications in the sections that follow. Finally, transfusion therapy in special circumstances is discussed.

Anemia. In the more severe sickle cell syndromes, hemoglobin concentrations typically range from 6-8 g/dL, whereas patients with the milder variants generally maintain hemoglobin concentrations of 9-11 g/dL. From the cardiorespiratory standpoint, sickle cell patients generally tolerate their chronic anemia rather well and do not routinely require transfusion. However, when acute complications intervene, causing a precipitous fall in hemoglobin levels, congestive heart failure or other cardiorespiratory compromise may ensue or pose an imminent danger. Urgent transfusion of red cells may then be required. The specific decision of whether to transfuse should be based on a comprehensive assessment of the clinical circumstance, taking into account such factors as the rate and extent of decline in hemoglobin concentration (a greater than 2-3 g/dL fall in hemoglobin levels, especially if abrupt, often merits red cell transfusion); the clinical status, including signs of actual or incipient cardiorespiratory failure; underlying pulmonary or cardiac abnormalities; and the prospects for spontaneous recovery of hemoglobin levels.

The physiologic goal of transfusion in this setting is to increase the oxygen-carrying capacity of the blood. However, the clinician should be aware that poor oxygen delivery to tissues in SCD has particular significance because hypoxemia and metabolic acidosis can trigger intravascular sickling, thus extending the clinical problem from anemia to sickle vaso-occlusion.

For the treatment of anemia alone, simple transfusion is generally adequate. The transfusion of 10-15 mL of red cells per kilogram can be expected to raise the hemoglobin by about 3-4 g/dL. In cases of severe anemia, however (ie, when hemoglobin levels are <5 g/dL), the uninterrupted transfusion of such volumes may pose a risk of volume overload, and, in these settings, the transfusion should be divided into two aliquots, administered slowly. For example, 5-7 mL of red cells per kilogram can be infused over 2-3 hours, and, after a pause of 1-2 hours, the dose can be repeated with red cells stored in the blood bank until immediately before infusion. There is also a potential advantage for using relatively fresh Red Blood Cells (RBCs) (those stored for less than 1 week), as the red cells are likely to have higher levels of 2,3-DPG and thereby have enhanced oxygen delivery to tissues compared with red cells that are stored for longer intervals. If necessary, a diuretic such as furosemide can also be administered. In urgent situations, an exchange transfusion may be required.

Because patients with SCD are generally well compensated at their baseline hemoglobin levels, it is usually sufficient to return to those levels with transfusion. If cardiac or pulmonary complications are present, however, higher hemoglobin endpoints for transfusion are justified.

Vaso-occlusion. The aim of transfusion in this setting is to halt or prevent intravascular sickling through the dilution or replacement of circulating sickle cells with normal, nonsickleable cells. Clinical experience has shown that transfused patients with SCD (who have mixtures of SS and normal, or AA, cells) are unlikely to develop vaso-occlusion if the relative fraction of sickle cells is less than 30-40%. This finding is supported by in-vitro data from Lessin et al,[12] who showed that the relative resistance to the flow of mixtures of AA and SS increases substantially when the fraction of SS cells exceeds 40%.

Blood flow is influenced not only by the relative percentages of sickle cells but also by the absolute concentration of sickle cells, or sickle hematocrit (the packed cell volume contributed only by SS cells), and the total hematocrit of the blood. Schmalzer et al[13] showed that in red cell suspensions with a fixed ratio of H_s/H_T (where H_s and H_T are the sickle and total hematocrits, respectively), the viscosity (η) rises with H_T at a given shear rate (Fig 2-1). This effect is most evident in pure SS suspensions ($H_s/H_T = 1.0$) and is least apparent in pure AA suspensions ($H_s/H_T = 0$). It is also more pronounced in deoxygenated suspensions compared with oxygenated ones.

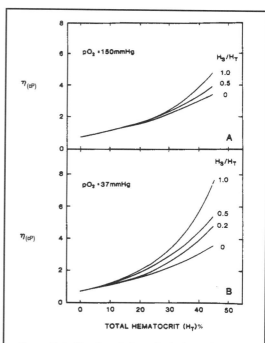

Figure 2-1. The rise of viscosity (η) as a function of H_T (total hematocrit), at fixed ratios of H_s (hematocrit of sickle cells)/H_T. **A**, Oxygenated red cell suspensions. **B**, Deoxygenated red cell suspensions. Adapted with permission from Schmalzer et al.[13]

The data from deoxygenated suspensions have been replotted to show the relationship between the viscosity and H_T at a fixed H_S (Fig 2-2); under these circumstances, any increment in H_T is due to the addition of normal red cells. The results show that the viscosity rises markedly with the addition of normal cells, and that this effect is accentuated when the starting content of sickle cells (H_S) is greatest. Unfortunately, these data mirror the clinical circumstance of simple transfusion in patients with SCD and alert us to the hazards of excessive transfusion.

Furthermore, at a constant H_S or H_S/H_T, the net oxygen delivery to tissues (H_T/η) declines as the H_T rises through the physiologic range of 20-40% (Fig 2-3). This shows that any advantage of increased oxygen-carrying capacity due to higher red cell mass (H_T) is potentially more than offset by the detrimental effect of higher viscosity, so that the net oxygen delivery to tissues declines. This effect, too, is more pronounced in mixtures of cells with a high sickle cell content.

These data highlight the rheologic advantages of exchange transfusion over simple transfusion in the management of patients with SCD. Both methods of transfusion achieve a relative enrichment of

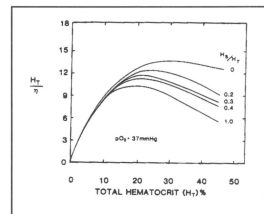

Figure 2-3. The change in H_T/η, a measure of net oxygen delivery to tissues, as a function of total hematocrit (H_T), at various ratios of H_S/H_T. Adapted with permission from Schmalzer et al.[13]

normal compared with sickle cells, but the exchange method alone is capable of lowering the HbS rapidly and limiting the rise in H_T, thereby helping to reduce viscosity and improve oxygen delivery to tissues maximally. Exchange transfusion therefore has an essential role in the treatment of severe anemia, significant hypoxemia, or other cardiopulmonary illness, and in the immediate prevention of treatment of vaso-occlusive complications in SCD. When such a hasty reduction in HbS concentration is not imperative, such as prior to elective surgery, repeated simple transfusions over a few weeks can accomplish the same goals as exchange transfusion but without the disadvantages of greater blood use and the increased risk inherent in the exchange procedure.

The distribution of HbS within red cells is also an important consideration. Specifically, in mixtures of AA and SS cells, only the latter have the capacity to sickle; in contrast, in compound heterozygous states such as HbSC disease, all cells possess HbS and, therefore, the potential to sickle under suitable physiologic conditions. When patients with compound heterozygous forms of SCD are being transfused, concerns for vaso-occlusion make it prudent to consider the percentage of *cells* that are

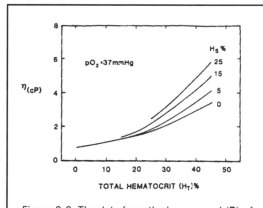

Figure 2-2. The data from the lower panel (**B**) of Fig 2-1 replotted to show the rise in viscosity (η) as a function of H_T (total hematocrit), at various sickle hematocrits (H_S). Adapted with permission from Schmalzer et al.[13]

sickleable, rather than the percentage of sickle hemoglobin. For example, if the goal of transfusion for a particular complication in patients with HbSS disease is to achieve a relative HbS concentration of less than 30%, that goal for HbSC patients should be adapted to mean achieving a result of less than 30% sickleable cells, or approximately 15% HbS.

Exchange transfusion may be accomplished through manual or automated techniques. Piomelli et al[14] have demonstrated that the efficiency of manual exchange transfusion compares with that of automated exchange, even when the aliquot volume is large; for reasons of safety, however, each aliquot should not exceed 10% of total blood volume. Whole blood or reconstituted RBCs are the preferred blood products for use in manual exchange transfusion because they allow a more gradual rise in the viscosity of the circulating blood through the course of the procedure.

Transfusion Therapy for Sickle Cell Complications

Current practice in the transfusion management of patients with SCD is largely based on in-vitro data and theoretical understanding of the disease process, experience with conventional treatment approaches, and, in too few instances, well-devised clinical trials. To a large extent, the lack of statistically compelling clinical information stems from the great logistic challenge of accruing sufficiently large numbers of patients, particularly when clinical trials ideally ought to be stratified to address each type of complication, subset of sickle patients (ie, sickle syndrome), and treatment approach under consideration.

At least neonates and young infants are spared the sequelae of SCD because of the preponderance of HbF during that period. As the synthesis of HbF begins to wane during the first several months of life, production of HbS rises, and infants with SCD become susceptible to its various complications. The various acute and chronic complications that may necessitate transfusion are listed in Table 2-1 according to their physiologic indications for treatment.[15]

Acute Complications

The pathognomonic acute clinical sequelae of SCD are the acute sickle cell "crises," including acute vaso-occlusive (pain), acute splenic sequestration, and aplastic crises, as well as other threatening clinical situations.

Acute vaso-occlusive (pain) crises. Acute painful crises account for the majority of hospitalizations of sickle cell patients in the United States.[16] Owing to abrupt sickle cell vaso-occlusion, these events may occur anywhere in the body but most commonly involve the musculoskeletal system or soft tissues. Approximately one-half of all HbSS patients between the ages of 6 and 18 months present with acute vaso-occlusive crises involving the metacarpal and/or metatarsal bones in painful episodes commonly termed "hand-foot syndrome." Like other pain crises, these events are typically self-limiting and spontaneously resolve within several days, but patients with pain crisis benefit from analgesia and brisk hydration. Simple transfusion of red cells has *no* proven role in this setting and should not be administered. Patients with repeated and debilitating pain crises may benefit from a limited (approximately 6-month) course of regular transfusion designed to suppress endogenous sickle red cell production and achieve a relative HbS concentration of 30-50%, but temptation to continue this remedy in an unlimited fashion should be strongly resisted because of the mounting risks of repeated transfusions (see below). In the very rare circumstance of acute, intractable pain crisis, a single-volume exchange transfusion, calculated to achieve a similar endpoint, may be considered.

Acute splenic sequestration crisis. In patients with SCD, the spleen ultimately becomes infarcted as a result of repeated, subclinical microocclusive events. Prior to reaching this condition and principally in early childhood, the spleen is subject to acute circulatory obstruction on the efferent side caused by the trapping of sickle cells. In about half of these instances, there is an antecedent, even trivial, history of viral infection, but often there is no apparent prodrome. While the affer-

Table 2-1. Acute and Chronic Complications of Sickle Cell Disease That May Require Red Cell Transfusion in Order to Correct Anemia or Counter Vaso-occlusion

	Anemia	Anemia and Vaso-occlusion	Vaso-occlusion
Acute	Aplastic crisis	Acute chest syndrome Acute splenic sequestration Acute papillary necrosis Sepsis	Stroke Priapism Intractable pain crisis

Chronic	Pregnancy
	Hematuria
	Chronic renal failure
	Cardiac failure
		Surgery
		Pregnancy-high risk
			Skin ulcer
			Prophylaxis for:
			  Stroke
			  Splenic sequestration
			  Angiography
			  Intractable pain

Used with permission from Sharon and Honig.[15]

ent side of the splenic circulation remains unobstructed, the rapidly progressive sequestration of red cells within the spleen may cause a precipitous fall in hemoglobin levels, followed by generalized circulatory collapse and even death.

Patients with classic acute splenic sequestration present with hypovolemic shock and peripheral circulatory failure, but even if they appear well compensated, these patients should be managed aggressively because of the catastrophic potential of this complication. The mainstay of treatment is prompt transfusion of Whole Blood or, if unavailable, RBCs. The former product is preferable because it is capable of correcting both the deficit of circulating red blood cells as well as that of intravascular volume, but its availability is generally limited. A suitable alternative is immediate resuscitation with crystalloid fluid, followed by the transfusion of RBCs. Simple transfusion calculated to return to baseline hemoglobin levels is generally sufficient; in fact, the posttransfusion hemoglobin levels are often higher than predicted, presumably

because trapped red cells are partially released from the spleen.

Up to 40-50% of patients with acute splenic sequestration suffer recurrences, and the mortality of the repeat episode is likely to be greater than that of the initial event.[17] If the first episode occurs in school-age years, splenectomy can be offered to prevent recurrence. On the other hand, initial presentation during childhood poses a difficult dilemma: surgical splenectomy at this stage carries a risk of postoperative sepsis, although fortunately this has been declining with preventive measures such as vaccination against Pneumococcus and penicillin prophylaxis. In such cases, it is reasonable to transfuse regularly for a limited time (perhaps a year) as a temporizing measure. Such a regimen, designed to maintain the HbS at less than 30%, is highly effective in preventing a recurrence during the period of regular transfusion and allows splenectomy to be performed at an age when it can be tolerated more safely, at least from the standpoint of infection. However, the clinician must weigh the risks associated with such a transfusion regimen against its potential benefits.

Aplastic crisis. This complication is characterized by a transient halt in erythropoiesis, caused in most, if not almost all, cases by parvovirus B19. Because the life span of sickle cells is so brief, even a temporary arrest in red cell production is capable of precipitously worsening the state of anemia. On the other hand, because spontaneous resolution of the underlying problem is typically forthcoming within a few days of presentation, decisions regarding transfusion should take into account the clinical state, hemoglobin level, and the outlook for prompt recovery; the latter can be ascertained from the reticulocyte count or, if necessary, examination of a marrow aspirate. If the transfusion of RBCs is deemed necessary, simple transfusion to achieve (near) baseline hemoglobin concentrations is sufficient. There is no evidence to prompt concern that transfusion will interfere with the process of spontaneous recovery. Health-care personnel are at risk for contracting nosocomial erythema infectiosum from patients with aplastic crises because the etiologic agent is common to both conditions.[18] Parvovirus B 19 has also been linked to aplastic crises in other congenital hemolytic anemias.

Stroke. Among the most feared and devastating of all complications suffered by sickle cell patients is stroke. Approximately 8-10% of these patients experience this complication, often during childhood. Most children present with signs of cerebral infarction, whereas older patients typically present with evidence of subarachnoid or cerebral hemorrhage. As with other, more common causes of cerebrovascular accident, clinical presentation often includes hemiplegia, seizures, coma, or even death. Occasionally, there is a history of antecedent headache or transient ischemic attacks, but, commonly, there is no harbinger. The large intracerebral arteries are typically involved in the catastrophic vasoocclusive event, but the pathophysiologic origin appears to be chronic, subclinical, micro-occlusive events within the vasa vasorum, their nutrient vessels. Repeated damage to the vasa vasorum appears to cause localized scarring, intimal hyperplasia, and progressive stenosis of the (arterial) lumen; ab-

normally adherent sickle cells might then be responsible for initiating vascular obstruction.[16]

The natural history of this complication is ominous. In the absence of further treatment, approximately 65-80% of patients who are stricken will suffer a recurrent event, usually within the first 2-3 years. Moreover, the morbidity and mortality associated with the subsequent events are likely to be greater than those experienced during the initial episode. Thus, the focus of management in stroke is not only to prevail through the acute event, but also to foil the likelihood of recurrence. Indeed, attention has recently been devoted to the question of whether the initial event itself might be thwarted.

Sickle cell patients in the acute phase of stroke should be treated with at least a single-volume exchange transfusion (60-70 mL/kg), aimed to reduce swiftly the relative concentration of HbS to less than 30%. In more severe cases, it may be desirable to achieve HbS levels of about 10% by using a double-volume exchange transfusion. The primary goal of the acute management is to minimize extension of the zone of ischemia; ideally, this might even aid in rescuing "borderline" areas that have undergone reversible ischemic changes. If angiography is planned, HbS levels below 20% should be attained in advance. (See the section on angiography below).

Currently, no sufficiently reliable test exists to discriminate those patients who are destined to have a recurrence from those who are likely to have a more benign course. Therefore, beyond the acute phase, all sickle cell stroke patients must be chronically transfused for at least 3-5 years to minimize the threat of recurrence. For the first several years, the goal should be to maintain peak (pretransfusion) HbS levels at less than 30-40%[19]; such a regimen is approximately 90% effective in reducing the incidence of stroke during the transfusion period. From the hematologic perspective, transfusion objectives can usually be accomplished by providing a simple RBC transfusion of 10-15 mL/kg every 3-4 weeks. After the first few years, it may be sufficiently safe and effective to raise the allowable threshold of HbS to 50%.[20] During the period of chronic transfusion, patients should be monitored with hemoglobin electrophoreses to measure the relative percentages of HbA and HbS, in addition to determinations of the hemoglobin and reticulocyte count. After these results are followed in an individual for some time, it is often possible to establish a relationship between the hemoglobin/reticulocyte results and the electrophoretic findings, thus obviating the need to obtain so often that latter, more costly and cumbersome test.[21]

The question of how long to transfuse sickle cell stroke patients is a vexing one. Unfortunately, commonly available tests (eg, radiographic findings) are an unreliable means by which to ascertain the adequacy of transfusion. Patients who have achieved radiographic (arteriographic) resolution of abnormalities during the course of transfusion still have suffered a recurrence of stroke after the transfusions have ceased, whereas other patients in whom transfusions were terminated despite the persistence of abnormalities have remained free of stroke.[19,22] Nevertheless, in most cases, it is prudent to assume that, regardless of its duration, once transfusion therapy ceases, the risk of recurrence again becomes unacceptably high. Ultimately, the decision regarding the duration of transfusion in these patients should depend on an assessment of the relative merits of continued transfusion—namely, the aversion of stroke and other vaso-occlusive complications vs the risks, including alloimmunization and iron overload (see below).

Although there are no commonly available methods to identify those sickle cell patients who are at the highest risk for developing stroke, recent reports indicate that specially adapted ultrasound methods to determine cerebral blood flow may be effective for this purpose. Children with SCD who have elevated cerebral blood flow as determined by Transcranial Doppler (TCD) ultrasonography seem to be at an increased risk for developing stroke. On the basis of this method of screening, the National Heart, Lung and Blood Institute sponsored a Stroke Prevention Trial in Sickle Cell Anemia ("STOP").[23] Investigators identified 130 children aged 2-16 years who had abnormal TCD studies and were, therefore, deemed to be at a high risk for stroke and

randomly assigned them to observation only (standard care), or to a regular transfusion regimen designed to maintain the Hb S at or less than 30%. At the end of the study period (ranging from about 1-2 ½ years), 10 out of 67 children who received standard care had developed stroke, compared to only one child out of 63 in the transfusion group.

These results are promising, but they do not address crucial questions. The fact that regular transfusion was highly effective in preventing stroke is hardly unexpected. The fundamental question raised by this study is whether TCD methodology is sufficiently sensitive and specific enough for the purpose of guiding transfusion recommendations in children with sickle cell disease. Unfortunately, this report does not contain all of the data that would help to address these questions. Approximately 2000 children with sickle cell disease were screened through use of the TCD technique for this study, and about 10% were found to have abnormal findings. The incidence of stroke in those who had normal studies, and were, therefore, excluded from the study, was not reported. Furthermore, while 10 patients out of 67 (15%) in the standard care group developed stroke during the trial period, the number of patients who would have developed stroke during a longer observation period is open to question. Information from pervious studies of TCD, as well as the current study, suggest that the risk of stroke in those patients who have abnormal TCD findings is approximately 10% per year over the first 2 years. Whether the annual risk of stroke declines with longer observation periods is open to question.

The first episode of stroke essentially serves as the screening tool to identify patients who merit long-term transfusion. Even this approach, which has the maximum possible sensitivity and specificity for selecting those patients who require regular transfusion (albeit at the cost of patients sustaining a first stroke), still subjects about one-third of patients to unnecessary long-term transfusion. The purpose of TCD screening is admittedly different, ie, to prevent the occurrence of *first* stroke, but even so, it would likely subject an even greater number of patients to unnecessary regular transfusion. Is this justifiable in the face of potentially serious side effects of chronic transfusion, such as alloimmunization and hemochromatosis? More information regarding the sensitivity and specificity of TCD screening would help to answer this question. The relative merits of each management approach appear difficult to compare at this point. Undoubtedly, should TCD-guided transfusion prove to be the superior approach, then the burden on transfusion facilities could increase dramatically in many regions, and the infrastructure for transfusion would have to be augmented.

Acute chest syndrome. The acute chest syndrome (ACS) is characterized by fever, cough, chest pain, and a new pulmonic infiltrate on chest roentgenogram, often accompanied by hypoxemia. In addition, leukocytosis, exacerbation of anemia, and alteration of the platelet count (to either higher or lower levels) often are seen. ACS is the second most frequent reason for hospitalization among patients with SCD, and it accounts for up to 25% of all deaths in this illness.[24]

The primary pathophysiologic process may be infection (pneumonia), or vaso-occlusion within the pulmonary vasculature, but, in either circumstance, the clinical presentation is often similar. Children are more likely than adults to have an infectious etiology,[25] but it may be difficult to ascertain in a particular case which process is predominant. This distinction is often clinically irrelevant, however, because either process is liable to evolve into the other. From a practical standpoint, the management is commonly directed at both processes. Pulmonary fat or marrow embolism has recently been recognized as an unexpectedly common finding in ACS, especially in severe cases.[25-27]

The finding of hypoxemia is particularly worrisome because it may presage a self-perpetuating cycle of hypoxemia, intrapulmonary sickling, and worsened hypoxemia. Transfusion should be considered whenever supplemental oxygen is required. In this setting, the transfusion of RBCs is essential to correct the anemia and to halt, or possibly reverse, the process of vaso-occlusion. Some have suggested that prompt transfusion has a beneficial impact on the clinical course of patients with

ACS.[28] When transfusion is provided on a timely basis, the clinical benefit achieved often far surpasses that which would have been anticipated on the basis of the transfused red cell volume alone; this observation supports the supposition that a dual, synergistic clinical benefit is realized after a transfusion in ACS.

An increased alveolar-arterial oxygen gradient may be a helpful predictor of clinical severity and the need for blood transfusion in these patients.[29] In milder or more slowly evolving clinical circumstances, it may be possible to use simple transfusion, but if clinical deterioration is rapid or the extent of hypoxemia severe, an exchange transfusion is warranted. In the more severe cases, a single-volume exchange transfusion intended to achieve an HbS level of 30% or less may be used.

Acute papillary necrosis. The renal medulla is prone to sickle cell vaso-occlusion because of the low flow characteristics of its vascular bed and its low oxygen tension. Mild medullary ischemia may cause asymptomatic microscopic hematuria, but severe ischemic damage can provoke renal papillary necrosis and gross hematuria. The recent incidence of renal papillary necrosis seems to be lower than that experienced before 1980. It is now believed that this complication was also precipitated by nephrotoxic drugs such as phenacetin and possibly acetaminophen,[30] which may have been used more indiscriminately in the past. When the loss of blood is prolonged or severe, the transfusion of RBCs may be required to correct the anemia; whether transfusion also helps to reverse the vaso-occlusive process has not been documented. Patients with sickle cell trait also may experience hematuria, but these patients rarely require transfusion.

End-stage renal disease. Patients with SCD experience progressive kidney damage resulting from the cumulative effects of micro-occlusive events within the renal medulla. Children often exhibit hyposthenuria, while increased renal blood flow and an increased glomerular filtration rate can be seen in adolescents. In adults, glomerulosclerosis and renal insufficiency may be seen by the third or fourth decade of life. Some patients develop end-stage renal disease requiring dialysis or renal transplantation. Nonsickle cell patients who develop chronic renal failure typically respond to recombinant erythropoietin, as discussed in Chapter 20, but sickle cell patients are comparatively unresponsive to this treatment and may require chronic transfusion.[30]

Priapism. As many as 40% of male sickle cell patients experience priapism, the unwanted, painful, and prolonged erection of the penis.[31] This complication is caused by obstructed venous outflow from the corpora cavernosa. The first episode may strike prepubertal or adolescent males, but postpubertal patients are particularly affected. Once stricken, individuals often experience recurrent episodes, which cause fibrosis of the corpora cavernosa, cessation of blood flow to this cavity, and, ultimately, erectile dysfunction.[32]

Conservative management with brisk IV hydration and analgesia is often the first approach used in cases of very recent onset, but this rarely suffices. If priapism has lasted more than a few hours (with or without an attempt at conservative management), or if the glans is so firm as to produce urinary obstruction, the prompt transfusion of RBCs should be considered. Simple transfusion may be adequate in uncomplicated cases,[33] but a single-volume exchange transfusion should be considered in severe or complicated cases (eg, when duration of the erection nears or exceeds 12 hours or when there is a significant past history of priapism). When successful, this remedy provides considerable relief from pain within a day, but complete detumescence may not occur for days or even weeks. If transfusion is unsuccessful in resolving priapism, it still will have been of benefit by preparing the patient for anesthesia and surgery. Creation of a shunt between the corpora cavernosa and corpora spongiosum has proven effective in reestablishing blood flow.[34]

Despite the potential benefits of exchange transfusion, a unique complication has been reported after its use in patients with priapism. At least eight such patients have suffered acute neurologic events, including stroke or seizure, after this treatment,[35,36] and the association of the two has been termed "ASPEN syndrome."[36] Severe headache

was a common presenting symptom in these patients. However, the hemoglobin concentration and relative levels of HbS were in desirable ranges (mean Hb=12.1 g/dL, mean HbS=27%),[35] so the etiology of this complication is enigmatic.

Hepatic crises. Sickle cell vaso-occlusion may occur within the liver, producing severe right-upper-quadrant pain, hyperbilirubinemia, and elevated levels of other liver functions. The clinical picture may resemble that of acute cholelithiasis. Severe vaso-occlusion within the liver has been reported to precipitate either acute or chronic liver failure, both of which may respond to exchange transfusion.[37,38] Chronic disease may, in addition, require regular transfusion over a longer term.

Sepsis and other serious illness. Acute septic illness may cause the inhibition of erythropoiesis, or increased hemolysis. In addition, the red cell T cryptantigen may be exposed during severe infections, leading to erythrocyte polyagglutination.[39] Red cell transfusion may be indicated during sepsis and other severe illnesses to provide increased oxygen-carrying capacity and to prevent generalized sickling that might develop because of associated hypoxemia or acidosis.

Skin ulcers. Adolescent and adult sickle cell patients are subject to chronic skin ulcers, particularly in the anterior tibial region and over the malleoli. If local, conservative treatment is unsuccessful or if a skin graft has been used for treatment, a limited transfusion program lasting up to several months may aid the healing process. The temptation to continue regular transfusions indefinitely should be avoided, however, because beyond a narrow time frame, the risks of chronic transfusion begin to outweigh its benefits for this indication.

Special Indications for Transfusion in Sickle Cell Disease

Pregnancy. During pregnancy, both the mother with SCD and her fetus are at increased risk of complications. The mother is subject to increased morbidity and even mortality due to a higher incidence of vaso-occlusive complications, including pain crises, ACS, and acute splenic sequestration; infectious complications, primarily urinary tract infections; worsening of anemia; and abruptio placenta, placenta previa, and toxemia. The fetus is at increased risk for spontaneous abortion, stillbirth, premature birth, and growth retardation. As recently as 1971, the maternal death rate in pregnancies of sickle cell mothers was reported to be as high as 6%, and the perinatal mortality rate was as high as 45%.[40] Not surprisingly, the focus of medical recommendations at that time was to prevent pregnancy. More recently, the maternal mortality rate has been reported as 2%, and the perinatal death rate as less than 10-25%, in pregnancies managed without prophylactic transfusion.[41-43] These improved results have stimulated a brisk debate regarding the optimal role of red cell transfusion in sickle cell pregnancy. Some have advocated initiating prophylactic transfusion therapy at the onset of pregnancy or at the start of the last trimester,[42,44] while others have recommended refraining from preventive red blood cell transfusion.[45]

In 1988, Koshy et al[46] reported the most extensive clinical trial conducted to date on transfusion in pregnant patients with SCD. Seventy-two pregnant patients with HbSS were randomly assigned to receive either prophylactic transfusion or transfusion for medical or obstetric complications. In addition, 66 patients with HbSC disease and 23 patients with HbS/β-thalassemia were assigned to the nonprophylactic transfusion group, presumably because their milder disease was not thought to justify the possibility of randomization to a mandatory transfusion group. Patients were ineligible for the study if they had major organ system damage, such as neurologic dysfunction, renal or liver disease, or multiple red cell alloantibodies. In this study, there was no significant difference in perinatal outcome between the prophylactic transfusion group and the group receiving transfusions for complications only. As expected, mothers who received prophylactic transfusion experienced fewer pain crises and other vaso-occlusive complications, but they received an average of 12 units of RBCs, whereas the emergency transfusion group received an average of 3 units each. Sixteen of 36 patients (44%) in this latter group ultimately required trans-

fusion on an emergency basis (consuming an average of 6.5 units each), as did 27% of the HbSC patients and 52% of the HbS/β-thalassemia patients. About one-quarter of all patients who received transfusions became alloimmunized in the course of the study.

These findings suggest that prophylactic transfusions do not have to be routinely provided to pregnant women with SCD who have no high-risk factors. Pathophysiologically, the study findings may be related to an apparent lack of improvement (ie, decrease) in uteroplacental resistance following transfusion in mothers with SCD.[47] Nevertheless, the conclusions derived from the study by Koshy et al[46] should be reserved because of the relatively small number of patients studied. In addition, vaso-occlusive sequelae targeting the placenta (eg, abruptio placenta and placenta previa) seem to develop early in pregnancy; thus, early and aggressive transfusion might be required to realize the full potential of preventive transfusion.

Prophylactic transfusion is recommended in pregnancies that bear high-risk factors such as multiple gestation or for mothers with a history of perinatal loss.[42] Additional indications for transfusion include, but are not limited to, toxemia, septicemia, acute renal failure, severe anemia (with hemoglobin 6 g/dL or more than 30% below baseline), hypoxemia, and ACS.[48] It is important to note that even when high-risk factors are not present and prophylactic transfusions are withheld, approximately one-quarter to one-half of pregnant mothers with SCD, including those with the milder syndromes, will require emergency transfusion eventually because of serious complications.[42,43,46] Under such circumstances, there should be no hesitation in providing this necessary treatment. The high incidence of emergency transfusion in seemingly routine cases should be a forceful reminder that great vigilance and meticulous obstetric care are mandatory in *all* cases.

In summary, both the pregnant mother with SCD and her fetus are at significant risk for serious complications. In the highest risk settings, there is consensus that prophylactic transfusion should be provided, perhaps even beginning in the first or second trimester. In standard risk cases, the benefits of prophylactic transfusion should be weighed against the costs and risks, particularly alloimmunization. In many routine cases, it may be possible to avoid preventive transfusion, but great care and vigilance are needed to recognize quickly the onset of complications that might benefit from timely transfusion.

Surgery. Surgery and the perioperative period pose special risks to patients with SCD, including sudden death, pulmonary infarction, infection, and pain crisis. Diminished perfusion or anesthesiologic accidents such as aspiration, difficult intubation, etc, can cause altered oxygenation, dehydration, hypothermia, and acidosis, which in turn can precipitate localized or generalized vascular obstruction. Various transfusion strategies have been advocated to prevent perioperative complications, but unfortunately, there is a dearth of rigorously conducted clinical trials that provide reliable guidance. The majority of reports regarding this subject are retrospective or anecdotal.

Several reports have asserted that beneficial results can be obtained without the regular use of prophylactic transfusion before surgery. In a group of 200 sickle cell patients who underwent surgery with general anesthesia, Homi et al[49] were able to avoid transfusion in about two-thirds of cases. In the remaining patients, transfusion was provided to raise the hemoglobin to baseline levels or to offset actual or anticipated blood loss. Six deaths occurred, all in the postoperative period. No details were provided regarding these patients' transfusion history, but five of the six had undergone emergency surgery and were in poor condition, even preoperatively. Bischoff et al[50] reported their experiences with 66 sickle cell patients (50 HbSS, 13 HbSC, and 3 HbS/β-thalassemia) who had undergone 82 surgical procedures. They found no meaningful differences in perioperative morbidity and mortality, regardless of the timing of transfusion in relation to surgery or of whether transfusion was provided at all. In a retrospective study reported by Griffin and Buchanan,[51] among 54 sickle cell patients who underwent 66 elective surgeries, transfusion was avoided in 57 (86%) of the proce-

dures. While there were no intraoperative complications, postoperative complications were experienced in 17 (26%) procedures, but no deaths occurred. In this study, the extent of surgery appeared to be an important risk factor for the development of complications. Ten of 20 patients who had major surgery, including laparotomy and thoracotomy, developed complications, whereas only 7 of 46 patients (15%) who had minor procedures developed similar difficulties. Tonsillectomy/adenoidectomy was responsible for nearly all the morbidity among those who had minor surgical procedures. In all settings, pulmonary complications were the most frequent, including ACS and atelectasis.

Other investigators have found preoperative transfusion to be beneficial. In a study of 32 patients who underwent 46 surgical procedures, Janik and Seeler[52] used simple preoperative red blood cell transfusions of 15-20 mL/kg to raise the hematocrit to at least 36% and lower the relative HbS concentration to 32-55%. None of these patients experienced any preoperative morbidity or mortality. Morrison et al[53] reported their experience with 42 patients who had preoperative exchange transfusions designed to achieve hematocrits greater than 35% and HbA concentrations greater than 40%. In this series, there were no deaths, and only minimal perioperative or postoperative complications occurred. In a group of 50 patients with SCD who underwent 67 surgical procedures, Fullerton et al[54] used simple preoperative transfusion in the initial portion of the study, and partial exchange transfusion in the latter phase. In all cases, the intent of transfusion was to raise the hemoglobin concentration to at least 11 g/dL, and lower the relative HbS concentration to less than 30%. All these patients had favorable perioperative experiences. Vitreoretinal surgery in sickle cell patients harbors an increased risk of anterior segment ischemia, but this can be successfully diminished by preoperative exchange transfusion.[55,56]

Conservative and aggressive transfusion regimens were compared prospectively by the Preoperative Transfusion in Sickle Cell Disease Study Group.[57] In their study, reported in 1995, 551 patients with HbSS disease who underwent a total of

604 elective operations were randomly assigned to either of these two transfusion approaches. The aggressive transfusion regimen was designed to achieve a preoperative hemoglobin concentration of 10 g/dL and a hemoglobin S concentration of 30% or less, while the conservative regimen aimed to attain a minimum hemoglobin of 10 g/dL regardless of the hemoglobin S percentage. The mean preoperative hemoglobin level was similar in both groups of patients: 11.0 g/dL in the aggressively transfused group (Group 1) compared with 10.6 g/dL in the conservatively transfused group (Group 2). However, Group 1 patients had a median preoperative HbS of 31%, compared with 59% in Group 2 patients. Although some overlap existed in the hematologic profiles of the two groups of patients, data were analyzed on an intent-to-treat basis. Perioperative complications arising up to 30 days after surgery were assessed. Cholecystectomy; ear, nose, and throat; and orthopedic procedures accounted for more than three-quarters of the operations performed. At least one serious or life-threatening postoperative complication—most commonly ACS—was experienced in about 20% of the procedures performed in each of the groups. The average duration of hospitalization was the same for both groups. There were two deaths among Group 1 patients and none among Group 2 patients. Both fatalities occurred in individuals who had prior histories of ACS and who suffered postoperative respiratory complications. The preoperative hemoglobin S was 30% or less in both cases. Patients in Group 1 had required an average of 5.0 RBC units to achieve pretransfusion goals, while an average of 2.5 units was needed in Group 2 patients. Ten percent of Group 1 patients developed new alloantibodies compared with only 5% of Group 2 patients.

The authors of this study concluded that an aggressive transfusion regimen offered no advantage over a conservative regimen in preventing perioperative complications, but the former approach was associated with twice the risk of transfusion-associated complications. Other tenable conclusions need to be considered, however. For example, the two transfusion regimens may not have differed substantially from each other, at least not from the physiologic perspective; this view is supported in part by the overlap in hematologic values of the two groups. In a similar vein, the aggressive transfusion regimen may not have been aggressive or intense enough to produce a measurable benefit in perioperative outcome, at least not when these patients were compared with the conservatively managed group. Regardless of the interpretation that one favors, the sobering finding of this study is that one-third of the patients in both groups experienced serious complications in the perioperative period.

The same study group also reported on the perioperative outcome of 364 patients with SCD who underwent cholecystectomy.[58] Patients who had been randomly assigned to either aggressive (Group 1) or conservative (Group 2) transfusion regimens and who were subjects in the initial study described above were included in this report. This second study also included two nonrandomized groups—patients who did not receive any prophylactic transfusion (Group 3) or who were transfused (Group 4). Group 3 patients had the highest vaso-occlusive (including pain and ACS) complication rate (32% vs 12-19% in Groups 1, 2, and 4). The total anesthesia time was unexpectedly shorter for those who had open cholecystectomy rather than laparoscopy. While the hospital stay was shorter in patients who had the laparoscopic procedure (6.8 vs 9.4 days), the overall complication rate was similar in the two groups (38% vs 40%). Thus, even the technical advance afforded by laparoscopy has not diminished the perioperative risks experienced by sickle cell patients.

These collective experiences in the perioperative management of patients with SCD prompt the following recommendations:

First, the preoperative transfusion of red blood cells has an essential role in the care of these patients, yet it is a complement to, not a substitute for ensuring optimal anesthesiologic and perioperative supportive care to avoid hypoxia, dehydration, acidosis, and hypothermia. Transfusions alone cannot be relied on to provide absolute protection in the operative period.

Second, the prophylactic transfusion of red blood cells is indicated whenever prolonged general anesthesia is used or anticipated (eg, in cases where there is a considerable likelihood that local anesthesia will not suffice). Indeed, there even appears to be a substantial risk of perioperative complications associated with procedures performed under regional anesthesia,[59] and transfusion may be required in many of these cases, too. In contrast, transfusion is rarely necessary for uncomplicated, minor procedures performed with brief inhalational anesthetic (eg, myringotomy tubes, some dental surgery). Tonsillectomy/adenoidectomy is *not* a trivial procedure and should be regarded as having at least a moderate risk level.[51,59]

Third, in the majority of cases, the hematologic goal of transfusion is to achieve a hemoglobin concentration of 10-12 g/dL; in some cases, it also may be desirable to achieve a relative HbS concentration of less than 30-40%. However, criteria for a more aggressive approach are not well established. The patient's clinical condition and past history, particularly that of pulmonary complications, should be taken into account. In certain types of surgery involving critical anatomic sites, such as cardiac, orthopedic, or neurosurgery, yet-even-more-intensive prophylactic transfusion regimens may be warranted.

The method of transfusion used, whether simple or partial exchange, is not as important as the hematologic endpoint. The choice of transfusion method depends mostly on the clinical urgency and time available prior to surgery. When time allows, repeated simple transfusion over 2-4 weeks will achieve the aforementioned goals and is technically the easiest. Additional merits include lower procedural risk and reduced total transfusion requirement and donor exposure. In emergency situations, however, a single-volume red-blood-cell exchange transfusion to achieve the above-stated goals will promptly prepare the patient for surgery.

Fourth, as noted previously, when an objective for transfusion is the lowering of the relative concentration of HbS, this should be interpreted in the compound heterozygous sickle cell syndromes to mean a lowering of the relative percentage of *sick-leable cells*. Hb S/β^0 thalassemia, however, has a hemoglobin pattern similar to that seen in HbSS disease, and in both cases the relative concentration of HbS and the percentage of sickleable cells are similar.

Fifth, patients with sickle cell trait usually do not require prophylactic transfusion, but in special circumstances—for example, open-heart surgery or orthopedic surgery requiring the application of a tourniquet—it may be necessary. In these procedures, generalized or regional stasis may allow even sickle trait cells to sickle.

Angiography. SCD patients who must undergo cardiac or cerebral angiography should have prophylactic transfusion to lower the relative concentration of HbS to less than 20%; this is because the high osmolarity of commonly used IV contrast agents may promote intravascular sickling.[60] In addition, adequate hydration and oxygenation must be ensured. Preparative transfusion is not required for IV urography, but vigorous hydration should be provided both during and after the procedure.

Transfusion-Related Complications and Selection of Donors

Alloimmunization. The sensitization to transfused red cell antigens (alloimmunization) is one of the major complications associated with transfusion in patients with SCD and should be one of the major components in weighing the risks vs benefits of transfusion in a particular clinical situation. This problem may lead to a bothersome and costly delay in procuring compatible blood, or even a life-threatening inability to obtain suitable blood for transfusion. Furthermore, alloimmunization is the basis for delayed hemolytic transfusion reactions, which in sickle cell patients may resemble painful vaso-occlusive crises and are frequently serious and occasionally lethal.[61] (See below.) Patients who are destined to be likely candidates for periodic transfusion should have extended red cell antigen phenotyping, as this will aid in compatibility testing if alloimmunization is suspected or develops.

The overall risk of alloimmunization in both adult and pediatric sickle cell patients is approximately 20-35%.[62-64] Predictably, patients who are transfused often are at somewhat greater risk for alloimmunization than those who are seldom transfused. Alloimmunization may develop early in the course of their transfusion history,[65] and these individuals are also more apt to develop multiple alloantibodies. From this standpoint, patients with SCD resemble the population at large: some transfusion recipients readily become alloimmunized and are termed "hyperresponders," but most do not become alloimmunized despite multiple transfusions.[66-68] To some extent, however, the risk of alloimmunization increases with progressive transfusion,[69] and one-half of those who become alloimmunized ultimately develop multiple alloantibodies.[62]

About one-half to two-thirds of the alloantibodies that develop in transfused sickle cell patients are directed at antigens of the Rh blood group system, the most common of these being anti-rh″(E).[63,66,67] Another 20% of the alloantibodies in these patients are anti-Kell (K) and anti-Kidd (Jkª and Jkᵇ).[67,70] Up to one-third of the alloantibodies are Lewis antibodies, but, as in the general population, these are not typically clinically significant.

Chronically transfused Black patients are at increased risk of alloimmunization compared with members of other racial groups. Whereas transfused patients with SCD have an alloimmunization rate of 30%, only about 5% of patients with thalassemia and 10% of patients who are transfused regularly for other conditions become alloimmunized. These findings are generally attributed to the greater disparity, with respect to race and red cell phenotype, that exists between blood donors and sickle cell recipients compared with other recipients.[62,63] In many urban areas, the donor pool is up to 95% White,[62,63] and these donors typically possess a variety of Rh, Duffy, Kell, and Kidd antigens that are not found often in the Black population. Orlina et al[63] have calculated that a Black recipient has a 33% chance of compatibility for these antigens with any individual from an all-Black pool of donors, yet only a 3% chance of matching with someone from a typical urban donor pool of 90% White and 10% Black. Other determinants, in addi-

tion to antigenic compatibility, play a role in the development of alloimmunization. The intrinsic antigenicity of individual red cell antigens is a significant factor. For example, about 70% of Blacks are Fy(a–b–), while more than 99% of Whites are positive for one or both antigens, yet the incidence of alloimmunization to these antigens in transfused Black patients is only about 15%.[67,70] Some researchers have proposed that Black patients with SCD might have a greater propensity toward alloimmunization than Blacks with other illnesses,[71] even though the two groups have a similar frequency of red cell antigens.[72] If this phenomenon exists, it might be explained by an altered immune state that sickle cell patients may have.

The optimal method for procuring and selecting blood donors for sickle cell patients remains controversial. Proposals have included suggestions according to the following criteria: 1) No special matching procedure, but simply using standard ABO and Rh typing.[65] This method is the easiest to use and is currently the most widely used, but it fully exposes recipients to the risks of alloimmunization. 2) Race. Although this method is unlikely to prevent alloimmunization, on the basis of statistical considerations, it would be predicted to at least delay its onset. This method reduces the time, effort, and expense required to find compatible donors, but it incurs a significant social cost[71] and would require extensive public education to be accepted. 3) Matching of extended red cell antigen profiles, including Kell and secondary Rh group antigens (eg, C and E).[62,68] This approach is the most costly, especially as it is applied unnecessarily to most individuals who are not destined to become alloimmunized; however, it provides the greatest possible benefit to those who would have suffered this significant complication. 4) Composite strategies, blending elements of the above approaches. For example, providing full phenotype matching after an initial antibody becomes detectable[73] targets only those who require the greatest care, but presumably does so at a stage before alloimmunization becomes a serious or insurmountable problem. Alternatively, technical advances may allow the rapid and convenient screening of units likely to be compatible for sickle cell recipients.[74] Increasing recruiting efforts for blood donation from minority groups would enhance the effectiveness of any of these approaches.

In addition to red cell alloimmunization, platelet alloimmunization has been reported in heavily transfused patients with SCD.[75] Approximately 85% of sickle cell patients who had received a lifetime total of 50 or more RBC transfusions were found to be alloimmunized to platelets, and, in at least half of these cases, the offending antibody had anti-HLA specificity. The incidence of platelet alloimmunization was concomitantly less in those who had received fewer RBC transfusions. Although the prevalence of red cell and platelet alloimmunization is quite high in frequently transfused sickle cell patients, there was a surprising lack of correlation in individuals between red cell and platelet alloimmunization. This suggests that propensity toward one form of alloimmunization does not augment the risk of developing the other form. The issue of platelet alloimmunization in transfused sickle cell patients is of particular concern in cases where marrow transplantation is being considered as a therapeutic option.

Delayed hemolytic transfusion reaction. This transfusion-associated complication occurs in about 5-20% of regularly transfused sickle cell patients, an incidence much higher than that found in other transfused populations.[76] It exhibits several unique features when manifested in patients with SCD and thus may constitute a distinctive syndrome in this setting.[77] Important characteristics include 1) severe pain, resembling sickle cell pain crisis; 2) marked reticulocytopenia; and 3) a posttransfusion hematocrit far *lower* than the pretransfusion level. Possible mechanisms for this outcome include the suppression of erythropoiesis, as evidenced by reticulocytopenia, together with hemolysis of donor red cells, sometimes, but not always, due to alloimmunization[78]; or destruction of autologous red cells, due to either standard autoimmune-mediated hemolysis or "bystander hemolysis."[76-78] In this latter process, there may be antigen-antibody interactions with transfused cells, but the principal consequence is complement activation and deposition on autologous cells, which are then subject to excessive hemolysis. Delayed hemolytic transfusion reactions are a particularly ominous threat as this potentially lethal complication is not necessarily prevented through the use of phenotypically matched blood.

Blood with sickle cell trait for patients without sickle cell disease. Blood with sickle cell trait (HbAS) has an oxygen-carrying capacity and is otherwise functionally comparable to normal blood, so that in most general, elective transfusion settings, it can be used safely. Sickle trait blood is also suitable for autologous transfusion, so long as the recipient has none of the risk factors cited above during the time of infusion.[79] However, it should be avoided in patients at high risk for hypoxemia or acidosis because even sickle trait blood may undergo sickling under such circumstances. For example, it should be avoided in the neonatal setting (especially for premature infants who are ventilator-dependent) and in patients with severe cardiopulmonary disease or shock. Unless special processing steps are used, blood with sickle trait should not be subject to frozen storage, as HbAS red cells may undergo excessive destruction during the deglycerolization process.[80]

Blood with sickle cell trait for patients with sickle cell disease. Blood with sickle cell trait is undesirable for use in sickle cell patients because the resulting mixture of HbAS and HbSS cells obfuscates results obtained by hemoglobin electrophoresis, which is commonly used to assess the progress of transfusion therapy. Furthermore, in the great majority of circumstances requiring transfusion in SCD, there is a danger of progressive sickling, which might be exacerbated rather than prevented by the infusion of sickle trait blood.

Thalassemias

The thalassemia syndromes, the most prevalent of all known genetic diseases, are most concentrated along an equatorial belt that extends from the Mediterranean basin and Africa to Southeast Asia. As is the case with sickle cell trait, the presence of the thalassemia trait condition has been regarded as conferring on affected individuals a protective influence against infection with falciparum malaria. In contrast to the qualitative hemoglobin disorders, which are characterized by structural change and for which SCD serves as a paradigm, the thalassemia syndromes are quantitative disorders of hemoglobin production. Although α-thalassemia is more prevalent worldwide, β-thalassemia has greater clinical significance, particularly in the United States, so greater emphasis is devoted to this disorder here.

Molecular Basis of the Thalassemia Syndromes

More than 100 mutations causing β-thalassemia have been identified, most of which are point mutations (ie, single DNA base substitutions) in or near the β-globin gene. The position of the mutation, or its molecular effect, is predictive of its clinical outcome. For example, "nonsense mutations" are single DNA base substitutions that create premature termination signals in place of codons for amino acids. Genes with this mutation produce no functional message and, in the case of the β-globin gene, no β^A-globin; they are designated β^0-thalassemia mutations. A nonsense mutation at β-39 is responsible for more than 90% of β-thalassemia mutations in Sardinians, and another at β-17 is the cause of one of the common forms of β-thalassemia in the Chinese. Additions or deletions of nucleotides in coding portions of genes (exons) produce frameshift mutations that also result in nonfunctional messenger RNA (mRNA) and the β^0-thalassemia phenotype. The adjacent δ-globin gene is occasionally affected by deletions, resulting in the hereditary persistence of HbF or $\delta\beta$-thalassemia. Almost half of all β-thalassemia mutations involve the splice site for the removal of intervening sequences, or introns, from precursor mRNA. Mutations that lie at the exact splice site prevent functional mRNA formation and also produce β^0-thalassemia. In contrast, mutations that are immediately adjacent to these splice sites cause diminished, but not absent, transcription of normal mRNA, and the result therefore is designated β^+-thalassemia. Similarly, mutations in the promoter region of the gene interfere with transcription and

also cause β^+-thalassemia. In β-thalassemia, the deficient production of β-chains results in the diminished formation of HbA; to some degree, there may be a compensatory increase in the production of HbF and HbA$_2$, but this process is always incomplete.

Many of the types of single-base pair substitutions that cause β-thalassemia have also been described for α-thalassemia, but these account for relatively few cases. The great majority of mutations causing α-thalassemia are fairly extensive deletions affecting one or both α-globin genes on chromosome 16.

A relatively uncommon but intriguing group of α- and β-thalassemia disorders is characterized not only by diminished production of the respective globin but also by structural abnormality as well.[81] HbE is a β-chain abnormality in which a nucleotide substitution causes the replacement of glutamate by lysine at the β-26 position and is prevalent in individuals from Southeast Asia. In addition to this structural change, however, the DNA substitution also causes the activation of an abnormal, or cryptic, splice site for precursor mRNA. When the normal splice site is read, β^E-globin is transcribed, but when the novel splice site is used, nonfunctional mRNA is synthesized. This results in an overall reduction of functional message and, hence, globin, produced by the affected chromosome. The most common α-globin structural mutation is hemoglobin Constant Spring, which is caused by a mutation affecting the translation termination codon of the α-globin genes. The result is transcription of an elongated mRNA, which produces an extended α-globin chain. The thalassemic features of this disorder probably stem from abnormal instability of the message as well as the globin.[81]

The β-globin gene exists as a single copy on chromosome 11, thus accounting for trait (heterozygous) and homozygous conditions. In contrast, there are two copies of α-globin on chromosome 16, and four clinical phenotypes are recognized. The loss of one functioning α-globin gene does not produce any obvious hematologic or clinical abnormality and, thus, is termed the *silent carrier* condition. The α-thalassemia trait is caused by the loss of two functioning genes and produces a hematologic picture similar to that seen in β-thalassemia trait, with mild anemia, mild-to-moderate microcytosis, and red cell dysmorphology. At birth, γ_4 tetramers, sometimes referred to as hemoglobin Barts, may be detected in small quantities (about 4-7% of total hemoglobin). Afterwards, minute amounts of β_4 tetramer, or HbH, may be found. HbH disease occurs with loss of function in three α-globin genes and typically causes moderate to severe anemia, severe microcytosis, prominent red cell dysmorphology, and mild chronic hemolysis, which may be acutely exacerbated by infections or exposure to oxidant drugs. This condition is readily evident at birth, and affected newborns have 20-30% Hb Barts; then, in their first year of life, HbH becomes the predominant hemoglobin species. The most severe form of α-thalassemia is caused by total absence of α-globin synthesis. Because all the hemoglobins normally present in newborns (A, A_2, and F) contain α-chains, none can be produced in fetuses with this disorder. Most affected fetuses succumb in utero with the syndrome of hydrops fetalis, characterized by massive hepatosplenomegaly, severe generalized edema, and heart failure. Fetuses that survive to birth rarely survive more than a few hours unless heroic measures are taken. The most severe forms of α-thalassemia, with three and four gene deletions, are restricted largely to individuals of East Asian descent.

Pathophysiology

The genetic abnormalities described thus far, causing decreased synthesis of the respective globins, account for only part of the anemia and pathophysiology encountered in the thalassemia syndromes. In β-thalassemia, a second and major component contributing to the pathogenesis of the disease is the imbalance in synthesis of α- and non-α-globin chains. The excess α-chains that remain uncombined are highly unstable and precipitate and ultimately become deposited on the red cell membrane. These damaged cells are subject to increased hemolysis, causing shortened red cell survival, and adding further to the severity of these patients' anemia.

Erythrocytes from individuals with thalassemia are significantly more susceptible to oxidative stress than are normal cells because they contain excess globin chains, elevated concentrations of nonheme iron, and comparatively low concentrations of hemoglobin.[82] In patients with β-thalassemia, the excess α-globin subunits are readily oxidized to methemoglobin in a process that simultaneously generates superoxide and other oxygen-free radicals. These oxygen-free radicals cause red cell injury through the production of additional methemoglobin, the formation of reversible and irreversible hemichromes, membrane lipid peroxidation, and oxidative damage to globins and cell membrane proteins. The latter effect produces abnormalities in cation exchange that significantly reduces red cell survival in these patients. These processes are summarized in Fig 2-4.[82]

Hemichromes are oxidative products of globin subunits that are soluble initially and can be returned to a fully functional state. However, if they are subjected to additional oxidative steps, they become irreversibly oxidized and insoluble and, as such, can be visualized after staining with supravital dye as Heinz bodies. Hemichromes seem to modify or even increase the antigenicity of the red cell membrane, and they also increase the binding of immunoglobin to the membrane. These changes promote phagocytosis and premature destruction of the red cells in which they occur. The oxidation of constituent lipids results in increased recognition by macrophages and the hastened breakdown of red cells. This process of the premature destruction of erythrocytes, even before their release from the marrow, is termed *ineffective erythropoiesis* and is a seminal finding in the severe thalassemias.

There is an analogous imbalance between α- and non-α-globin chains in the more severe forms of α-thalassemia (eg, HbH disease). In this instance, β_4- and γ_4-chain homotetramers undergo oxidation to hemichromes, which then precipitate, causing red cell membrane damage and premature destruction. Differences in the hemolytic processes in α- and β-thalassemia have been reviewed.[83] In addition, it is important to recognize that HbH does not display a Bohr effect and is wholly ineffective as

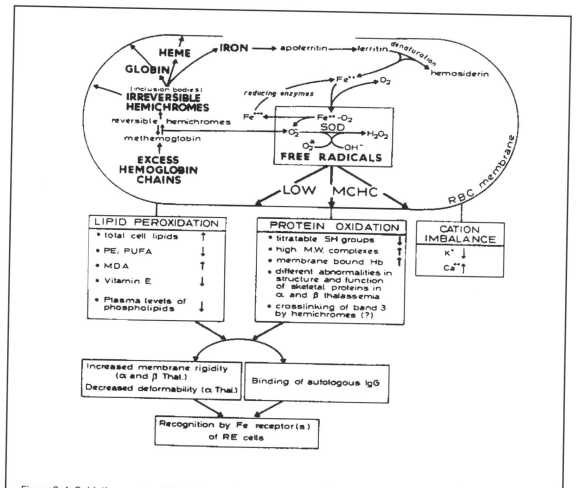

Figure 2-4. Oxidative events within thalassemic red cells that contribute to membrane damage and shortened red cell survival. Used with permission from Shinar and Rachmilewitz.[82]

a carrier of oxygen under typical physiologic conditions. In individuals with high HbH concentrations, the total hemoglobin concentration may therefore be a misleading indicator of the oxygen-carrying capacity of the blood.

Clinical Features of the Thalassemia Syndromes

The clinical picture of β-thalassemia begins to develop at several months of age, when the waning production of HbF is normally replaced by a rising synthesis of HbA. An intense erythropoietic drive,

mediated by erythropoietin, attempts to compensate for the worsening anemia, but this is largely a futile process because of the phenomenon of ineffective erythropoiesis. Marrow cavities expand in the drive to increase circulating red cell mass, and, in the untreated child, characteristic bony deformities develop. As cortices of long bones become thin, they become prone to pathologic fracture. In addition, abnormal marrow spaces develop in the skull and face, producing a characteristic facial appearance caused by maxillary hypertrophy, dental overbite, and frontal bossing. The liver and spleen become enlarged as they are recruited to become sites of extramedullary hematopoiesis and are stimulated to undergo reticuloendothelial expansion. Because of the rapid rate of hemolysis, jaundice and eventually cholelithiasis commonly develop. Impaired growth is seen frequently. Eventually, congestive heart failure becomes a major threat that arises, not only from the severity of the anemia, but also from augmentation of the circulating plasma volume that is associated with shunting a large portion of the cardiac output through expanded marrow cavities and the enlarged liver and spleen. In milder forms of the disease, there is a correspondingly slower progression of symptoms and complications and increased duration of survival. Individuals with β-thalassemia trait have a mild hypochromic, microcytic anemia but are not clinically impaired.

As noted previously, the extent of clinical disease in those with α-thalassemia depends on the number of genes affected. The two-gene deletion produces a hematologic picture resembling that seen in β-thalassemia trait, but clinical disease potentially severe enough to require transfusion arises with the deletion of three genes (HbH disease); hydrops fetalis, with four genes absent, is generally regarded as being too severe to permit long-term viability. Because the α-globin gene is fully expressed at the time of birth, the hematologic profiles of the various syndromes are manifest at that time.

Transfusion Therapy for Severe Thalassemia Syndromes

The mainstay of therapy for the severe β-thalassemia syndromes is the periodic transfusion of RBCs. The goals of transfusion in this setting are now recognized as being twofold: to correct the anemia and to suppress ineffective erythropoiesis, thereby avoiding its deleterious consequences. Early transfusion protocols sought to maintain hemoglobin concentrations in the range of 6-8 g/dL and were successful at alleviating the immediate consequences of anemia. However, they were ineffective in suppressing erythropoiesis and preventing the sequelae of marrow expansion, as well as the concomitantly increased gastrointestinal absorption of iron. In 1964, Wolman[84] reported an innovative approach in the management of these patients. He found that patients who were transfused to maintain hemoglobin levels of at least 8.5-10.5 g/dL had obtained superior results compared with those who had received less-intensive transfusion therapy. Patients who were maintained at the higher hemoglobin levels had greater suppression of their erythropoietic drive and more successful prevention of the adverse sequelae of ineffective erythropoiesis. Furthermore, these patients had improved growth patterns and cardiac performance. Subsequent regimens sought to maintain yet higher hemoglobin concentrations, achieving minimum levels of about 9.5-10.0 g/dL, and the results of these trials showed some further improvement in clinical outcome. This approach is now termed "hypertransfusion" and typically consists of transfusing 10-20 mL of red blood cells per kilogram every 2-4 weeks. Filters to render the transfusate leukocyte-reduced should be used routinely to minimize the risk of febrile transfusion reactions to which these multitransfused patients may be particularly susceptible.

Regular transfusions should be initiated as soon as significant anemia becomes apparent and the diagnosis is established. In severe β-thalassemia major, this routinely occurs in the first year of life. In infants, the advent of progressive anemia is accompanied by growth delay. Timely institution of hypertransfusion helps to avert marrow hypertrophy and its sequelae,[85] and normal growth and cardiac function can be maintained as long as transfusion-associated complications, such as hemosiderosis, are adequately addressed. If there is any uncertainty as to whether a patient may have a milder *thalassemia intermedia* syndrome, which characteristically does not require periodic transfusions, such an individual may be observed closely and his or her transfusions delayed until the clinical picture becomes clearer.

Some clinicians have had favorable experiences with, and advocate, even more intensive transfusion regimens ("supertransfusion"), which aim to maintain a minimum hematocrit of at least 35%.[86] However, this practice has not been universally embraced.[87] To some extent, the goal for any individual patient should be individualized on the basis of an assessment of the potential benefits of more aggressive transfusion vs the risks, which include hemosiderosis and immune and infectious complications.

As noted previously, massive splenomegaly is commonly found in untreated, severe β-thalassemia major. Although regular transfusions help to limit the contribution of extramedullary hematopoiesis to this finding, reticuloendothelial expansion may be diminished, but not prevented, by this treatment. Thus, even appropriately managed patients can develop significant hypersplenism. In patients so affected, transfusion requirements often increase progressively. When the transfusion requirement exceeds 200 mL/kg/per year, splenectomy is advised because it has been shown to reliably reduce the transfusion requirement by 25-75%.[88-90] This benefit appears to be enduring.[91]

Transfusion with a selected population of young red cells ("neocytes") offers the advantages of enhanced survival of transfused blood, diminished overall iron load,[92-93] and can now be accomplished expeditiously using commercial systems (Neocel, Medsep Corp, Covina, CA).[94] However, the potential benefits are tempered by the serious disadvantages of exposure to an increased number of donors and higher direct preparation costs.

In the case of β-thalassemia, transfusion is likely to be required only in the homozygous condition. However, pregnant individuals with heterozygous β-thalassemia may have exacerbations of anemia, and they too may benefit from transfusion therapy. In α-thalassemia, patients with HbH disease who are in otherwise good health usually do not require regular transfusions, but, during periods of oxidative stress, RBC transfusion may be necessary. Splenectomy should be considered only in the uncommon circumstance of frank hypersplenism.

Hemosiderosis

The benefits of regular transfusion therapy are acquired at a cost. The complications of transfusion, such as alloimmunization or infection, are chance occurrences and depend on the individual characteristics of donor units. On the other hand, *every* milliliter of transfused RBCs contains approximately 1 mg of elemental iron; the accumulation of iron is an inexorable consequence of long-term transfusion, for the body has no suitable means to excrete excess iron. Signs of clinical toxicity are likely to become evident when the total body iron burden reaches 400-1000 mg/kg of body weight, and these levels may be achieved after just several years of regular transfusion; levels beyond this range are often lethal.[95] The primary sites of potentially lethal iron toxicity are the heart and liver, but endocrine abnormalities are commonly observed as well.

Iron overload can be treated or even prevented with the faithful administration of the iron-chelating agent deferoxamine. This agent has a high affinity and specificity for iron and achieves its elimination as a bound complex in the urine. Unfortunately, the only effective method currently available for administration is through parenteral routes. Most commonly, it is administered subcutaneously overnight via a portable infusion pump. Most authorities recommend instituting therapy with this agent when a total of approximately 25 units of RBCs has been transfused, the serum ferritin has reached about 1000 ng/mL, or the patient is about 3-5 years of age.[96] When deferoxamine is used regularly, net iron loss can be achieved even while transfusion therapy remains ongoing.[97-98] However, this medication has several unfavorable characteristics: its requirement for parenteral administration impedes compliance; it is very expensive; and it may cause neurotoxicity, particularly visual and auditory disturbances. These flaws must be endured, however, until a superior substitute is found.

Disorders of Red Cell Enzymes

Numerous erythrocyte constituents, including hemoglobin and a variety of cell membrane components, must be maintained in the reduced state, and this essential task is accomplished by the pentose phosphate shunt. In contrast, the glycolytic pathway is the source of metabolic energy for the erythrocyte. Assorted enzyme deficiencies have been reported in both pathways, and chronic hemolytic anemia is the most common clinical consequence in these cases, with the exception of deficiencies in phosphofructokinase, triosephosphate isomerase, and phosphoglycerate kinase, which display multisystemic symptoms. Most enzyme deficiencies affecting these two pathways are inherited in an autosomal recessive fashion, but G6PD deficiency (affecting the pentose phosphate shunt) and phosphoglycerate kinase (affecting the glycolytic pathway) are inherited in an X-linked fashion. G6PD deficiency and pyruvate kinase deficiency are the most common enzyme disorders encountered that cause chronic hemolytic anemia, and they are discussed here.

G6PD deficiency is most common in people from the same geographic areas harboring the malaria parasite that was referred to previously, and it may be inherited simultaneously with the hemoglobin disorders endemic in those areas. Two main clinical forms have been described: an African variant, designated Gd^{A-}, and a Mediterranean form, Gd^{Mediterranean}. Both types are characterized by an accelerated age-related decrease in the red cell activity of the enzyme. In the African form, the decline in enzyme activity with age is gradual, so, at any given time, only a small fraction of the circulating red cells is significantly deficient in enzyme activity. In contrast, there is much lower enzyme activity in the Mediterranean variety, and nearly all the circulating red cells are affected. Erythrocytes that are deficient in G6PD are highly vulnerable to oxidant stress, which typically is precipitated by infections and certain drugs and chemicals. In red cells that are incapable of handling such a metabolic stress, the hemoglobin precipitates and forms Heinz bodies. These precipitates become deposited on the red cell membrane and are removed by the spleen, but, eventually, the membrane sustains irreparable damage and the cell becomes subject to premature destruction. Under normal, well-compensated circumstances, both variants of G6PD deficiency exhibit little, if any, hematologic abnormality, but, when faced with an acute oxidant stress, the two forms exhibit strikingly differ-

ent responses. Patients with the African form sustain just a limited degree of hemolysis, but patients with the Mediterranean form may suffer a profound, life-threatening hemolytic crisis. In such instances, the transfusion of RBCs may be vital and life-saving. In less obvious cases, decisions regarding transfusion should take into account the absolute level of hemoglobin, the apparent rate of hemolysis, and the projected decline in hemoglobin concentration.

Pyruvate kinase deficiency exists primarily in individuals of northern European origin. Two characteristic metabolic abnormalities associated with this deficiency are decreased red cell concentrations of adenosine triphosphate and increased concentrations of 2,3-DPG.[99] Through mechanisms that are not well understood, erythrocytes from individuals with pyruvate kinase deficiency undergo premature destruction in the spleen, liver, and marrow, which causes varying degrees of anemia. The clinical expression of this deficiency varies considerably: some cases present in the neonatal period with an acute anemia requiring exchange transfusion, while other cases remain undetected well through adulthood. In most cases, the hemoglobin concentration ranges from 8-12 g/dL, but acute exacerbation of the anemia may arise during pregnancy or infection. The transfusion of RBCs may be helpful during these periods but is rarely required on a chronic basis. Splenectomy is often effective in diminishing the rate of hemolysis in these patients, helping the hemoglobin concentration to rise about 1-3 g/dL above preoperative levels, and it may eliminate or at least reduce the need for additional transfusion.[99]

Disorders of Red Cell Membranes

The primary functions of the red cell membrane are to maintain structural integrity and to regulate ion transport and water permeability. The most common disorders of the red cell membrane include hereditary spherocytosis and hereditary elliptocytosis. Hereditary spherocytosis is seen most frequently in people of northern European extraction, while hereditary elliptocytosis is more widespread.

Several variants have been reported for each of these disorders, but, in nearly all cases, there is an autosomal dominant mode of inheritance.

Chronic hemolysis is a characteristic finding in both disorders, but the severity varies considerably, even within each entity. In milder cases, hemolysis is mild and well compensated, but, in more severely affected individuals, there may be conspicuous anemia. Hemolysis occurs within the spleen as the misshapen and inflexible red cells in these disorders attempt to traverse the spleen's tortuous circulation, acquire cumulative structural and/or metabolic defects ("splenic conditioning"), and are destroyed prematurely. Especially in cases of hereditary spherocytosis, splenectomy is often effective in decreasing the rate of hemolysis and alleviating the anemia, even while the morphologic abnormality persists. Prior to splenectomy, patients with these membrane disorders are at risk for contracting aplastic crisis owing to parvovirus infection, in a manner comparable to that described for SCD. In hereditary spherocytosis, hemolysis may be exacerbated by infection, strenuous exercise, or pregnancy. Regardless of the etiology, transfusion is indicated if the exacerbation of anemia is protracted or severe.

Conclusion

The transfusion of red blood cells is an essential therapy for congenital hemolytic anemias. However, the many indications for their use in this setting are not always well established or uniformly accepted. In any particular clinical circumstance, the clinician needs to consider the physiologic goal of treatment, and whether the transfusion of red cells is the best method to achieve that goal. Similar considerations also will help to determine the amount and frequency of transfusion therapy.

References

1. Ballas SK, Mohandas N. Pathophysiology of vaso-occlusion. Hematol Oncol Clin N Am 1996;10:1221-39.

2. Bookchin RM, Lew VL. Pathophysiology of sickle cell anemia. Hematol Oncol Clin N Am 1996;10:1241-53.

3. Hofrichter J, Ross PD, Eaton WA. A physical description of hemoglobin S gelation. In: Hercules JI, Cottam GL, Waterman MR, Schechter AN, eds. Proceedings of the Symposium on Molecular and Cellular Aspects of Sickle Cell Disease. DHEW publication (NIH) 76-1007. Bethesda: US Department of Health, Education and Welfare, 1976:185-224.

4. Nagel RL, Fabry ME, Kaul DK, et al. Known and potential sources for epistatic effects in sickle cell anemia. Ann N Y Acad Sci 1989; 565:228-38.

5. Hebbel RP. Beyond hemoglobin polymerization: The red blood cell membrane and sickle cell disease pathophysiology. Blood 1991;77: 214-37.

6. Hebbel RP. The sickle erythrocyte in double jeopardy: Autoxidation and iron decompartmentalization. Semin Hematol 1990;27:51-69.

7. Powars DR, Chan L, Schroeder WA. The influence of fetal hemoglobin on the clinical expression of sickle cell anemia. Ann N Y Acad Sci 1989:565:262-78.

8. Powars DR, Meiselman HJ, Fisher TC. β^S-gene-cluster haplotypes modulate hematologic and hemorheologic expression in sickle cell anemia. Am J Pediatr Hematol Oncol 1994;16:55-61.

9. Pagnier J, Mears JG, Dunda-Belkhodja O, et al. Evidence for the multicentric origin of the sickle cell hemoglobin gene in Africa. Proc Natl Acad Sci U S A 1984;81:1771-3.

10. Powars DR. β^S-gene-cluster haplotypes in sickle cell anemia. Hematol Oncol Clin N Am 1991;5:475-93.

11. Nagel RL. Severity, pathobiology, epistatic effects, and genetic markers in sickle cell anemia. Semin Hematol 1991;28:180-201.

12. Lessin LS, Kurantsin-Mills J, Klug PP, et al. Determination of rheologically optimal mixtures of AA and SS erythrocytes. Blood 1977;50 (Suppl 1):111.

13. Schmalzer EA, Lee JO, Brown AK, et al. Viscosity of mixtures of sickle and normal red cells at varying hematocrit levels. Transfusion 1987;27:228-33.

14. Piomelli S, Seaman C, Ackerman K, et al. Planning an exchange transfusion in patients with sickle cell syndromes. Am J Pediatr Hematol Oncol 1990;12:268-76.

15. Sharon BI, Honig GR. Management of congenital hemolytic anemia. In: Rossi EC, Simon TL, Moss GS, eds. Principles of transfusion medicine. Baltimore: Williams & Wilkins, 1991:136.

16. Bunn HF, Forget BG. Hemoglobin: Molecular, genetic and clinical aspects. Philadelphia: WB Saunders, 1986:515-27.

17. Powell RW, Levine GL, Yang YM, et al. Acute splenic sequestration crisis in sickle cell disease: Early detection and treatment. J Pediatr Surg 1992;27:215-9.

18. Bell LM, Naides SJ, Stoffman P, et al. Human parvovirus B19 infection among hospital staff members after contact with infected patients. N Engl J Med 1989;321:485-91.

19. Russel MO, Goldberg HI, Hodson A, et al. Effect of transfusion therapy on arteriographic abnormalities and on recurrence of stroke in sickle cell disease. Blood 1984;63:162-9.

20. Cohen AR, Martin MB, Silber JH, et al. A modified transfusion program for prevention of stroke in sickle cell disease. Blood 1992;79:1657-61.

21. Quattlebaum TG, Pierce MM. Estimates of need for transfusion during hypertransfusion therapy in sickle cell disease. J Pediatr 1986;109:456-9.

22. Miller ST, Rao SP, Jensen D, et al. Is chronic transfusion necessary to prevent recurrent stroke in children with sickle cell disease? Ann N Y Acad Sci 1989;565:435-7.

23. Adams RJ, McKie VC, Hsu L, et al. Prevention of a first stroke by transfusions in children with sickle cell anemia and abnormal results on transcranial doppler ultrasonography. N Engl J Med 1998;339:5-11.

24. Dreyer ZE. Chest infections and syndromes in sickle cell disease of childhood. Semin Respir Infect 1996;11:163-72.

25. Vichinsky EP, Styles LA, Colengelo LH, et al. ACS in sickle cell disease: Clinical presentation and course. Blood 1997;89:1787-92.

26. Emre U, Miller S, Gutierez M, et al. Effect of transfusion in ACS of sickle cell disease. J Pediatr 1995;127:901-4.

27. Castro O. Systemic fat embolism and pulmonary hypertension in sickle cell disease. Hematol Oncol Clin N Am 1996;10:1289-303.

28. Mallouh AA, Asha M. Beneficial effect of blood transfusion in children with sickle cell chest syndrome. Am J Dis Child 1988;142:178-82.

29. Emre U, Miller ST, Rao S, et al. Alveolararterial oxygen gradient in ACS of sickle cell disease. J Pediatr 1993;123:272-5.

30. Wong W, Elliot-Mills D, Powars D. Renal failure in sickle cell anemia. Hematol Oncol Clin N Am 1996;10:1321-31.

31. Emond AM, Holman R, Hayes RJ, et al. Priapism and impotence in homozygous sickle cell disease. Arch Intern Med 1980;140:1434-7.

32. Powars DR, Johnson CS. Priapism. Hematol Oncol Clin N Am 1996;10:1363-72.

33. Seeler RA. Intensive transfusion therapy for priapism in boys with sickle cell anemia. J Urol 1973;110:360-1.

34. Hamre MR, Harmon EP, Kirkpatrick DV, et al. Priapism as a complication of sickle cell disease. J Urol 1991;145:1-5.

35. Rackoff WR, Ohene-Frempong K, Month S, et al. Neurologic events after partial exchange transfusion for priapism in sickle cell disease. J Pediatr 1992;120:882-5.

36. Siegel JF, Rich MA, Brock WA. Association of sickle cell disease, priapism, exchange transfusion and neurological events: ASPEN syndrome. J Urol 1993;150:1480-2.

37. O'Callaghan A, O'Brien SG, Ninkovic M, et al. Chronic intrahepatic cholestasis in sickle cell disease requiring exchange transfusion. Gut 1995;37:144-7.

38. Betrosian A, Balla M, Kafiri G, et al. Case report: Reversal of liver failure in sickle cell vaso-occlusive crisis. Am J Med Sci 1996;311: 292-5.

39. Weisz-Carrington P. Principles of clinical immunohematology. Chicago: Year Book Medical Publishers, 1986:183.

40. Fort AT, Morrison JC, Berreras L, et al. Counseling the patient with sickle cell disease about reproduction: Pregnancy outcome does not justify the maternal risk! Am J Obstet Gynecol 1971;111:324-7.

41. Powars DR. Sandhu M. Niland-Weiss J, et al. Pregnancy in sickle cell disease. Obstet Gynecol 1986;67:217-28.

42. Seoud MAF, Cantwell C, Nobles G, Levy DL. Outcome of pregnancies complicated by sickle cell and sickle-C hemoglobinopathies. Am J Perinatol 1994;11:187-91.

43. Howard RJ, Tuck SM, Pearson TC. Pregnancy in sickle cell disease in the UK: Results of a multicentre survey of the effect of prophylactic blood transfusion on maternal and fetal outcome. Br J Obstet Gynecol 1995;102: 947-51.

44. Cunningham FG, Pritchard JA, Mason R. Pregnancy and sickle cell hemoglobinopathies: Results with and without prophylactic transfusions. Obstet Gynecol 1983;62: 419-24.

45. Charache S, Scott J, Niebyl J, et al. Management of sickle cell disease in pregnant patients. Obstet Gynecol 1980;55:407-10.

46. Koshy M, Burd L, Wallace D, et al. Prophylactic red-cell transfusions in pregnant patients with sickle cell disease. N Engl J Med 1988; 319:1447-52.

47. Howard RJ, Tuck SM, Pearson TC. Blood transfusion in pregnancies complicated by maternal sickle cell disease. Effect on blood rheology and uteroplacental Doppler velocimetry. Clin Lab Haematol 1994;16:253-9.

48. Koshy M, Burd L. Management of pregnancy in sickle cell syndromes. Hematol Oncol Clin N Am 1991;5:585-96.

49. Homi J, Reynolds J, Skinner A, et al. General anesthesia in sickle cell disease. Br Med J 1979;1:1599-601.

50. Bischoff RJ, Williamson A, Dalali MJ, et al. Assessment of the use of transfusion therapy perioperatively in patients with sickle cell hemoglobinopathies. Ann Surg 1988;207:434-8.

51. Griffin TC, Buchanan GR. Elective surgery in children with sickle cell disease without preoperative blood transfusion. J Pediatr Surg 1993;28:681-5.

52. Janik J, Seeler RA. Perioperative management of children with sickle hemoglobinopathy. J Pediatr Surg 1980;15:117-20.

53. Morrison JC, Whybrew WD, Bucovaz ET. Use of partial exchange transfusion preoperatively in patients with sickle cell hemoglobinopathies. Am J Obstet Gynecol 1978;132:59-63.

54. Fullerton MW, Philippart AI, Sarnaik S, et al. Preoperative exchange transfusion in sickle cell anemia. J Pediatr Surg 1981;16:297-300.

55. Ryan SJ, Goldberg MF. Anterior segment ischemia following scleral buckling in sickle cell hemoglobinopathy. Am J Ophthalmol 1971;72:35-50.

56. Jampol LM, Green JL, Goldberg MF, et al. An update on vitrectomy surgery and retinal detachment repair in sickle cell disease. Arch Ophthalmol 1982;100:591-3.

57. Vichinsky EP, Haberkern CM, Neumayr L, et al. A comparison of conservative and aggressive transfusion regimens in the perioperative management of sickle cell disease. N Engl J Med 1995;333:206-13.

58. Haberkern C, Neumayr LD, Orringer AP, et al. Cholecystectomy in sickle cell anemia patients: Perioperative outcome of 364 cases from the National Preoperative Transfusion Study. Blood 1997;89:1533-42.

59. Koshy M, Weiner SJ, Miller ST, et al. Surgery and anesthesia in sickle cell disease. Blood 1995;86:3676-84.

60. Stockman JA, Nigro MA, Mishkin MM, et al. Occlusion of large cerebral vessels in sickle-cell anemia. N Engl J Med 1972;287:846-9.

61. Milner PF, Squires JE, Larison PJ, et al. Post-transfusion crises in sickle cell anemia: Role of delayed hemolytic transfusion reactions to transfusion. South Med J 1985;78:1462-8.

62. Vichinsky EP, Earles A, Johnson RA, et al. Alloimmunization in sickle cell anemia and transfusion of racially unmatched blood. N Engl J Med 1990;322:1617-21.

63. Orlina AR, Sosler SD, Koshy M. Problems of chronic transfusion in sickle cell disease. J Clin Apheresis 1991;6:234-40.

64. Sosler SD, Jilly BJ, Saporito C, et al. A simple, practical model for reducing alloimmunization in patients with sickle cell disease. Am J Hematol 1993;43:103-6.

65. Blumberg N, Ross K, Avila E, et al. Should chronic transfusions be matched for antigens other than ABO and Rho (D)? Vox Sang 1984; 47:205-8.

66. Orlina AR, Unger PJ, Koshy M. Post-transfusion alloimmunization in patients with sickle cell disease. Am J Hematol 1978;5: 101-6.

67. Coles SM, Klein HG, Holland PV. Alloimmunization in two multitransfused patient populations. Transfusion 1981;21:462-6.

68. Ambruso DR, Githens JH, Alcorn R, et al. Experience with donors matched for minor blood group antigens in patients with sickle cell anemia who are receiving chronic transfusion therapy. Transfusion 1987;27:94-8.

69. Rosse WF, Gallagher D, Kinney TR, et al. Transfusion and alloimmunization in sickle cell disease. Blood 1990;76:1431-7.

70. Alarif L, Castro O, Ofosu M, et al. HLA-B35 is associated with red cell alloimmunization in sickle cell disease. Clin Immunol Immunopathol 1986;38:178-83.

71. Charache S. Problems in transfusion therapy. N Engl J Med 1990;322:1666-8.

72. Patten E, Patel SN, Soto B, et al. Transfusion management of patients with sickle cell disease. Ann N Y Acad Sci 1989;565:446-8.

73. Ness PM. To match or not to match: The question for chronically transfused patients with sickle cell anemia (editorial). Transfusion 1994;34:558-60.

74. Sandler SG, Mallory D, Wolfe JS, et al. Screening with monoclonal anti-Fy3 to provide blood for phenotype-matched transfusions for patients with sickle cell disease. Transfusion 1997;37:393-7.

75. Friedman DF, Lukas MB, Jawad A, et al. Alloimmunization to platelets in heavily transfused patients with sickle cell disease. Blood 1996;88:3216-22.

76. Garratty G. Severe reactions associated with transfusion of patients with sickle cell disease (editorial). Transfusion 1997;37:357-61.

77. Petz LD, Calhoun L, Shulman IA, et al. The sickle cell hemolytic transfusion reaction syndrome. Transfusion 1997;37:382-92.

78. King KE, Shirey RS, Lankiewicz MW, et al. Delayed hemolytic transfusion reactions in sickle cell disease: Simultaneous destruction of recipients' red cells. Transfusion 1997;37: 376-81.

79. Romanoff ME, Woodward DG, Bullard WG. Autologous blood transfusion in patients with sickle cell trait. Anesthesiology 1988;68: 820-1.

80. Walker RH, ed. Technical manual. 11th ed. Bethesda, MD: American Association of Blood Banks, 1993:118.

81. Adams JG, Coleman MB. Structural hemoglobin variants that produce the phenotype of thalassemia. Semin Hematol 1990;27:229-38.

82. Shinar E, Rachmilewitz EA. Oxidative denaturation of red cells in thalassemia. Semin Hematol 1990;27:70-82.

83. Shinar E, Rachmilewitz EA. Differences in the pathophysiology of hemolysis of α- and β-thalassemic red blood cells. Ann N Y Acad Sci 1990;612:118-26.

84. Wolman IJ. Transfusion therapy in Cooley's anemia: Growth and health as related to long-range hemoglobin levels. Ann N Y Acad Sci 1964;119:736-47.

85. Piomelli S, Danoff SJ, Becker MH, et al. Prevention of bone malformations and cardiomegaly in Cooley's anemia by early hyper-

transfusion regimen. Ann N Y Acad Sci 1969; 165:427-36.

86. Propper RD, Button LN, Nathan DG. New approaches to the transfusion management of thalassemia. Blood 1980;55:55-60.

87. Piomelli S. The management of patients with Cooley's anemia: Transfusions and splenectomy. Semin Hematol 1995;32:262-8.

88. Cohen A, Markenson AL, Schwartz E. Transfusion requirements and splenectomy in thalassemia major. J Pediatr 1980;97:100-2.

89. Piomelli S, Loew T. Management of thalassemia major (Cooley's anemia). Hematol Oncol Clin N Am 1991;5:557-69.

90. Rebulla P, Modell B. Transfusion requirements and effects in patients with thalassaemia major. Lancet 1991;337:277-80.

91. Cohen A, Gayer R, Mizanin J. Long-term effect of splenectomy on transfusion requirements in thalassemia major. Am J Hematol 1989;30:254-6.

92. Piomelli S, Seaman C, Reibman J, et al. Separation of younger red cells with improved survival in vivo: An approach to chronic transfusion therapy. Proc Natl Acad Sci U S A 1978; 75:3474-8.

93. Berdoukas VA, Kwan YL, Sansotta ML. A study on the value of red cell exchange transfusion in transfusion dependent anaemias. Clin Lab Haematol 1986;8:209-20.

94. Collins AF, Goncalves-Dias C, Haddad S, et al. Comparison of a transfusion preparation of newly formed red cells and standard washed red cell transfusion in patients with homozygous β-thalassemia. Transfusion 1994;34: 517-20.

95. Gordeuk VR, Bacon BR, Brittenham GM. Iron overload: Causes and consequences. Annu Rev Nutr 1987;7:485-508.

96. Giardina PJ, Grady RW. Chelation therapy in β-thalassemia: The benefits and limitations of desferrioxamine. Semin Hematol 1995;32: 304-12.

97. Cohen A, Martin M, Schwartz E. Depletion of excessive liver iron stores with deferoxamine. Br J Haematol 1984;58:369-73.

98. Wolfe L, Olivieri N, Sallan D, et al. Prevention of cardiac disease by subcutaneous deferoxamine in patients with thalassemia major. N Engl J Med 1985;312:1600-3.

99. Tanaka KR, Zerez CR. Red cell enzymopathies of the glycolytic pathway. Semin Hematol 1990;27:165-85.

In: Mintz PD, ed.
Transfusion Therapy: Clinical Principles and Practice
Bethesda, MD: AABB Press, 1999

3

Transfusion Therapy in Autoimmune Hemolytic Anemia

LEIGH C. JEFFERIES, MD, AND ANNE F. EDER, MD, PhD

 AUTOIMMUNE HEMOLYTIC ANE-mia (AIHA) encompasses a group of disorders distinguished by the physical properties of the autoantibody mediating the red cell destruction. On the basis of either the optimal temperature at which these autoantibodies react with red cells or their association with various drugs, these acquired anemias include warm autoimmune hemolytic anemia (WAIHA), cold autoimmune hemolytic anemia (cold agglutinin disease, or CAD), paroxysmal cold hemoglobinuria (PCH), or drug-induced hemolytic anemia (Table 3-1). The annual incidence of AIHA is estimated to be 1 in 80,000 persons,[1] with the warm autoantibody type comprising 41-70%; CAD, 16-32%; PCH, 2%; drug-induced hemolytic anemia, 12-18%; and mixed warm and cold AIHA,

7%.[2,3] This chapter reviews the pathogenesis and clinical features of each type, emphasizes the serologic findings that contribute to establishing the diagnosis, and discusses the practical considerations governing blood product transfusion in AIHA.

Warm Autoimmune Hemolytic Anemia

WAIHA is the most common form of AIHA accounting for up to 70% of cases.[2] Warm-type autoantibodies most often belong to the IgG class and bind erythrocytes optimally at 37 C. Rarely, IgA and IgM warm autoantibodies may accompany IgG or, even less commonly, occur alone.[4] The immunologic mechanisms leading to the development of red cell autoantibodies and their structural analysis

Leigh C. Jefferies, MD, Associate Director, Blood Bank/Transfusion Medicine Section, and Anne F. Eder, MD, PhD, Assistant Instructor, Department of Pathology and Laboratory Medicine, University of Pennsylvania School of Medicine, Philadelphia, Pennsylvania

Table 3-1. Classification of Autoimmune Hemolytic Anemia

Warm autoimmune hemolytic anemia
    Primary (idiopathic)
    Secondary
        Lymphoproliferative diseases
        Autoimmune disorders (systemic
            lupus erythematosus and others)
        Other malignancies and miscellane-
            ous diseases
Cold autoimmune hemolytic anemia
    Primary (idiopathic)
    Secondary
        Lymphoproliferative diseases
        Infections (*Mycoplasma* pneumonia,
            infectious mononucleosis)
        Miscellaneous diseases
Paroxysmal cold hemoglobinuria
    Associated with tertiary syphilis
    Postviral infection
Drug-induced hemolytic anemia
    Drug-adsorption (hapten) type
    Drug-dependent (immune complex)
      type
    Autoantibody type

have been reviewed.[5,6] The vast majority of warm autoantibodies belong to the IgG1 subclass. IgG1 and IgG3 are more efficient in activating complement than other subclasses of immunoglobulins. Pathogenic warm autoantibodies bind to the red cell surface and activate complement,[7] a process that rarely leads to completion of the complement cascade and intravascular hemolysis. More commonly, complement is present on the red cell as C3b or C3d owing to C3b inactivator, with degradation of C3b to C3d. Extravascular destruction occurs because of the interaction of macrophages with IgG or C3b receptors.[8] Macrophages in the spleen, and to a lesser extent in the liver and marrow, may ingest an opsonized red cell or produce

spherocytes by removing a portion of the red cell membrane. Spherocytes are particularly susceptible to extravascular osmotic lysis in splenic sinusoids.[9]

Clinical Presentation, Laboratory Findings, and Treatment

WAIHA is often associated with lymphoproliferative disorders, particularly B-cell lymphomas and chronic lymphocytic leukemia, systemic lupus erythematosus, and other autoimmune diseases, as well as malignant tumors.[3] As many as 60% of cases, however, are not associated with any apparent underlying disorder and are considered idiopathic or primary.[1,2] Idiopathic WAIHA is seen most frequently in individuals after their fourth or fifth decade, whereas the incidence of secondary WAIHA reflects the age distribution of the underlying disease.

The onset of anemia in WAIHA may be gradual with minimal symptoms or rapid with life-threatening hemolysis. Fatigue, pallor, palpitations, dyspnea, and congestive heart failure may be evident. Splenomegaly may result from the chronic hemolytic process or may be due to an underlying lymphoproliferative disorder. Findings associated with underlying disease such as systemic lupus erythenatosus may be present. The severity of disease reflects properties of the red cell autoantibodies, such as their serum titer, avidity for the red cell, and ability to fix complement.[10]

Laboratory findings depend on the degree as well as the site of hemolysis. Hallmarks of intravascular hemolysis include increased serum lactic dehydrogenase and unconjugated bilirubin, increased urinary bilinogen, and decreased or absent serum haptoglobin. In the presence of severe hemolysis, hemoglobinuria and hemoglobinemia may be present.[11] Extravascular hemolysis results in the formation of spherocytes and fragmented red cells. The presence of spherocytes indicates ongoing red cell destruction mediated by phagocytic cells in the spleen, liver, and marrow. Additional findings on the peripheral blood smear may include reticulocytosis, polychromasia, and nucleated red cells, and examination of a marrow biopsy may reveal erythroid hyperplasia with megaloblastoid features as well as findings associated with underlying lymphoproliferative or collagen vascular diseases.

For patients with unstable WAIHA, either idiopathic or secondary, corticosteroids are the mainstay of therapy. Permanent remissions, however, are infrequent in adults. Additional treatment modalities in these cases include splenectomy, immunosuppressive therapy, plasma exchange, Vinca alkaloids, danazol, and intravenous γ-globulin.[5,12-15] The need for transfusion therapy depends on the degree of hemolysis and the ability of the patient to tolerate anemia.

Serologic Evaluation

The selection of blood for transfusion to patients with WAIHA poses special challenges not encountered in the routine setting. Communication between the clinical and transfusion services is essential to patient care, and a general understanding of serologic evaluation is important to facilitate the interaction. Routine serologic evaluation involves the determination of red cell phenotype, a serum antibody detection test (indirect antiglobulin test [IAT]), and donor unit crossmatch. Additional testing in cases of AIHA includes evaluation of the patient's red cells for bound antibody.[16] A summary of the serologic tests that may be used to evaluate AIHA (warm and cold) is provided in Table 3-2. Aspects of the patient's transfusion history as well as the medical indication for transfusion will influence the strategy for pretransfusion testing for patients with WAIHA (Fig 3-1).

Determination of the Red Cell Phenotype

Determination of the patient's ABO group and Rh type usually presents no special difficulties in pa-

---

Table 3-2. Serologic Evaluation—Pretransfusion Testing

Routine pretransfusion testing
  ABO, Rh determination of patient
  Antibody detection test (indirect antiglobulin test): detects clinically significant
    alloantibodies in patient serum
  Crossmatch: tests patient serum with donor RBCs to ensure compatibility
  Direct antiglobulin test*: detects IgG and/or complement on patient RBCs
  Elution of bound IgG: detects alloantibody if patient has been recently transfused

Additional serologic evaluation for autoimmune hemolytic anemia (warm and cold)
  Absorption of patient serum with RBCs: separates alloantibodies from autoantibody
  Determination of thermal amplitude of autoantibody
  Confirmation of isotype of autoantibody
  Phenotyping of patient RBCs: determines alloantibodies that patient is capable of producing[†]
  Direct antiglobulin test: detects IgG and/or complement on patient RBCs
  Elution of RBC-bound IgG for characterization if antibody detection test results are negative

---

*Usually, the direct antiglobulin test is performed as part of pretransfusion testing only if the antibody detection test is positive.

†Phenotyping of patient RBCs may not be necessary for initial transfusion if evaluation for alloantibodies is definitive.

RBCs = red blood cells

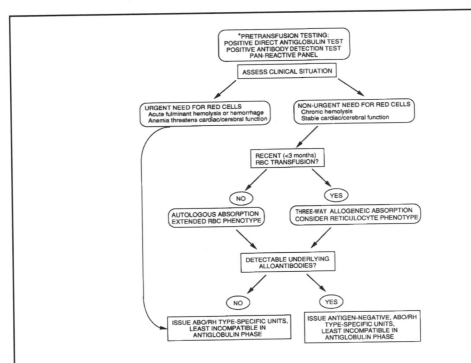

Figure 3-1. The approach to serologic evaluation and transfusion of patients with warm-type autoimmune hemolytic anemia is influenced by the urgency of transfusion and the transfusion history. RBC = red blood cell

*In some cases, the antibody detection test results may be negative or rarely may show specificity for a particular red cell antigen (eg, panel not panreactive), and the direct antiglobulin test results may rarely be negative on routine testing.

tients with WAIHA because the patient's red cells do not agglutinate spontaneously in vitro at room temperature. Knowledge of the other antigens expressed on the red cells, such as Rh, Kell, Kidd, Duffy, and MNSs antigens, may be useful in the management of a patient with AIHA, especially when the patient requires repeated transfusions. Individuals usually will not generate antibodies directed against antigens that are expressed on their own red cells. Alloantibodies may arise when an individual is sensitized to a foreign red cell antigen following transfusion or pregnancy. The value of an extended phenotype is greatest when techniques to identify serum alloantibodies cannot be performed or completed before urgent transfusion. Thus, red cell units that lack those antigens against which the patient could have produced a clinically

significant antibody can be selected for transfusion. If the patient's cells are coated with autoantibody, phenotyping may not be possible for all antigens; however, special techniques allow the autoantibody to be removed without altering antigen expression.[17,18] Moreover, if a patient has received red cell transfusions recently, the patient's red cells will have to be separated from transfused red cells before phenotyping can be performed.[19(pp625-7)] This strategy depends on such methods as density gradient centrifugation to separate the patient's reticulocytes from older, allogeneic red cells.

Serum Evaluation for Red-Cell-Specific Antibodies

Although warm autoantibodies do not usually interfere with ABO and Rh typing, they often compl cate evaluation of serum reactivity. The antibody detection test, also known as the indirect Coombs test or IAT, is used to detect clinically significant red cell antibodies in the patient's serum (Fig 3-2). Serum reactivity is determined by incubating the patient's serum with a phenotypically defined panel of group O red cells, adding antihuman IgG to crosslink membrane-bound IgG, and assessing hemagglutination. If red cell alloantibodies are present, blood chosen for transfusion should lack the respective antigen to prevent alloimmune-mediated hemolysis.[2,19(p365)] The antibody detection test detects autoantibodies as well as alloantibodies.

In approximately 80% of cases of AIHA, autoantibodies are not only bound to patients' red cells but also circulate in the serum.[20] Most autoantibodies also react with all other donor and reagent red cells. Red cell alloantibodies occur in 20-38% of patients with AIHA who have a history of transfusion or pregnancy.[21,22] Thus, the patient's antibody detection test results may be positive owing to autoantibody, one or more alloantibodies, or both auto- and alloantibodies. The strength and pattern of the reactivity of the serum with the panel reagent red cells may provide a critical clue to the identity of the underlying alloantibody. For example, if the serum produces strong hemagglutination of all Kell positive cells but weak hemagglutination of all other panel cells and the patient's own red cells, this pattern suggests the presence of anti-Kell alloantibody and autoantibody with no definable specificity.

Several techniques are used to identify red cell alloantibodies directly when an autoantibody is also present.[19(p664-7)] These adsorption protocols involve preferentially removing the autoantibody from the serum by incubations with red cells before

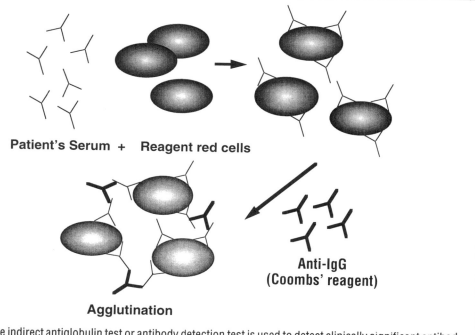

Patient's Serum + Reagent red cells

**Anti-IgG
(Coombs' reagent)**

Agglutination

Figure 3-2. The indirect antiglobulin test or antibody detection test is used to detect clinically significant antibodies with red cell specificity in the patient's serum. Reagent red cells are incubated with the patient's serum and washed to remove unbound globulins. Antihuman globulin is added, causing agglutination of the antibody-coated red cells.

evaluating the serum for the presence of alloantibodies. If a patient has not received red cell transfusions in the previous 3 months, autologous adsorption of the serum may be performed with the patient's own red cells. After bound autoantibody is removed, the red cells are incubated with serum to remove any additional circulating autoantibody.[17,18] Alloantibodies are not absorbed onto the patient's red cells by this procedure and remain in the serum, allowing for further identification. In anticipation of continued transfusions, it is prudent to store the patient's own red cells at the time of the first transfusion episode, so that they may be used for future autologous adsorptions.

Alternatively, if the patient has been transfused recently and the circulating red cells are not a homogeneous population of the patient's own cells, adsorption can be carried out with allogeneic red cells of known, specific phenotypes. If the patient's extended red cell phenotype is known, antigenically matched red cells are used for adsorbing red cell autoantibodies from serum. Often, the patient's red cell phenotype has not been determined prior to the first transfusion, in which case another technique, the three-way differential allogeneic adsorption, is performed. Red cells are selected for this differential adsorption such that the most important clinically significant alloantibodies, such as those directed against Kell, Kidd, Duffy, and Rhesus antigens, can be identified in the adsorbed aliquots of the patient's serum. Red cells from three different donors are used to adsorb the serum in parallel. The antigen distribution on these three donors is such that at least one is negative for the DCcEe, MNSs, Fy^a, Fy^b, JK^a, Jk^b, and K antigens. The adsorbed serum samples are tested against informative panel cells so that the specificity of underlying alloantibodies may be assigned. With all these techniques, multiple adsorptions may be necessary to remove the autoantibody completely, depending on its titer in the patient's serum. Therefore, this step may represent the most time-consuming portion of the serologic evaluation prior to transfusion.

In contrast to serum alloantibodies, red cell autoantibodies in WAIHA typically react with all red cells and have no definitive specificity. In a significant proportion of cases, the autoantibody binds all red cells except those with the rare Rh_{null} phenotype that lack Rh antigens.[20,23] In some rare cases, the undiluted autoantibody can be shown to have relative specificity within the Rh system, with preferential binding to such antigens as e or another Rh system antigen. For example, such relative specificity would be evidenced by agglutination of R_1R_1 (CDe/CDe) cells at higher serum dilutions compared with R_2R_2 (cDE/cDE) cells, which do not express the e antigen. However, absent or weak reactivity of autoantibodies with Rh_{null} red cells is not necessarily indicative of specificity to an Rh antigen because these cells also have other surface antigen deficiencies, including LW, Fy, and glycophorin expression.[24] Specificities of IgG autoantibodies for other blood group antigens (eg, Kell, Gerbich, U, Vel, etc) have been described in rare cases.[20,25] Alternatively, the specificity of warm autoantibodies may be due to the senescent red cell antigen, a degradation product of band 3 that emerges as the red cell ages.[26,27]

Red Cell Evaluation for Bound Ig and/or Complement

The most important assay for distinguishing AIHA from other forms of hemolytic anemia is the direct antiglobulin test (DAT) or direct Coombs test, which detects IgG and complement components bound to the red cell membrane (Fig 3-3). Antibodies directed against IgG or C3d are incubated with the patient's red cells and evaluated for their ability to cause hemagglutination. The rabbit or murine antiglobulin reagents must contain antibodies against the most common subclasses of IgG observed in WAIHA (IgG1 and IgG3) and against C3d.[28] Initial screening with a reagent containing a mixture of these antibodies should be followed by confirmation of positive results with reagents specific for IgG and C3d. In rare instances, antisera specific for IgA and IgM may be used. While the titer of serum autoantibody and strength of the DAT do not always predict the severity of the disease, patients with severe autoimmune hemolysis usually have strongly positive results on DATs.

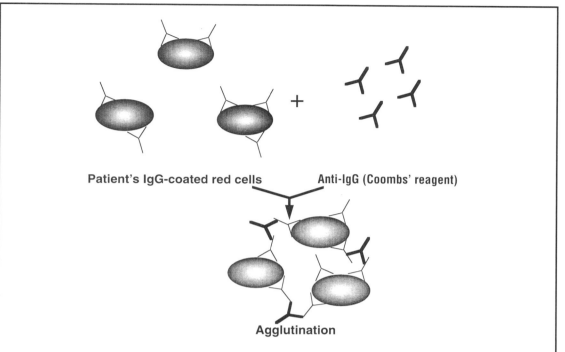

Patient's IgG-coated red cells   **Anti-IgG (Coombs' reagent)**

Agglutination

Figure 3-3. The direct antiglobulin test demonstrates in-vivo coating of red cells with antibody (as shown) and/or complement, depending on the specificity of the antihuman globulin reagent. Washed red cells are agglutinated by antihuman globulin. The strength of the observed agglutination is proportional to the amount of antibody or complement on the red cells.

In one study of WAIHA, red cells in 67% of cases were coated with IgG alone, 24% had both IgG and complement, 7% had only complement, and 1% were negative.[3] DAT results in patients with clinical evidence of autoimmune hemolysis may be due to the rare occurrence of IgA or IgM autoantibodies, low-affinity IgG autoantibodies, or surface concentrations of IgG antibodies below the threshold of detection for the routine DAT.[29] More sensitive tests using radiolabeled or fluoroscein-labeled anti-IgG (Coombs' reagent) may detect red-cell-bound autoantibodies in some of these cases.[24,30] Conversely, a positive DAT result is not always indicative of autoimmune hemolysis. Approximately 1 in 10,000 normal donors has detectable IgG on his or her red cells, and some healthy individuals have detectable C3d on their red cells. Other causes of false-positive tests include hypergammaglobuline-

mia, medications that cause the nonspecific attachment of plasma proteins to the red cell surface, and the collection of samples from intravenous lines containing low-ionic-strength saline solutions.[25(p72)31,32] Consequently, interpretation of the DAT result requires correlation with the patient's clinical condition.

Further characterization of IgG bound to the red cell may be important in certain circumstances. The IgG may be eluted from the surface of the red cell and studied in parallel with the patient's serum.[19(pp655-9)] An eluate reactive with screening cells supports the diagnosis of AIHA whereas a non-reactive eluate suggests a drug-induced or other disease-related cause of the positive DAT finding. This observation is particularly useful because, in some cases of WAIHA, the autoantibodies may be entirely adsorbed onto the surface of circulating red cells with none detectable in the patient's serum. The reactivity of the eluate with all reagent red cells would confirm the presence of autoantibodies. Detailed characterization of the specificity of the eluted antibodies does not affect clinical management and is rarely indicated unless clinical and laboratory data suggest the simultaneous occurrence of a delayed hemolytic transfusion reaction. For example, a patient with WAIHA and a history of favorable responses to red cell transfusions may demonstrate a decrement in hematocrit and other signs of hemolysis 3-7 days following a recent transfusion. This clinical scenario could be consistent with either autoimmune or alloimmune hemolysis. To evaluate for the presence of an alloantibody in an eluate that also contains an autoantibody, the same allogeneic absorption techniques described for serum may be performed with the eluate. Identification of an alloantibody in the eluate would suggest a delayed transfusion reaction as a cause for hemolysis rather than an autoimmune hemolytic process.[33] A summary of the typical serologic findings in AIHA is provided in Table 3-3.

Selection of Blood for Transfusion in Warm Autoimmune Hemolytic Anemia

The final step in selecting blood for transfusion is the crossmatch that involves incubating the patient's serum with donor red cells and evaluating for agglutination as an indication of compatibility. If alloantibodies are identified in the antibody detection test, red cell units lacking the corresponding red cell antigen are selected for crossmatch. In contrast, the serum autoantibodies identified by pretransfusion testing typically bind all donor red cells, rendering all units incompatible. Therefore, in the great majority of cases, no special selection of donor units is possible to avoid reactivity with the autoantibody. In these cases, several donor units should be evaluated for their compatibility with the patient's serum, and those demonstrating the least degree of incompatibility in vitro should be chosen for transfusion. Although such selection of least-incompatible units is logical and practiced widely,

there is no evidence for the improved survival i vivo of weakly reactive units compared with mor strongly reactive units.

If the autoantibody has relative specificity for single antigen such as an Rh determinant, bloo lacking that antigen may have prolonged surviv compared with the patient's own red cells.[2,34-38] Se lecting such antigen-negative units may be advan tageous, but this practice is not accepted unive sally because relatively few patients have bee evaluated and the benefit of such practice may b marginal. Regardless, transfusion of blood of the pa tient's Rh phenotype has been advocated to avoi later development of Rh alloantibodies.

In-vivo compatibility testing, using test aliquo of ^{51}Cr-labeled red cells, provides crude estimate of the survival of transfused red cells in the periph eral circulation.[39-41] In general, the survival greater than 85% of labeled red cells at 1 hour ma preclude rapid hemolysis and acute symptomati transfusion reactions; however, it may not predi red cell survival at 24 hours adequately.[41] Con versely, shortened survival of red cells, less tha 70% in 24 hours, does not necessarily contraind cate transfusion that may alleviate severe anem temporarily.[40] Thus, the survival of a test volume red cells may not predict the utility of transfusio accurately and has questionable practical value i this setting.

From a practical perspective, communicatio between the clinician and the blood bank or facilit performing pretransfusion testing is crucial for th optimal management of cases of WAIHA. Becaus the serologic evaluation likely will be tim consuming, notification of the potential need fo transfusion and initiation of workup should occu as soon as transfusion is considered. The results evaluations performed at other facilities, such a prior identification of alloantibodies and/or dete mination of the patient's red cell phenotype, ma expedite the preparation of blood for transfusion The knowledge of recent transfusions is also im perative to determine which serologic procedure such as autologous absorption and red cell phen typing or three-way differential allogeneic adsor tion, should be performed.

Table 3-3. Serologic Findings in Autoimmune Hemolytic Anemia

Classification	Warm		Cold	Paroxysmal Cold Hemoglobinuria
Autoantibody	IgG		IgM	IgG biphasic
Indirect antiglobulin test (serum reactivity)	Reactive	(80%)	Nonreactive by prewarm method	Nonreactive
Direct antiglobulin test (red cell bound)	IgG	(67%)	C3d	C3d
	IgG+C3d	(24%)		
	C3d	(7%)		
	Negative	(1%)		
Eluate	Panagglutinin		Nonreactive	Nonreactive

Practical Aspects of Transfusion in Warm Autoimmune Hemolytic Anemia

Unique risks are encountered during the transfusion of patients with WAIHA. First, the presence of the autoantibody complicates pretransfusion testing and may mask the presence of coexisting alloantibodies. This increases the risk of an alloantibody-induced hemolytic transfusion reaction. Second, the autoantibody itself may cause the decreased survival of transfused cells. However, the survival of transfused red cells is likely to be as good as that of the patient's own red cells, resulting in at least temporary alleviation of symptomatic anemia without causing acute symptomatic transfusion reactions.

Although hemolytic transfusion reactions occur infrequently,[42] the risk is particularly significant in those patients with severe ongoing hemolytic anemia for whom transfusion may be associated with worsening hemolysis and clinical deterioration.[37,43] For these patients, the risk may be aggravated by transfusions of large volumes of red cells; consequently, the minimum volume of red cells that will confer clinical benefit should be transfused. The signs and symptoms of anemia can usually be alleviated with relatively small quantities of red cells such as one-half to one unit.[44] The volume transfused should represent the least amount required to maintain adequate oxygen supply and should be transfused slowly. The maximum allowable infusion time is 4 hours per unit or portion thereof.[19(p456)] The possibility of high-output cardiac failure and circulatory overload, as well as the potential for hemolytic transfusion reaction, warrant close observation during transfusion. Signs and symptoms of exacerbated hemolysis occurring during or soon after transfusion should be reviewed with the transfusion service. While these findings may be unavoidable because of the presence of the autoantibody, they may reflect an ABO-incompatible transfusion resulting from clerical error or alloimmune hemolysis resulting from the presence of undetected alloantibodies.

Not all transfusion reactions are due to auto- or alloantibody-mediated hemolysis; however, the signs and symptoms of hemolytic reactions cannot be clinically distinguished from those of nonhemolytic reactions. Febrile, nonhemolytic reactions may also be manifested by fever, chills, or rigors but are not associated with serologic evidence of antibody-mediated hemolysis following transfusion. Because the transfusion should be discontinued if the patient experiences any untoward effects, life-saving transfusions for patients with WAIHA may be unnecessarily delayed if the nature of the reaction is subsequently determined to be a benign, febrile, or mild allergic reaction. To minimize the risk of febrile, nonhemolytic transfusion reaction during transfusion therapy for WAIHA, leukocyte reduction may be used. Additional benefits of leukocyte reduction include the decreased risk of alloimmunization to HLA and platelet antigens and the decreased risk of cytomegalovirus transmission. Leukocyte-reduced blood components are also indicated for patients who likely will require multiple red cell and platelet transfusions, such as those patients who are undergoing marrow transplantation for hematologic malignancies and those who have experienced febrile transfusion reactions previously. Fever and/or chills observed during or soon after a transfusion of leukocyte-reduced blood would be due more likely to a serologic problem such as ABO incompatibility or autoimmune or alloimmune hemolysis, than to a febrile, nonhemolytic transfusion reaction. These symptoms should alert the clinician to request further investigation by the transfusion service.

The decision to initiate transfusion therapy in WAIHA should consider multiple factors, including the patient's clinical status, the potential benefit of transfusion, the potential response to other therapeutic modalities, and the status of the serologic evaluation and pretransfusion testing (Fig 3-1). Severe but stable anemia at initial presentation is often well tolerated and may respond during the first week of therapy to corticosteroids, thus obviating the need for transfusion.[11] Patients with chronic stable anemia may be considered for periodic transfusion to relieve symptoms. The frequency of transfusions will depend on the rate of hemolysis and the degree of suppression of erythropoiesis by transfusion. Urgent transfusion may be necessary in patients with acute fulminant hemolysis or progressively severe anemia. When cardiac or cerebral function may be compromised, transfusion is warranted without delay, before all the serologic tests are completed.

Cold Autoantibodies and Cold Agglutinin Disease

Cold autoantibodies react most strongly with red cells at 0-5 C; however, they become clinically significant only when their thermal range of reactivity extends to at least 28-31 C. Depending on the ambient conditions, these temperatures may be encountered in the microvasculature of distal extremities. Although many individuals have demonstrable cold agglutinins in their sera, only a small subset experience cold autoantibody hemolytic disease, or CAD. Cold agglutinins may also assume clinical significance in the setting of iatrogenic hypothermia, such as cold cardioplegia used in cardiopulmonary bypass surgery.[45] The management of patients with cold agglutinins undergoing cardiopulmonary bypass surgery is discussed in Chapter 9.

Pathogenic cold autoantibodies are distinguished from benign ones by their ability to activate complement on the surface of red cells and mediate intravascular and extravascular hemolysis, resulting in the clinical manifestations of CAD. The IgM autoantibody binds red cells in the cool peripheral circulation, where it activates complement to the stage of C3b. Upon returning to warmer visceral circulation, the IgM dissociates from the red cell membrane. The C3b-coated red cells are cleared to some extent in the liver while the C3b inactivator system degrades C3b into C3dg, C3d, or both on many red cells. These red cells tend to have a near-normal survival in vivo and account for the often mild anemia of chronic disease.[46-48] Autoantibodies with a broad range of thermal amplitude or impairment of the regulatory C3b inactivator system may cause more severe hemolytic anemia.

Clinical Presentation, Laboratory Findings, and Treatment

CAD occurs as a chronic condition associated with B-cell neoplasms such as lymphoma, Waldenstrom's macroglobulinemia, or chronic lymphocytic leukemia, or as a transient condition following infections such as *Mycoplasma* pneumonia or infectious mononucleosis.[47,49] Because of these disease associations, secondary CAD is more likely a chronic disease in older individuals and an acute condition in young individuals. The chronic form is usually characterized by a mild to moderate stable anemia, which depends upon the capacity of the cold agglutinins to cause the activation of complement on the red cell surface. Cold exposure precipitates acrocyanosis of the distal extremities owing to the agglutination of red cells by autoantibody and may be associated with intravascular hemolysis and sudden decrease in hematocrit.

Laboratory findings of hemolysis are usually not striking. The possibility of a B-cell neoplasm should be investigated before initiating therapy for chronic CAD because certain chemotherapeutic agents may benefit patients with secondary forms of CAD. When associated with B-cell neoplasms, serum protein electrophoresis will likely identify the cold agglutinin as monoclonal IgM. With idiopathic chronic CAD, the anemia is generally mild and the avoidance of cold may prevent exacerbations. Prednisone or splenectomy are rarely beneficial.[50(p672),51] However, the recognition of patients with IgG-IgM mixed cold agglutinins or patients with low-titer, high-thermal-amplitude cold agglutinins is important because these patients may respond to corticosteroids.[52-54] Plasma exchange to remove circulating cold agglutinins may be useful in severe exacerbations.[55] Because IgM remains almost entirely in the intravascular space, the exchange of one plasma volume removes approximately 67% of the circulating cold agglutinin.

Transient CAD associated with infectious diseases is typically abrupt in onset, with occasionally severe anemia occurring in the second or third week of the illness. The cold agglutinins are usually IgM (although IgG and IgA cold agglutinins are sometimes also present) and are polyclonal. Supportive measures include hydration to promote renal blood flow, avoidance of cold temperatures, and occasionally transfusion. The hemolytic anemia usually resolves spontaneously in a few weeks.[47,49,56]

Serologic Evaluation

Determination of the Red Cell Phenotype

In CAD, difficulties with ABO and Rh typing may be encountered because of spontaneous autoagglutination of the patient's red cells mediated by the polyvalent IgM autoantibody at room temperature. The interfering serum reactivity may be eliminated by prewarming the sample to 37 C before testing or by using various reagents to abolish autoagglutination. Unreliable reverse typing with patient serum also may be resolved by using prewarmed serum and cells or adsorbed serum.[2,19] Because, usually, identification of serum alloantibodies can be accomplished in CAD by maintaining samples at 37 C or by controlling the reaction temperature, it is usually not necessary to perform extended red cell phenotyping to predict alloantibody formation in these patients.

Serum Evaluation for Red-Cell-Specific Antibodies

Parameters used to characterize cold autoantibodies include titer, thermal amplitude, isotype, and serologic specificity. In most patients with chronic CAD, the titer of the autoantibody is very high, detectable at dilutions of 1:1,000 or higher at 4 C, whereas, in healthy individuals, nonpathogenic IgM cold agglutinins usually do not exceed a titer of 1:64 at 4 C.[2,50(p460)] Therefore, dilution studies may be used as an initial screen to detect pathogenic cold agglutinins. For example, a 1:50 dilution of serum may be used as the screening threshold for further investigation of possible cold agglutinins. The thermal amplitude of the autoantibody may predict the pathogenicity of the antibody more accurately than the titer in serum.[47,52] Thermal amplitude may

be determined by evaluating the agglutination of reagent red cells at temperatures ranging from 4 C to 37 C. Cold-type autoantibodies react more strongly with red cells at 0-5 C than at higher temperatures. Hemagglutination disappears as the temperature rises toward 37 C, although in some cases the thermal amplitude is relatively high, within the range of 31-37 C. Such studies may be helpful in those relatively uncommon cases of low-titered cold agglutinins to corroborate the potential pathogenic nature of the autoantibody. Of particular interest, patients with low-titer cold agglutinins may respond to corticosteroid therapy.[52]

Cold agglutinins typically have specificity for the Ii blood group system, carbohydrate antigens closely related to ABO and Lewis blood groups, and rarely for other carbohydrate antigens such as Pr, Gd, Sa, Lud, and Fl.[56,57] The distinction of relative i vs I specificity, or the recognition of one of these other red cell antigens by the cold agglutinin, is generally academic because the specificity does not affect clinical management or the selection of blood for transfusion. Regardless, cold agglutinin specificity may be determined by comparing the reactivity of the serum with red cells from newborns, who express primarily the i antigen, with that observed with red cells from adults, who express primarily the I antigen. Alternatively, enzyme-treated red cells and rare adult red cells that lack the I antigen may be used to define the specificity. In most cases of chronic CAD and transient CAD associated with *Mycoplasma* pneumonia, the autoantibody has anti-I specificity, whereas in cases of transient CAD associated with infectious mononucleosis, the antibody usually has anti-i specificity.[47] These tests, however, are not sufficiently sensitive or specific to establish or confirm the diagnosis of these infectious diseases.

While cold agglutinins are usually of the IgM isotype, in rare instances, IgG or IgA autoantibodies are also present. Because patients with IgG cold agglutinins may respond to corticosteroids or splenectomy, the isotype may be confirmed by performing a DAT to evaluate the patient's red cells for cell-bound IgG or by using sulfhydryl reagents such as dithiothreitol to treat the patient's serum before serologic testing.[54,58,59] Dithiothreitol or other reducing agents disrupt the disulfide bonds of IgM tetramers, thereby eliminating the ability of the cold autoantibody to agglutinate red cells spontaneously.

An important step in the serologic evaluation of CAD is to identify any coexisting red cell alloantibodies. Fortunately, the cold agglutinin is not likely to interfere with the antibody detection test. Because of the cold reactivity, the autoantibody in CAD may be undetected when the antibody detection test or IAT is performed with prewarmed samples at 37 C. This allows the detection of other IgG alloantibodies without interference of the cold agglutinin. Alternatively, autoabsorption in the cold with patient or allogeneic red cells will remove the cold reactive autoantibody, leaving any alloantibodies in the absorbed serum for further identification.[19(pp661-2)]

Red Cell Evaluation for Bound Ig and/or Complement

DAT results are typically positive for bound C3d and negative for bound IgG. Because only complement is present on red cells, eluates are usually nonreactive. In those uncommon cases of mixed IgG-IgM CAD, the direct antiglobulin test may be useful in determining if IgG antibody is present on red cells.

Selection of Blood for Transfusion in Cold Agglutinin Disease

For patients with CAD, blood selected for transfusion ideally should lack any red cell antigens corresponding to serum alloantibodies in the patient. This depends upon identifying alloantibodies accurately while avoiding interference from cold autoantibody, either by the use of prewarming methods or by adsorption techniques described previously. When crossmatching is performed at 37 C, only antibodies with a broad thermal range and reactivity at a physiologic temperature will interfere with compatibility testing. Compatibility at this temperature, however, does not ensure completely

normal survival of transfused cells because the cold agglutinin may cause complement activation in cooler areas of the circulation. Following transfusion, red cells may undergo a phase of destruction until they have acquired resistance to complement-mediated lysis.[37] As with WAIHA, transfusion in CAD should be approached with caution; however, it should not be withheld if clinically indicated.

A few investigators have compared the survival of rare i donor units with that of I donor units (virtually all donor units) in patients with CAD, but results have not been consistent.[60,61] Red cells from i adults are seldom available, and the transfusion of adult I red cells usually results in an appropriate increase in hematocrit. Therefore, selection of rare units is not generally recommended.

Practical Aspects of Transfusion in Cold Agglutinin Disease

For simple transfusions, the advantage of warming transfused blood has not been demonstrated clearly, and transfusion specialists have provided conflicting recommendations.[37,44,50(p676)] The use of an in-line blood warmer may be of value in CAD; however, more emphasis has been placed on warming the patient. Procedures requiring systemic hypothermia, such as cardiopulmonary bypass, may lead to complement activation and hemolysis. Cold cardioplegia may cause intracoronary hemagglutination with ischemia or infarction.[62,63] Asymptomatic patients with low-titer (<32), low-thermal-amplitude (<28 C) cold agglutinins can undergo hypothermic cardiopulmonary bypass without increased risk of hemolysis.[64] However, recommendations for preoperative screening for significant cold agglutinins in patients undergoing cardiac surgery are controversial.[45] Most transfusion services do not routinely evaluate patients scheduled for cardiopulmonary bypass for clinically significant cold agglutinins but will perform serologic studies (eg, thermal amplitude titration) for patients with symptomatic CAD. Several different intraoperative techniques have been used during cardiothoracic surgery to prevent hemolysis.[65,66] In some cases, these have been used in conjunction with preoperative plasmapheresis. When plasmapheresis is used, warming of the extracorporeal circuit may be beneficial.[55] The clinical management of such patients is discussed in Chapter 9.

Leukocyte-reduced blood components may be used for transfusion to patients with cold AIHA to minimize the risk of febrile transfusion reactions and prevent unnecessary delays in transfusion therapy due to the investigation of adverse reactions. However, because alloantibodies are not as difficult to identify in patients with cold-type compared with warm-type AIHA, this practice may be overly cautious. Moreover, washing red cells to remove residual plasma is not generally indicated in these cases. Washed red cells may be indicated in cases of severe allergic reactions or in cases of posttransfusion purpura when antigen-negative or autologous units are not available.[67] Some early investigators speculated that washing might remove complement and result in the improved survival of transfused cells in patients with CAD.[68] However, serum complement is usually not strikingly reduced in patients with warm or cold AIHA[2] and the practice of washing is not generally recommended.

Autoimmune Hemolytic Anemia with Both Cold and Warm Autoantibodies

Approximately 7-8% of all AIHAs have serologic findings characteristic of both warm and cold red cell autoantibodies.[69-71] Patients with mixed-type AIHA usually present with acute hemolysis. The incidence of systemic lupus erythematosus in patients with mixed-type AIHA ranges from 25-42% in different series. The initial response to corticosteroid therapy may be dramatic; however, many patients have chronic hemolysis.[70,71]

Serologic evaluation shows both warm-reactive IgG autoantibodies as well as cold-reactive IgM autoantibodies. In contrast to typical CAD, the IgM autoantibodies usually are low in titer (<1:64 at 4 C) but have broad thermal amplitude, with reactivity up to 37 C.[70] The DAT results are positive for both IgG and C3d on the patient's red cells, and the eluate contains the IgG autoantibody as expected. The cold-reactive IgM autoantibody may have

anti-I or anti-i specificity, or no apparent specificity, and the IgG autoantibody may be indistinguishable from specificities seen with typical WAIHA. As with WAIHA or CAD, it is important to identify the underlying red cell alloantibodies as part of the pretransfusion testing using the techniques described above. The potential risks of transfusion discussed previously are similar for mixed-type AIHA.

Paroxysmal Cold Hemoglobinuria

PCH, the rarest form of AIHA, was described originally in the early 1900s in adults with syphilis who experienced acute episodes of hemolysis. Today, PCH is predominantly a self-limiting disease in children, associated with *Mycoplasma* pneumonia, upper respiratory viral syndromes, or other bacterial or viral infection. Constitutional symptoms, such as the sudden onset of shaking chills, back and leg pain, abdominal cramps, and fever, as well as hemoglobinuria, hemoglobinemia, jaundice, and other laboratory findings of severe hemolytic anemia, may be evident.[35,72] Generally, the treatment is supportive; glucocorticoids and splenectomy are usually not effective. If the hemolysis is severe, the patient should be well hydrated to maintain renal perfusion and function. Fulminant hemolysis may require transfusion therapy.

Serologic Evaluation

The biphasic nature of hemolysis in PCH was attributed by Donath and Landsteiner in 1904 to a cold-reacting autohemolysin and a lytic, warm-reacting factor. The diagnostic assay for the autoantibody still bears their names.[73] The Donath-Landsteiner assay involves incubating the patient's serum with normal red cells and normal serum as a source of complement, first at 4 C and then at 37 C, to reveal the presence of the IgG autoantibody responsible for PCH. The biphasic hemolysin binds to red cells in the cold and fixes the early components of complement. The complement cascade is completed upon warming the coated red cells, resulting in hemolysis. The DAT typically reveals only complement coating of patient red cells because the IgG autoantibody reacts with red cells in colder areas of the body and detaches from the red cell surface at warmer temperatures. Consequently, eluates prepared from patients with PCH are nonreactive, as with CAD.

Because the Donath-Landsteiner test and the DAT are not performed routinely as parts of the pretransfusion testing, diagnosis requires clinical correlation and communication with the transfusion service.

Selection of Blood for Transfusion in Paroxysmal Cold Hemoglobinuria

Because the causative autoantibody rarely causes hemagglutination above 4 C, random donor red cells will be compatible with patient sera when tested by routine crossmatch procedures. The most common autoantibody has specificity for the P antigen, a globoside, and reacts with all red cells except those of the very rare p or P^k phenotypes. Rare examples of anti-I, anti-i, and anti-Pr biphasic hemolysins have been reported.[74-76] There is some evidence that p red cells survive better than P-positive red cells; however, the incidence of p blood is approximately 1 in 200,000.[77,78] Patients would likely require transfusion before such blood could be located. Because P-positive red cells do not necessarily precipitate hemolysis, the transfusion of red cells of common P types should not be withheld if transfusion is urgently needed. While there is an absence of extensive data, several reports suggest the use of in-line blood warmers for the transfusion of patients with this diagnosis.[78,79] As with other types of AIHA, leukocyte-reduced red cell units should be transfused to patients with PCH to reduce the risk of febrile, nonhemolytic transfusion reactions that could needlessly confound the clinical picture and delay medically necessary therapy. Some investigators report the use of washed blood[72]; however, controlled comparisons using washed vs unwashed blood have not been made, and this practice is not recommended at this time.

Drug-Induced Hemolytic Anemias

Drug-induced hemolytic anemias constituted 12-18% of AIHA cases when high-dose penicillin and α-methyldopa were commonly used.[2,3] Declining use of these therapeutics has decreased the prevalence of this diagnosis; however, the list of drugs implicated in autoimmune hemolysis is extensive and continues to grow (Table 3-4).[19] In a patient with unexplained hemolysis, a complete medication history should be taken and each drug considered carefully as a possible etiology. Evidence that the drug is responsible for immune hemolysis should include serologic and clinical data. Serologic investigation into drug-induced hemolytic anemia involves direct antiglobulin testing and evaluation of serum reactivity in the presence and absence of the drug or metabolite. Difficulties in interpreting the clinical relevance of the serologic data arise because many drugs elicit positive results on a DAT; however, only some drugs cause hemolytic anemia. The presence of antibody, even on the surface of the patient's cells, does not necessarily indicate red cell destruction. In addition, appropriate controls often are not included in the serologic workup, complicating interpretation.[80] Clinical evidence supporting the diagnosis of drug-induced hemolytic anemia includes the association of hemolysis with the initiation of therapy and resolution with discontinuation of the drug. Proof also requires the recurrence of hemolysis when the drug is reintroduced to the patient.[80] In the interest of patient safety, this final criterion is rarely met.

Three mechanisms that may cause a positive DAT result and possible hemolysis are drug adsorption, drug-dependent antibody (formerly immune complex formation), and autoimmune induction. A unifying theory of the mechanism underlying drug-induced antibody reactions has been proposed based on the specificity of the antibody generated by the interaction of the drug with the red cell.[25] Antibodies directed solely against the drug or hapten bound to the surface of the red cell result in the in-vitro reactions typical of a drug adsorption reaction; those directed against a combination of the drug and membrane components produce in-

Table 3-4. Drugs Reported to Cause Hemolytic Anemia*

Hapten	Drug Dependent		Autoantibody
Penicillin	Stibophen	Acetaminophen	∝-methyldopa
Cephalothin	Quinine	Streptomycin	Mefenamic acid
Cephaloridine	Quinidine	Hydralazine	L-dopa
Ampicillin	Phenacetin	Probenecid	Procainamide
Methicillin	Hydrochlorothiazide	Sulfinylurea derivative	Ibuprofen
Carbenicillin	Rifampin	Chlorinated hydrocarbon	Thioridazine
	p-aminosalicylic acid	insecticide	
	Dipyrone	Carbimazole	
	Antihistamines	Cianidanol	
	Sulfonamides	Cephalosporin	
	Isoniazid	Nomifensine	
	Chlorpromazine	5-fluorouracil	
	Pyramidon	Tolmetin	
	Melphalan	Fenoprofen	
	Insulin	Sulindac	
	Tetracycline		

*Modified from Vengelen-Tyler.[19(pp399-407)]

vitro reactions associated with the drug-dependent or immune complex mechanism, and those directed against primarily membrane components produce in-vitro reactions associated with autoantibodies. Finally, some drugs, especially first-generation cephalosporins, alter the red cell membrane such that serum proteins, including immunoglobulins, adhere nonspecifically to the cell surface, resulting in a positive DAT finding.[81,82] This reaction does not involve an immune response to the drug and is not associated with hemolysis.

The drug adsorption mechanism results in drug antibodies, which react with the drug when it is bound to the red cell membrane. Penicillin represents the classic example of a drug that may cause extravascular hemolysis by this mechanism. For hemolytic anemia to develop, intravenous doses of 10 million units or more per day for several days are necessary. Approximately 3% of patients receiving intravenous penicillin in these doses will show a positive DAT result, but hemolytic anemia is much less common. When hemolysis occurs, the implicated antibody is an IgG antibody that recognizes the benzylpenicilloyl determinant or other metabolite of penicillin.[83] The hemolytic anemia usually occurs a week after antibiotic therapy is initiated and it subsides within days after the drug is discontinued. In low doses, penicillin may evoke development of low-avidity IgM penicillin antibodies that cause a positive DAT result but not hemolytic anemia.

When the drug-dependent (immune complex) mechanism is involved, immune complexes initiate complement activation on the red cell surface and may lead to intravascular hemolysis, resulting in hemoglobinemia, hemoglobinuria, and renal failure. Only small concentrations of a drug are required to initiate hemolysis once an individual has been sensitized and demonstrates the drug antibody. Hemolysis resolves shortly after the drug has been discontinued. Some studies have suggested that the binding of these immune complexes to red cells may be specific for blood group antigens. For example, drug-dependent antibodies associated with rifampicin, nitrofurantoin, and dexchlorpheniramine reacted with cells rich in I antigen, and an antibody associated with chlorpropamide reacted only with Jk^a+ red cells.[84,85]

The third mechanism involves the development of autoantibodies that react with intrinsic red cell antigens and do not react with the drug in vitro. The drug traditionally associated with this mechanism is α-methyldopa.[86] Some 20% of patients treated with this drug develop a positive DAT result while 0.5-1.0% develop hemolytic anemia. With α-methyldopa, the DAT is dose-dependent, becomes weaker after the drug is discontinued, but may continue to yield positive results for up to 2 years.[82,87] The serologic findings of this type of drug-induced AIHA are indistinguishable from those of WAIHA. The mechanism by which drugs lead to autoantibody development is not known; however, this may involve effects on immunoregulatory T cells or alteration in the intrinsic red cell anti-

gen.[82,88] Because α-methyldopa is rarely prescribed today, hemolytic anemia attributed to this drug has greatly decreased. The use of newer drugs, such as nomifensine, can result in AIHA by this mechanism.[82,89,90]

Serologic Evaluation

Serologic findings in cases of drug-induced hemolytic anemias depend on the mechanism of immune destruction (Table 3-5). For cases involving the adsorption mechanism, the DAT results are positive for IgG or sometimes IgG and complement.[82] Results of the IAT, or antibody screen, are negative unless the reagent red cells are coated with the implicated drug. The diagnosis is conclusive when both the eluate and the patient's serum react with drug-coated cells. When the drug-dependent (immune complex) mechanism is responsible for hemolytic anemia, the serologic findings are similar, except that the DAT usually detects complement alone on the red cells. The patient's serum reacts with red cells only in the presence of the offending drug, and the eluate from the pati-

Table 3-5. Serologic Findings in Drug-Induced Autoimmune Hemolytic Anemia

Classification	Drug Adsorption (hapten)	Drug Dependent (immune complex)	Autoantibody
Drug prototype	Penicillin	Quinidine	Methyldopa
IAT (serum reactivity)	Nonreactive, unless reagent red cells are **coated** with drug	Reactive, in the **presence** of drug	Reactive, in the **absence** of drug
DAT (red cell bound)	IgG sometimes IgG + C3d	C3d	IgG
Eluate	Nonreactive, unless reagent red cells are **coated** with drug	Nonreactive, even in the **presence** of drug	Reactive, in the **absence** of drug

IAT = indirect antiglobulin test; DAT = direct antiglobulin test

ent's red cells usually does not react with normal red cells.[91,92] If drug-dependent antibodies are suspected but evaluation with the parent drug does not support the diagnosis, metabolites present in the urine or serum of individuals after ingestion of the drug could be tested.

With the autoimmune mechanism, the serologic findings resemble those of WAIHA. The DAT results are positive for IgG, although weak complement binding has been reported also. Antibodies in the serum and on the red cells are indistinguishable from those found in WAIHA, and the eluate reacts with normal cells without the presence of a drug.

Selection of Blood for Transfusion in Drug-Induced Hemolytic Anemias

If transfusion is necessary for cases of drug-induced hemolytic anemias, routine pretransfusion testing to identify red cell alloantibodies and to supply ABO/Rh-compatible blood usually does not present special difficulties. The survival of transfused red cells may not be normal if the drug or immune complexes are still present. However, if a drug such as α-methyldopa has evoked an autoantibody that is present in the serum, serologic evaluation to identify the underlying alloantibodies will require additional procedures, and all donor units will be incompatible. If the autoantibody is not associated with hemolytic anemia and the patient's own cells have normal survival, there is evidence that the transfused cells will also have normal survival.[41,82]

Summary

Warm-, cold-, biphasic, or drug-induced antibodies are responsible for the clinical manifestations of WAIHA, CAD, PCH, and drug-induced hemolytic anemia, respectively. If AIHA is suspected, the clinical history should be communicated to the transfusion service because specific tests to confirm these diagnoses are not performed routinely and additional tests may be required to select appropriate blood for transfusion. Serologic evaluation in these cases includes red cell typing, a serum reactivity screen, and donor unit crossmatch. The DAT

to detect bound IgG and/or complement on the surface of the patient's red cells distinguishes autoimmune from other types of hemolysis. The presence of autoantibodies may interfere in one or more of these tests. If the autoantibody interferes in the antibody detection test, procedures such as autoadsorption or three-way allogeneic adsorption may be necessary to identify, underlying red cell alloantibodies prior to transfusion. Although transfused red cells may not have normal survival in patients' with red cell autoantibodies, transfusion may provide temporary benefit. The decision to transfuse should consider the severity of anemia, the risk of withholding transfusion, and the potential benefit of alternative therapy.

References

1. Pirofsky B. Autoimmunization and the autoimmune hemolytic anemias. Baltimore, MD: Williams and Wilkins, 1969:22.
2. Petz LD, Garratty G. Acquired immune hemolytic anemias. New York: Churchill Livingstone, 1980:28-37.
3. Sokol RJ, Hewitt S, Stamps BK. Autoimmune haemolysis: An 18-year study of 865 cases referred to a regional transfusion centre. Br Med J 1981;282:2023-7.
4. Sokol RJ, Booker DJ, Stamps R, et al. IgA red cell antibodies and autoimmune hemolysis. Transfusion 1997;37:175-81.
5. Schwartz RS, Berkman EM, Silberstein LE. The autoimmune hemolytic anemias. In: Hoffman R, Benz EJ, Shattil SJ, et al, eds. Hematology: Basic principles and practice. New York: Churchill Livingstone, 1995:710-29.
6. Siegel DL, Silberstein LE. Structural analyses of red blood cell autoantibodies. In: Garratty G, ed. Immunobiology of transfusion medicine. New York: Marcel Dekker, Inc., 1994: 387-99.
7. Huber H, Douglas SD, Nusbacher J, et al. IgG subclass specificity of human monocyte receptor sites. Nature 1971;229:419-20.
8. Schreiber AD, Frank MM. Role of antibody and complement in the immune clearance

and destruction of erythrocytes, II: Molecular nature of IgG and IgM complement-fixing sites and effects of their interaction with serum. J Clin Invest 1972;51:583-9.

9. Lo Buglio AF, Cotran RS, Jandl JH. Red cells coated with immunoglobulin G: Binding and sphering by mononuclear cells in man. Science 1967;158:1582-5.

10. Borsos T, Rapp HJ. Complement fixation on cell surfaces by 1S and 7S antibodies. Science 1965;150:505-6.

11. Pirofsky B. Clinical aspects of autoimmune hemolytic anemia. Semin Hematol 1976;13: 251-65.

12. Ahn YS, Harrington WJ, Mylvaganam R, et al. Danazol therapy for autoimmune hemolytic anemia. Ann Intern Med 1985;102:298-301.

13. Besa EC. Rapid transient reversal of anemia and long-term effect of maintenance intravenous immunoglobulin for autoimmune hemolytic anemia in patients with lymphoproliferative disorders. Am J Med 1988;84:691-8.

14. Kutti J, Wadenvik H, Safai-Kuttis, et al. Successful treatment of refractory autoimmune hemolytic anemia by plasmapheresis. Scand J Haematol 1984;32:149-52.

15. Murphy S, LoBuglio AF. Drug therapy of autoimmune hemolytic anemia. Semin Hematol 1976;13:323-34.

16. Sokol RJ, Booker DJ, Stamps R. Investigation of patients with autoimmune haemolytic anaemia and provision of blood for transfusion. J Clin Pathol 1995;48:602-10.

17. Branch DR, Petz LD. A new reagent (ZZAP) having multiple applications in immunohematology. Am J Clin Pathol 1982;78:161-7.

18. Edwards JM, Moulds JJ, Judd WJ. Chloroquine dissociation of antigen-antibody complexes: A new technique for typing red blood cells with a positive direct antiglobulin test. Transfusion 1982;22:59-61.

19. Vengelen-Tyler V, ed. Technical manual. 12th ed. Bethesda, MD: American Association of Blood Banks, 1996.

20. Issitt PD, Pavone BG, Goldfinger D, et al. Anti-Wr[b] and other autoantibodies responsible for positive direct antiglobulin test in 150 individuals. Br J Haematol 1976;34:5-18.

21. Laine ML, Beattie KM. Frequency of alloantibodies accompanying autoantibodies. Transfusion 1985;25:545-6.

22. Wallhermfechtel MA, Pohl BA, Chaplin H. Alloimmunization in patients with warm autoantibodies. Transfusion 1984;24:482-5.

23. Weiner W, Vox GH. Serology of acquired hemolytic anemias. Blood 1963;22:607-13.

24. Gilliland BC. Autoimmune hemolytic anemia. In: Rossi EC, Simon TL, Moss GS, eds. Principles of transfusion medicine, 2nd ed. Baltimore, MD: Williams and Wilkins, 1996: 101-20.

25. Garratty G. Target antigens for red cell-bound autoantibodies. In: Nance SJ, ed. Clinical and basic science aspects of immunohematology. Arlington, VA: American Association of Blood Banks, 1991:33-72.

26. Branch DR, Shulman IA, Sy Siok Hian AL, et al. Two distinct categories of warm autoantibody reactivity with age-fractionated red cells. Blood 1984;63:177-80.

27. Kay MMB. Senescent cell antigen: A red cell aging antigen. In: Garratty G, ed. Red cell antigens and antibodies. Arlington, VA: American Association of Blood Banks, 1986:35-82.

28. Chaplin H, Monroe MC. Comparisons of pooled polyclonal rabbit anti-human C3d with four monoclonal mouse anti-human C3ds, II: Quantitation of RBC bound C3d, and characterization of antiglobulin agglutination reactions against RBC from 27 patients with autoimmune hemolytic anemia. Vox Sang 1986;50:87-93.

29. Gilliland BC, Baxter E, Evans RS. Red cell antibodies in acquired hemolytic anemia with negative antiglobulin serum tests. N Engl J Med 1971;285:252-6.

30. Salama A, Mueller-Eckhardt C, Bhakdi S. A two-stage immunoradiometric assay with ^{125}I-staphylococcal protein A for the detection of antibodies and complement of human blood cells. Vox Sang 1985;48:239-45.

31. Geisland JR, Milam JD. Spuriously positive direct antiglobulin tests caused by silicone gel. Transfusion 1980;20:711-3.

32. Judd WJ, Butch SH, Oberman HA, et al. The evaluation of a positive direct antiglobulin test in pretransfusion testing. Transfusion 1980; 20:17-23.

33. Pineda AA, Taswell HF, Brzica SM Jr. Delayed hemolytic transfusion reaction: An immunologic hazard of blood transfusion. Transfusion 1978;18:1-7.

34. Bell CA, Zwicker H, Sacks HJ. Autoimmune hemolytic anemia: Routine serologic evaluation in a general hospital population. Am J Clin Pathol 1973;60:903-11.

35. Habibi B, Homberg JC, Schaison G, et al. Autoimmune hemolytic anemia in children: A review of 80 cases. Am J Med 1974;56: 61-9.

36. Mollison PL. Measurement of survival and destruction of red cells of haemolytic syndromes. Br Med Bull 1959;15:59-67.

37. Mollison PL. Red cell incompatibility in vivo. In: Mollison PL, Engelfriet CP, Contreras M, eds. Blood transfusion in clinical medicine. London: Blackwell Scientific Publications, 1993:434-97.

38. Salmon C. Autoimmune hemolytic anemia. In: Back JF, Sivenson RS, Schwartz RS, eds. Immunology. New York: John Wiley and Sons, 1978:675-98.

39. Chaplin H. Special problems in transfusion management of patients with autoimmune hemolytic anemia. In: Bell CA, ed. A seminar on laboratory management of hemolysis. Washington, DC: American Association of Blood Banks, 1979:135.

40. Mayer K, Bettigole RE, Harris JP, et al. Test in vivo to determine donor compatibility. Transfusion 1968;8:28-32.

41. Silvergleid AJ, Wells RP, et al. Compatibility test using [52]chromium-labeled red blood in crossmatch positive patients. Transfusion 1978;18:8-14.

42. Salama A, Berghöfer H, Mueller-Eckhardt C. Red blood cell transfusion in warm-type auto-immune haemolytic anaemia. Lancet 1992; 340:1515-7.

43. Petz LD. Blood transfusions in acquired hemolytic anemia. In: Petz LD, Swisher SN, Kleinman S, et al, eds. Clinical practice of transfusion medicine. 3rd ed. New York: Churchill Livingstone, 1996:469-99.

44. Rosenfield RE, Jagathambal K. Transfusion therapy for autoimmune hemolytic anemia. Semin Hematol 1976;13:311-21.

45. Agarwal SK, Ghosh PK, Gupta D. Cardiac surgery and cold-reactive proteins. Ann Thorac Surg 1995;60:1143-50.

46. Atkinson JP, Frank MM. Studies on the in vivo effects of antibody: Interaction of IgM antibody and complement in the immune clearance and destruction of erythrocytes in man. J Clin Invest 1974;54:339-48.

47. Pruzanski W, Shumack KH. Biologic activity of cold-reacting autoantibodies (first of two parts). N Engl J Med 1977;297:538-42.

48. Schreiber AD, McDermott PB. Effect of C3b inactivator on monocyte-bound C3-coated human erythrocytes. Blood 1978;52:896-904.

49. Rosenfield RE, Schmidt PH, Calvo RC, et al. Anti-i, a frequent cold agglutinin in infectious mononucleosis. Vox Sang 1965;10:631-4.

50. Dacie JV. The autoimmune haemolytic anaemias. Part II. London: J and A Churchill, 1962.

51. Schubothe H. The cold hemagglutinin disease. Semin Hematol 1966;3:27-47.

52. Schreiber AD, Herskovitz BS, Goldwein M. Low-titer cold-hemagglutinin disease: Mechanism of hemolysis and response to corticosteroids. N Engl J Med 1977;296:1490-4.

53. Silberstein LE, Berkman EM, Schreiber AD. Cold hemagglutinin disease associated with IgG cold-reactive antibody. Ann Intern Med 1987;106:238-42.

54. Szymanski IO, Teno R, Rybak ME. Hemolytic anemia due to a mixture of low-titer IgG lambda and IgM lambda agglutinins reacting optimally at 22 C. Vox Sang 1986;51:112-6.

55. Andrzejewski C, Gault E, Briggs M, et al. The benefit of a 37 C extracorporeal circuit in plasma exchange therapy for selected cases with cold agglutinin disease. J Clin Apheresis 1988;4:13-7.

56. Roelcke D. Cold agglutination: Antibodies and antigens. Clin Immunol Immunopathol 1974;2:266-80.

57. Roelcke D, Kreft H. Characterization of various anti-Pr cold agglutinins. Transfusion 1984;24:210-3.

58. Moore JA, Chaplin H. Autoimmune hemolytic anemia associated with an IgG cold incomplete antibody. Vox Sang 1973;24:236-45.

59. Silberstein LE, Shoenfeld Y, Schwartz RS, et al. A combination of IgG and IgM autoantibodies in chronic cold agglutinin disease: Immunologic studies and response to splenectomy. Vox Sang 1985;48:105-9.

60. Van Loghem JJ, Peetom F, Vander Hart M, et al. Serological and immunochemical studies in hemolytic anemia with high-titer cold agglutinins. Vox Sang 1963;8:33-46.

61. Woll JE, Smith CM, Nusbacher J. Treatment of acute cold agglutinin hemolytic anemia with transfusion of adult i RBCs. JAMA 1974; 299:1779-80.

62. Diaz JH, Cooper ES, Ochsner JL. Cold hemagglutination pathophysiology, evaluation and management of patients undergoing cardiac surgery with induced hypothermia. Arch Intern Med 1984;144:1639-41.

63. Wertlake PJ, McGinnis MH, Schmidt PJ. Cold antibody and persistent hemolysis after surgery under hypothermia. Transfusion 1969;9: 70-3.

64. Moore RA, Geller EA, Mathews ES, et al. The effect of hypothermic cardiopulmonary bypass on patients with low-titer, nonspecific cold agglutinins. Ann Thorac Surg 1984;37: 233-8.

65. Landymore R, Isom W, Barlam B. Management of patients with cold agglutinins who require open heart surgery. Can J Surg 1984; 266:79-80.

66. Park JV, Weiss CI. Cardiopulmonary bypass and myocardial protection management problems in cardiac surgical patients with cold autoimmune disease. Anesth Analg 1988;67: 75-8.

67. Yap PL, Pryde EAD, McClelland DBL. IgA content of frozen-thawed-washed red blood cells and blood products measured by radioimmunoassay. Transfusion 1982;22:36-8.

68. Evans RS, Turner E, Bingham M, Woods R. Chronic hemolytic anemia due to cold agglutinins. II. The role of C in red cell destruction. J Clin Invest 1968;47:691-701.

69. Kaji E, Miura Y, Ikemoto S. Characterization of autoantibodies in mixed-type autoimmune hemolytic anemia. Vox Sang 1991;60:45-52.

70. Shulman I, Branch DR, Nelson JM, et al. Autoimmune hemolytic anemia with both cold and warm autoantibodies. JAMA 1985; 253:1746-8.

71. Sokol RJ, Hewitt S, Stamps BK. Autoimmune haemolysis: Mixed warm and cold antibody type. Acta Haematol 1983;69:266-74.

72. Heddle NM. Acute paroxysmal cold hemoglobinuria. Transfus Med Rev 1989;3: 219-29.

73. Donath J, Landsteiner K. Uber paroxysmale Haemoglobinurie. Munchen Med Wochenschr 1904;51:1590-3.

74. Judd WJ, Wilkinson SL, Issitt PD, et al. Donath-Landsteiner hemolytic anemia due to an anti-Pr-like biphasic hemolysin. Transfusion 1986;26:423-5.

75. Shirey RS, Park K, Ness PM, et al. Anti-i biphasic hemolysin in chronic paroxysmal cold hemoglobinuria. Transfusion 1986;26:62-4.

76. Worlledge SM, Rousso C. Studies on the serology of paroxysmal cold haemoglobinuria (PCH) with special reference to its relationship with the P blood group system. Vox Sang 1965;10:293-8.

77. Nordhagen R, Stensvold, Winsnes A, et al. Paroxysmal cold haemoglobinuria: The most frequent acute autoimmune haemolytic anaemia in children? Acta Paediatr Scand 1984; 73:258-62.

78. Rausen AR, Levine R, Hsu TCS, et al. Compatible transfusion therapy for patients with PCH. Pediatrics 1975;55:275-8.

79. Johnsen HE, Brostrphom K, Madsen M. Paroxysmal cold haemoglobinuria in children: 3 cases encountered within a period of 7 months. Scand J Haematol 1978;20:413-6.

80. Garratty G. Drug-induced immune cytopenia (guest editorial). Transfus Med Rev 1993;7:213-4.

81. Danielson DA, Douglas SW III, Herzog P, et al. Drug-induced blood disorders. JAMA 1984;252:3257-60.

82. Petz LD, Branch DR. Drug-induced immune hemolytic anemia. In: Chaplin H, ed. Methods in hematology: Immune hemolytic anemias. New York: Churchill Livingstone, 1985:47-94.

83. White JM, Brown DL, Hepner GW, et al. Penicillin-induced hemolytic anemia. Br Med J 1968;3:26-9.

84. Duran-Suarez JR, Martin-Vega C, Argelagues E, et al. Red cell I antigen as immune complex receptor in drug-induced hemolytic anemia. Vox Sang 1981;41:313-5.

85. Sosler SD, Behzad O, Garratty G, et al. Acute hemolytic anemia associated with a chlorpropamide-induced apparent auto-anti-Jk^a. Transfusion 1984;24:206-9.

86. Petz LD. Drug-induced autoimmune hemolytic anemia. Transfus Med Rev 1993;7:213-4.

87. Branch DR, Gallagher MT, Shulman IA, et al. Reticuloendothelial cell function in alpha-methyldopa-induced hemolytic anemia. Vox Sang 1983;45:278-87.

88. Kirtland HH, Mohler DN, Horwitz DA. Methyldopa inhibition of suppressor-lymphocyte function. A proposed cause of autoimmune hemolytic anemia. N Engl J Med 1980;302:825-32.

89. Scott GL, Myles AB, Bacon PA. Autoimmune haemolytic anaemia and mefenamic acid therapy. Br J Med 1968;3:543-5.

90. Territo MC, Peters RW, Tanaka KR. Autoimmune hemolytic anemia due to levodopa therapy. JAMA 1973;226:1347-8.

91. Croft JD, Swisher SN, Gilliland BC, et al. Coombs' test positivity induced by drugs: Mechanisms of immunologic reactions and red cell destruction. Ann Intern Med 1968;68:176-87.

92. Worlledge SM. Immune drug-induced hemolytic anemias. Semin Hematol 1973;10:327-44.

In: Mintz PD, ed.
Transfusion Therapy: Clinical Principles and Practice
Bethesda, MD: AABB Press, 1999

4

Platelet Transfusion Therapy

JAY H. HERMAN, MD

 THE RELATIONSHIP BETWEEN THE hemostatic effect of platelet transfusion and the need to achieve a sustained rise in platelet count has been known for some time, as reflected in an early editorial by Dr. C. L. Conley.[1] He pointed out that "hemostatic effects are demonstrable only when the transfused platelets are viable and remain in the circulation of the recipient in sufficient numbers to maintain an adequate platelet count.... It is now apparent that the problems concerned with the transfusion of platelets are in many ways analogous to those of red cell transfusion."[1(p636)]

There are scant recent data and only a handful of earlier studies to help guide the ever-growing practice of platelet transfusion. Despite the large amount of money, blood donations, and medical resources devoted to this practice, zealously held beliefs about what product to choose, which patients will benefit, how many platelets to transfuse and when, and how often platelets are indicated are supported too frequently by anecdote and extrapolation rather than by controlled scientific study.

Platelet Products

There are two basic types of platelet components available for transfusion: pooled platelet concentrates derived from whole blood donation, properly called Platelets but often called random-donor platelets (RDPs); and platelets derived from volunteer donor cytapheresis, properly called Platelets, Pheresis but often called single-donor platelets (SDPs).[2] The production costs for apheresis platelets are much higher than for whole blood-derived concentrates and depend on the recruitment of donors willing to devote hours to the process, often at fixed collection sites rather than at more convenient bloodmobiles. This common terminology may lead physicians to feel that SDPs are better than

Jay H. Herman, MD, Director, Transfusion Medicine, Temple University Hospital and Professor, Department of Pathology and Laboratory Medicine, Temple University School of Medicine, Philadelphia, Pennsylvania

RDPs. However, unless they are selected as matched products for a patient, SDPs are still "random," and, conversely, RDPs can be crossmatched before pooling and so may not be random at all.

For some time, Platelets have been prepared from Whole Blood collected during regular blood donations. Most commonly in the United States, platelet-rich plasma is prepared through the centrifugation of Whole Blood followed by a further concentration once the packed red cells have been separated. The preparation of Platelets from buffy coat preparations of Whole Blood have gained popularity in many parts of Europe. The citrated anticoagulants currently in use provide excellent platelet recovery, function, and survival, whichever method is used.[3] The American Association of Blood Banks *Standards for Blood Banks and Transfusion Services*[4] and US Food and Drug Administration (FDA) regulations[5] stipulate that there must be at least 5.5×10^{10} platelets in no less than 75% of Platelets. Currently, an average unit (U) of Platelets derived from Whole Blood contains approximately 8×10^{10} platelets. Platelets are usually suspended in 45-65 mL of fresh plasma containing about 10^8 leukocytes.

Numerous devices are licensed for the preparation of Platelets, Pheresis. Although these devices differ in operation, donor management, final product plasma volume, and leukocyte content, the differences should have little bearing on the ordering practices of most physicians as long as the platelet content is adequate. Most of these devices separate platelets from the other formed blood elements according to the sedimentation or flow characteristics of anticoagulated donor blood processed through the instrument. This allows the equivalent of many units of Platelets to be collected in 2 hours or less with minimal loss of red cells or plasma. Yields vary widely because of both donor-dependent and device parameters,[6] but the average platelet content of most apheresis products is about 4×10^{11} platelets, with a minimum of 3.0×10^{11} in at least 75% of the products, according to AABB *Standards* and FDA guidelines. Acid-citrate-dextrose is the only anticoagulant that is licensed for the preparation of platelets in the United States.

Attention must be directed to the large variation in platelet content of the various products because this affects transfusion dose and outcome, the main topic of this chapter. Table 4-1 details the chief dif-

Table 4-1. Platelet Product Contents

	Platelets, Pheresis (SDPs)	Platelets (RDPs) (Single Unit)	Platelets (RDPs) Pool (5 Units)
Platelets			
Minimum	$>3.0 \times 10^{11}$	$>5.5 \times 10^{10}$	—
Average	$\sim 4.2 \times 10^{11}$	$\sim 7\text{-}9 \times 10^{10}$	$\sim 4 \times 10^{11}$
Leukocytes	$10^7 - 10^5 *$	$\sim 8 \times 10^7$	$\sim 4 \times 10^8$
Red cells	Rare	Usually <1 mL	<5 mL
Volume (mL)	200-300	45-60	~300
Matching potential	Yes	Yes (often impractical)	No

*Some devices consistently collect products with fewer than 10^6 leukocytes.

SDPs = single-donor platelets; RDPs = random-donor platelets

ferences between Platelets, Pheresis and Platelets. There is no standardized platelet content or volume for these products, given that donors have wide biologic variation in platelet count and the efficiency of collection also varies greatly.

Each type of platelet product has advantages and disadvantages, summarized in Table 4-2. It is important for physicians treating a bleeding patient to realize that insistence upon one type of product or another may create delays in platelet transfusion. This is due to the difficulty in maintaining an adequate platelet inventory because both types of products have limited storage capabilities.[7] Constant agitation of platelets is required to prevent activation through clumping and to facilitate gas exchange through the permeable plastic containers. This retards the development of acidosis in the storage container caused by platelet metabolic byproducts. Maintenance of pH has been shown to be the most critical factor for platelet viability. It is also known that platelets will activate and become damaged unless kept in a controlled, stable, thermal environment of 22 ± 2 C. Transporting and storing platelets—even to parts of the hospital, such as the operating room or intensive care units, where they may be held for some time before transfusion—require proper attention to these needs to avoid the degradation of platelet quality.

Although platelets have been shown to maintain viability for up to 7 days, growing concern about bacterial contamination (introduced at collection from either skin flora or asymptomatic donor bacteremia)[8] led the FDA to limit the shelf life of Platelet units to 5 days. This short shelf life means that Platelet units are often unavailable because it is impractical for many blood banks to have an inventory of unassigned Platelet units unless their daily platelet transfusion volume is sufficiently large to avoid outdating. Platelet inventories are often depleted on Mondays and days following holidays because of the unavailability of donors on weekends.

Platelets are often transfused regardless of their ABO type because ABO antigens are only weakly expressed on platelets. Most adults have soluble A or B antigenic substances in their blood that are capable of neutralizing the antibodies in small amounts of ABO-incompatible plasma (such as one platelet transfusion). For smaller patients or for repeated transfusions, ABO-compatible platelets are recommended to avoid any risk of hemolysis induced by ABO-incompatible plasma. Passenger red cells in the platelets may lead to alloimmunization to red cell antigens, making adherence to Rh compatibility important when females of child-bearing potential are being transfused.

Table 4-2. Platelet Product Comparison

	Single-Donor Platelets	Random-Donor Platelets
Advantages	Single donor exposure	Dose escalation possible
	Patient matching possible	Maximal availability
	Low red blood cell and white blood cell content	Blood collection coproduct
Disadvantages	Limits platelet dose	Multiple donor exposures
	Limited availability	Matching often impractical
	Inconvenient for donor	Higher red blood cell and white blood cell content

Once platelet concentrates are pooled into a transfer bag to achieve an adequate transfusion dose, this becomes an "open" system with a 4-hour expiration from the time of pooling. It is unfortunate that Platelets are often wasted because of a lack of understanding that when orders are received to prepare them, the Platelets must either be used or discarded within 4 hours. Often, Platelets, Pheresis units are stored in two plastic bags, which are then pooled for transfusion upon order. Although this is a closed system, one bag has insufficient surface area to support platelet viability for the entire product beyond 24 hours.

The current risk of acquiring a transfusion-transmitted disease is exceedingly small, but it seems intuitively obvious that the incidence of such disease would be affected by limiting patients to fewer donor exposures, thereby minimizing the likelihood of encountering an infectious unit that managed to elude all established safeguards of modern blood donation. However, an older study of oncology patients before the advent of hepatitic C virus screening found little effect on the rate of posttransfusion hepatitis when apheresis platelets were used rather than pooled concentrates.[9] This was presumably related to the evidence from transfusion-transmitted disease studies that the curve of donor exposures plotted against the risk of hepatitis reached a plateau after a finite number of transfusions.[10,11] Most platelet recipients are exposed to numerous transfusion events, and it had been suggested that donor limitation might not help prevent posttransfusion hepatitis in these patients.[12] Yet even if this were true, the initiation of hepatitis C virus testing has certainly lowered the transfusion risk dramatically and has raised the point at which the risk of hepatitis reaches this plateau. Many still choose apheresis platelets for their patients for this reason.

There is a commonly held belief that limiting donor exposure through the use of unmatched Platelets, Pheresis rather than pools of Platelets will prevent primary HLA alloimmunization. However, this has been shown not to be true.[13,14] In these studies, there was no dose-response relationship between the number of transfusions of pooled Platelets and HLA alloimmunization. The development of the alloimmune refractory state was found to be recipient dependent. Most patients became alloimmunized early in their transfusion history, and this alloimmunization was unaffected by underlying diagnosis or therapy. While limiting donor exposure through the use of apheresis platelets may delay an anamnestic response in already sensitized patients,[15] later studies, a number of which used pooled Platelets, have clearly linked the reduction of primary alloimmunization to leukocyte reduction rather than to donor limitation.[16-21] It appears that the mechanism of primary alloim- munization depends on the transfusion of donor leukocytes that have intact Class II HLA antigens. The Class I antigens found on platelets are weak immunogens.[22] Most recently, a carefully controlled, multicenter, randomized trial of leukocyte reduction clearly showed that apheresis platelets were no better than leukocyte-reduced pools in preventing primary alloimmunization.[23] Leukocyte reduction of platelets and the provision of cytomegalovirus-reduced risk components are discussed in Chapter 16. The management of transfusion reactions is addressed in Chapter 18.

Indications for Platelet Transfusion

Platelets should be thought of not as hemostatic agents but as human biologic products designed for deficit replacement therapy. For someone else's platelets to be of benefit, patients should be deficient in their own platelet number and/or function.

There are a number of recognized indications for platelet transfusion. The most frequently encountered are the treatment of thrombocytopenic bleeding and the prevention of spontaneous hemorrhage associated with low platelet counts; the next section covers in detail the platelet transfusion threshold for these indications. Platelets are also used to provide "coverage" for invasive procedures during thrombocytopenia. Some studies indicate that invasive procedures are safe when the platelet count is at least 50,000/μL,[24,25] and the inference is that transfusion to this level is indicated. Even higher levels may be appropriate if there is no opportunity to achieve direct hemostasis. However, some procedures can be carried out even in the presence of severe thrombocytopenia if hemostasis can be controlled directly. Prophylactic transfusion prior to invasive bedside procedures is discussed in Chapter 8.

Dilutional thrombocytopenia often accompanies massive transfusion when fluids and stored red cells devoid of platelets are used in large quantities. Following replacement of 1 blood volume, the platelet concentration is reduced by almost half. However, profound thrombocytopenia and abnormal bleeding usually do not develop, and transfusion is not indicated just because the platelet count is low.[26] Platelets should be reserved for patients who have bleeding disproportionate to the level of thrombocytopenia or who reveal a diffuse bleeding diathesis. These conditions may be evidence of a coagulopathy or perhaps are related to the effects of perfusion disturbances on the microvasculature. The management of platelet transfusion in surgery and trauma is discussed in Chapter 9.

Less commonly, platelets have been used to correct thrombocytopathic conditions associated with von Willebrand's disease, congenital platelet defects, and acquired platelet defects such as the aspirin effect, cardiopulmonary bypass, or uremia. The chief difficulty for many of these indications, aside from the paucity of data in support of efficacy, is that the transfused platelets will typically be affected as well as the patient's own platelets. The platelet count often falls after cardiopulmonary bypass, and an associated platelet function defect has been described.[27,28] Prospective studies have shown no benefit from the prophylactic administration of platelet transfusions to such patients,[29] and thus it seems prudent to reserve platelet transfusion for those patients with unexpected or disproportionate bleeding. There have been some reports that "fresh" whole blood is important for hemostasis in this setting, presumably from platelets that have not been subjected to storage.[30,31] The transfusion and pharmcologic management of acquired disorders of hemostasis are discussed in Chapter 7, and the treatment of congenital coagulation disorders is addressed in Chapter 6.

Splenomegaly may cause thrombocytopenia from excessive sequestration, but the platelet count rarely falls much below 40,000/μL. Because a disproportionate number of transfused platelets will become sequestered also, platelet transfusion is rarely useful (or necessary) in this setting.

For immune thrombocytopenic purpura, platelet transfusion is generally not useful because the autoantibody shortens the survival of transfused platelets as it does the patient's own platelets. When hemorrhagic emergencies do occur in such cases, hypertransfusion of platelets can result in transient rises in the platelet count that may have some clinical benefit. In a similar manner, platelets may be used in the treatment of clinical conditions, such as disseminated intravascular coagulation, liver disease, and liver transplantation, that are associated with a consumptive coagulopathy. The effectiveness of this has not been widely studied, and unless a sustained increment in platelet count is observed, it is difficult to support the continued transfusion of platelets in this setting. Some diseases associated with increased platelet activation and consumption, such as heparin-induced thrombocytopenia and thrombotic thrombocytopenic purpura, may be worsened by platelet transfusion.[32,33]

Transfusion Threshold and Prophylactic Transfusion

An early study shed light on the relationship between bleeding and thrombocytopenia.[34] In this study of acute leukemia patients, hemorrhage was associated with low or falling platelet counts below 20,000/μL, and the lower the platelet count, the greater the frequency of hemorrhage. However, these authors have subsequently reminded us that most of the patients in the study were receiving aspirin, and the data need to be viewed with that in mind. There was no threshold for the risk of bleeding, with a linear relationship of bleeding to platelet count. Both the frequency and the severity of hemorrhage increased in association with lower platelet counts. The presence of other clinical factors also influenced bleeding, in that precipitating events, which alone would have failed to cause hemorrhage, regularly resulted in hemorrhage when coupled with thrombocytopenia.

A number of clinical factors are said to affect platelet recovery and survival: fever, perhaps from the underlying cause rather than the elevated temperature itself; infection, especially sepsis; consumptive processes such as disseminated intravascular coagulation; splenomegaly; concomitant administration of amphotericin; and immune-mediated processes such as alloimmunization, autoimmunity, and drug antibody.[35-37] Anatomic lesions or mucositis, anemia, and high leukocyte counts are additional factors that predispose a patient to bleed even if the response to platelet transfusion is unaffected.

The practice of prophylactic transfusion to treat amegakaryocytic thrombocytopenia grew from findings such as these. One of the few studies available in support of the use of platelet transfusion to prevent rather than treat bleeding reported 56 pediatric leukemia patients who were to receive transfusion at a dose of $4 U/m^2$ when their platelet counts fell below $20,000/\mu L$ or when significant hemorrhage was noted.[38] The patients receiving prophylactic transfusion had about twice the number of transfusion events, but only three of 25 patients had one bleeding episode each in the prophylactic group while eight of 21 patients had 27 bleeding episodes in the therapeutic group ($p<0.00001$). However, overall survival was not different in the two groups.

A study that helped determine the threshold for spontaneous hemorrhage was reported by Slichter and Harker.[39] Twenty aplastic anemia patients with no additional clinical risk factors underwent ^{51}Cr-labeled autologous red blood cell survival studies to detect spontaneous occult fecal blood loss at various platelet counts in the absence of platelet or red cell transfusion. Normal blood loss (<5 mL/day) was seen at platelet counts greater than $10,000/\mu L$ while an increased blood loss (9 ± 7 mL/day) was noted at counts between 5000-$10,000/\mu L$ and a marked blood loss (50 ± 20 mL/day) was seen at counts below $5000/\mu L$.

Using data such as these, several groups have advocated altering the common practice of prophylactic transfusion to reflect both our current understanding of a much lower baseline threshold of bleeding and the presence of clinical risk factors.[40] In one of the earliest studies, constant clinical assessment for risk factors was coupled with a "sliding scale" for the transfusion trigger, starting at platelet counts of $5000/\mu L$ or lower.[41] There was a lower incidence of bleeding at all triggers when compared with bleeding in a historical control group while overall platelet use was decreased.

Under this stringent policy, minor hemorrhage was common but the incidence of major hemorrhage was low: 3% of patients had lethal bleeding in the stringent group and significant central nervous system (CNS) sequelae were seen in an additional 1%. Most major hemorrhages were due to immune refractoriness or profound thrombocytopenia when numerous clinical risk factors were present and were comparable in incidence to that in historical controls who had been transfused when standard transfusion triggers were in use. A number of recent studies have reported similar findings in both leukemia and stem cell transplantation patients.[42-44]

A practical approach to prophylactic transfusion that incorporates much of this information has been advanced by Schiffer.[45] He points out that experienced oncologists can identify most patients at risk of hemorrhage without stringent criteria, given the subjective nature of the assessment of risk factors. While some patients need platelet counts maintained at high levels, and a few can avoid any transfusion safely, even at counts of $5000/\mu L$, most patients fall in between and need to have their threshold and target increment individualized. Factors such as lack of readily available physician assessment in hospitals without house staff, lack of accessible platelet inventories, and scheduling problems inherent in outpatient treatment can interfere with the application of a rigorous transfusion algorithm.

Assessment and Dose

Both hemorrhage itself and the underlying conditions that cause the bleeding may increase platelet consumption and appreciably shorten platelet survival. It is a historical truism that the hemostatic goal of platelet transfusion therapy is to raise the circulating platelet count because sustained levels above 40,000/µL are correlated directly with the likelihood of hemostasis.[35]

Once the indication and threshold have been decided and platelets have been transfused, assessment of the response is usually based on measurement of the post-transfusion count. A "pharmacologic" model that accounts for the pre- and posttransfusion counts, the blood volume of the patient, and the survival of the transfused platelets is useful when deciding on platelet dose and frequency of transfusion.[46] Apheresis platelet concentrates are often substituted for the customary pooled platelet product, commonly 6 or 8 units of whole blood-derived Platelets. This may cause difficulty in assessing the response to transfusion if the apheresis concentrate used has a low yield of platelets, given that some plateletpheresis centers distribute concentrates with 3.0×10^{11} platelets per product or lower. Based on the average content of platelets in whole blood-derived platelet concentrates, 3.0×10^{11} platelets per product would be equivalent to about only a "four pack."

It is useful to assess the efficacy of platelet transfusions by the effect they have on clinical bleeding, but only if the bleeding is caused predominantly by a platelet deficit. Obviously, if bleeding is present, cessation of hemorrhage is the therapeutic endpoint for platelet transfusion. However, in the absence of observable hemorrhage, most physicians determine whether platelet transfusions are successful by observing the measured increment in posttransfusion platelet count compared with pretransfusion values.

Arriving at dose calculations is relatively simple. The volume of distribution for transfused platelets is about half again as great as the patient's blood volume, and so for an average patient with a blood volume of 2.5 L/m^2, the volume of distribution for platelets will be 3.75 L/m^2. For Platelets that contain about 8×10^{10} platelets each, the infusion of 1 unit of Platelets theoretically should raise the platelet count by about 21,000/µL for each square meter of body surface area. In actuality, platelet transfusions often result in only about half of the expected increments because of the clinical factors stated above. Allowing for this, a dose of 5 pooled units of Platelets would be calculated to raise the platelet count from 10,000/µL to 40,000/µL in a patient whose body surface area is 2 m^2.

A number of common platelet-dosing algorithms have been advanced to make ordering easier; all are expected to achieve an "adequate" transfusion response (Table 4-3). The higher platelet

Table 4-3. Standard Platelet Doses

Patient	Dose
Infants	10 mL of platelet concentrate for every kilogram of body weight
Children	1 unit of Platelets (random donor platelets) for every 10-15 kg body weight
Adults	5-8 units of pooled Platelets (random donor platelets) or 1 unit of Platelets, Pheresis, regardless of platelet content

content in recent whole blood-derived platelets has led to "standard" pools of 5 or even 4 units of Platelets, again given to patients regardless of body size (and hence regardless of blood volume). Additionally, the platelet content of many apheresis platelets has been reduced because of shorter collection times (to improve donor recruitment) and the practice of "splitting" the collection into two separate products, each with half of the platelets collected. The motivation for this splitting of an apheresis donation has been attributed to dose standardization and efforts to improve Platelets, Pheresis availability, but the practice also seeks better cost recovery because full price is usually charged for each half-product. It should be pointed out that platelets are the only transfusion product with such commonly used standard doses. These standard doses negate the ability to adjust the platelet dose on the basis of clinical need, as is done for Red Blood Cells, Fresh Frozen Plasma, Cryoprecipitated AHF, and plasma derivatives.

The concept of correcting the observed increment in platelet count, as opposed to achieving the expected rise in platelet count, as a way of judging the success of a transfusion, has now become accepted as a "gold standard" in transfusion medicine. The corrected count increment (CCI) adjusts the observed raw increment in platelet count for the platelet content of the transfusion and the body surface area in square meters of the patient (as an approximation of blood volume). It is most useful when measured as a peak level within minutes to 1 hour of the transfusion in order to discriminate between immune destruction and a pathologic consumption.[47] A poor platelet increment obtained within this time frame tends to reflect immune destruction, whereas poor platelet counts obtained at a later time after transfusion tend to indicate a pathologic consumptive process. Another formula, the percent platelet recovery, adjusts the platelet increment for the calculated blood volume of the patient. The CCI and percent platelet recovery calculation methods are given in Fig 4-1. The platelet increment is measured by subtracting the post-transfusion platelet count from the pretransfusion count, which has been preferably obtained close to the transfusion event to avoid inaccurate sampling. The pretransfusion count has been shown to drift further downward if there is a significant delay before transfusion, and this can obscure a successful increment. In one study of stem cell transplantation patients with relatively uncomplicated thrombocytopenia, the mean rate of reduction in the platelet count was $740/\mu L$ per hour in adults and $820/\mu L$ per hour in pediatric patients.[48]

On the basis of studies of prophylactic transfusions and normal volunteers, the expected CCI in a successful transfusion should be between 10,000 and 20,000, although clinical factors in bleeding patients may blunt this response. Platelet transfusion failures are usually defined as CCIs of less than 7500 at 1 hour. Consistent failure to achieve expected CCIs defines the platelet refractory state. Many recommend the use of matched platelets to improve posttransfusion platelet recovery if a low 1-hour CCI indicates that an immune-mediated cause of platelet transfusion failure is likely.[36,49-50]

Corrected count increment (CCI):

$$\frac{(\text{Platelet increment}) \times (\text{body surface area in square meters})}{\text{Number of platelets transfused } (\times 10^{11})}$$

Percent platelet recovery:

$$\frac{(\text{Platelet increment}) \times (\text{weight in kilograms}) \times (\text{blood volume as 75 mL/kg}) \times 100 \text{ (for percent)}}{(\text{Platelet count of transfused product}) \times (\text{volume of product in milliliters})}$$

Figure 4-1. Methods for platelet increment correction.

As already mentioned, a wide biologic variation of platelet transfusion response has been observed, so "failure" is difficult to define. It is often set at 50% of whatever value was expected, but other definitions of refractoriness to platelet transfusion have been published, especially in the stem cell transplantation population.[51] Sequestration of transfused platelets in the spleen and other organs is said to account for 30-40% of the platelets in commonly used doses. This sequestration of platelets may be increased, sometimes without overt splenomegaly.

It is critically important to appreciate that because the number of platelets transfused is factored into the calculation, the CCI does not indicate in any way that a satisfactory posttransfusion platelet *count* has been achieved. If a clinically inadequate dose of platelets has been given, the CCI may still be high.

A study by Hanson and Slichter[52] made some interesting observations on the recovery and survival of platelets after transfusion. Sixteen normal volunteers and 27 stable thrombocytopenic patients underwent radiolabeled platelet survival studies, with a random, fixed number of nonrecovered platelets, about 7100/µL each day. It is postulated that this number of platelets is needed to maintain vascular integrity. Median platelet survival was 7.0 days when the platelet count was 50,000-100,000/µL compared with 5.1 days when counts were lower. Posttransfusion recovery and survival of labeled autologous platelets were reduced when the platelet count was below 50,000/µL, and survival curves were even steeper at lower platelet counts.

Surprisingly, there have been relatively few studies of platelet dose. Those that exist have tried to define platelet dose and expected response to transfusion, but differences in transfusion products and clinical settings may lead to questions of their applicability. However, the original study of platelet transfusion by Freireich et al may still be applicable.[35] Less than 6-hour-old platelet-rich plasma prepared by plateletpheresis with a median platelet dose of $2.55 \times 10^{11}/m^2$ was transfused on a schedule to 28 pediatric leukemia patients with median pretransfusion platelet counts of 6000/µL. The median increment when the dose was less than $1.25/m^2$ was 12,000/µL, while the median increment at doses greater than $4.5/m^2$ was 60,000/µL. Survival of transfused platelets was curvilinear, depending on how high the platelet transfusion increment raised the platelet count and whether fever or sepsis was present. The incidence of hemorrhage was linear, from less than 20% at platelet counts above 40,000/µL to more than 80% at platelet counts of 2000/µL, while platelet transfusion reduced bleeding significantly, especially major hemorrhage.

Another early study providing data relating to dose was published by Djerassi and colleagues.[53] Platelet concentrates from acid citrate dextrose Whole Blood less than 3 hours old, with doses calculated by body weight, were transfused on schedule to 25 pediatric leukemia patients with median pretransfusion platelet counts of 25,000/µL. Hemostasis correlated with increments greater than 20,000/µL, and 84% of bleeding episodes stopped when this increment was achieved, whereas only 33% stopped at lower increments (p<0.01). Doses of 0.04 U/lb were less likely to raise the platelet count by more than 20,000/µL than were doses of 0.08 U/lb (p<0.01), although the 0.04 U/lb dose represented the commonly recommended dose of 1 U/10 kg. Platelet transfusion survival in bleeding patients was shorter (2-3 days) compared with normal platelet survival.

In the past few years, interest in defining the proper dose for platelet transfusion has been renewed. As the number of platelet transfusion recipients grows and the cost of blood products rises, many transfusion services have tried to lower the standard dose of platelets to conserve this resource effectively. In one study that compared different dosing strategies in prophylactic transfusion, nine acute myelogenous leukemia patients received prophylactic apheresis platelet transfusions at a median dose of 2×10^{11} during remission induction and of 4×10^{11} during consolidation several weeks later; the transfusion threshold used was 20,000/µL.[54] The sequential study design did not control for clinical differences between induction and consolidation, and there was no randomization or crossover. There was a similar number of transfusions in both arms of the study, resulting in more platelets being used for patients in the higher-dose arm during consolidation; however, the duration of thrombocytopenia was longer. The interval between transfusions was greater for higher-dose (median 4.4 days) than for lower-dose (3.03 days) transfusions, thus explaining the similar number of transfusions in both study arms. A similar effect was seen on posttransfusion increment and survival, with the higher dose giving a median 14-hour CCI of 5820 and a median 38-hour CCI of 3750 compared with 4660 and 2480, respectively, for the lower dose. The decline in raw platelet counts was steeper for the lower-dose (47%) than for the higher-dose products (36%).

A retrospective, multiple regression study by Bishop and colleagues on the causes of platelet refractoriness has served as a landmark in the study of refractoriness but was unable to address the effect of dose because the same dose (six pooled Platelets) was used for all transfusions.[36] Interestingly, this study found that the single most significant factor associated with refractoriness to platelet transfusion was marrow transplantation, although only 39 of the 941 transfusions were to marrow transplant recipients.

This effect of transplantation on platelet transfusion outcome was evident in a similar, retrospective, multiple regression analysis of refractoriness in a pure stem cell transplantation population.[55] A high incidence of refractoriness was seen in 526 platelet transfusions in 66 marrow or peripheral blood stem cell transplant recipients, with almost two-thirds (64%) of patients having 1 hour CCIs less than 7500 and 40% having CCIs less than 5000. This refractoriness was often transient, and most patients had consistent, measurable platelet increments despite low CCIs. Independent factors associated with lower CCIs were having lymphocytotoxic antibody, being male, having a body surface area greater than 1.7 m^2, having had a prior pregnancy, and having an ABO mismatch (A into O). Many factors identified in previous studies of leukemia patients, including infection, drugs, condi-

tioning regimen, prior transfusion, and age of platelets, were not independently predictive of platelet transfusion failure in the marrow transplantation setting. Although some researchers have reported that "fresh" platelets are more effective for some patients, especially those with infection, this effect is seen primarily if the platelets have been stored for less than 1 day.[56] In the above mentioned study, the youngest platelets were at least 2 days old, and the effect of storage may have been present already. No dose effect was evident when a subset of apheresis platelets with recorded platelet content was analyzed separately, but there was marked clustering of platelet content around the median, which may have obscured any dose effect. Refractoriness to platelet transfusions is also discussed in Chapter 12.

Most transplantation centers can readily identify patients who exhibit poor CCIs despite no definable risk factors but who can achieve higher CCIs with higher corrected count increments with higher doses of platelets. Perhaps the fixed platelet loss defined by Hanson and Slichter[52] is increased in these patients, or else there is a greater degree of sequestration. It is intriguing to try to link this to the diffuse endothelial cell injury induced by the transplantation preparative regimens.

A number of recent abstracts not yet published as full reports have begun to address the lack of data regarding the effect of platelet dose on transfusion outcome. A study comparing higher yield apheresis platelets with more conventional platelet products found that higher sustained increments were achieved with unsplit, higher-dose apheresis platelets than with standard-dose products.[57] However, higher doses were just as ineffective as standard doses in treating platelet refractoriness. The patients in this study were predominantly acute leukemia patients.

In a nonrandomized, noncrossover study, escalated doses of platelets were given to similar patients receiving prophylactic transfusion.[58] A direct and almost linear relationship was seen between platelet dose and posttransfusion increment when dose cohorts separated into 4, 6, and 8 × 10^{11} platelets per concentrate were used. Higher doses also had a direct effect on the interval between transfusion, indicating that higher doses could prolong that interval. These effects were especially true for the pediatric patients studied.

Another study took a different approach and looked at total platelet usage at one institution when the standard dose of pooled platelets was cut from 1 U/10 kg to 1 U/12 kg to reflect the higher platelet content of the whole blood-derived platelets now available.[59] This reduction of standard dose did not prolong the mean transfusion interval when it was applied to all platelet recipients as a group, and it also decreased the mean number of platelets transfused overall. However, the effect of this standard dose on individual patient response was not studied.

Most of the available data have focused on acute leukemia patients and the use of products and transfusion regimens that may not reflect current practice in support of hematopoietic stem cell transplantation. Our group designed a randomized, crossover, blinded study to investigate the economic and clinical consequences of reduced platelet dose for prophylactic transfusion in a pure transplantation setting. The results of the completed study, reported to date in abstract form only, are summarized below.[60]

Apheresis platelets were segregated according to platelet content into high-third (HD) and lower-third (LD) dose cohorts of routinely available products from the local blood center, with HD and LD platelets transfused in random sequential pairs to the same patient; the median content for HD platelets was 4.9×10^{11} and for LD platelets was 3.1×10^{11}. The randomized, double-blind, multiple crossover design controlled for clinical risk factors and patient variables, while no changes were made in transfusion parameters such as the platelet count threshold of 15,000/μL. Only sequential prophylactic transfusions were studied; intervening therapeutic transfusions for bleeding or to cover procedures excluded the HD/LD paired transfusions and refractory patients were removed from the study. The results of 79 paired transfusions to 46 patients revealed that HD platelets had a time to next transfusion of 3.03 days compared with 2.16

days for LD platelets in the same patient (p<0.01), with disproportionate differences in median platelet increments: 31,000/μL for HD compared with 17,000/μL for LD (p<0.0001). The age of the platelets had no effect on increment or platelet survival (from day 2 through day 5), but ABO mismatch (A into O) affected increment (p<0.05). Multiple regression analysis of 74 patient variables identified no other patient factors as having a significant independent effect on platelet response. A cost analysis model applied to these data found that the number of platelet transfusions to the patients in this study would have been significantly reduced, along with the cost of transfusion (p=0.05), if only HD transfusions had been given.[61]

These recent studies indicate that the response to platelet transfusion may be affected by certain factors that would seem to make higher, rather than lower, doses of platelets a better choice for prophylactic transfusion, especially during stem cell transplantation. Whether the dose-response relationship for platelet transfusion is truly nonlinear with respect to escalated doses, as many of these studies suggest, requires further data.

Conclusion

A recent review article by Strauss[62] evaluated much of the preceding information and offered recommendations for appropriate platelet dosing in the setting of amegakaryocytic, thrombocytopenic bleeding. These are summarized in Table 4-4. For CNS or life-threatening bleeding, higher posttransfusion target platelet counts (eg, 75,000-100,000/μL) are typically used.

These recommended doses should be adjusted for the patient's size with the use of current platelet content data for both pools and apheresis platelets. Standard doses are convenient *starting* points for platelet transfusion in most patients if they increase the platelet count enough to produce the desired clinical outcome. Adjustments to dose and frequency of transfusion are often required because of coexisting clinical factors. More data are needed in diverse clinical settings to determine the appropriate threshold, dose, and frequency of platelet trans-

Table 4-4. Platelet Transfusion Recommendations[62]

Prophylactic platelet transfusion*:

Target platelet count	> 25,000/μL
Dose[†]	> 4×10^{11} platelets
Threshold[‡]	< 10,000/μL

Therapeutic platelet transfusion[§]:

Target platelet count	> 40,000/μL
Dose[†]	> 6×10^{11} platelets
Threshold	Individualized

*To prevent spontaneous hemorrhage in amegakaryocytic, thrombocytopenic patients.
[†]For patients weighing more than 55 kg.
[‡]Unless clinical risk factors are present.
[§]For non-central nervous system, non-life-threatening hemorrhage in amegakaryocytic, thrombocytopenic patients.

fusion. Until these studies are completed, extrapolation from the few reports reviewed in this chapter will have to suffice.

References

1. Conley CL. Blood platelets and platelet transfusions. Arch Intern Med 1961;107:635-8.

2. Herman JH. Single-donor (apheresis) vs pooled platelet concentrates. In: Kurtz SR, Brubaker DB, eds. Clinical decisions in platelet therapy. Bethesda, MD: American Association of Blood Banks, 1992:19-30.

3. Moroff G, Holme S. Concepts about current conditions for the preparation and storage of platelets. Transfus Med Rev 1991;5:48-59.

4. Menitove JE, ed. Standards for blood banks and transfusion services. 18th ed. Bethesda, MD: American Association of Blood Banks, 1997:16.

5. Code of federal regulations. 21 CFR 640.24(c). Washington, DC: US Government Printing Office, 1998 (revised annually).

6. Bertholf MF, Mintz PD. Comparison of plateletpheresis using two cell separators and identical donors. Transfusion 1989;29:521-3.

7. Murphy S. Platelet storage for transfusion. Semin Hematol 1985;22:165-77.

8. Braine HG, Kickler TS, Charache P, et al. Bacterial sepsis secondary to platelet transfusion: An adverse effect of extended storage at room temperature. Transfusion 1986;26:391-3.

9. Schiffer CA, Slichter SJ. Platelet transfusion from single donors. N Engl J Med 1982; 307:245-8.

10. Aach RD, Szmuness W, Mosley JW, et al. Serum alanine aminotransferase of donors in relation to the risk of non-A, non-B hepatitis in recipients. N Engl J Med 1981;304:989-94.

11. Sirchia G, Giovanetti AM, Parravicini A, et al. Prospective evaluation of posttransfusion hepatitis. Transfusion 1991;31:299-302.

12. Bove JR. Transfusion-associated hepatitis and AIDS. N Engl J Med 1987;317:242-5.

13. Dutcher JP, Schiffer CA, Aisner J, Wiernik PH. Long-term follow-up of patients with leukemia receiving platelet transfusion: Identifica-

tion of a large group of patients who do not become alloimmunized. Blood 1981;58: 1007-11.

14. Dutcher JP, Schiffer CA, Aisner J, Wiernik PH. Alloimmunization following platelet transfusion: The absence of a dose-response relationship. Blood 1980;57:395-8.

15. Gmür J, von Felton A, Osterwalder B, et al. Delayed alloimmunization using random single-donor platelet transfusion: A prospective study in thrombocytopenic patients with acute leukemia. Blood 1983;62:473-9.

16. Eernisse JG, Brand A. Prevention of platelet refractoriness due to HLA antibodies by administration of leukocyte-poor blood components. Exp Hematol 1981;9:77-83.

17. Sniecinski I, O'Donnell MR, Nowicki B, Hill LR. Prevention of refractoriness and HLA-alloimmunization using filtered blood products. Blood 1988;71:1402-7.

18. Andreu G, Dewailly J, Leberre C, et al. Prevention of HLA alloimmunization with leukocyte-poor packed red cells and platelet concentrates obtained by filtration. Blood 1988;72:964-9.

19. Saarinen UM, Kekomäki R, Siimes MA, Myllyla G. Effective prophylaxis against platelet refractoriness in multitransfused patients by use of leukocyte-free blood components. Blood 1990;75:512-7.

20. Oksanen K, Kekomäki R, Ruutu T, et al. Prevention of alloimmunization in patients with acute leukemia by use of white cell-reduced blood components—a randomized trial. Transfusion 1991;31:588-94.

21. van Marwijk Kooy MM, van Prooijen HC, Moes M, et al. Use of leukocyte-depleted platelet concentrates for the prevention of refractoriness and primary HLA alloimmunization: A prospective, randomized trial. Blood 1991;77:201-5.

22. Meryman HT. Transfusion-induced alloimmunization and immunosuppression and the effects of leukocyte depletion. Transfus Med Rev 1989;3:180-93.

23. Trial to Reduce Alloimmunization to Platelets (TRAP) Study Group. Leukocyte reduction and ultraviolet B irradiation of platelets to prevent alloimmunization and refractoriness to platelet transfusions. N Engl J Med 1997;337: 1861-9.

24. McVay PA, Toy PTCY. Lack of increased bleeding after liver biopsy in patients with mild hemostatic abnormalities. Am J Clin Pathol 1990;94:747-53.

25. McVay PA, Toy PTCY. Lack of increased bleeding after paracentesis and thoracentesis in patients with mild coagulation abnormalities. Transfusion 1991;31:164-71.

26. Reed LR, Ciavarella D. Heimbach DM, et al. Prophylactic platelet administration during massive transfusion. Ann Surg 1986;203:40.

27. Addonizio VP. Platelet function in cardiopulmonary bypass and artificial organs. Hematol Oncol Clin North Am 1990;4:145-55.

28. Campbell FW. The contribution of platelet dysfunction to postbypass bleeding. J Cardiothorac Vasc Anesth 1991;5:8-12.

29. Simon TL, Aki Bechara F, Murphy W. Controlled trial of routine administration of platelet concentrates in cardiopulmonary bypass surgery. Ann Thorac Surg 1984;37:359.

30. Mohr R, Good DA, Yelling A, et al. Fresh blood units contain large potent platelets that improve hemostasis after open heart operations. Ann Thorac Surg 1992;53:650-4.

31. Manno CS, Hedberg KW, Bunin GR, et al. Comparison of the hemostatic effects of fresh whole blood, stored whole blood and components after open heart surgery in children. Blood 1991;77:930-6.

32. Harkness DR, Byrnes JJ, Lian EC, et al. Hazard of platelet transfusion in thrombotic thrombocytopenic purpura. JAMA 1981;246:1931-3.

33. Gordon LI, Kwaan HC, Rossi EC. Deleterious effects of platelet transfusion and recovery thrombocytosis in patients with thrombotic microangiopathy. Semin Hematol 1987;24: 194-201.

34. Gaydos LA, Freireich EJ, Mantel N. The quantitative relation between platelet count and

hemorrhage in patients with acute leukemia. N Engl J Med 1962;266:905-9.

35. Freireich EJ, Kliman A, Gaydos LA, et al. Response to repeated platelet transfusion from the same donor. Ann Intern Med 1963;59: 277-87.

36. Bishop JF, McGrath K, Wolf MM, et al. Clinical factors influencing the efficacy of pooled platelet transfusions. Blood 1988;71:383-7.

37. Bishop JF, Matthews JP, McGrath K, et al. Factors influencing 20-hour increments after platelet transfusion. Transfusion 1991;31: 392-6.

38. Murphy S, Litwin S, Herring LM, et al. Indications for platelet transfusion in children with acute leukemia. Am J Hematol 1982;12:347-56.

39. Slichter SJ, Harker LA. Thrombocytopenia: Mechanisms and management of defects in platelet production. Clin Hematol 1978;7: 523-40.

40. Beutler E. Platelet transfusions: The 20,000/μL trigger. Blood 1993;81:1411-3.

41. Gmür J, Burger J, Schanz U, et al. Safety of stringent prophylactic platelet transfusion policy for patients with acute leukemia. Lancet 1991;338:1223-6.

42. Gil-Fernandez JJ, Alegre A, Fernandez-Villalta MJ, et al. Clinical results of a stringent policy on prophylactic platelet transfusion: Nonrandomized comparative analysis in 190 bone marrow transplant patients from a single institution. Bone Marrow Transplant 1996;18: 931-5.

43. Heckman KD, Weiner GJ, Davis CS, et al. Randomized study of prophylactic platelet transfusion threshold during induction therapy for adult acute leukemia: 10,000/μL versus 20,000/μL. J Clin Oncol 1997;15: 1143-9.

44. Rebulla P, Finazzi G, Marangoni F, et al. A multicenter randomized study of the threshold for prophylactic platelet transfusions in adults with acute myeloid leukemia. N Engl J Med 1997;337:1870-5.

45. Schiffer CA. Prophylactic platelet transfusions. Transfusion 1992;32:295-8.

46. Heyman MR, Schiffer CA. Platelet transfusion therapy for the cancer patient. Semin Oncol 1990;17:198-209.

47. Daly PA, Schiffer CA, Aisner J, Wiernik PH. Platelet transfusion therapy: One hour posttransfusion increments are valuable in predicting the need for HLA-matched preparations. JAMA 1980;243:435-8.

48. Del Rosario MLU, Kao KJ. Determination of the rate of reduction in platelet counts in recipients of hematopoietic stem and progenitor cell transplant: Clinical implications for platelet transfusion therapy. Transfusion 1997;37: 1163-8.

49. Moroff G, Garratty G, Heal JM, et al. Selection of platelets for refractory patients by HLA matching and prospective crossmatching. Transfusion 1992;32:633-9.

50. Friedberg RC, Donnelly SF, Boyd JC, et al. Clinical and blood bank factors in the management of platelet refractoriness and alloimmunization. Blood 1993;81:3428-34.

51. Benson K, Fields K, Hiemenz J, et al. The platelet refractory bone marrow transplant patient: Prophylaxis and treatment of bleeding. Semin Oncol 1993;20:102-9.

52. Hanson SR, Slichter SJ. Platelet kinetics in patients with bone marrow hypoplasia: Evidence for a fixed platelet requirement. Blood 1985;66:1105-9.

53. Djerassi I, Farber S, Evans AE. Transfusions of fresh platelet concentrates to patients with secondary thrombocytopenia. N Engl J Med 1963;268:221-6.

54. Yata Y, Baba M, Oshima T. On the optimal use of platelets and the transfusion regimen for leukemia patients. Jpn J Transfus Med 1990; 36:784-7.

55. Klumpp TR, Herman J, Innis S, et al. Factors associated with response to platelet transfusion following hematopoietic stem cell transplantation. Bone Marrow Transplant 1996; 17:1035-41.

56. Norol F, Kuentz M, Cordonnier C, et al. Influence of clinical status on the efficiency of

stored platelet transfusion. Br J Haematol 1994; 86:125-9.

57. Kiss JE, Steer K, Triulzi DJ, Winkelstein A. Transfusion response to "standard" dose and high-yield single donor platelets (abstract). Transfusion 1993;33(Suppl):4S.

58. Norol F, Duedari N, Kuentz M, et al. Comparison of different doses of platelet transfusion (abstract). Blood 1995;86(Suppl):353a.

59. Menitove JE, Hertenstein EG, Tse LC. Decreasing platelet concentrate dose: Impact on platelet transfusion interval (abstract). Blood 1996;88(Suppl):333a.

60. Herman JH, Klumpp TR, Christman RA, et al. The effect of platelet dose on the outcome of prophylactic platelet transfusion (abstract). Transfusion 1995;35(Suppl):46S.

61. Ackerman SJ, Klumpp TR, Herman JH, et al. Cost analysis of higher-dose versus lower-dose single-donor platelet transfusions in peripheral blood stem cell and bone marrow transplant patients (abstract). Blood 1996;88 (Suppl):333a.

62. Strauss RG. Clinical perspectives of platelet transfusion: Defining the optimal dose. J Clin Apher 1995;10:124-7.

In: Mintz PD, ed.
Transfusion Therapy: Clinical Principles and Practice
Bethesda, MD: AABB Press, 1999

5

Granulocyte Transfusion Therapy

RONALD G. STRAUSS, MD

CURRENT LEUKAPHERESIS TECH-nology permits the collection of large numbers of polymorphonuclear cells (PMNs), or neutrophils, from healthy donors as a standard blood component (Granulocytes, Pheresis) to support patients with neutropenia or PMN dysfunction who have developed infections. This chapter analyzes the use of PMN transfusions—called granulocyte transfusions by convention—as an adjunct to antimicrobial drugs in either the treatment or the possible prevention of certain types of infections.

Serious and repeated infections with bacteria, yeast, and fungus continue even today to be a consequence of severe neutropenia (<0.1 × 10⁹/L blood PMNs) or PMN dysfunction (eg, chronic granulomatous disease). In the National Institutes of Health 1997 multicenter TRAP study (Trial to Reduce Alloimmunization to Platelets), 7% of adult patients with acute nonlymphocytic leukemia died of infection during their first remission induction therapy despite the use of modern antibiotic therapy.[1] In a 1996 study of patients given intense chemotherapy, some of whom also received transfusions of autologous hematopoietic stem cells, 7.6% of patients suffered systemic fungal infections.[2] Unless severe neutropenia is reversed fairly quickly, the mortality of systemic infections approaches 100%.

Previous attempts to prevent infections in severely neutropenic patients using prophylactic granulocyte transfusions achieved only modest success (ie, the rates of certain infections were reduced, but granulocyte transfusions failed to prevent all infections), and the transfusions were toxic and expensive. Similarly, the use of therapeutic granulocyte transfusions to treat infections in neutropenic patients has diminished strikingly over the past several years despite many reports that have demonstrated its efficacy in certain experimental

Ronald G. Strauss, MD, Medical Director, DeGowin Blood Center, University of Iowa Hospitals and Clinics, and Professor of Pathology and Pediatrics, University of Iowa College of Medicine, Iowa City, Iowa

and clinical settings.[3] This lack of enthusiasm for granulocyte transfusions can be explained, at least in part, by a diminished need for PMN replacement owing to 1) the availability of more effective antimicrobial drugs to prevent and treat infections and 2) the development of recombinant hematopoietic cytokines and peripheral blood progenitor cell (PBPC) transfusions to hasten marrow recovery and shorten the duration of severe neutropenia following myeloablation.

Recombinant cytokines, such as granulocyte colony-stimulating factor (G-CSF) and granulocyte-macrophage colony-stimulating factor (GM-CSF), are glycoprotein growth factors that enhance the production, differentiation, and function of myeloid cells.[4,5] G-CSF has revolutionized the collection of PMNs for granulocyte transfusion therapy and of hematopoietic progenitor cells for transplantation.[5] Both G-CSF and GM-CSF have been given to patients to accelerate marrow recovery following chemotherapy, to reduce the rate of developing infections, and to diminish the need for prolonged hospitalization.[4] In contrast to this success in preventing neutropenic infections, the role of G-CSF and GM-CSF as treatment for already established infections is not as firmly documented. Regardless, these cytokines frequently are prescribed for patients with neutropenia and severe infections, and it seems reasonable to consider adding therapeutic granulocyte transfusions when severe bacterial, yeast, or fungal infections progress despite the use of antibiotic plus cytokine therapy.

Both the preference to use combination antibiotic therapy and cytokines to treat infected neutropenic patients and the reluctance to prescribe granulocyte transfusions have been reinforced by knowledge that leukapheresis products collected for granulocyte transfusions historically contained woefully inadequate numbers of PMNs. However, granulocyte transfusion therapy is entering a new era. It is now possible to collect relatively large numbers of PMNs from normal donors stimulated with G-CSF and corticosteroids using modern leukapheresis techniques. This fact, along with the historical success of granulocyte transfusion in treating bacterial infections even when PMNs

were given in relatively low doses,[3] suggests that critical reassessment of therapeutic granulocyte transfusion is warranted. Further, the possible role of prophylactic granulocyte transfusion also needs to be reassessed because of the relatively rapid engraftment following the use of PBPC transfusion when compared with either autologous or allogeneic marrow transplantation. Thus, it is reasonable to hypothesize that severe neutropenia following intense myeloablative therapy might even be eliminated by prophylactic granulocyte transfusion, particularly when used with peripheral blood progenitor cell transfusions.

Therapeutic Granulocyte Transfusions

Overview of Therapeutic Granulocyte Transfusions in Neutropenia

Thirty-four papers that reported the use of therapeutic granulocyte transfusion in severely neutropenic patients ($<0.5 \times 10^9$/L blood PMNs) were reviewed in 1997.[6] Patients were tabulated (Table 5-1) according to the index infection that prompted granulocyte transfusion therapy, and each patient was counted only once. (Eg, patients with septicemia were listed only in the septicemia section, even if they had another infection such as pneumonia. As an exception, all patients with invasive fungal infections (sepsis, pneumonia, sinusitis, etc) were grouped into one category. All patients given granulocyte transfusions for a designated type of infection were listed under the "Treated" heading. Of the treated patients, those for whom the actual course and mortality of the index infection could be clearly documented were listed again under the "Evaluable" heading. Granulocyte transfusion therapy was deemed successful if so stated by the authors. Several of the 34 reports described uncontrolled studies of small numbers of patients with a diversity of underlying diseases, types of infections, antimicrobial therapies, and granulocyte transfusion management strategies (ie, variable dose and

Table 5-1. Infections Treated With Granulocyte Transfusion in 34 Studies of Neutropenic Patients*

Type of Infection	Treated	Evaluable	Success Rate
Bacterial septicemia	298	206	127/206 = 62%
Sepsis organism unspecified	132	39	18/39 = 46%
Invasive fungus and yeast	83	77	28/77 = 36%
Pnemonia	115	11	7/11 = 64%
Localized infections	143	47	39/47 = 83%
Fever etiology unknown	184	85	64/85 = 75%

*Individual references are cited in Strauss.[6]

quality of PMNs), as well as varying definitions of success. Because of these confounding factors, no definitive conclusions could be drawn, and data were combined merely to document the breadth of experience reported.

To obtain more definitive information regarding efficacy, seven controlled studies[7-13] of therapeutic granulocyte transfusions were analyzed in more detail (Table 5-2). In these studies, the response of infected neutropenic patients to treatment with antibiotics plus granulocyte transfusions (the study group) was compared with that of comparable patients given antibiotics alone and evaluated concurrently (the control group). Three of the studies reported a significant benefit overall for granulocyte transfusions.[7-9] In two additional studies,[10,11] the overall success of granulocyte transfusions was not demonstrated, but certain subgroups of patients were found to benefit significantly (amounting to partial success for the therapy). For example, in the first controlled study,[11] many patients received an inadequate dose of granulocytes by current standards, and overall success was not demonstrated. However, when the 39 patients in the transfusion group are subdivided, 100% of the patients survived if they received granulocyte transfusions on at least four occasions, as did 80% of those receiv-

ing at least three granulocyte transfusions, compared with only 30% survival among the control subjects. In the other study that found partial success,[10] no advantage for granulocyte transfusions could be demonstrated when all of the patients were analyzed. However, when the subgroup of patients with persistent marrow failure was analyzed separately (ie, those with marrow recovery were excluded), 75% of those receiving granulocyte transfusions responded favorably, compared with only 20% of the control subjects. Thus, some measure of success for granulocyte transfusions was evident in five of the seven controlled studies (ie, three overall[7-9] and two partial[10,11]). However, this was counterbalanced by four studies that were negative in some respect (two overall[12,13] and two partial[10,11]).

An explanation of these inconsistent results is evident on critical analysis of the adequacy of granulocyte transfusion support (Table 5-2). Patients in the three successful controlled trials generally received higher doses of PMNs, and donors were selected to be leukocyte compatible.[7-9] In contrast, the two negative controlled studies can be criticized legitimately in light of current technology. The dose of PMNs transfused (0.4-0.5×10^{10}) was extremely low.[12,13] This daily dose is approxi-

Table 5-2. Seven Controlled Studies of Therapeutic Granulocyte Transfusion in Neutropenic Patients

| | Transfusion Group | | | | | Control Group | | |
| | | | | Matching* | | | | |
Reference	Patients	Survival	Dose × 10^{10}	HLA	WBC	Patients	Survival	Success
Higby et al[7]	17	76%	2.2 (F)	No	Yes	19	26%	Yes
Vogler et al[8]	17	59%	2.7 (C)	Yes	Yes	13	15%	Yes
Herzig et al[9]	13	75%	1.7 (F) 0.4 (C)	No	Yes	14	36%	Yes
Alavi et al[10]	12	82%	5.9 (F)	No	No	19	62%	Partial
Graw et al[11]	39	46%	2.0 (F) 0.6 (C)	No	Yes	37	30%	Partial
Winston et al[12]	48	63%	0.5 (C)	No	No	47	72%	No
Fortuny et al[13]	17	78%	0.4 (C)	No	Yes	22	80%	No

*Donor-recipient compatibility was enhanced by HLA matching or white blood cell crossmatch.
F = filtration leukapheresis; C = centrifugation leukapheresis.

mately one-tenth the number of PMNs that currently can be transfused (5-7 × 10^{10}), and it is not surprising that granulocyte transfusions were unsuccessful when given in such a grossly inadequate fashion. As another factor, investigators in one of the two negative studies[12] made no provisions for the possibility of leukocyte alloimmunization, and they selected donors without attempting to improve leukocyte compatibility. Finally, the control subjects responded reasonably well to antibiotics alone in both of the negative studies,[12,13] making it difficult to demonstrate a statistically significant advantage for the addition of granulocyte transfusions.

The preceding analysis is qualitative and suffers from the imprecision of combining data from studies that, although controlled, were not truly comparable (ie, that were not uniform in such factors as patient's clinical status, the selection of control subjects, granulocyte transfusion dose, compatibility etc). In 1996, data from the seven controlled granulocyte transfusion trials were analyzed quantitatively by formal meta-analysis,[14] and many of the impressions of the preceding qualitative analysis were confirmed—specifically, that the dose of PMNs transfused and the survival rates of nontransfused control subjects were primarily responsible for the differing success rates of the reported studies. In clinical settings in which the survival rate of nontransfused control subjects was low, study subjects were found to have benefited from adequate doses of granulocytes. On the basis of the results of the meta-analysis, the authors concluded that severely neutropenic patients with infection known to carry a high mortality rate be considered for granulocyte transfusions given in an adequate dose.[14]

Therapeutic Granulocyte Transfusions in Specific Clinical Settings

Bacterial Sepsis

Bacterial sepsis was the most common infection for which granulocyte transfusions were prescribed in the 34 studies described above (Table 5-1). Most neutropenic patients with bacterial sepsis, who experience marrow recovery during the early days of infection, will respond to antibiotics alone.[3,6] Most patients with newly diagnosed acute leukemia experience successful induction chemotherapy and will fit into this category of relatively brief severe neutropenia without a need for granulocyte transfusions. In contrast, patients with persistent neutropenia due to continuing marrow failure may develop sepsis and benefit from granulocyte transfusions added to antibiotic therapy.[3] Examples are patients with relatively high-risk leukemia (eg, those who are elderly at the initial diagnosis or those with relapsed leukemia who are undergoing investigational chemotherapy) and recipients of hematopoietic progenitor cell grafts in whom hematopoietic recovery sometimes may be delayed for at least 2-3 weeks.

Yeast and Fungal Infections

Currently, yeast and fungal infections pose difficult problems. Occasional case reports, experimental studies in animals, and experience in treating patients with chronic granulomatous disease[15,16] support the success of granulocyte transfusions in some patients with yeast and fungal infections. In addition, an uncontrolled study of 15 patients[17] documented a 60% favorable response when granulocytes collected from donors stimulated with G-CSF were given to neutropenic patients with fungal infections—a rate of success higher than expected per usual clinical experience. In contrast, a large clinical study[18] comparing infected marrow transplant patients given granulocyte transfusions (n = 50) with those treated without granulocyte transfusions (n = 37) found no benefit for granulocyte transfusions in treating fungal and yeast infections. This last study, a retrospective review, was not designed to provide definitive answers.[18] Patients were not randomly selected for therapy; instead, the decision to use granulocyte transfusions was determined per individual physician preferences, making it impossible to exclude selection bias. Clinical heterogeneity was not balanced as neither patient's characteristics nor the types of infections being treated were distributed evenly between the granulocyte transfusion and no-granulocyte transfusion arms of the study. The dose of PMNs transfused was known for only 15% of the administered transfusions and likely was quite low because of suboptimal collection techniques. Thus, granulocyte transfusion therapy is promising but not proved for yeast and fungal infections in neutropenic patients.

Neonatal Infections

Neonates (infants within the first month of life) may suffer life-threatening bacterial infections related, at least in part, to neutropenia and PMN dysfunction.[19,20] Neutropenia must be viewed differently in neonates than in older patients, in whom granulocyte transfusions are usually considered when the blood PMN count falls to below 0.5 $\times 10^9$/L. In contrast, absolute blood PMN counts falling to only 3.0 $\times 10^9$/L in neonates might prompt consideration for granulocyte transfusions. The blood neutrophil count varies greatly during the first days of life, and a transient neutrophilia with absolute PMN counts of 10-25 $\times 10^9$/L is commonly seen in healthy neonates. Sepsis should be suspected in any sick neonate with an absolute PMN count of less than 3.0×10^9/L during the first week of life. The mechanism of neutropenia cannot always be identified, but in some infants a marked decrease in the marrow PMN storage pool can be demonstrated.[19,20] For example, metamyelocytes and segmented PMNs account for 26-65% of all nucleated cells in normal marrow, but in some neonates with sepsis, they will account for less than 10% of nucleated marrow cells.

Several investigators have reported the use of granulocyte transfusions to treat neonatal sepsis.[21] Of the six controlled studies,[22-27] four[22-25] demonstrated a significant benefit from granulocyte transfusions (Table 5-3). However, these studies can be criticized for their small size and faulty design, and for the heterogeneity of both the patients and the quality of granulocyte transfusions. Thus, the use of granulocyte transfusions for neonatal sepsis remains controversial, and many neonatologists prefer alternative therapies such as intravenous immunoglobulin (IVIG). Although this use is debated, some rationale exists for prescribing physiologic doses of IVIG to neonates with a birth weight below 1.5 kg because these infants are born before the bulk of maternal IgG is transported across the placenta and often are hypogammaglobulinemic. Most prophylactic studies evaluating the use of IVIG to prevent infections have found little or only modest benefit,[19] with a few studies suggesting efficacy.[28-30] In contrast, several therapeutic studies reported benefit for adding IVIG to antibiotics during the treatment of neonatal infections.[19] However, the data are inconsistent and insufficient to justify the routine use of IVIG as standard therapy to prevent and/or treat infections in preterm infants. Moreover, caution is warranted because, at high doses, IVIG has been demonstrated to impair body defense mechanisms and to increase susceptibility to fatal infections.[31-33]

Recombinant cytokines offer another alternative to granulocyte transfusions for neonatal sepsis. In neonates, studies of cytokine production have yielded conflicting results, with investigators finding values reported that are higher than, equal to, or lower than adult values. Generally, G-CSF and GM-CSF levels are lower in preterm than in term neonates, and the ability of preterm leukocytes to increase production further when stimulated is diminished. Some investigators found plasma G-CSF levels to be markedly elevated in neonates with infection,[34-36] but others found G-CSF messenger

Table 5-3. Six Controlled Trials of Granulocyte Transfusions for Neonatal Infections

Reference	Randomized	Neonates Transfused	Survival (%)	Neonates Not Transfused	Survival (%)
Laurenti et al[22]	No	20	90*	18	28
Christensen et al[23]	Yes	7	100*	9	11
	No†	–	–	10	100
Cairo et al[24]	Yes	13	100*	10	60
Cairo et al[25]	Yes‡	21	95*	14	64
Baley et al[26]	Yes	12	58	13	69
Wheeler et al[27]	Yes	4	50	5	40
	No†	–	–	11	91

*Survival rate of transfused infants was significantly better than that of nontransfused infants.

†Nontransfused infants were not randomized because all had adequate marrow storage pools.

‡Expanded version of study reported earlier by Cairo et al.[24]

RNA expression and protein production to be decreased in neonatal leukocytes, particularly in activated cells.[37,38] In a randomized controlled study,[39] 42 neonates with presumed bacterial sepsis received three doses of either G-CSF or placebo. Therapy with G-CSF significantly increased the marrow PMN storage pool, blood PMN counts, and expression of PMN membrane C3bi. In a similar randomized study of GM-CSF,[40] 20 preterm neonates within 72 hours of birth received either GM-CSF or placebo for 7 days; GM-CSF increased marrow PMNs, blood PMNs, and C3bi receptor expression. However, the efficacy of these agents to diminish infections and the potential for adverse effects have not been defined. Thus, as is the case for granulocyte transfusions and IVIG, the role of recombinant cytokines in the treatment of neonatal infections is unclear, and none can be recommended as standard or routine neonatal practice. Moreover, supportive care with antibiotics provides adequate therapy for most neonates. Thus, attention should be focused on prompt diagnosis of infection and optimal antibiotic therapy. If the outcome of standard supportive therapy is less than optimal, additional therapies such as granulocyte transfusions, IVIG, and recombinant cytokines must be explored.

Recommendations for Therapeutic Granulocyte Transfusion Practice

To determine the optimal role for therapeutic granulocyte transfusions, individual physicians must survey the outcome of life-threatening bacterial, yeast, and fungal infections in their own high-risk patients (eg, neonates and patients with severe neutropenia or PMN dysfunction disorders). If infections in these patients respond promptly to antibiotics alone (ie, if they result in acceptable morbidity) and survival approaches 100%, granulocyte transfusions are unnecessary and should not be used because the number of demonstrable benefits would not outweigh the potential risks. However, if significant numbers of infected high-risk patients fail to respond to antibiotics alone, the addition of granulocyte transfusions should be considered, along with other modifications of therapy (eg, selection of different antibiotics; closer monitoring of antibiotic blood levels; and administration of IVIG, G-CSF or other recombinant cytokines, and immune modulating agents). Once the decision to use therapeutic granulocyte transfusions has been made, the transfusions must be given effectively. Recommendations for PMN collection and transfusion are discussed later in this chapter.

Prophylactic Granulocyte Transfusions

Existing reports of 12 controlled trials (Table 5-4) indicate that prophylactic granulocyte transfusions historically were of marginal value[41-52] (also, Cooper MR, personal communication). Overall, benefits seemed few, while risks and expenses were substantial. However, some measure of success was found in seven of the 12 studies.[41-47] The remaining five studies failed to show a benefit for prophylactic granulocyte transfusions.[48-52] Yet, in none of these five negative studies were large numbers of PMNs obtained from matched donors and transfused daily (Table 5-4). Thus, in a situation analogous to that of the negative therapeutic granulocyte transfusion trials, the failure of prophylactic granulocyte transfusions might be explained, at least on the basis of clinical or qualitative analysis, by inadequate transfusion therapy.

In 1997, data from eight of the controlled prophylactic granulocyte transfusion trials were analyzed quantitatively by formal meta-analysis,[53] and many of the impressions of the preceding qualitative analysis were confirmed—specifically, that variability in the dose of PMNs transfused, inconsistent attempts to provide leukocyte-compatible granulocyte transfusions, and the varying duration of severe neutropenia were primarily responsible for the differing success rates in the reported studies. It was recommended that, in the design of future trials of prophylactic granulocyte transfusions, provision should be made to transfuse high doses of compatible PMNs.[53]

Clearly, prophylactic granulocyte transfusions cannot be recommended at this time as standard or

Table 5-4. Twelve Controlled Studies of Prophylactic Granulocyte Transfusions in Neutropenic Patients

| Reference | Dose $\times 10^{10}$ | Frequency | Matching | | Success |
			HLA	WBC	
Mannoni et al[41]	2.1	Daily	No	Yes	Yes
Gomez-Villagran et al[42]	1.2	Daily	No	Yes	Yes
Clift et al[43]	1.5 - 2.2	Dally	Yes	Yes	Yes
Strauss et al[44]	0.7	Daily	No	No	Partial
Hester et al[45]	1.6	Daily	Yes	No	Partial
Buckner et al[46]	NR	Daily	Yes	No	Partial
Curtis et al[47]	0.07	NR	Yes	No	Partial
Schiffer et al[48]	1.2	Alternate Days	No	No	No
Sutton et al[49]	0.9	Daily	No	No	No
Ford et al[50]	1.5	Alternate Days	No	No	No
Cooper et al[51]	2.6	Twice Weekly	Yes	Yes	No
Winston et al[52]	1.2	Daily	No	No	No

WBC = white blood cell; NR = not reported.

routine therapy for severely neutropenic patients. However, consideration should be given to the critical investigation of prophylactic granulocyte transfusions, particularly in marrow transplant patients. Progressive infections with yeast and fungus occur often in marrow transplant recipients because these patients are severely neutropenic for 1-3 weeks, exhibit PMN dysfunction for several weeks, and manifest defective cellular and humoral immunity for months following transplantation. Altered immunity is particularly profound, and infections pose a major threat when T lymphocytes in the marrow are depleted to diminish graft-vs-host disease. In one study of such patients,[54] 10% of 1186 marrow transplant patients developed a noncandidal fungal infection, with only 17% of the infected patients surviving.

Marrow transplantation is undergoing marked technological changes with both autologous and allogeneic transplantation being supplanted by transfusion of PBPCs collected following cytokine (usually G-CSF) stimulation. This technique is used increasingly because it is convenient and economical, and, most important, because it leads to relatively rapid engraftment.[55-57] Recovery to a blood PMN count of at least 0.5 $\times 10^9$/L occurs within 7-14 days after transfusion of PBPCs. In some patients, the period of severe neutropenia ($<0.1 \times 10^9$/L) persists only a few days, particularly when G-CSF is given to the patients following myeloablation. In the future, donors of PBPCs may be stimulated with recombinant cytokines other than G-CSF alone, such as stem cell factor[58] or interleukin-7,[59] and the period of severe neutropenia may be shortened even more by transfusion of PBPCs collected under these conditions. Thus, the complete elimination of severe neutropenia using this transplantation-plus-prophylactic-granulocyte transfusion approach is a distinct possibility that deserves careful study. However, as a cautionary note, its elimination during the first few days after transplantation may not be sufficient to improve early mortality rates. This is because many other factors not directly related to neutropenia may lead to patient's deaths. In a study of 2276 marrow transplant patients, mortality was no different when patients with blood PMNs below $100/\mu L$ at days 10-14 after transplantation were compared to patients with blood PMNs equal to or greater than $100/\mu L$ at the same point in time.[60] This was confirmed in another report of 712 marrow recipients when blood leukocyte counts were studied beginning on day 2 after transplantation.[61] Severe neutropenia persisting beyond 12-14 days after transplantation was related to mortality, and, eventually, granulocyte transfusions and recombinant cytokines may prove to be more useful at later times after transplantation than for early intervention.

Allogeneic PBPC donors receive G-CSF daily for 4-7 days and undergo leukapheresis to collect sufficient progenitor cells for transplantation/transfusion, which is usually performed on days 5-7. Donor blood PMN counts increase—often to more than $50 \times 10^9/L$—with G-CSF stimulation, and extraordinarily large doses of PMNs for granulocyte transfusions can be collected on the days following progenitor cell leukapheresis. Alternatively, marrow can be collected in the conventional way, with G-CSF administration and PMN collections beginning after marrow transplantation.[57] Obviously, systematic studies are needed to define the optimal G-CSF dose and schedule; the proper timing of leukapheresis procedures, first to collect PBPCs for transplantation and then to collect PMNs for granulocyte transfusions; the coordination of myeloablation, marrow, or PBPC collection, storage, and transplantation with subsequent PMN collection and transfusion; and the potential risks and inconveniences to the donor of prolonged G-CSF stimulation and multiple collection procedures. Preliminary studies have been reported to establish the feasibility and develop methods.[57] However, the efficacy of prophylactic granulocyte transfusions used as part of this approach—PBPC transplantation followed by PMN transfusion—vs PBPC transplantation followed by cytokine therapy of the patient without granulocyte transfusions must be investigated by properly designed randomized trials.

Collection and Transfusion of Neutrophil Concentrates

Donor Stimulation

A major limitation of granulocyte transfusion efficacy has been the inability to transfuse satisfactory numbers of adequately functioning PMNs. To ensure an adequate number and quality of PMNs, granulocyte concentrates must be collected from stimulated donors by leukapheresis (automated cell separators) using an erythrocyte-sedimenting agent such as hydroxyethyl starch.[62] The bloodstream of an average-sized adult contains $2\text{-}4 \times 10^{10}$ PMNs. Under steady-state conditions, about 6×10^{10} PMNs are produced daily, but with the stress of a severe bacterial infection, the marrow of an otherwise healthy adult will produce between 10^{11} and 10^{12} PMNs in 24 hours. Granulocyte concentrates collected from healthy donors who are not stimulated with corticosteroids or G-CSF will contain between 0.2 and 0.8×10^{10} PMNs—about 1% of a healthy marrow's output under the stress of infection. Because donor PMNs are collected with about 40-50% efficiency, it is unlikely that leukapheresis technology can be improved to a degree that will markedly increase PMN yields. Hence, donor stimulation is mandatory to achieve even the hope of a reasonable PMN dose per granulocyte transfusion.

Donor stimulation with properly timed corticosteroids (≥ 4 hours before leukapheresis) will increase the yield to about 2×10^{10} PMNs.[63] Stimulation with G-CSF alone or in combination with corticosteroids will produce higher but variable PMN yields, depending on the G-CSF dose and schedule of administration. Yields of $4\text{-}7 \times 10^{10}$ PMNs are achieved regularly, and posttransfusion blood PMN counts often increase to more than $1 \times 10^9/L$, with PMNs persisting in the recipient's bloodstream for more than 24 hours following the granulocyte transfusion.[57,64-66] For optimal donor stimulation, G-CSF is given subcutaneously at a dose of 300-600 μg (usually 5 μg/kg donor body weight) 12 hours before leukapheresis, with corticosteroids given orally as dexamethasone (8-12 mg) or prednisone (60 mg), according to a variety of schedules but usually approximately 12 hours before leukapheresis.[6,65,67]

Although G-CSF and corticosteroids are known to inhibit PMN functions, they have relatively minor effects at the doses administered to donors for PMN collection.[68] The functional properties of PMNs collected from donors stimulated with a single dose of G-CSF appear to be normal.[66,68] When these cells are transfused, they exhibit a prolonged intravascular survival.[57,69] This prolonged survival may relate to multiple factors, including a shift of an increased proportion of young cells from the marrow into the circulation, an alteration in expression of several membrane proteins associated with PMN adherence and egress from the circulation, and possibly specific antiapoptotic effects of G-CSF.[68,70] Some studies have suggested that G-CSF-mobilized PMNs exhibit decreased migration to tissue sites.[68] However, studies with indium-labeled cells indicate that they migrate satisfactorily to sites of inflammation and infection.[69]

The ability to collect and store PMNs may differ when donors are stimulated and used only once during a course of granulocyte transfusion therapy rather than stimulated and used repeatedly for collection. PMNs collected after several days of G-CSF stimulation are qualitatively different than PMNs collected after a single dose of G-CSF:[68] They are younger, exhibit increased metabolic activity and different surface marker expression, may have enhanced antifungal properties, and may not have the same separation characteristics and functions.[68] Because the functional properties and, possibly, the efficacy and toxicity of PMNs will differ when collected under conditions of single vs repeated G-CSF and corticosteroid stimulation, additional studies are needed to define optimal donor stimulation. Moreover, the relative efficacy of granulocyte transfusions collected from G-CSF plus corticosteroid-stimulated donors, compared with either therapy with antibiotics alone or antibiotics plus granulocytes collected from donors stimulated only with corticosteroids, has not been established by randomized trials. Only patients in uncontrolled or preliminary studies have been reported.[17,57,64,69,71]

Hydroxyethyl Starch

The optimal type of hydroxyethyl starch for PMN collection is controversial. In an uncontrolled multicenter trial, pentastarch appeared to be an efficacious and safe erythrocyte-sedimenting agent for use during centrifugation leukapheresis.[63] Its efficacy seemed established because PMN concentrates, prepared by a variety of centrifugation leukapheresis techniques in four cytapheresis centers, were found to contain quantities of leukocytes comparable to concentrates prepared previously (historical controls) at participating centers using hetastarch. Most concentrates contained at least 2×10^{10} PMNs, if collected by a continuous flow device (8 L of blood processed) from donors properly stimulated with steroids.

In 1995, the efficacy of pentastarch for PMN collection was challenged. In two studies,[72,73] the effects of pentastarch and hetastarch on the donors' erythrocyte sedimentation rates were compared, and pentastarch was thought to exert lesser effects on these rates than hetastarch. Consequently, pentastarch was predicted by a granulocyte collection efficiency equation to be less effective in enhancing PMN yields. This prediction was supported later by a controlled clinical trial[74] in which steroid-stimulated donors underwent paired PMN collections—separated by 2 weeks to 7 months—during which they received 500 mL of either 10% pentastarch or 6% hetastarch. Approximately 7 L of donor blood were processed at a 1:13 starch:donor blood ratio. In 92% of the donors, hetastarch procedures were more efficient. The PMN yield (mean ± SD) was $2.3 \pm 0.7 \times 10^{10}$ with hetastarch versus $1.4 \pm 0.076 \times 10^{10}$ with pentastarch.

It is unclear why pentastarch performed so poorly in these studies[72-74] when compared with performance results in the initial multicenter trial[63] and with data from the DeGowin Blood Center (Table 5-5). The pentastarch solutions studied by both centers appear to have similar biochemical properties, but true identity cannot be established. In particular, information about the C2/C6 hydroxyethylation ratio—a property that can influence erythrocyte sedimentation[75]—is not given in any report, and the possibility that different pentastarch solutions were studied by the different groups cannot be excluded. Until the issue is resolved, it is prudent for each center preparing granulocyte concentrates to perform continuing quality assessment of its leukapheresis program. The average PMN yield obtained by processing

10 L of donor blood following corticosteroid stimulation and using pentastarch at a 1:13 starch:donor blood ratio should be between 1.5 and 2.5×10^{10}; after G-CSF stimulation with or without corticosteroids, the PMN yield should be between 4 and 7 $\times 10^{10}$. If this is achieved, it seems reasonable to use pentastarch because of its more rapid elimination from the bloodstream and its lesser effects on coagulation.[76]

Transfusing Neutrophil Concentrates

Historically, a major criticism of granulocyte transfusion therapy has been the relatively small doses of PMNs available in granulocyte concentrates. Thus, the feasibility of stimulating normal donors with G-CSF and corticosteroids to obtain markedly greater numbers of PMNs for transfusion has renewed interest in this therapy both as a treatment for infections in neutropenic patients and as a means to diminish the risks of infection in a prophylactic setting. However, other medical advances—including the treatment of patients with G-CSF and other recombinant cytokines, the availability of more effective antimicrobial agents, and the use of PBPC transfusions—have reduced the likelihood of progressive and unresponsive infections in severely neutropenic patients. Thus, it is ironic that now, when more effective doses of PMNs could be transfused, their need can be questioned. Nonetheless, defining the appropriate role of granulocyte transfusions offers an exciting area for investigation and possible clinical application.

Until definitive information is available, the following plan is recommended for therapeutic granulocyte transfusion therapy.

- Consider granulocyte transfusions for severe bacterial, yeast, or fungal infections in neutropenic patients ($<0.5 \times 10^9$/L blood) when the infection progresses or fails to resolve despite optimal antibiotics. When tissue infections are being monitored roentgenographically, findings may be quite ambiguous and misleading, depending on the blood PMN count.[77]
- Collect PMNs ($4\text{-}7 \times 10^{10}$) from allogeneic blood donors as follows:

Table 5-5. Granulocyte Units at the DeGowin Blood Center, University of Iowa Hospitals and Clinics*

Yield $\times 10^{10}$	Prednisone (n=353)	Prednisone+ G-CSF (n=113)
Total leukocytes		
Mean ± SD	2.15 ± 1.15	7.04 ± 3.04
Median	1.97	7.05
Neutrophils		
Mean ± SD	1.53 ± 1.10	5.79 ± 2.70
Median	1.40	5.57

*Donors were stimulated with either prednisone alone (60-mg total dose given orally as 20 mg approximately 12, 10, and 4 hours before beginning leukapheresis) or prednisone (as described) plus granulocyte colony-stimulating factor (G-CSF) given subcutaneously as 300 μg approximately 12 hours before beginning leukapheresis. Each leukapheresis procedure is performed by continuous flow centrifugation, using hetastarch or pentastarch at a 1:13 starch:donor blood ratio, until 10 L of donor blood is processed.

1. Stimulate neutrophilia by giving the donor 300-600 µg G-CSF subcutaneously 12 hours before beginning leukapheresis plus corticosteroid either as 8-12 mg of dexamethasone orally 12 hours before leukapheresis or as 60 mg of oral prednisone taken as 20 mg approximately 12, 10, and 4 hours before beginning leukapheresis.
2. Process 10 L of donor blood using a continuous flow blood separator with citrated hydroxyethyl starch (hetastarch or pentastarch) solution infused throughout the entire collection at a starch:donor blood ratio of 1:13.

- Transfuse one PMN concentrate (4-7 × 10^{10} PMNs) daily until either the marrow recovers (blood PMNs 0.5 × 10^9/L without granulocyte transfusions) or the infection is clinically resolved. As a practical point, determining marrow recovery may be difficult. Transfused PMNs, when collected from G-CSF and corticosteroid-stimulated donors and given at doses of 4-7 × 10^{10} PMNs, may elevate the recipient's blood PMN count to 1-4 × 10^9/L for several hours after infusion. Thus, accurately distinguishing transfused PMNs from those produced endogenously during marrow recovery is challenging, and marrow recovery must be based on a sustained increase in blood PMN counts after granulocyte transfusions are discontinued.

Prophylactic granulocyte transfusions, although of great interest and potential benefit, must be considered investigational at this time. Too many questions pertaining to both efficacy and potential toxicity remain unanswered to recommend a plan of clinical practice at this time.

References

1. The Trial to Reduce Alloimmunization to Platelets Study Group. Leukocyte reduction and ultraviolet B irradiation of platelets to prevent alloimmunization and refractoriness to platelet transfusions. N Engl J Med 1997;337:1861-9.
2. Peters BG, Adkins DR, Harrison BR, et al. Antifungal effects of yeast-derived rhu-GM-CSF in patients receiving high-dose chemotherapy given with or without autologous stem cell transplantation: A retrospective analysis. Bone Marrow Transplant 1996;18:93-102.
3. Strauss RG. Therapeutic granulocyte transfusions in 1993. Blood 1993;81:1675-8.
4. Gabrilove J. The development of granulocyte colony-stimulating factor and its various clinical applications. Blood 1992;80:1382-7.
5. Anderlini P, Przepiorka D, Champlin R, Körbling M. Biologic and clinical effects of granulocyte colony-stimulating factor in normal individuals. Blood 1996;88:2819-25.
6. Strauss RG. Granulocyte transfusions. In: McLeod BC, Price TH, Drew MJ, eds. Apheresis: Principles and practice. Bethesda, MD: AABB Press, 1997:195-209.
7. Higby DJ, Yates JW, Henderson ES, Holland JF. Filtration leukapheresis for granulocytic transfusion therapy. N Engl J Med 1975;292:761-6.
8. Vogler WR, Winton EF. A controlled study of the efficacy of granulocyte transfusions in patients with neutropenia. Am J Med 1977;63:548-55.
9. Herzig RH, Herzig GP, Graw RG Jr, et al. Successful granulocyte transfusion therapy for gram-negative septicemia. N Engl J Med 1977;396:701-5.
10. Alavi JB, Root RK, Djerassi I, et al. A randomized clinical trial of granulocyte transfusions for infection in acute leukemia. N Engl J Med 1977;296:706-11.
11. Graw RG Jr, Herzig G, Perry S, Henderson IS. Normal granulocyte transfusion therapy. N Engl J Med 1972;287:367-76.
12. Winston DJ, Ho WG, Gale RP. Therapeutic granulocyte transfusions for documented infections: A controlled trial in 95 infectious granulocytopenic episodes. Ann Intern Med 1982;97:509-15.
13. Fortuny IE, Bloomfield CD, Hadlock DC, et al. Granulocyte transfusion: A controlled study in patients with acute non-lymphocytic leukemia. Transfusion 1975;15:548-58.

14. Vamvakas EC, Pineda AA. Meta-analysis of clinical studies of efficacy of granulocyte transfusions in the treatment of bacterial sepsis. J Clin Apheresis 1996;11:1-9.

15. Yomtovian R, Abramson J, Quie P, McCullough J. Granulocyte transfusion therapy in chronic granulomatous disease; report of a patient and review of the literature. Transfusion 1981;21:739-44.

16. Buescher ES, Gallin JI. Leukocyte transfusion in chronic granulomatous disease; persistence of transfused leukocytes in sputum. N Engl J Med 1982;307:800-4.

17. Hester JP, Dignani MC, Anaisse EJ, et al. Collection and transfusion of granulocyte concentrates from donors primed with granulocyte stimulating factor and response of myelosuppressed patients with established infection. J Clin Apheresis 1995;10:188-93.

18. Bhatia S, McCullough JJ, Perry EH, et al. Granulocyte transfusions: Efficacy in fungal infections in neutropenic patients following bone marrow transplantation. Transfusion 1994; 34:226-31.

19. Strauss RG. Granulopoiesis and neutrophil function in the neonate. In: Stockman JA, Pochedly C, eds. Developmental and neonatal hematology. New York: Raven Press, 1988; 88-98.

20. Rosenthal J, Cairo MS. Neonatal myelopoiesis and immunomodulation of host defenses. In: Petz LD, Swisher SN, Kleinman S, et al, eds. Clinical practice of transfusion medicine. 3rd ed. New York: Churchill Livingstone, 1996: 685-704.

21. Strauss RG. Current status of granulocyte transfusions to treat neonatal sepsis. J Clin Apheresis 1989;5:25-30.

22. Laurenti F, Ferro R, Isacchi G, et al. Polymorphonuclear leukocyte transfusion for the treatment for sepsis in the newborn infant. J Pediatr 1981;98:118-23.

23. Christensen RD, Rothstein G, Anstall HB, Bybee B. Granulocyte transfusions in neonates with bacterial infection, neutropenia, and depletion of mature marrow neutrophils. Pediatrics 1982;70:1-6.

24. Cairo MS, Rucker R, Bennetts GA, et al. Improved survival of newborns receiving leukocyte transfusions for sepsis. Pediatrics 1984; 74:887-92.

25. Cairo MS, Worcester C, Rucker R, et al. Role of circulating complement and polymorphonuclear leukocyte transfusion in treatment and outcome in critically ill neonates with sepsis. J Pediatr 1987;110:935-41.

26. Baley JE, Stork EK, Warkentin PI, Shurin SB. Buffy coat transfusions in neutropenic neonates with presumed sepsis: A prospective, randomized trial. Pediatrics 1987;80:712-20.

27. Wheeler JC, Chauvenet AR, Johnson CA, et al. Buffy coat transfusions in neonates with sepsis and neutrophil storage pool depletion. Pediatrics 1987;79:422-5.

28. Haque KN, Zaidi MH, Haque SK, et al. Intravenous immunoglobulin for prevention of sepsis in preterm and low birth weight infants. Pediatr Infect Dis 1986;5:622-7.

29. Chirico G, Rondini G, Plebani A, et al. Intravenous gammaglobulin therapy for prophylaxis of infection in high-risk neonates. J Pediatr 1987;110:437-40.

30. Conway S, Ng P, Howel D, et al. Prophylactic intravenous immunoglobulin in preterm infants: A controlled trial. Vox Sang 1990;59: 6-11.

31. Cross AS, Siegel G, Byrne WR, et al. Intravenous immune globulin impairs anti-bacterial defenses of a cyclophosphamide-treated host. Clin Exp Immunol 1989;76:159-63.

32. Weisman LE, Weisman E, Lorenzetti PM. High intravenous doses of human immune globulin suppress neonatal group B streptococcal immunity in rats. J Pediatr 1989;115: 445-9.

33. Cross AS, Alving BM, Sadoff JC, et al. Intravenous immune globulin: A cautionary note. Lancet 1984;1:912-3.

34. Bedford-Russell AR, Davies EG, McGuigan S, et al. Plasma granulocyte-colony stimulating

factor concentrations (G-CSF) in the early neonatal period. Br J Haematol 1994;86:642-6.

35. Gessler P, Kirchmann N, Kientsch-Engel R, et al. Serum concentrations of granulocyte colony-stimulating factor in healthy term and preterm neonates and in those with various diseases including bacterial infections. Blood 1993;82:3177-9.

36. Ohls RK, Li Y, Abdel-Mageed A, et al. Neutrophil pool sizes and granulocyte colony-stimulating factor production in human mid-trimester fetuses. Pediatr Res 1995;37:806-9.

37. Schibler KR, Liechty KW, White WL, Christensen RD. Production of granulocyte colony-stimulating factor in vitro by monocytes from preterm and term neonates. Blood 1993;82:2478-82.

38. Min Lee S, Knoppel E, van de Ven C, Cairo MS. Transcriptional rates of granulocyte-macrophage colony-stimulating factor genes in activated cord versus adult mononuclear cells: Alteration in cytokine expression may be secondary to posttranscriptional instability. Pediatr Res 1993;34:560-4.

39. Gillan ER, Christensen RD, Suen Y, et al. A randomized, placebo-controlled trial of recombinant human granulocyte colony-stimulating factor administration in newborn infants with presumed sepsis: Significant induction of peripheral and bone marrow neutrophilia. Blood 1994;94:1427-30.

40. Cairo MS, Christensen R, Sender LS, et al. Results of a phase I/II trial of recombinant human granulocyte-macrophage colony-stimulating factor in very low birthweight neonates: Significant induction of circulatory neutrophils, monocytes, platelets, and bone marrow neutrophils. Blood 1995;86:259-63.

41. Mannoni P, Rodet M, Vernant JP, et al. Efficiency of prophylactic granulocyte transfusions in preventing infections in acute leukemia. Blood Transfus Immunohaematol 1979;22:503-8.

42. Gomez-Villagran JL, Torres-Gomez A, Gomez-Garcia P, et al. A controlled trial of prophylactic granulocyte transfusions during induction chemotherapy for acute nonlymphoblastic leukemia. Cancer 1984;54:734-8.

43. Clift RA, Sanders JE, Thomas ED, et al. Granulocyte transfusions for the prevention of infection in patients receiving bone-marrow transplants. N Engl J Med 1978;298:1052-6.

44. Strauss RG, Connett JE, Gale RP, et al. A controlled trial of prophylactic granulocyte transfusions during initial induction chemotherapy for acute myelogenous leukemia. N Engl J Med 1981;305:597-603.

45. Hester JP, McCredie KB, Freireich EJ. Advances in supportive care: Blood component transfusions. In: Care of the child with cancer. Atlanta, GA: American Cancer Society, 1979:93-7.

46. Buckner CD, Clift RA, Thomas ED, et al. Early infections complications in allogenic marrow transplant recipients with acute leukemia: Effects of prophylactic measures. Infection 1983;11:243-7.

47. Curtis JE, Hasselback R, Bergsagel DE. Leukocyte transfusions for the prophylaxis and treatment of infections associated with granulocytopenia. Can Med Assoc J 1977;117:341-6.

48. Schiffer CA, Aisner J, Daly PA, et al. Alloimmunization following prophylactic granulocyte transfusion. Blood 1979;54:766-70.

49. Sutton DMC, Shumak KH, Baker MA. Prophylactic granulocyte transfusions in acute leukemia. Plasma Ther Transfus Technol 1982;3:45-52.

50. Ford JM, Cullen MH, Roberts MM, et al. Prophylactic granulocyte transfusions: Results of a randomized controlled trial in patients with acute myelogenous leukemia. Transfusion 1982;22:311-5.

51. Cooper MR, Heise E, Richards F, et al. A prospective study of histocompatible leukocyte and platelet transfusions during chemotherapeutic induction of acute myeloblastic leukemia. In: Goldman JM, Lowenthal RM, eds. Leukocytes: Separation, collection and transfusion. San Diego: Academic Press, 1981:436-9.

52. Winston DJ, Ho WG, Young LS, Gale RP. Prophylactic granulocyte transfusions during hu-

man bone marrow transplantation. Am J Med 1982;68:893-900.

53. Vamvakas EC, Pineda AA. Determinants of the efficacy of prophylactic granulocyte transfusions: A meta-analysis. J Clin Apheresis 1997; 12:74-81.

54. Pirsch JD, Maki DG. Infectious complications in adults with bone marrow transplantation and T-cell depletion of donor marrow. Ann Intern Med 1986;104:619-24.

55. Urbano-Ispizua A, Salano C, Brunets S, et al. Allogeneic peripheral blood progenitor cell transplantation: Analysis of short-term engraftment and acute GVHD incidence in 33 cases. Bone Marrow Transplant 1996;18:35-40.

56. Schwella N, Siegert W, Beyer J, et al. Autografting with blood progenitor cells: Predictive value of preapheresis blood cell counts on progenitor cell harvest and correlation of the reinfused cell dose with hematopoietic reconstitution. Ann Hematol 1995;71:227-34.

57. Adkins D, Spitzer G, Johnson M, et al. Transfusions of granulocyte-colony-stimulating factor-mobilized granulocyte components to allogeneic transplant recipients: Analysis of kinetics and factors determining posttransfusion neutrophil and platelet counts. Transfusion 1997;37:737-48.

58. Broudy VC. Stem cell factor and hematopoiesis. Blood 1997;90:1345-64.

59. Grzegorzewski KJ, Komschlies KL, Franco JL, et al. Quantitative and cell-cycle differences in progenitor cells mobilized by recombinant human interleukin-7 and recombinant human granulocyte colony-stimulating factor. Blood 1996;88:4139-48.

60. Offner F, Schoch G, Fisher LD, et al. Mortality hazard functions as related to neutropenia at different times after marrow transplantation. Blood 1996;88:4058-62.

61. Mehta J, Powles R, Horton C, et al. Leukocyte recovery and early treatment-related mortality after bone marrow transplantation (letter). Blood 1997;89:4237-8.

62. Strauss RG, Rohert PA, Randels MJ, Winegarden D. Granulocyte collection. J Clin Apheresis 1991;6:241-5.

63. Strauss RG, Hester JP, Vogler WR, et al. A multi-center trial to document the efficacy and safety of a rapidly excreted analogue of hydroxyethyl starch for leukapheresis; with a note on steroid stimulation. Transfusion 1986; 26:258-62.

64. Bensinger WI, Price TH, Dale DC, et al. The effects of daily recombinant human granulocyte colony stimulating factor administration on normal granulocyte donors undergoing leukapheresis. Blood 1993;81:1883-8.

65. Liles WC, Huang JE, Llewellyn C, et al. A comparative trial of granulocyte colony-stimulating factor and dexamethasone, separately and in combination, for the mobilization of neutrophils in the peripheral blood of normal volunteers. Transfusion 1997;37: 182-8.

66. Caspar CB, Seger RA, Burger J, Gmur J. Effective stimulation of donors of granulocyte transfusions with recombinant methionyl granulocyte colony-stimulating factor. Blood 1993;81:2866-71.

67. Leitman SF, Oblitas JM. Optimization of granulocytapheresis mobilization regimens using granulocyte colony-stimulating factor (G-CSF) and dexamethasone (Dexa) (abstract). Transfusion 1997;37:67S.

68. Price TH, Chatta GS, Dale DC. Effect of recombinant granulocyte colony-stimulating factor on neutrophil kinetics in normal young and elderly humans. Blood 1996;88:335-40.

69. Adkins D, Goodgold H, Hendershott L, et al. Indium-labeled white blood cells apheresed from donors receiving G-CSF localize to sites of inflammation when infused into allogeneic bone marrow transplant recipients. Bone Marrow Transplant 1997;19:809-14.

70. Kerst JM, de Haas M, van der Schoot CE, et al. Recombinant granulocyte colony-stimulating factor administration to healthy volunteers: Induction of immunophenotypically and functionally altered neutrophils via

an effect on myeloid progenitor cells. Blood 1993;82:3265-72.

71. Bowdon R, Price T, Boeckh M, et al. Phase I/II study of granulocyte transfusions from G-CSF-stimulated unrelated donors for treatment of infections in neutropenic blood and marrow transplant (BMT) patients (abstract). Blood 1997;90(Suppl 1):435a.

72. Lee JH, Cullis H, Leitman SF, Klein HG. Efficacy of pentastarch in granulocyte collection by centrifugal leukapheresis. J Clin Apheresis 1995;10:198-202.

73. Lee JH, Klein HG. The effect of donor red cell sedimentation rate on efficiency of granulocyte collection by centrifugal leukapheresis. Transfusion 1995;35:384-8.

74. Lee JH, Leitman SF, Klein HG. A controlled comparison of the efficacy of hetastarch and pentastarch in granulocyte collections by centrifugal leukapheresis. Blood 1995;86:4662-6.

75. Treib J, Haass A, Pindur G, et al. HES 200/0.5 is not HES 200/0.5: Influence of the C2/C6 hydroxyethylation ratio of hemorheology, coagulation and elimination kinetics. Thromb Haemost 1995;74:1452-6.

76. Strauss RG. Volume replacement and coagulation: A comparative review. J Cardiothorac Anesth 1988;2(Suppl 1):24-32.

77. Pestalozzi BC, Krestin GP, Schanz U, et al. Hepatic lesions of chronic disseminated candidiasis may become invisible during neutropenia. Blood 1997;90:3858-64.

In: Mintz PD, ed.
Transfusion Therapy: Clinical Principles and Practice
Bethesda, MD: AABB Press, 1999

6

Treatment of Congenital Coagulopathies

JEANNE M. LUSHER, MD

 MANAGEMENT OF THE CONGENItal coagulopathies, particularly hemophilia A, hemophilia B, and von Willebrand disease (vWD), has changed considerably in recent years. The availability of hepatitis A and B vaccines and of safer products (virus-attenuated plasma-derived clotting factor concentrates, recombinant products, and synthetic agents such as desmopressin acetate) has resulted in more aggressive treatment regimens as well as in prophylactic regimens aimed at the prevention of debilitating joint disease. For persons who develop inhibitor antibodies against Factor VIII, it is now common to use large daily doses of Factor VIII to induce immune tolerance. Cryoprecipitates, once regarded as the treatment of choice for persons with hemophilia A and vWD, are no longer recom-

mended for these disorders, being considered less safe than currently available clotting factor concentrates.[1]

In the United States as well as in several other countries, surveillance of persons with hemophilia for blood-borne viral infections has been ongoing for over a decade. There have been no new cases of human immunodeficiency virus (HIV) infection attributable to clotting factor in North America since 1987, and documented instances of the transmission of hepatitis by clotting factor have been quite rare in recent years.[2] While there is concern that certain nonenveloped viruses, such as human parvovirus B19 and hepatitis A virus, can still be transmitted by some plasma-derived clotting factor concentrates,[3] and questions as to whether the agent causing new variant Creutzfeldt-Jakob disease

Jeanne M. Lusher, MD, Marion I. Barnhart Hemostasis Research Professor, and Distinguished Professor of Pediatrics, Wayne State University School of Medicine and Co-Director, Division of Hematology/Oncology, Children's Hospital of Michigan, Detroit, Michigan

might be as well, the products available today are considerably safer than ever before. As a result, the experts on bleeding disorders are focusing on improving treatment regimens; the development of new, "second-generation" recombinant products, and the possibility of a cure for both hemophilia A and B through gene therapy.

A well-organized network of comprehensive hemophilia treatment centers in the United States provides diagnostic services; consultation; management by specialized, highly experienced teams of professionals; and patient education. The National Hemophilia Foundation (116 West 32nd Street, New York, NY 10001) provides a vast array of services, including educational materials, updated treatment recommendations, and scientific programs. Educational materials and other current information can be obtained by calling the foundation's toll free number, 1-800-42-HANDI.

Treatment of Hemophilia A and Hemophilia B

General Principles

Hemophilia A (Factor VIII deficiency) and hemophilia B (Factor IX deficiency) are both inherited as X-linked recessive traits and thus affect males almost exclusively. Because both disorders have the same clinical presentation (bleeding into joints, muscles, and other soft tissues), specific factor assays are the only way to differentiate between them. There are differing degrees of severity; as a general rule, however, all affected members of a kindred will have the same degree of severity. Severe hemophilia is defined as 0.01 U/mL or less of Factors VIII or IX; moderate hemophilia, as 0.01-0.05 U/mL; and mild hemophilia, as 0.05-0.30 U/mL. (It has been determined that 1.0 unit of Factors VIII or IX is the amount of Factor VIII or IX in one milliliter of pooled normal human plasma.) Approximately two-thirds of persons with hemophilia have severe disease, while approximately 15% have moderate disease and approximately 20% have mild disease. Individuals with severe hemophilia have more frequent bleeding episodes, which may be spontaneous or result from trivial injuries. Those with mild hemophilia generally bleed only following a significant injury, surgery, or invasive dentistry.

In approximately one-third of newly diagnosed infants or young children, there is no family history of hemophilia and the disorder has resulted from a spontaneous mutation in the Factor VIII or IX gene.[4-6] Thus, bleeding from head trauma, circumcision, or other invasive procedure at birth with no family history of bleeding disorders does not exclude the possibility of severe hemophilia. Neither Factor VIII nor IX cross the placenta; thus, a child who inherits the gene for hemophilia can bleed from head trauma during delivery or from circumcision or other trauma. Avoidance of vacuum suction or prolonged labor is recommended to prevent neonatal intracranial hemorrhage or large cephalhematoma.[7,8] If intracranial hemorrhage is suspected, appropriate replacement therapy (with clotting factor) should be given promptly, *before* imaging studies are performed.

Acute joint bleeding, intramuscular bleeding, or head injury in an infant, child, or adult with hemophilia should be treated *immediately.* The aim is to increase the patient's Factor VIII (or IX) level to a safe range to stop the bleeding. For severe bleeding episodes, the treatment should aim for a higher circulating Factor VIII (or IX) level (see Table 6-1).

Just prior to any surgical procedure, invasive dentistry, or lumbar puncture, the patient's Factor VIII (or IX) level should be increased to a safe range by an infusion of a Factor VIII or IX concentrate (or desmopressin acetate in the case of mild hemophilia A) (see the section on dosage.)

At the regional comprehensive hemophilia treatment centers, the education of patients and their families is of utmost importance; this includes an understanding of the disease, symptoms, signs of early hemorrhage, and their own treatment (product and dosage). Many patients are on home treatment, having been taught to self-infuse (or infuse their child), calculate dosage, maintain treatment logs, and call the hemophilia center for serious bleeding episodes or for bleeding that fails to respond to the usual treatment.

Table 6-1. Dosage Guidelines for Treatment of Bleeding in Severe and Moderately Severe Hemophilia A and B Without Inhibitors

Type of Bleeding	Desired Factor Level (%)	Factor VIII Dose* (Units/kg)	Factor IX Dose* (Units/kg)	Duration of Treatment (Days)	Ancillary Treatment[†]
Persistent or profuse epistaxis	20-30	10-15	20-30	1-2	Local pressure
Oral mucosal bleeding (including tongue, mouth lacerations)	20-30	10-15	20-30	1-2	Avoidance of trauma that would dislodge clot; antifibrinolytic agent for 7-10 days; nothing by mouth; sedation in small children with tongue laceration
Acute hemarthrosis	30-50	15-25	30-50	1-3	Non-weight-bearing on affected joint
Intramuscular hemorrhage	30-50	15-25	30-50	2-5	Non-weight-bearing
Iliopsoas or other retroperitoneal bleeding	30-50	15-25	30-50	3-10	Bed rest
Retropharyngeal bleeding	40-50	20-25	40-50	3-4	Antifibrinolytic agent for 7-10 days
Intracranial hemorrhage	80-100	40-50	80-100	10-14[‡§]	
Surgery	80-100	40-50	80-100	10-14[‡] (shorter duration for minor procedures)	
Gastrointestinal bleeding	30-50	15-25	30-50	2-3	Increased fluids, orally or intravenously (avoid antifibrinolytic agents!)
Persistent painless gross hematuria[‖]	30-50	15-25	30-50	1-2	

* After calculating dosage, give to nearest vial without discarding clotting factor.

[†] Approximately 25% of HIV-infected hemophiliacs have had some degree of thrombocytopenia. If severe, Zidovudine or other agents such as Intravenous Immune Globulin (IVIG) may be helpful in increasing the platelet count.

[‡] Continuous infusion is preferable to avoid dangerously low trough levels. Following a bolus dose, Factor VIII or Factor IX is given at a dose of 3-4 U/kg/hour, with subsequent dosing dependent on circulating plasma level.

[§] This should be followed with a 6-12-month period of prophylaxis when feasible to prevent recurrent intracranial hemorrhage.

[‖] Painless, spontaneous gross hematuria generally requires no treatment (other than increasing fluid intake to maintain renal output). If it persists for more than 3 or 4 days, however, treat with clotting factor.

Hemophilia A

Hemophilia A is considerably more common than hemophilia B, accounting for 80-85% of cases of hemophilia. Various products are licensed and available for the treatment or prevention of bleeding; these include plasma-derived Factor VIII concentrates of varying degrees of purity (as defined by the specific activity of Factor VIII in the final product, excluding albumin, which is added as a stabilizer), recombinant Factor VIII concentrates, and the synthetic agent desmopressin. (As noted earlier, cryoprecipitates are no longer recommended as they are considered to be less safe in terms of the potential transmission of blood-borne viruses.)

Plasma-Derived Factor VIII Concentrates

A listing of plasma-derived Factor VIII concentrates that are currently licensed and available in the United States appears in Table 6-2A. These concentrates are prepared from pooled plasma derived from large numbers of donors (often > 60,000). In addition to rigorous donor screening, these products are subjected to virus inactivation processes (pasteurization and/or solvent/detergent treatment), ultrafiltration, or immunoaffinity purification. However, even with these improved techniques, there is still a risk of the transmission of certain viruses, particularly the nonlipid enveloped viruses, hepatitis A virus and human parvovirus B19.[2,3,9-12] Also, despite lack of evidence that the agent causing Creutzfeldt-Jakob disease can be transmitted by plasma products, a large number of product withdrawals because of donors later identified as having Creutzfeldt-Jakob disease has been cause for concern. Nonetheless, the plasma-derived Factor VIII concentrates currently available in the United States are no doubt much safer than ever before.

These concentrates vary in their specific activity of Factor VIII (units per milligram of protein) (see Tables 6-2B and 6-2C). The so-called ultrapure concentrates listed in Table 6-2B have higher specific activity. Yet, there is very little evidence to support the claim that Factor VIII concentrates of higher specific activity are better than intermediate-purity Factor VIII concentrates. Some studies of HIV-infected patients showed a slower decline in CD4 cell counts in those using ultrapure Factor VIII concentrates than in those using intermediate-purity products; however, there is no evidence that use of the higher purified concentrates prolongs life.[13-15]

Recombinant Factor VIII Products

In view of concerns about the viral safety of plasma-derived concentrates in the 1970s and 1980s, there was considerable excitement surrounding the development of recombinant clotting factor concentrates (see Table 6-2A). The breakthrough for hemophilia A came when scientists at Genentech (Berkeley, CA) and Genetics Institute (Cambridge, MA) simultaneously announced the successful cloning of the Factor VIII gene and the expression of its product, human Factor VIII. These achievements were detailed in a series of articles that appeared in a single issue of the journal *Nature*, in 1984.[16-18] Purification and scale-up then occurred in a remarkably short period, and pre- licensure clinical trials in persons with hemophilia A began in 1987. Baxter's (Glendale, CA) recombinant Factor VIII, Recombinate, was licensed by the Food and Drug Administration in late 1992, and Bayer Corporation's (West Haven, CT) Kogenate was licensed in early 1993. These same products are also sold by Centeon (King of Prussia, PA) under different trade names (see Table 6-2A).

Because of the size and complexity of the Factor VIII gene and the complexities of expression of Factor VIII, mammalian cells must be used. Recombinant Factor VIII is produced in well-characterized hamster cell lines (Recombinate in Chinese hamster ovary [CHO] cells and Kogenate in baby hamster kidney cells).[19] In the production of Recombinate, the CHO cells are transfected with the gene for human von Willebrand factor (vWF) as well as the gene for human Factor VIII; however, vWF is removed in the purification process and does not appear in the final product.[19]

The currently licensed recombinant Factor VIII preparations contain pasteurized human serum al-

Table 6-2. Therapeutic Products for Hemophilia A That Are Licensed in the United States

*A. Recombinant Factor VIII Products**

Product Name	Manufacturer	Method of Virus Depletion or Inactivation	Specific Activity[†] (IU/mg protein) Final Product	Specific Activity[†] (IU/mg protein) Discounting Albumin	Hepatitis Safety Studies in Humans With this Product
Recombinate	Baxter	Immunoaffinity chromatography	1.65 - 19	> 3000	Yes
Kogenate	Bayer	Immunoaffinity chromatography	8 - 30	> 3000	Yes
Bioclate	Baxter (distributed by Centeon)	Immunoaffinity chromatography	1.65 - 19	> 3000	Yes
Helixate	Bayer (distributed by Centeon)	Immunoaffinity chromatography	8 - 30	> 3000	Yes

*Recombinant clotting factor preparations are referred to as "ultrapure."

[†]The degree of product purity is reflected by the specific activity of Factor VIII (units/milligram protein). Because most Factor VIII concentrates, including recombinant Factor VIII, have human serum albumin added as a stabilizer, most persons look at the specific activity discounting albumin. The specific activity is determined from in-process material prior to the addition of albumin.

(continued)

Table 6-2. Therapeutic Products for Hemophilia A That Are Licensed in the United States (continued)

B. *Immunoaffinity Purified (Very High Purity) Factor VIII Products Derived From Human Plasma* *

Product Name	Manufacturer	Method of Virus Depletion or Inactivation	Specific Activity[†] (IU/mg protein) Final Product	Specific Activity[†] (IU/mg protein) Discounting Albumin	Hepatitis Safety Studies in Humans With This Product	Hepatitis Safety Studies in Humans With Another Product, but Similar Virus Inactivation Method
Monoclate P	Centeon	1. Immunoaffinity chromatography 2. Pasteurization (60 C, 10 hours)	Approx. 5 - 10	> 3000	Yes	Yes
Hemofil M	Baxter	1. Immunoaffinity chromatography 2. Solvent/detergent (TNBP/Triton X-100) 3. Heat (25 C, ≥ 10 hours)	Approx. 2 - 11	> 3000	Yes	No
Monarc M	Manufactured by Baxter for American Red Cross from American Red Cross - collected plasma	1. Immunoaffinity chromatography 2. Solvent/detergent (TNBP/Triton X-100) 3. Heat (25 C, ≥ 10 hours)	Approx. 2 - 11	> 3000	No	Yes

TNBP = tri(N-butyl)phosphate

*Immunoaffinity purified products are referred to as "very high purity" or "ultrapure" products.

[†]The degree of product purity is reflected by the specific activity of Factor VIII (units/milligram protein). Because most Factor VIII concentrates, including recombinant Factor VIII, have human serum albumin added as a stabilizer, most persons look at the specific activity discounting albumin.

Table 6-2. Therapeutic Products for Hemophilia A That Are Licensed in the United States (continued)

C. Intermediate-Purity and High-Purity Factor VIII Products Derived From Human Plasma (Contain von Willebrand factor)

Product Name	Manufacturer	Method of Virus Depletion or Inactivation	Specific Activity* (IU/mg protein) Final Product	Specific Activity* (IU/mg protein) Discounting Albumin	Hepatitis Safety Studies in Humans with this Product	Hepatitis Safety Studies in Humans with Another Product, but Similar Virus Inactivation Method
Alphanate	Alpha Therapeutics	1. Immunoaffinity chromatography 2. Solvent/detergent: tri(N- butyl)phosphate [TNBP] and polysorbate 80 3. Heat (80 C, 72 hours)	Approx. 8 - 30	Corrected specific activity of 477	No	Yes
Koāte-HP	Bayer	Solvent/detergent (TNBP and polysorbate 80)	Approx. 9 - 22	50	No	Yes
Humate-P	Centeon Pharma (Marburg, Germany)	Pasteurization (60 C, 10 hours)	Approx. 1 - 2	—	Yes	No

*The degree of product purity is reflected by the specific activity of Factor VIII (units/milligram protein). Because most Factor VIII concentrates, including recombinant Factor VIII, have human serum albumin added as a stabilizer, most persons look at the specific activity discounting albumin.

bumin, which is used in the cell culture medium and is also added as a stabilizer. While pasteurized human serum albumin has an excellent track record of safety, recombinant Factor VIII preparations now in development will be truly albumin free. Two new, not yet licensed, recombinant Factor VIII preparations (Bayer's Kogenate SF and Genetics Institute's B-domainless recombinant Factor VIII, ReFacto) still use human serum albumin in the cell culture medium but do not add it as a stabilizer.

The design of so-called second-generation recombinant Factor VIII products is based on the current knowledge of Factor VIII structure and function. The full-length Factor VIII molecule consists of a light chain (containing domains A3, C1, and C2) and various heavy chain derivatives (containing domains A1, A2, and B). The heavily glycosylated B-domain appears to be dispensable for the hemostatic activity of Factor VIII.[20] B-domain-deleted Factor VIII has greater stability, is less prone to proteolytic degradation, and needs no albumin for stabilization. Produced by Pharmacia in Stockholm, Sweden, the B-domainless recombinant-VIII SQ, ReFacto, has been in prelicensure clinical trials since 1993. This product is essentially identical to plasma-derived Factor VIII in terms of structural and functional properties and vWF binding kinetics.[19-21] Lyophilized recombinant-VIII SQ is stabilized with sugars, amino acids, and polysorbate 80. It contains no vWF, and no albumin is added to the final product. To date, clinical trials data indicate that the product is effective, safe, and no more immunogenic than other Factor VIII preparations. It should be noted, however, that following the infusion of ReFacto, one-stage Factor VIII assays of patient samples give values that are about 50% less than chromogenic assay values.[19]

The main advantage of these recombinant Factor VIII preparations is viral safety. Overall, recombinant clotting factor concentrates appear to be the safest form of treatment. Recombinant technology also offers the promise of unlimited supply; however, at present, worldwide demands for recombinant Factor VIII far exceed supply. The main disadvantage of recombinant Factor VIII (as well as of other recombinant clotting factor concentrates) is

cost: these products are generally more costly than their plasma-derived alternatives. Although recombinant Factor VIII preparations have been used in humans for more than a decade without any unusual complications, as with any new technology, continued surveillance for any unexpected long-term complications is warranted.

Desmopressin (1-deamino-8-D-arginine vasopressin or DDAVP)

For persons with mild hemophilia A, as well as for carrier females who have very low levels of Factor VIII, desmopressin is the treatment of choice. This synthetic agent can be given parenterally or by intranasal spray (Table 6-3).[22-24] The drug effects a rapid release of vWF and Factor VIII from storage sites. (It is thus ineffective in severe hemophilia A, as there is no Factor VIII in body stores to be released.) The recommended IV dosage is 0.3 µg/kg body weight (maximum dose 20 µg); if necessary, doses can be repeated every 12-24 hours. However, many persons with mild hemophilia exhibit tachyphylaxis (diminishing response) when repeat doses are given at frequent intervals.[25] If this occurs and there is a clinical need for continued hemostatic levels of Factor VIII, one should switch to a Factor VIII concentrate.

With the recommended IV dose of desmopressin (0.3 µg/kg), recipients will have an average threefold (range 2-12 ×) increase over baseline Factor VIII levels. The degree of response is generally reproducible in individuals; that is, if a person has a fourfold increase in Factor VIII on one occasion, it is likely that he or she will again have a fourfold increase if given desmopressin some months later.[26]

Side effects of desmopressin are generally minor, being limited to facial flushing and a feeling of facial warmth. However, the drug is a potent antidiuretic agent, and there is a slight risk of hyponatremia and water intoxication with convulsions. This risk can generally be avoided by limiting fluid intake for 12-18 hours after administering desmopressin, by not giving hypotonic IV fluids postoperatively, and by monitoring fluids and electrolytes in postoperative patients. In view of an increased

Table 6-3. Desmopressin Formulations Useful in Mild Hemophilia A* and in von Willebrand Disease†

Product Name	Manufacturer	Distributed in US by	Formulation	Recommended Dosage and Administration
Desmopressin‡ (injection)	Ferring AB (Malmö, Sweden)	Rhône-Poulenc Rohrer	For parenteral (IV) or SQ use, 4 µg in a 10-mL vial or 15 µg in a 1-mL vial	1. 0.3 µg/kg mixed in 30 mL normal saline solution, infused slowly over 30 minutes intravenously 2. 0.4 µg/kg subcutaneously. May repeat after 24 hours.
Stimate (nasal spray)	Ferring AB	Centeon	Nasal spray, 1.5 mg/mL. The metered dose pump delivers 0.1 mL (150 µg) per actuation. The bottle contains 2.5 mL with spray pump capable of delivering 25 150-µg doses or 12 300-µg doses.	In patients weighing <50 kg, one spray in one nostril (delivers 150 µg). For those weighing >50 kg, give one spray in *each nostril* (total dose 300 µg). May repeat after 24 hours.

*Desmopressin will be useful in persons with mild hemophilia A (as well as in carrier females with low levels of Factor VIII) whenever it is judged that an approximate threefold (range 2-12 x) increase in Factor VIII will be sufficient to control or prevent bleeding.

†Desmopressin is the treatment of choice for persons with Type 1 von Willebrand disease. It *may* also be effective in some persons with Type 2A von Willebrand disease.

‡Caution: Desmopressin is a potent antidiuretic agent. Fluids should be restricted for 12-18 hours following administration to prevent hyponatremia and water intoxication (see text).

likelihood of fluid balance problems in the very young and the elderly, the drug should be used with caution in these extremes of age. Desmopressin is not recommended for children under 2 years of age. Also, in view of sporadic reports of coronary or cerebrovascular thrombosis in association with the use of IV desmopressin, it seems prudent to avoid the use of this drug in persons with known risk factors for such complications.[27]

Desmopressin can also be used intranasally.[22,24] For hemostatic purposes, the intranasal dose is 15 times larger than that recommended for diabetes insipidus. A multidose intranasal spray formulation (Stimate nasal spray, Ferring AB, Malmo, Sweden) includes a metered dose spray pump that delivers 150 μg per activation (spray) of the pump. The recommended dosage is one spray for patients weighing less than 50 kg and two sprays (one in each nostril) for those weighing more than 50 kg. This form is ideal for home and outpatient use both for the treatment of bleeding as well as for prophylaxis before invasive dentistry. As with the IV form of the drug, patients should be cautioned about the risks of fluid overload and advised to limit fluids for 12-18 hours after using Stimate nasal spray.

Dosage and Administration of Factor VIII Concentrates

The dose of Factor VIII to be given depends on the type and severity of the patient's bleeding and the desired circulating level of Factor VIII. For practical purposes of calculation, the dose is based on the knowledge that the infusion of 1 U/kg body weight will increase the patient's plasma level by 0.02 U/mL (2%). Thus, the Factor VIII dosage in units/per kilogram equals the desired percentage of Factor VIII increase, divided by two. For example, to raise the patient's Factor VIII level by 50%, the dose of Factor VIII would be 25 U/kg. Further bolus doses (if deemed necessary) are generally given based on Factor VIII's half-life of 8-12 hours. (For example, in the above-mentioned situation in which the patient's Factor VIII level was raised to 50%, to keep that level above 20%, repeat bolus doses should be given every 12 hours.)

Factor VIII can also be given by continuous infusion.[28-32] This mode of administration is often used in operative and postoperative situations, and for the treatment of central nervous system (CNS) hemorrhage or other very serious bleeding episodes such as compartment syndrome. Continuous infusion avoids the possibility of dangerously low trough levels and reduces the amount of clotting factor required to maintain a certain level (thereby permitting considerable economic savings).[28-32] This probably results from optimal saturation produced in most peripheral body compartments when clotting factor is given by continuous infusion. Continuous infusion of reconstituted (but not further diluted) Factor VIII concentrates can be done using a minipump. A small amount of heparin (1-5 U/mL) may be used to prevent thrombophlebitis.[32]

Prophylaxis vs Episodic Treatment

Episodic ("on demand") treatment for acute bleeding episodes has been the mainstay of management in the United States (and most other countries). In general, treatment with an appropriate dose of clotting factor should be given immediately in order to prevent continued bleeding into a joint, muscle, the CNS, or other hazardous area (eg, retropharyngeal). If an acute hemarthrosis is treated early, often one dose of clotting factor will suffice and less blood will accumulate in the joint space. A physician should never wait until severe joint pain and swelling have occurred! As noted earlier, if intracranial hemorrhage is suspected, treatment should be given immediately, *before* imaging studies or neurosurgery consultation are obtained.

The concept of routine *prophylactic administration* of clotting factor is aimed at preventing chronic, progressive, debilitating joint disease. If each episode of joint bleeding is not treated promptly, large amounts of blood accumulate within the joint space. The blood serves as an irritant to the synovial membrane, resulting in the proliferation of vascular synovial tissue into the joint space. When this occurs, even routine use of the joint can lead to synovial trauma, and a vicious cycle of rebleeding ensues into the so-called target joint. Ultimately there is greater synovial proliferation and thickening, and finally erosion of underlying cartilage and bone.[33] Because this process often begins in early childhood in persons with severe hemophilia and because it is often very difficult for the parents of young children to recognize joint bleeding, there has been considerable interest in beginning prophylaxis at 1-2 years of age. Prof. I.M. Nilsson and her colleagues in Sweden were the first to use prophylaxis in hemophilic children and now have more than 30 years' experience with it.[34-36] The aim is to prevent chronic, debilitating joint disease by giving Factor VIII concentrates every other day (or three times per week)—in essence, converting severe hemophilia to a milder form of the disease. In view of the excellent results with prophylaxis in Sweden, and with the availability of much safer clotting factor concentrates in recent years, others are recommending this approach. In early 1994, the US National Hemophilia Foundation's Medical and Scientific Advisory Council recommended that prophylaxis be considered optimal care for children with severe hemophilia A and B.[37] The recommended dosage of Factor VIII for prophylaxis is 25-40 U/kg body weight given every other day (or at least three times per week), and of Factor IX is 25-40 U/kg given twice weekly (in view of the longer half-life of Factor IX). Whenever feasible, such prophylaxis should be done by venipuncture. If one must use a central venous catheter, all possible complications, as well as the need for a surgical procedure to insert the catheter, education in the care and use of the line, etc, should be discussed with the child's family.[37] The main complication is line sepsis.[38-40] The rate of complications has been lower with ports than with external central venous catheters; thus, most clinicians now recommend a port if prophylaxis cannot be done by venipuncture. Starting with patients in early childhood, Swedish physicians have continued prophylaxis into young adult life, and most of their patients have excellent joint function and excellent orthopedic and radiographic scores.[34]

Prophylaxis can also be used in older children and adults (who were not on prophylaxis since early childhood) to prevent frequent rebleeding into a target joint. Generally, this type of prophylaxis is given daily or every other day, but only for a certain period of time (approximately 3 months).

Development of Inhibitor Antibodies in Hemophilia A

An inhibitor antibody should be suspected if a patient's bleeding fails to respond to an appropriate dose of clotting factor. The presence of an inhibitor can be documented by an inhibitor assay (see below); Factor VIII recovery and half-life will also be abnormally low. While previous surveys and estimates had indicated that 12-15% of persons with severe and moderately severe hemophilia A developed Factor VIII inhibitors,[41] more recent prospective studies have documented a much higher incidence. In a German study of a group of previously untreated patients with severe and moderate hemophilia A, each patient was followed with inhibitor assays after every 11 exposure days (defined as a day on which a patient received one or more doses of Factor VIII concentrate). Although various products were used, most received intermediate-purity, plasma-derived Factor VIII concentrates. In this cohort, 35% developed inhibitors; in those children with severe hemophilia, 51% developed inhibitors.[42]

In the prelicensure clinical trials with recombinant Factor VIII products (Bayer's Kogenate,[43] Baxter's Recombinate,[44] and Pharmacia's ReFacto,[45]) frequent prospective monitoring for inhibitors was done over an extended period. In clinical trials with each of these recombinant Factor VIII products, no new inhibitors developed in previously treated subjects; however, in studies of previously untreated patients, inhibitors developed in 25-32% of the patients after a median of 10-11 exposure days. Interestingly, in each of these trials, approximately one-third of the inhibitors were transient, disappearing within weeks or months despite continued on-demand treatment with recombinant Factor VIII.[43-45] From these (and other) prospective studies, it is clear that most inhibitors occur early in life, after relatively few exposures to Factor VIII, if one is carefully looking for them with frequent inhibitor assays. Among the nontransient inhibitors, genetic factors appear to play a role. Certain abnormalities in the Factor VIII gene, such as stop codons, frameshift mutations, and large deletions, are associated with a higher frequency of inhibitors. Additionally, in each of several studies, there was a higher percentage (about 50%) of inhibitors in African-American (or Black) children than in Caucasians.[43,44,46] There is also a familial predilection for inhibitor development; that is, if one hemophilic child has developed a high-titer inhibitor, his hemophilic brother is more likely to develop one as well. This is also true of affected grandsons—that is, if a hemophilic grandfather has developed a high-titer inhibitor, his hemophilic grandsons are more likely to develop a high-titer inhibitor.

While inhibitors can develop in later childhood, adolescence, or adult life, most develop relatively early in life, within the first 50 exposure days to Factor VIII (median 10-11 days).

Laboratory Detection and Measurement of Inhibitors

The recommended test for the detection and measurement of Factor VIII (and IX) inhibitors is the Bethesda assay.[47] This quantitative test is based on measurement of the amount of Factor VIII inactivated by patient plasma in an incubation mixture over 2 hours at 37 C. An inhibitor unit is called a Bethesda unit (BU), defined as the amount of inhibitor that would inactivate half the Factor VIII in the incubation mixture. Most inhibitors developing in hemophiliacs have simple, first-order reaction kinetics, and unitage in BUs can be read from a graph.[47,48] In general, a value of 0.6 BU or greater is considered positive.

In an attempt to separate true inhibitors from laboratory aberrations in the case of very-low-level inhibitor values (eg, those between 0.6 and 1.5 BU), a modification of the original Bethesda method has been recommended. In the so-called Nijmegen modification,[49] the system is buffered. According to several reports, many low-level inhibitors (as measured by the standard Bethesda assay) are negative by the Nijmegen method.

The Bethesda assay can also be modified to measure the degree to which the patient's inhibitor inactivates porcine Factor VIII, by using porcine Factor VIII as the source of Factor VIII. While there is species cross-reactivity in Factor VIII inhibitors, those developing in humans generally inactivate human Factor VIII to a greater extent than they inactivate porcine Factor VIII. Thus, porcine Factor VIII has often been effective in controlling bleeding in hemophilic patients whose inhibitor has little or no cross-reactivity with porcine Factor VIII.[50-53] Many hemophilia centers routinely monitor their inhibitor patients' antiporcine levels as well as their antihuman Factor VIII levels (in BUs) and thus know whether porcine Factor VIII is likely to be effective in the case of serious injury or for emergency surgery.

Management of the Patient With an Inhibitor

If a patient has a very low titer inhibitor (in the range of 0.6-3.0 BU), hemostasis may be achievable with (human) Factor VIII concentrates in the usual or slightly increased dosage.[53] Such low-titer inhibitors may disappear over time, may persist as low-titer inhibitors, or may increase to higher levels. In those patients with higher-titer inhibitors or in low-titer inhibitor patients who do not have an adequate clinical response to human Factor VIII concentrates, another approach must be used. For the treatment of bleeding, several alternative agents can be tried, including 1) prothrombin complex concentrates (PCCs), both "standard" and activated (APCCs); 2) porcine Factor VIII; and 3) recombinant Factor VIIa (Table 6-4). These products have proved to be life-saving in many patients with high-titer inhibitors; however, each has its limitations. Additionally, one can attempt to eradicate the inhibitor by using an immune tolerance induction (ITI) regimen.

Prothrombin complex concentrates. PCCs were first used to treat bleeding in inhibitor patients in the early 1970s.[54,55] It soon became apparent that, while often somewhat effective, PCCs

---

Table 6-4. Therapeutic Products for Use in Persons With Inhibitors

A. Products That May Be Useful in Controlling or Preventing Bleeding in Persons With Hemophilia A and Factor VIII Inhibitors*

1. Prothrombin Complex Concentrates (PCCs)
   - Konyne 80 (Bayer)
   - Proplex T (Baxter)
   - Profilnine SD (Alpha)
   - Bebulin VH (Baxter-Immuno)
2. Activated Prothrombin Complex Concentrates (APCCs)
   - Autoplex T (Nabi)
   - FEIBA VH (Baxter-Immuno)
3. Porcine Factor VIII
   - Hyate:C (Speywood)
4. Recombinant Factor VIIa
   - NovoSeven (Novo Nordisk)

B. Products That May Be Useful in Controlling or Preventing Bleeding in Persons With Hemophilia B and Factor IX Inhibitors*

1. PCCs (see above listing)
2. APCCs (see above listing)
3. Recombinant Factor VIIa[†]

---

*See text for dosage, dosage frequency, patient selection, and potential complications of products.

[†]In hemophilia B patients who have inhibitors to Factor IX and anaphylactic reactions to Factor IX-containing products, recombinant Factor VIIa is the treatment of choice.

---

were not nearly as effective as was Factor VIII in a noninhibitor patient. Soon thereafter, two purposely activated PCCs (APCCs) (Immuno's FEIBA and Baxter's Autoplex) were developed to be used only in inhibitor patients. These more costly products seemed to be somewhat more effective than standard PCCs; however, the APCCs are not predictably effective and are still less effective than is Factor VIII in a noninhibitor patient.[56-58] It also should be noted that there is no readily available laboratory test for monitoring the effectiveness of these so-called bypassing agents (PCCs and APCCs), and there is no general agreement concerning their mode of action.[41] Nonetheless, the PCCs and APCCs have been the mainstay of treatment for inhibitor patients for almost three decades, and many inhibitor patients are on home treatment with them.

The recommended dosage is 50-75 U/kg per dose. While the unit systems differ depending on the product (ie, with PCCs, the units used for calculation are Factor IX units; for FEIBA, the units are FEIBA units; for Autoplex, the units are Factor VIII correctional units), the calculation is the same for each. Depending on the product and the type and extent of bleeding, repeat doses are given at 8-, 12-, or 24-hour intervals. The use of large, repetitive (> 3) doses of PCCs for a bleeding episode should be avoided, as there have been approximately 20 published cases of acute myocardial infarction in young persons with inhibitors who were receiving PCCs.[59,60] Thus, inhibitor patients on home treatment with PCCs should be advised to call their physician before using a third or fourth dose for a joint or soft tissue hemorrhage.

Porcine Factor VIII concentrates. This product is manufactured by Speywood (Wrexham, UK) under the trade name Hyate:C. Used in the United States since the early 1980s, this product has an excellent record of viral safety. Patients who are likely to have a good therapeutic response to Hyate:C are those with little or no cross-reactivity to porcine Factor VIII as measured in the modified Bethesda assay. The recommended initial dosage is 100 Factor VIII U/kg body weight; subsequent dosing depends on the patient's circulating Factor VIII level. Often, a better therapeutic response is noted on the second day of treatment with Hyate:C. This product has proven to be quite effective in properly selected patients (again, those with low cross-reactivity to porcine Factor VIII).[50-53,61] It has been life- or limb-saving in inhibitor patients with traumatic intracranial hemorrhage or compartment syndrome and has often proven to be effective in maintaining hemostasis during and following surgical procedures.

Disadvantages include the product cost and the fact that it is a foreign species protein. Thus, there is a risk of allergic reactions, sometimes (although rarely) severe. Such reactions often can be prevented or minimized by infusing the product slowly. In addition, many (but certainly not all) patients will ultimately develop a high-titer inhibitor to porcine Factor VIII. While older porcine Factor VIII preparations, produced in the 1950s, often resulted in severe thrombocytopenia, this has been far less of a problem with Hyate:C (which contains very little porcine vWF).[62]

Recombinant Factor VIIa. This product, produced by Novo-Nordisk Pharmaceuticals (Gentofte, Denmark), is licensed in European countries and in Canada but not currently in the United States. This recombinant product is produced in Chinese hamster ovary cells; no human or animal proteins are used in its manufacture (nor are they added later).[19] Recombinant Factor VIIa (NovoSeven) was first used in 1988 in a high-titer inhibitor patient undergoing open synovectomy in

Sweden; hemostasis was judged excellent both intra- and postoperatively.[63] In subsequent years, recombinant Factor VIIa has been used in compassionate-use protocols in several countries[64-66] and in an open-label home treatment study in the United States.[67] The product appears to be safe and effective. Although some patients have responded to smaller doses, the recommended dose is 90 µg/kg body weight. Because of its very short half-life,[66,68] repeat doses (when necessary) should be given at 2- to 3-hour intervals. As with other therapeutic products used to stop bleeding, treatment with recombinant Factor VIIa is more likely to be effective when administered early, and with fewer doses of the product.[69]

While a shortening of the prothrombin time is usually seen following the infusion of recombinant Factor VIIa, there is no readily available laboratory test for monitoring the patient's response. (Factor VIIa assays can be done but are generally limited to highly specialized research laboratories). If given by continuous infusion, as postoperatively, one can monitor the patient's Factor VII level. A plasma level of ≥10 Factor VII U/mL is usually hemostatically effective. The main disadvantages of NovoSeven are its cost (where licensed and commercially available) and its short half-life.

Attempts to eradicate Factor VIII inhibitors: immune tolerance induction regimens. In the mid-1970s, Prof. H.H. Brackmann, in Bonn, Germany, developed an ITI regime, which came to be known as "the Bonn regimen."[70] This regimen was very intensive and costly, incorporating very large doses of Factor VIII given twice daily, plus FEIBA. While effective in eradicating inhibitors in many of Prof. Brackmann's patients, this regimen did not become popular elsewhere because of its cost and its rigorous demands on patients and physicians. It often took many months or years to accomplish its purpose. Additionally, by the early 1980s, many were worried about acquired immunodeficiency syndrome and were often decreasing treatment with clotting factor concentrates.

With the introduction of much safer, virus-attenuated plasma-derived concentrates and recombinant products, other groups began trying lesser modifications of the original Bonn protocol. Some groups found that 50 Factor VIII U/kg given once daily was often effective within a matter of months.[71] Others used even less, with some success.[72] ITI is now being used in many US hemophilia centers, with the knowledge that it is far preferable to get rid of the patient's inhibitor so that he or she can again be treated with the usual doses of Factor VIII for bleeding episodes (or for prophylaxis). While there is no generally agreed-upon "best" regimen, most clinicians use Factor VIII alone (ie, without corticosteroids or immunosuppressive drugs), either daily or twice weekly. Starting dosages vary from 50 to 200 Factor VIII U/kg per day, generally depending on the patient's historic maximum inhibitor titer. When the inhibitor titer becomes negative and Factor VIII recovery and modified half-life become normal or near-normal, doses of Factor VIII are decreased. There is an International Immune Tolerance Registry[73] as well as a North American ITI registry, and a German registry; these are aimed at collecting information that can be analyzed to determine predictors of success as well as the regimens most likely to be effective. Among patients with hemophilia A, 75-80% are reported to have had a good response.

Hemophilia B

While hemophilia B (Factor IX deficiency) is clinically indistinguishable from hemophilia A, there are some important differences in treatment, incidence of inhibitors,[74] and complications. Several types of Factor IX concentrates are licensed and available for the treatment and prevention of bleeding in persons with hemophilia B (Table 6-5). These include PCCs (Factor IX complex concentrates) and highly purified Factor IX concentrates (both plasma-derived and recombinant products). There is no synthetic agent that will rapidly increase Factor IX levels; that is, there is no equivalent of desmopressin for persons with mild hemophilia B. Factor IX is a much smaller molecule than Factor VIII, and it diffuses from the intravascular to extravascular space. Dosage calculations differ as well (see below and Table 6-1).

Therapeutic Products for Hemophilia B

Prothrombin complex concentrates. PCCs were first introduced in the United States in the late 1960s. These products contain not only Factor IX, but also Factors II, VII, and X; proteins C and S; and varying amounts of partially activated clotting factors. Soon after their introduction, thrombotic complications associated with their use began to be reported. Most, but not all, of these occurred in immobile postoperative patients or in patients with hepatocellular dysfunction.[75-79] Recommendations to add heparin to reconstituted PCC prior to use did not prevent this complication; however, precautions published in a number of reports no doubt resulted in the more judicious use of PCCs in certain high-risk situations.[50] Nonetheless, thrombotic complications continued to be reported.[59]

While PCCs are effective and reasonably safe in terms of virus transmission, their use should be avoided in certain situations. These include surgical situations (particularly orthopedic procedures), crush injuries, hepatic dysfunction, large intramuscular hemorrhages, in infants, and in persons with a history of thrombosis following the use of a PCC. In such cases, a high-purity, coagulation Factor IX concentrate is recommended.[50,80]

High-purity (coagulation) Factor IX concentrates. In the early 1990s, plasma-derived coagulation Factor IX concentrates became available in the United States.[50] These products contain Factor IX almost exclusively, and there have been no reports of thrombotic complications with their use. These high-purity Factor IX concentrates include Mononine (Centeon), Alpha Nine SD (Alpha Therapeutics, Los Angeles, CA), and Immunine (Immuno AG, Vienna, Austria).[81-83]

In February 1997, a recombinant Factor IX product (BeneFix, Genetics Institute, Cambridge, MA) was licensed for use in the United States. This product is produced in Chinese hamster ovary cells and contains no human or animal proteins.[19] Following the infusion of BeneFix, recovery is lower than is achieved with plasma-derived Factor IX. On average, 1 IU of BeneFix per kilogram of body weight increases the circulating Factor IX by 0.8

Table 6-5. Factor IX Concentrates for Use in Persons With Hemophilia B

Product Name	Manufacturer	Method of Virus Depletion or Inactivation	Specific Activity (IU/mg protein), Final Product	Hepatitis Safety Studies in Humans With This Product	Hepatitis Safety Studies in Humans With Another Product, but Similar Virus Inactivation Method
A. Factor IX Complex Concentrates Derived From Human Plasma					
Konȳne 80	Bayer	Dry heat (80 C, 72 hours)	Approx. 1.25	No	Yes
Proplex T	Baxter	Dry heat (68 C, 144 hours)	Approx. 3.9	No	No
Profilnine SD	Alpha Therapeutics	Solvent/detergent (TNBP and polysorbate 80)	Approx. 4.5	No	Yes
Bebulin VH	Immuno (Vienna, Austria) (distributed by Baxter-Immuno)	Vapor heat (10 hours, 60 C, 1190 mbar pressure plus 1 hour, 80 C, 1375 mbar)	Approx. 2	Yes	No
B. Coagulation Factor IX Products Derived From Human Plasma					
AlphaNine SD	Alpha Therapeutics	1. Dual-affinity chromatography 2. Solvent/detergent (TNBP and polysorbate 80) 3. Nanofiltration	Approx. 229 ± 23 (22)	Yes	Yes
Mononine	Centeon	1. Immunoaffinity chromatography 2. Sodium thiocyanate 3. Ultrafiltration	> 160	Yes	No
C. Recombinant Factor IX Products					
BeneFix	Genetics Institute	1. Affinity chromatography 2. Ultrafiltration	> 200	Yes	No

TNBP = tri(N-butyl)phosphate

IU/mL (rather than by 1.0 IU/mL; see below).[84] Individual variations should be noted, however, as some patients have lower and some have higher recovery values. Each patient's recovery following a test dose while not bleeding should be determined, as recovery values are fairly reproducible in individuals over time. (On average, children have lower recovery values than do adults.) Test results can then be used to calculate the patient's dose. BeneFix appears to be both effective and safe in patients with hemophilia B.

Dosage and administration of Factor IX concentrates. As is the case in hemophilia A, the dose of Factor IX to be given depends on the type and severity of the patient's bleeding and the desired Factor IX level (see Table 6-1). Dosage is based on the knowledge that the infusion of 1 U/kg body weight will increase the patient's plasma level by 0.01 U/mL (1%). Thus, if a circulating level of 0.50 U/mL (50%) is desired, the dose of Factor IX would be 50 U/kg. (As noted above, in the case of BeneFix, recovery is generally lower than it is with plasma-derived Factor IX concentrates). The half-life of Factor IX is longer than that of Factor VIII, being approximately 18 hours. Thus, repeat bolus doses (if necessary) are generally given once daily.

Factor IX can also be given by continuous infusion[85] with the use of a minipump. Continuous infusion is often used in intra- and postoperative patients or for CNS hemorrhage—situations in which dangerously low trough levels of Factor IX should be avoided.

Prophylaxis vs Episodic Treatment

The principles outlined for hemophilia A apply here, too. Episodic (on demand) treatment for acute bleeding episodes is the mainstay of treatment, and treatment should be given immediately for bleeding into joints, muscles, the CNS, or other hazardous areas.

Prophylaxis (as in young children to prevent chronic, debilitating joint disease) can be given less often in view of the longer half-life for Factor IX than for Factor VIII. The recommended dose is 25-50 Factor IX U/kg, given twice weekly.[37] As is the

case for hemophilia A, prophylaxis can also be used in older children and adults (who are not already on prophylaxis) to prevent frequent rebleeding into a target joint. Here, prophylaxis is generally given every other day for approximately 3 months.

Development of Inhibitor Antibodies in Hemophilia B

Inhibitor antibodies to Factor IX occur less often than they do to Factor VIII, being reported in 1-3% of persons with hemophilia B.[74] Most occur in persons with severe hemophilia B, and most (but not all) develop in childhood after relatively few exposures to Factor IX. As is the case for hemophilia A, genetic factors appear to play a role, with certain Factor IX gene defects (ie, large deletions) being associated with a higher rate of inhibitor formation.[74]

In roughly half of the hemophilia B patients with inhibitors, anaphylaxis (or severe allergic reactions) has occurred on the infusion of Factor IX.[86] (This does not occur with Factor VIII inhibitors.) In most of the reported cases of this association (anaphylaxis and inhibitor detection), these reactions have occurred early in life, after relatively few exposures to Factor IX. No one brand or type of Factor IX concentrate has been implicated. Rather, the severe allergic-type reactions occur in certain individuals with the infusion of any Factor IX-containing product. Unless the patient can be desensitized, the only appropriate treatment for bleeding episodes is Factor VIIa (NovoSeven).[86]

Management of Factor IX Inhibitors

As in the case of Factor VIII inhibitors, management can be divided into the treatment of bleeding episodes and attempts to eradicate the inhibitor. Therapeutic options for the treatment of bleeding are somewhat more limited than they are for Factor VIII inhibitors. That is, porcine Factor VIII cannot be used, nor can PCCs and APCCs in patients with severe allergic reactions to Factor IX-containing products.

PCCs and APCCs (FEIBA VH and Autoplex T) bypass the need for Factor IX as well as for Factor

VIII and are at least somewhat effective in controlling bleeding. The recommended dosage and administration are the same as they would be for Factor VIII inhibitors; 50-75 U/kg per dose, with repeat bolus doses given at 8-12 hours, if necessary (Table 6-4). The same cautions apply with PCCs here as they do with Factor VIII inhibitor patients: frequent repeated large doses should be avoided in view of reported cases of acute myocardial infarction.

Recombinant Factor VIIa (NovoSeven) has proved to be quite effective in preventing or controlling bleeding in hemophilia B patients with Factor IX inhibitors, just as it has been in patients with Factor VIII inhibitors. The recommended dosage is 90 μg/kg body weight, with repeat doses being given every 2-3 hours, as necessary (see the above section on its use in Factor VIII inhibitor patients). NovoSeven, which contains no Factor IX, is clearly the product of choice for hemophilia B patients with inhibitors who have severe allergic reactions to Factor IX-containing products.[86] However, NovoSeven is not yet licensed in the United States. It is, however, available on a compassionate-use basis for such patients.

Attempts to Eradicate Factor IX Inhibitors:
Immune Tolerance Induction Regimens

ITI regimens have not been as successful in suppressing or eradicating Factor IX inhibitors as they have Factor VIII inhibitors. In the North American ITI Registry, approximately 50% of patients have had a good response (vs 75-80% of those with hemophilia A and Factor VIII inhibitors). The response rate is even poorer in patients who have had severe allergic reactions to Factor IX, have been desensitized, and then started on an ITI regimen. Not only do few such patients have a good response, but also several have developed nephrotic syndrome approximately 8-9 months after starting ITI.[87]

von Willebrand Disease

vWD is by far the most common of the hereditary disorders of coagulation, affecting an estimated 1-2% of the population.[88,89] It is worldwide in distribution and affects all racial groups. This disorder was first described in 1926 by a Scandinavian physician, Dr. Erik von Willebrand of Helsinki, Finland. von Willebrand studied a large group of interrelated people living on one of the Åland Islands in the Gulf of Bothnia, many of whom had recurrent epistaxis, gum bleeding, and other types of mucous membrane bleeding. While the bleeding tendency affected both males and females, it was often more problematic in young women, many of whom had menorrhagia. Five young women had bled to death during menstrual periods, one during her first period. von Willebrand noted that affected individuals had normal numbers of platelets but had prolonged bleeding times.[90] For a number of years thereafter, the diagnosis of vWD was based on the finding of a prolonged bleeding time, normal platelet count, and an autosomal dominant inheritance pattern in a person with mucous membrane-type bleeding.

As our understanding of hemostasis advanced, so did our understanding of vWD. It is now known that the basic defect in vWD is in vWF, a large, multimeric plasma glycoprotein[91] that is synthesized in endothelial cells and in megakaryocytes. vWF has two major biologic functions. First, it is necessary for platelet adhesion to injury sites in the vessel wall, where rapid blood flow creates high wall shear forces. Second, it protects Factor VIII from rapid proteolytic degradation in the circulation by forming a complex with Factor VIII and thereby stabilizing it.

vWF circulates as a series of multimers of increasing size, the largest having a molecular weight of 20 million daltons.[92] Protomers of approximately 500,000 daltons make up the multimers, and each protomer is made up of two identical subunits of 220,000 daltons. The repeating structure is important, as it provides a large number of repeated binding sites, allowing vWF to serve as a bridge both between platelets and between platelets and vessel wall injury sites. The multimeric structure of vWF can be visualized after electrophoresis of plasma in agarose gels. Multimeric analysis is used to diagnose the variant forms of vWD that lack the high molecular-weight multimers. Because of their increased size and large number of binding sites, these multimers have greater functional activity and thus are the most effective multimers in hemostasis.

It is important to note that vWD is characterized by either a quantitative or a qualitative defect in vWF. If an individual lacks vWF, his or her platelets will not adhere to injury sites in the vessel wall, and bleeding will continue. Additionally, even though the person is able to synthesize normal amounts of Factor VIII, with no vWF to complex with (and protect) the Factor VIII, it will be rapidly destroyed in the circulation, resulting in a subnormal Factor VIII level.

In endothelial cells, vWF is stored in Weibel-Palade bodies; in platelets, it is stored in alpha granules, from which it is released when platelets undergo the release reaction. Platelets contain even larger vWF multimers than those seen in plasma. The release of these hemostatically important large multimers from platelets at the site of vessel wall injury is no doubt of hemostatic importance.

Normal vWF has two binding domains for Factor VIII and also has two platelet binding domains. In one of the variant forms of vWF, called the Normandy variant, the abnormal vWF produced does not bind Factor VIII. This results in very low levels of Factor VIII, considerably out of proportion to the decrease in vWF.[93] An erroneous diagnosis of hemophilia A may be made, unless the patient is a female or the inheritance pattern appears to be autosomal. In another interesting variant form, Type 2M vWD, there is an abnormal binding site for platelet glycoprotein 1B, which results in reduced ristocetin cofactor activity. vWF multimers are normal in Type 2M.[94]

vWD Types 1, 2, and 3

vWD Type I is the most common type, accounting for approximately 80% of persons with vWD. Affected individuals have subnormal levels of vWF, but the vWF they produce is structurally and functionally normal. Levels of vWF, vWF antigen, and Factor VIII will be proportionately decreased; for example, all three tests may be 30% of normal. On agarose gels, the multimeric structure of vWF is normal.

In contrast, in the Type 2 variants, which account for approximately 20% of cases of vWD, the affected individual produces a vWF that is structurally and functionally abnormal. Levels of vWF and vWF antigen may be either decreased or normal. The Type 2 variants are characterized by an absence of the largest multimers in plasma. In some of these variants, the multimeric structure of vWF is also abnormal in platelets. Among the Type 2 variants, the most common subtypes are 2A and 2B. In Type 2A (more common than 2B), only the smallest vWF multimers are identified on sodium dodecyl sulfate gels. This results in a marked reduction in ristocetin cofactor activity, with a lesser reduction in vWF antigen (vWF:Ag). Types 2A and 2B can easily be distinguished by performing platelet aggregation using varying concentrations of ristocetin. In Type 2A, platelet agglutination does not occur on the addition of standard amounts of ristocetin, whereas, in Type 2B, platelet agglutination occurs at very low concentrations of ristocetin, at concentrations too low to induce aggregation in normal individuals or in persons with Type 1 or Type 2A vWD (see Fig 6-1). This is because the abnormal multimers produced in vWD 2B have a heightened affinity for platelets.

In Type 3, which is rare but is the most severe form of vWD, vWF, vWF antigen, and Factor VIII are all extremely low, generally less than 3% of normal, and the bleeding time is quite prolonged. Affected individuals are either homozygous or doubly heterozygous, having inherited a gene for vWD from each parent. In addition to severe mucous membrane bleeding, affected individuals often bleed into joints and soft tissues.

The reason that it is important to determine the *type* of vWD a person has is that treatment differs depending on the type (see below). Recommended diagnostic tests and results are listed in Table 6-6.

A number of things can influence vWF levels in normal individuals as well as in persons with Types 1 and 2 vWD. One of these is the person's ABO blood group. Normal individuals who are blood

| Test | von Willebrand Variants | | | | | | |
	Type 1	Type 2A	Type 2B	PT-vWD	Type 2N	Type 2M	Type 3
vWF antigen	↓	↓	± ↓	± ↓	↓	↓	Absent
Ristocetin cofactor	↓	↓↓↓	± ↓	± ↓	↓	↓↓↓	Absent
Factor VIII	↓	Normal	Normal	Normal	↓↓	Normal	Absent
RIPA	± ↓	↓↓	Normal	Normal	Normal	↓	Absent
RIPA-LD	Absent	Absent	Increased	Increased	Absent	Absent	Absent
Frequency	70-80%	10-12%	3-5%	0-1%	1-2%	1-2%	1-3%
Multimeters:							

Figure 6-1. Summary of variants of von Willebrand disease. The abbreviations are ristocetin-induced platelet aggregation (RIPA) and platelet aggregation to low doses of ristocetin (RIPA-LD). The von Willebrand disease variants are types 1, 2A, 2B, 2N, and 3 and platelet-type von Willebrand disease (PT-vWD). The lower portion of the figure illustrates the multimeters of von Willebrand factor (vWF) that are identified by sodium dodecyl sulfate agarose gel electrophoresis of vWF for each of these variants. Used with permission from Montgomery RR.[96]

group O have lower levels of vWF than do those who are of blood group AB. Group O individuals have mean levels of vWF of 74.8%, whereas AB individuals have mean values of 123.3%.[95,96] Additionally, vWF behaves as an acute-phase reactant protein and is thus elevated in collagen vascular disorders, postoperatively, and whenever endothelial cells are stimulated, such as in disseminated intravascular coagulation. vWF is also elevated in hyperthyroidism, in the third trimester of pregnancy, and in stressful situations.

Treatment of vWD

vWD Type 1

In the most common form of vWD (Type 1), the treatment of choice is desmopressin. When given parenterally or intranasally, this synthetic agent effects a rapid release of vWF from its storage sites.[97]

In Type 1, what vWF the individual is able to produce is structurally and functionally normal. Thus when desmopressin is given, structurally and functionally normal vWF will be released from the stores, its levels will increase, bleeding will cease, and the bleeding time will be transiently corrected. Factor VIII levels will also rise, as the patient's Factor VIII is being protected from rapid proteolytic degradation by adequate levels of vWF.

As noted under the treatment of (mild) hemophilia A, desmopressin can be given IV or by intranasal spray (Table 6-3). The drug is generally given IV pre- and postoperatively, as its effects will then be almost immediate. The recommended IV dosage is 0.3 µg/kg body weight (maximum recommended dose 20 µg); doses can be repeated, if necessary, every 12-24 hours. If repeat doses are given this often, however, some individuals will have tachyphylaxis as the stores are depleted. This phenomenon is less of a problem in vWD than it is in

---

Table 6-6. Recommended Diagnostic Tests for Suspected von Willebrand Disease

- Activated partial thromboplastin time (APTT)
- Bleeding time (modified Ivy bleeding time, template method)
- Factor VIII assay
- Ristocetin cofactor assay
- vWF antigen assay
- Multimeric analysis of von Willebrand Factor (by sodium dodecyl sulfate agarose gel electrophoresis)*
- Ristocetin-induced platelet aggregation using varying concentrations of ristocetin

---

Note: The diagnosis of von Willebrand disease cannot be ruled out by the presence of a normal APTT and normal bleeding time! These screening tests may yield normal results in persons with mild to moderate von Willebrand disease.

*This test is generally available only in highly specialized research laboratories.

vWF = von Willebrand factor

---

mild hemophilia A, however, and many Type 1 vWD patients will continue to have a good hemostatic response to daily doses of desmopressin.[25] If they do not, they should be given a Factor VIII concentrate (see below).

For home or outpatient use, the highly concentrated intranasal spray formulation of desmopressin is ideal.[98] Patients should be instructed in the use of Stimate nasal spray (and given a test dose) before being sent home with it. Dosage is the same as for mild hemophilia A—namely, one spray in one nostril for persons weighing less than 50 kg, and two sprays (one in each nostril) for those weighing more than 50 kg. The intranasal spray formulation is often very useful in women with Type 1 vWD who have menorrhagia. Here, it is used at the onset of menses and again the following day, if necessary. Stimate nasal spray can also be used prior to invasive dentistry, prior to sports activities such as field hockey (to prevent excessive bruising and bleeding), and to treat minor bleeding episodes at home.

For the side effects of desmopressin and recommended precautions, see the earlier section on desmopressin under hemophilia A.

If a person with Type 1 vWD does not respond to desmopressin or is being scheduled for major surgery in which higher, sustained levels of vWF are desired, he or she should be given a plasma-derived Factor VIII concentrate that contains the hemostatically important higher-molecular-weight multimers of vWF.[99] These products include Humate-P (Centeon), Koate-HP (Bayer Corp.), and Alphanate (Alpha Therapeutics Corp.) (Note that a recombinant Factor VIII preparation or an ultrapure plasma-derived Factor VIII concentrate should *not* be used to increase vWF, as these products contain no or very little vWF). While there is no consensus concerning dosage, some general guidelines are provided in Table 6-7.

vWD Types 2 and 3

In persons with Type 2A vWD, desmopressin may be somewhat effective, particularly for minor bleeding episodes. It is recommended that a test dose be given in a nonbleeding state to see if desmopressin corrects the bleeding time. For those patients who do not have an adequate response to desmopressin and for those with vWD Types 2B and 3, one of the above-noted plasma-derived Factor VIII concentrates (rich in the higher-molecular-weight multimers of vWF) should be used (see Table 6-7).

In calculating dosage, there is no generally agreed-upon method. Because the Factor VIII concentrates licensed in the United States do not have their vWF content listed on the label or package insert, most in th e United States physicians calculate dosage on the basis of Factor VIII content. Similarly, most monitor patients by measuring plasma Factor VIII levels (plus clinical evaluation for bleeding). While many physicians obtain daily ristocetin cofactor assays in postoperative patients, results are generally not back soon enough to use for that day's clinical dosing. Other products for vWD are available in certain other countries, and some of these, as well as Humate-P, have vWF content (in ristocetin

cofactor units) listed on the label in those countries. It is hoped that this will soon be the case in the United States as well. The Subcommittee on von Willebrand factor of the International Society of Thrombosis and Haemostasis is addressing the issues of laboratory standardization of ristocetin cofactor assays and the advantages and disadvantages of labeling Factor VIII concentrates with their vWF content.

Many physicians treating vWD patients feel that for major surgery, it is most important to correct the patient's Factor VIII level, whereas for mucous membrane bleeding, correction of the bleeding time is most important.

Alloantibodies (inhibitors directed against vWF)

Alloantibodies, usually directed against vWF, are a rare complication of replacement therapy in per-

---

Table 6-7. General Guidelines for Treatment of von Willebrand Disease, Types 2 and 3 and Type 1 When Desmopressin Is Not Sufficient Therapy or Cannot Be Used*

A. For major surgery:
  - Maintain Factor VIII level and ristocetin cofactor (R:Co) level[†] ≥ 50% for 7-10 days (usually give a Factor VIII concentrate in a dosage of 20-40 U/kg once or twice daily)
B. For minor surgery:
  - Maintain Factor VIII level and R:Co level[†] ≥50% for 1-3 days
  - Then maintain Factor VIII level >20-30% for additional 4-7 days
C. For dental extraction (permanent teeth):
  - Give a single large infusion to obtain peak of 50-60% Factor VIII (and R:Co)
  - Also give an antifibrinolytic agent for 7 days, starting the day before extraction
D. Intracerebral, gastrointestinal, or mucosal bleeding:
  - Maintain Factor VIII level and R:Co level[†] >50% for 10 days (usually give Factor VIII concentrate in a dosage of 40 U/kg once or twice daily)

---

*While desmopressin is the treatment of choice for persons with Type 1 von Willebrand disease, those with Types 2 and 3 should receive a plasma-derived Factor VIII concentrate rich in the hemostatically important high-molecular-weight multimers of von Willebrand factor (eg, Humate-P, Alphanate, Koāte-HP).

†Currently, none of the Factor VIII concentrates marketed in the United States has R:Co units on the label. Thus, dosage is calculated on the basis of Factor VIII content. While many physicians obtain assays of R:Co in patients' plasma, results are seldom available in time to adjust that day's dosage. Thus, most physicians use Factor VIII assays and the patient's clinical condition as guides for follow-up dosing.

sons with severe (Type 3) vWD. There appears to be a familial tendency to develop antibodies, and those with deletions in the vWF gene are at greater risk.

Adjunctive Therapy

For oral surgical procedures or other bleeding in the oropharynx, an antifibrinolytic agent (see below) should be used, along with desmopressin or Factor VIII concentrate.

For menorrhagia, estrogen-containing contraceptives increase Factor VIII and vWF and are often of therapeutic benefit. If they are not or if they are contraindicated, Stimate nasal spray should be tried.

Other Hereditary Disorders of Blood Coagulation

Hereditary deficiencies of the other clotting factors (eg, fibrinogen; prothrombin; Factors V, VII, X, XI, XII, and XIII; Fletcher factor, etc) occur but most are rare,[100] and not all are associated with increased bleeding (ie, deficiencies of Factor XII, prekallikrein, high-molecular-weight kininogen, and some cases of Factor XI deficiency are not). All of these disorders are transmitted as autosomal recessive traits. For some of these rare deficiency states, a clotting factor concentrate is licensed and commercially available in the United States. These deficiencies and their treatment are summarized in Table 6-8.

For patients with hereditary deficiencies of Factors II (prothrombin), VII, or X, a PCC can be used to prevent or control bleeding because the PCCs contain not only Factor IX, but also Factors II, VII, and X. In the case of Factor VII deficiency, both a plasma-derived Factor VII concentrate (produced by Immuno in Vienna, Austria) and a recombinant Factor VIIa concentrate (NovoSeven) are available in Europe, but neither product is licensed in the United States. These Factor VII concentrates are preferable to PCCs in the treatment of bleeding in persons with Factor VII deficiency as higher levels can be obtained. It should be noted that PCCs vary considerably (by brands as well as from lot to lot) in their Factor VII content.

Factor XI deficiency, which occurs most commonly in persons of Ashkenazi Jewish descent,[101] may or may not be associated with a bleeding tendency. In certain families with certain Factor XI genotypes, a bleeding tendency and excessive bleeding with surgery occur, whereas in other families there may be little or no bleeding. This often has little relationship to the patient's Factor XI level. While plasma-derived Factor XI concentrates are manufactured in the UK (BioProducts Laboratory Factor XI concentrate) and in France (LFB's Hemoleven),[101] there is no licensed Factor XI concentrate for use in the United States. Thus, Fresh Frozen Plasma (FFP) is generally used if treatment is judged necessary.

In the rare persons with hereditary α-1 antiplasmin deficiency and in those with hereditary plasminogen activator inhibitor deficiency, the fibrinolytic balance is tipped in the direction of excessive fibrinolysis. Following injury or surgery, rapid clot lysis can result in large ecchymoses and hematomas. Treatment, as necessary, with an antifibrinolytic agent such as epsilon amino caproic acid (Amicar; Immunex Corp., Seattle, WA) should be tried.[100]

For deficiency states associated with bleeding for which there is no concentrate available, FFP should be used in a dosage of 5-20 mL/kg body weight. Dosage and dosage frequency depend on the severity of bleeding, the hemostatic level, and the biologic half-life of the clotting factor that is deficient. For example, Factor XIII (fibrin stabilizing factor) has a long half-life of 5-7 days, and only 2-3% of it is needed for hemostasis. Factor V, on the other hand, has a much shorter half-life, and 25% (or greater) of it is needed for hemostasis.[100] However, for many bleeding episodes, one dose of FFP will suffice. Because there is obvious concern about the possible transmission of blood-borne viruses with the use of FFP, two variations have been licensed. One is "FFP donor retested" and the other is solvent/detergent-treated plasma.[102] In the former, FFP is held in quarantine for at least 112 days; the donor then returns and his or her initially collected FFP is released for use only if repeat tests for infec-

Table 6-8. Rare Hereditary Disorders of Coagulation

Clotting Factor That Is Deficient or Abnormal	Hemostatic Level	Half-Life in Circulation	Clinical States	Inheritance Pattern	Available Therapeutic Products	Dosage
Factor I (Fibrinogen)	50-70 mg/dL	3-4 days	- Afibrinogenemia	Autosomal recessive	Cryoprecipitate	1.5 bags/10 kg (usually one dose will suffice)
			- Hypofibrinogenemia	Autosomal dominant	Cryoprecipitate	1 bag/10 kg (usually one dose)
			- Dysfibrinogenemias (some associations with hemorrhage, some have no symptoms, and some are associated with venous or arterial thrombosis)	Usually autosomal dominant	Cryoprecipitate	
Factor II (Prothrombin)	20 U/dL (20%)	60 hours	- Hypoprothrombinemia	Autosomal recessive	Prothrombin complex concentrates (PCCs) or Fresh Frozen Plasma (FFP)	15-20 mL FFP/kg initially, then 15 mL/kg every 36-48 hours
			- Dysprothrombinemias	Autosomal recessive		
Factor V	0.25 U/mL (25%)	16 hours		Usually autosomal recessive (in some families, combined with Factor VIII)	FFP (less than 1-2 months old as Factor V is labile in frozen plasma)	20 mL/kg initially, then 10 mL/kg every 12-24 hours
Factor VII	0.10-0.20 U/mL	3-6 hours	Hemorrhagic symptoms highly variable, but may be severe	Autosomal recessive	FFP Plasma-derived Factor VII concentrate (not licensed in US) Recombinant Factor VIIa (not licensed in US) PCC (Factor VII content varies!)	FFP 10 mL/kg every 12 hour 90 µg/kg every 2-3 hours

Table 6-8. Rare Hereditary Disorders of Coagulation (continued)

Clotting Factor That is Deficient or Abnormal	Hemostatic Level	Half-Life in Circulation	Clinical States	Inheritance Pattern	Available Therapeutic Products	Dosage
Factor X	25-30 U/dL	30 hours	Factor X deficiency Dysfunctional Factor X (acquired deficiency may be seen in amyloidosis)	Autosomal recessive Autosomal recessive	FFP or Certain PCCs (assay their Factor X content, as this varies with the PCC and is not on the label)	For minor bleeding, FFP 20 mL/kg initially, then 6 mL/kg every 12 hours For major bleeding, PCCs
Factor XI	20 U/dL (20%) but quite variable!	2-1/2 - 3 days	Variable clinical manifestations; may be minimal, or more severe mucous membrane bleeding	Autosomal recessive (most commonly seen in persons of Ashkenazi Jewish ancestry)	FFP (Factor XI concentrates are produced in Europe, not licensed in US)	When necessary, 15-20 mL FFP/kg, then 7.5-10mL/kg every 12-24 hours. Antifibrinolytic agents postoperatively if surgery involves mucosal surfaces.
Factor XII	None needed clinically		No excessive bleeding; *may* be a slight tendency to venous thrombosis	Autosomal recessive	None needed	None
Factor XIII (Fibrin stabilizing factor)	0.02-0.03 U/mL (2-3%)	7-10 days	Intracranial hemorrhage; delayed bleeding after trauma; poor wound healing	Autosomal recessive (very rare)	Cryoprecipitate FFP Concentrates available in Europe	1 bag/10 kg every 7 days
Prekallikrein	None needed clinically		No excessive bleeding	Autosomal recessive or autosomal dominant	None needed	None
High-molecular-weight kininogen	None needed clinically		No excessive bleeding	Autosomal recessive or autosomal dominant	None needed	None

(continued)

Table 6-8. Rare Hereditary Disorders of Coagulation (continued)

Clotting Factor That is Deficient or Abnormal	Hemostatic Level	Half-Life in Circulation	Clinical States	Inheritance Pattern	Available Therapeutic Products	Dosage
α-2 antiplasmin		3 days	α-2 antiplasmin deficiency (results in excessive fibrinolysis), mucocutaneous bleeding, joint bleeding, delayed or recurrent bleeding	Autosomal recessive	Antifibrinolytic agents •epsilon amino caproic acid •tranexamic acid	75 mg/kg every 6 hours 25 mg/kg every 8 hours
Plasminogen activator inhibitor (PAI-1)			PAI-1 deficiency (results in excessive fibrinolysis; recurrent bleeding after surgery or trauma)	Autosomal recessive	Antifibrinolytic agents •epsilon amino caproic acid •tranexamic acid	75 mg/kg every 6 hours 25 mg/kg every 8 hours

tious disease markers are negative. The 112-day hold period is believed to exceed the infectious "window period" in at least 95% of blood donors for HIV-1 and HIV-2, hepatitis B virus, and hepatitis C virus. "FFP donor retested" is a single-donor product. Solvent/detergent-treated plasma (PLAS+SD, V.I., Technologies, Melville, NY) is an ABO group-specific product, produced from pools of no more than 2500 volunteer donors.[102] This product is discussed in greater detail in Chapter 7. Both of these products can be used in place of FFP and both would appear to be safer. (Both are more costly than FFP as well.)

Afibrinogenemia or dysfibrinogenemia can be treated with cryoprecipitate, or with FFP, such as "FFP donor retested." To raise the fibrinogen level in an afibrinogenemic patient to a hemostatic level of 100 mg/dL, approximately 1.5 bags of Cryoprecipitated AHF per 10 kg body weight should be given. Because of the long half-life, repeat doses can be given every 3-4 days.

Other Considerations

Use of Antifibrinolytic Agents in Persons With Congenital Coagulopathies

In certain situations, antifibrinolytic agents are useful adjuncts to treatment with clotting factor concentrates or desmopressin. They are particularly useful in bleeding in the oral cavity (eg, tongue or mouth lacerations, teeth extractions, tonsillectomy), as tissues of the oropharynx are rich in fibrinolytic substances. Thus, rapid clot lysis and rebleeding may occur if an antifibrinolytic drug is not used as adjunctive treatment. Epsilon amino caproic acid (Amicar) or tranexamic acid (Cyklokapron, Pharmacia & Upjohn, Kalamazoo, MI) should be given for 7-10 days. Both are available in oral and parenteral forms. The recommended dosage for epsilon amino caproic acid is 75 mg/kg body weight every 6 hours, and for tranexamic acid, 25 mg/kg body weight, three times daily.

For dental extractions or mouth lacerations, these agents can also be used locally as a mouthwash. Sindet-Pederson and colleagues recommend the use of a mouthwash consisting of 10% tranexamic acid for injection, diluted with sterile water.[103] Others have used the parenteral form of epsilon aminocaproic acid in similar fashion.

Analgesic Agents

In an individual with a congenital coagulopathy or other underlying bleeding disorder, drugs that interfere with platelet function, particularly aspirin (and all aspirin-containing compounds), should be avoided. Acetaminophen (Tylenol) is a useful alternative for pain or fever. Many of the nonsteroidal anti-inflammatory drugs (eg, Motrin, Pharmacia & Upjohn, Kalamazoo, MI; Voltaren, Geigy, Summit, NJ; and Indocin, Merck & Co., Inc., West Point, PA) also interfere with platelet function, but by a different mechanism than aspirin.[104]

References

1. National Hemophilia Foundation Medical and Scientific Advisory Council (MASAC). Recommendations concerning the treatment of hemophilia and related bleeding disorders. Medical Advisory No. 301. New York: National Hemophilia Foundation, Nov. 1997.

2. Lee CA. Transfusion-transmitted disease. Baillieres Clin Haematol 1996;9:369-94.

3. Lusher JM, Kessler CM, Laurian Y, Pierce G. Viral contamination of blood products. Lancet 1994;344:405-6.

4. Giannelli F, Green PM. The molecular basis of haemophilia A and B. Baillieres Clin Haematol 1996;9:211-28.

5. Green PM, Naylor JA, Giannelli F. The hemophilias. Adv Genet 1995;32:99-139.

6. Lakich D, Kazazian HH, Antonarakis SE, Gitschier J. Inversions disrupting the Factor VIII gene as a common cause of severe hemophilia A. Nat Genet 1993;5:236-41.

7. Kadir RA, Economides DL. Obstetric management of carriers of haemophilia. Haemophilia 1997;3:81-6.

8. Kletzel M, Miller CH, Becton DL, et al. Post delivery head bleeding in hemophilic neonates. Am J Dis Child 1989;143:1107-10.

9. Peerlinck K, Vermylen J. Acute hepatitis A in patients with haemophilia A. Lancet 1993; 341:179.

10. Williams MD, Cohen B, Beddal AC, et al. Transmission of parvovirus B19 by coagulation factor concentrates. Vox Sang 1990;58: 177-81.

11. Azzi A, Ciappi S, Zakrzewska K, et al. Human parvovirus B19 infection in hemophiliacs first infused with two high-purity virally attenuated factor VIII concentrates. Am J Hematol 1992;39:228-30.

12. Mannucci PM, Gdovin S, Gringeri A, et al. Transmission of hepatitis A to patients with hemophilia by factor VIII concentrates treated with organic solvent and detergent to inactivate viruses. Ann Intern Med 1994; 120:1-7.

13. Mannucci PM, Brettler DB, Aledort LM, et al. Immune status of human immunodeficiency virus seropositive and seronegative hemophiliacs infused for 3.5 years with recombinant Factor VIII. Blood 1994;83:1958-62.

14. Hilgartner MW, Buckley JD, Operskalski EA, et al. Purity of factor VIII concentrates and serial CD4 counts. Lancet 1993;341:1373-4.

15. Seremetis SV, Aledort LM, Bergman GE, et al. Three-year randomized study of high-purity or intermediate purity factor VIII concentrates in symptom-free HIV-seropositive haemophiliacs: Effects on immune status. Lancet 1993;342:7000-3.

16. Vehar GA, Keyt B, Eaton D, et al. Structure of human factor VIII. Nature 1984;312:337-42.

17. Toole JT, Knopf JL, Wozney JM, et al. Molecular cloning of a cDNA encoding human antihemophilic factor. Nature 1984;312:342-7.

18. Wood WI, Capon DJ, Simonsen CC, et al. Expression of active human factor VIII from recombinant DNA clones. Nature 1984;312: 330-7.

19. Lusher JM. Recombinant clotting factor concentrates. Baillieres Clin Haematol 1996;9: 291-303.

20. Kaufman RJ, Pipe SW, Tagliavacca L, et al. Biosynthesis, assembly and secretion of coagulation Factor VIII. Blood Coagul Fibrinolysis 1997;8(Suppl 2):S3-14.

21. Fijnvandraat K, Berntorp E, ten Cate JW, et al. Recombinant B-domain deleted Factor VIII (r-VIII SQ): Pharmacokinetics and initial safety aspects in hemophilia A patients. Thromb Haemost 1997;77:298-302.

22. Nilsson IM, Lethagen S. Current status of DDAVP formulation and their use. In: Lusher JM, Kessler CM, eds. Hemophilia and von Willebrand's disease in the 1990s. Amsterdam: Elsevier Scientific Publications, 1991: 443-53.

23. Mannucci PM. Desmopressin: A nontransfusional hemostatic agent. Ann Rev Med 1990; 41:55-64.

24. Lethagen S, Ragnarson-Tenvall G. Self-treatment with desmopressin intranasal spray in patients with bleeding disorders. Effects on bleeding symptoms and socioeconomic factors. Ann Hematol 1993;66: 257-60.

25. Mannucci PM, Bettega D, Cattaneo M. Patterns of development of tachyphylaxis in patients with haemophilia and von Willebrand disease after repeated doses of desmopressin (DDAVP). Br J Haematol 1992;82:87-93.

26. Lusher JM. Response to 1-deamino-8-D-arginine vasopressin (DDAVP) in von Willebrand disease. Haemostasis 1994;24:276-84.

27. Lusher JM. Myocardial infarction and stroke: Is the risk increased by desmopressin? In: Mariani G, Mannucci PM, Cattaneo M, eds. Desmopressin in bleeding disorders. NATO ASI Series A: Life Sciences. New York: Plenum Press, 1993:42:347-53.

28. Schulman S, Martinowitz U. Design and assessment of clinical trials on continuous infusion. Blood Coagul Fibrinolysis 1996;7 (Suppl 1):S7-9.

29. Morfini M, Messori A, Longo G. Factor VIII pharmacokinetics: Intermittent infusion versus continuous infusion. Blood Coagul Fibrinolysis 1996;7(Suppl 1):S11-4.

30. Goldsmith JC. Rationale and indications for continuous infusion of antihemophilic factor (Factor VIII). Blood Coagul Fibrinolysis 1996;7(Suppl 1):S3-6.

31. Bona RD, Weinstein RA, Weisman SJ, et al. The use of continuous infusion of factor concentrates in the treatment of hemophilia. Am J Hematol 1989;32:8-13.

32. Martinowitz U, Schulman S. Continuous infusion of factor concentrates: Review of use in hemophilia A and demonstration of safety and efficacy in hemophilia B. Acta Haematol 1995;94(Suppl 1):35-42.

33. Arnold WD, Hilgartner MW. Hemophilic arthropathy. Current concepts of pathogenesis and management. J Bone Joint Surg Am 1977;59:287-305.

34. Nilsson IM, Berntorp E, Ljung R, et al. Prophylactic treatment of severe hemophilia A and B can prevent joint disability. Semin Hematol 1994;31(Suppl 2):5-9.

35. Petrini P, Lindvall N, Egberg N, Blombäck M. Prophylaxis with factor concentrates in preventing hemophilic arthropathy. J Pediatr Hematol Oncol 1991;12:280-7.

36. Berntorp E. The treatment of haemophilia, including prophylaxis, constant infusion and DDAVP. Baillieres Clin Haematol 1996;9:259-71.

37. National Hemophilia Foundation Medical and Scientific Advisory Council (MASAC). Recommendations concerning prophylaxis. Medical Bulletin No. 193, Chapter Advisory No. 197. New York: National Hemophilia Foundation, 1994.

38. Ragni MV, Hord JD, Blatt J. Central venous catheter infection in haemophiliacs undergoing prophylaxis or immune tolerance with clotting factor concentrates. Haemophilia 1997;3:90-5.

39. Warrier I, Baird-Cox K, Lusher JM. Use of central venous catheters in children with haemophilia: One haemophilia treatment centre's experience. Haemophilia 1997;3:194-8.

40. Perkins JL, Johnson VA, Osip JM, et al. The use of implantable venous access devices (IVADs) in children with hemophilia. J Pediatr Hematol Oncol 1997;19:339-44.

41. Lusher JM. Factor VIII inhibitors: Etiology, characterization, natural history and management. Ann N Y Acad Sci 1987;509:89-102.

42. Ehrenforth S, Kreuz W, Scharrer I, et al. Incidence of factor VIII and factor IX inhibitors in haemophiliacs. Lancet 1992;339:594-8.

43. Lusher JM, Arkin S, Abildgaard CF, et al. Recombinant factor VIII for the treatment of previously untreated patients with hemophilia A. N Engl J Med 1993;328:453-9.

44. Bray GL, Gomperts ED, Courter S, et al. A multicenter study of recombinant factor VIII (Recombinate): Safety, efficacy, and inhibitor risk in previously untreated patients with hemophilia A. Blood 1994;83:2428-35.

45. Lusher JM, Courter S, Spira J, et al. Safety, efficacy and inhibitor development in previously untreated patients (PUPs) treated exclusively with recombinant B-domain deleted Factor VIII (r-VIII SQ): 3 study years (abstract). Haemophilia 1998;4:227.

46. Addiego J, Kasper C, Abildgaard CF, et al. Frequency of inhibitor development in haemophiliacs treated with low-purity factor VIII. Lancet 1993;342:462-4.

47. Kasper CK, Aledort LM, Counts RB, et al. Proceedings: A more uniform measurement of factor VIII inhibitors. Thromb Diath Haemorrh 1975:34:612.

48. Kasper CK. Laboratory diagnosis of factor VIII inhibitors. In: Acquired hemophilia. Continuing Education Monograph, Los Angeles: Orthopaedic Hospital Publications, 1993;11-23.

49. Verbruggen B, Novakova I, Wessels H, et al. The Nijmegen modification of the Bethesda assay for Factor VIII:C inhibitors: Improved specificity and reliability. Thromb Haemost 1995;73:247-51.

50. Kasper CK, Lusher JM, and the Transfusion Practices Committee. Recent evolution of clotting factor concentrates for hemophilia A and B. Transfusion 1993;33:422-34.

51. Brettler DB, Forsberg AD, Levine PH, et al. The use of porcine factor VIII concentrate (Hyate:C) in the treatment of patients with inhibitor antibodies to factor VIII: A multicenter US experience. Arch Intern Med 1989;149:1381-5.

52. Kernoff PBA. The clinical use of porcine Factor VIII. In: Kasper CK, ed. Recent advances in hemophilia care. New York: Alan R. Liss, 1990:47-56.

53. Lusher JM, Warrier I. The role of prothrombin complex concentrates and factor VIII concentrates (human and porcine) in management of bleeding episodes in inhibitor patients. In: Lusher JM , Kessler CM, eds. Hemophilia and von Willebrand's disease in the 1990s. Amsterdam: Elsevier Scientific Publications 1991:271-7.

54. Penner JA, Kelly PE. Management of patients with factor VIII or factor IX inhibitors. Semin Thrombos Hemost 1975;1:386-99.

55. Kurczynski EM, Penner JA. Activated prothrombin complex concentrate for patients with factor VIII inhibitors. N Engl J Med 1974;291:164-7.

56. Lusher JM, Shapiro SS, Palascak JE, et al. Efficacy of prothrombin complex concentrates in hemophiliacs with antibodies to factor VIII: A multicenter therapeutic trial. N Engl J Med 1980;303:421-5.

57. Sjamsodein LJ, Heignen L, Mauser- Bunschoten E, et al. The effect of activated prothrombin complex concentrate (FEIBA) on joint and muscle bleeding in patients with hemophilia A and antibodies for factor VIII: A double-blind clinical trial. N Engl J Med 1981; 305:717-21.

58. Lusher JM, Blatt PM, Penner JA, et al. Autoplex versus Proplex: A controlled, double-blind study of effectiveness in acute hemarthrosis in hemophiliacs with inhibitors to factor VIII. Blood 1983;62:1135-8.

59. Lusher JM. Thrombogenicity associated with factor IX complex concentrates. Semin Hematol 1991;28(Suppl 6):3-4.

60. Chavin SI, Siegel DM, Rocco TA Jr, Olson JP. Acute myocardial infarction during management with an activated prothrombin complex concentrate in a patient with factor VIII deficiency and factor VIII inhibitor. Am J Med 1988;85:245-9.

61. Lusher JM, Giangrande PLF, Ewenstein B, et al. Efficacy, safety and treatment cost considerations. Haemophilia 1997;3(Suppl 3); 12-7.

62. Hay CRM, Lozier JN, Lee CA, et al. Safety profile or porcine factor VIII and its use as hospital and home therapy for patients with haemophilia A and inhibitors. Thromb Haemost 1996;75:25-9.

63. Hedner U, Glazer S, Pingel K, et al. Successful use of recombinant factor VIIa in patients with severe hemophilia A during synovectomy. Lancet 1988;2:1193.

64. Hedner U, Glazer S, Falch J. Recombinant activated factor VII in the treatment of bleeding episodes in patients with inherited and acquired bleeding disorders. Transfus Med Rev 1993;7:78-83.

65. Hedner U, Glazer S. Management of hemophilia patients with inhibitors. Hematol Oncol Clin North Am 1992;6:1035-6.

66. Lusher JM, Roberts HR, Hedner U. Recombinant Factor VIIa (NovoSeven): Summary of world wide clinical experience. Blood Coagul Fibrinolysis 1998;9:119-28.

67. Key N. Efficacy of recombinant factor VIIa (F VIIa) when administered in the home to control joint, muscle and mucocutaneous bleeds in hemophiliacs with inhibitors (abstract). Thrombos Haemost 1997;162(Suppl):51.

68. Lindley CM, Sawyer WT, Macik G, et al. Pharmacokinetics and pharmacodynamics of recombinant Factor VIIa. Clin Pharmacol Ther 1994;55:638-48.

69. Lusher JM. Recombinant activated factor VII for treatment of intramuscular haemorrhages: A comparison of early versus late

treatment. Blood Coagul Fibrinolysis 1998; 9(Suppl 1):111-4.

70. Brackmann HH. Induced immune tolerance in factor VIII inhibitor patients. Prog Clin Biol Res 1984;150:181-95.

71. Ewing NP, Sanders NL, Dietrich SL, et al. Induction of immune tolerance to factor VIII in hemophiliacs with inhibitors. JAMA 1988; 259:65-85.

72. van Leeuwen EF, Mauser-Bunschoten EP, van Kijken PJ, et al. Disappearance of factor VIII:C antibodies in patients with haemophilia A upon frequent administration of factor VIII in intermediate or low dose. Br J Haematol 1986;64:291-7.

73. Mariani G, Ghirardini A, Bellocco R. Immune tolerance in hemophilia. Principal results from the international registry. Thromb Haemost 1994;72:155.

74. High KA. Factor IX: Molecular structure, epitopes, and mutations associated with inhibitor formation. In: Aledort L, Hoyer L, Lusher J, et al, eds. Inhibitors to coagulation factors. New York: Plenum Publications, 1995:79-86.

75. Blatt PM, Lundblad RL, Kingdon HS, et al. Thrombogenic materials in prothrombin complex concentrates. Ann Intern Med 1974; 81:766-70.

76. Cederbaum AI, Blatt PM, Roberts HR. Intravascular coagulation with use of human prothrombin complex concentrates. Ann Intern Med 1976;84:683.

77. Kasper CK. Clinical use of prothrombin complex concentrates: Report of thromboembolic complications. Thromb Diath Haemorrhagica 1975;33:640-4.

78. White GC, Roberts HR, Kingdon HS, Lundblad RL. Prothrombin complex concentrates: Potentially thrombogenic materials and clues to the mechanism of thrombosis in vivo. Blood 1977;49:159-70.

79. Lusher JM. Prediction and management of adverse events associated with the use of factor IX complex concentrates. Semin Hematol 1993;30(Suppl 1):36-40.

80. National Hemophilia Foundation Medical and Scientific Advisory Committee (MASAC). Recommendations concerning the use of coagulation factor IX products in persons with hemophilia B. Medical Bulletin. New York: National Hemophilia Foundation, May 29, 1992.

81. Lusher JM. Factor IX concentrates. In: Forbes CD, Aledort L, Madhok R, eds. Haemophilia. London: Chapman & Hall, 1997: 203-11.

82. Mannucci PM, Bauer KA, Gringeri A, et al. No activation of the common pathway of the coagulation cascade after a highly purified factor IX concentrate. Br J Haematol 1991; 79:606-11.

83. Shapiro A. New Factor IX concentrates. J Pediatr Hematol Oncol 1994;1:479-90.

84. BeneFix, Package insert. Cambridge, MA: Genetics Institute, 1997.

85. Schulman S, Gitel S, Zivelin A, et al. The feasibility of using concentrates containing factor IX for continuous infusion. Haemophilia 1995;1:103-10.

86. Warrier I, Ewenstein B, Koerper MA, et al. Factor IX inhibitors and anaphylaxis in hemophilia B. J Pediatr Hematol Oncol 1997; 19:23-7.

87. Ewenstein B, Takemoto C, Warrier I, et al. Nephrotic syndrome as a complication of immune tolerance in hemophilia B. Blood 1997;89:1115-6.

88. Rodeghiero F, Castaman G, Dini E. Epidemiologic investigation of the prevalence of von Willebrand's disease. Blood 1987;69:454.

89. Lusher JM, Sarnaik I. Hematology. JAMA (Contempo Issue) 1996;275:1814-5.

90. von Willebrand EA. Hereditar pseudohemofili. Finska Lak Handl 1926;68:87.

91. Ruggeri ZM, Zimmerman TS. von Willebrand factor and von Willebrand's disease. Blood 1987;70:895.

92. Zimmerman T, Ruggeri ZM. von Willebrand's disease. Hum Pathol 1987;18:110.

93. Gaucher C, Jorieux S, Mercier B, et al. The "Normandy" variant of von Willebrand's dis-

ease: Characterization of a point mutation in the von Willebrand factor gene. Blood 1991; 77:1937-41.

94. Mancuso DJ, Kroner PA. Type 2M: Milwaukee-1 von Willebrand disease: An inframe deletion in the Cys^{509}-Cys^{695} loop of the vWF A1 domain causes deficient binding of vWF to platelets. Blood 1996;88:2559-68.

95. Gill JC, Endres-Brooks J, Bauer PJ, et al. The effect of ABO blood group on the diagnosis of von Willebrand's disease. Blood 1987;69:1691-5.

96. Montgomery RR, Gill JC, Scott JP. Hemophilia and von Willebrand disease. In: Nathan DG, Oski SH, eds. Nathan and Oski's hematology of infancy and childhood. 5th ed. Philadelphia: WB Saunders, 1998:1631-59.

97. Rodeghiero F, Castaman G, Mannucci PM. Clinical indications for desmopressin (DDAVP) in congenital and acquired von Willebrand disease. Blood Rev 1991;5:155-61.

98. Lethagen S. Self-treatment with desmopressin intranasal spray in patients with bleeding disorders: Effect on bleeding symptoms and socio-economic factors. Ann Hematol 1993;66:257-60.

99. Rodeghiero F, Castaman G, Meyer D, Mannucci PM. Replacement therapy with virus-inactivated plasma concentrates in von Willebrand disease. Vox Sang 1992;62:193-9.

100. Bauer KA. Rare hereditary coagulation factor abnormalities. In: Nathan DG, Oski SH, eds. Nathan and Oski's hematology of infancy and childhood. 5th ed. Philadelphia: WB Saunders, 1998:1660-75.

101. Smith JK. Factor XI deficiency and its management. Haemophilia 1996;2:128-36.

102. Klein HG, Dodd RY, Drik WH, et al. Current status of solvent/detergent-treated frozen plasma. Transfusion 1998;38:102-7.

103. Sindet-Pederson S, Ingerslev J, Ramström G, Blombäck M. Management of oral bleeding in haemophilic patients. Lancet 1988;2:566.

104. Shattil SJ, Bennett JS. Acquired qualitative platelet disorders due to diseases, drugs and foods. In: Beutler E, Lichtmann MA, Coller BS, Kipps TJ, eds. Williams hematology. 5th ed. New York: McGraw-Hill, Inc.,1995:1386-400.

In: Mintz PD, ed.
Transfusion Therapy: Clinical Principles and Practice
Bethesda, MD: AABB Press, 1999

7

Treatment of Acquired Disorders of Hemostasis

JOHN E. HUMPHRIES, MD

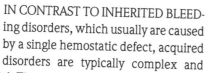 IN CONTRAST TO INHERITED BLEED-
ing disorders, which usually are caused
by a single hemostatic defect, acquired
disorders are typically complex and
multifactorial. This chapter reviews the hemostatic
defect(s), coagulation laboratory abnormalities,
and treatment of the more common acquired
bleeding disorders, including liver disease, uremia,
vitamin K deficiency, oral anticoagulation, and disseminated intravascular coagulation (DIC). In addition, because of their potentially life-threatening
nature, two less common disorders, acquired hemophilia A and acquired von Willebrand's disease
(vWD), are covered.

Determining the optimal therapeutic strategy
for the treatment or prevention of bleeding in a patient with a hemostatic disorder requires careful
determination of the specific hemostatic defect or
defects along with some estimation of the severity
of the disorder. The availability of a clinical laboratory that performs round-the-clock, basic hemostasis testing, including testing of the prothrombin
time (PT), activated partial thromboplastin time, fibrinogen concentration, D-dimer titer, and perhaps
the bleeding time, is essential to the diagnosis and
management of acquired hemostatic disorders.
The laboratory that also provides rapid turnaround
specialty assays, including those for Factor VIII activity, von Willebrand factor (vWF) ristocetin cofactor activity, and antithrombin activity, further enhances the clinician's capacity to manage these
complicated patients. That said, for disorders such
as liver disease, uremia, and DIC, there are disap-
pointingly few clinical studies that clearly demonstrate that the extent of abnormal hemostasis test
results (eg, PT and bleeding time) correlates well

*John E. Humphries, MD, Associate Professor and Associate Director, Special Coagulation Laboratory, Departments of
Internal Medicine and Pathology, University of Virginia Health Sciences Center, Charlottesville, Virginia*

with either spontaneous bleeding or bleeding with invasive procedures. Furthermore, clinical trials showing that the correction of the defects stops or prevents bleeding with invasive procedures are also in short supply. Therefore, this presentation is based on available published information in combination with this author's clinical experience. The recommendations herein should be viewed as general guidelines; each patient must be managed as an individual, with his or her specific clinical disorder and particular set of hemostatic defects factored in as determined by laboratory abnormalities in combination with the extent of active bleeding or type of invasive procedure planned for that patient. A review and discussion of the published studies concerning blood component therapy prior to invasive procedures are found in Chapter 8.

Blood Components and Products

Treatment of acquired bleeding disorders often requires the use of more than one modality. Obviously, accurate diagnosis of the bleeding disorder is critical to the effective treatment of active bleeding and the prevention of bleeding with surgical interventions. Once the blood components and products necessary to replace the missing factor(s) or other blood components are defined, their administration is often an essential part of the treatment plan. Discussed in this section are Plasma, Platelets, cryoprecipitate, and factor concentrates.

Plasma

Plasma is available as Fresh Frozen Plasma (FFP) and Pooled Plasma, Solvent/Detergent-Treated (PLAS+SD, V.I. Technologies, Melville, NY).

PLAS+SD is derived from blood collected from volunteer donors. The plasma from no more than 2500 donations is pooled and treated with the solvent, tri(n-butyl) phosphate (1%), and the detergent, Triton X-100 (1%). This product is provided in 200 mL doses. The solvent-detergent treatment signifiantly inactivates lipid-enveloped viruses, but nonlipid-enveloped viruses, such as hepatitis A and

parvovirus B-19, are not inactivated. The solvent and detergent are removed after treatment. PLAS+SD contains no less than 0.7 units/mL each of factors V, VII, X, XI, and XIII and no less than 1.8 mg/mL of fibrinogen. The product lacks the largest vWF mulimeters. The indications for PLAS+SD are those for which FFP is indicated. In this chapter, when FFP is noted as an appropriate treatment, PLAS+SD is an acceptable alternative. Clinicians and transfusion medicine specialists will need to decide whether to use single donor, nonvirally inactivated FFP or pooled, treated PLAS+SD. The cost of the latter to one hospital with which the author is familiar is approximately three times as high as the cost of FFP.

A unit of Fresh Frozen Plasma (FFP) is prepared from 1 unit of Whole Blood, frozen within 8 hours of phlebotomy and stored at -18 C for up to 1 year. An average unit of FFP contains 1 U/mL of all clotting factors. FFP is useful in the correction of coagulation factor deficiencies that are multiple or for which no factor concentrates are available. The frequency of FFP administration will depend on the half-life of the coagulation factor being replaced (see Table 7-1). Because acquired disorders such as liver disease often involve a deficiency of more than one coagulation factor, factor concentrates are usually insufficient to correct the coagulation defect. However, the correction of coagulation factor deficiency due to multiple factor deficiencies usually is indicated only for the treatment of bleeding or prior to an invasive procedure when the PT is at least 1.5 times the mean of its normal range (about 18 seconds).[1,2] The administration of 10-20 mL/kg of FFP usually will increase the level of the coagulation proteins by 20-30%.[3] Without the use of plasmapheresis, it is difficult to achieve greater increases in the factor levels. For the coagulation factors with longer half-lives, daily infusions of FFP for several days can produce greater increases; however, with liver disease or vitamin K deficiency, Factor VII, which has a half-life of only 6-7 hours, can be corrected with FFP by 20-30% at most without risking volume overload, and that correction will usually be brief.

Table 7-1. Fresh Frozen Plasma

Coagulation Factor	Concentration	Half-Life (Hours)
Fibrinogen	200 - 450 mg/dL	100 - 150
Prothrombin (Factor II)	1 U/mL	50 - 80
Factor V	1 U/mL	12 - 24
Factor VII	1 U/mL	6
Factor VIII	1 U/mL	12
Factor IX	1 U/mL	24
Factor X	1 U/mL	30 - 60
Factor XI	1 U/mL	40 - 80
Factor XIII	1 U/mL	150 - 300
von Willebrand Factor	1 U/mL	24

Cryoprecipitate

Cryoprecipitate is formed by slowly thawing FFP at 1-6 C and collecting the precipitated proteins, yielding approximately 10-15 mL per unit of plasma.[4] This product is enriched for Factor VIII, vWF, fibrinogen, and, to a lesser extent, Factor XIII (see Table 7-2). Unlike cryoprecipitate, concentrates of Factor VIII and Factor VIII/vWF are readily available and undergo virus inactivation procedures; therefore, cryoprecipitate has a role only in the treatment of inherited or acquired hypofibrinogenemia, dysfibrinogenemia, or Factor XIII deficiency. Because acquired, clinically significant Factor XIII deficiency is quite rare, it is not covered further in this chapter.

Platelets

Platelet concentrates, either from a single-donor apheresis unit or pooled from multiple donors, are used to treat thrombocytopenia or platelet dysfunction. In those disorders with platelet destruction (eg, immune thrombocytopenic purpura) or in which the milieu rapidly renders the platelets dysfunctional (eg, uremia), other modalities are preferred over platelet concentrates unless the bleeding is life-threatening. Platelet concentrates are discussed in detail in Chapter 4.

Factor Concentrates

Concentrates of Factor VIII, Factor IX, and Factor VIII/vWF are available in the United States for use in the management of inherited or acquired hemophilia A, hemophilia B, and vWD. A concentrate of porcine Factor VIII is useful in the management of patients with alloantibodies or autoantibodies to Factor VIII who cannot be managed with the use of human Factor VIII infusions. In addition, prothrombin complex concentrates that contain Factor IX along with the other vitamin K-dependent coagulation factors are available. Depending on the manufacturer, the prothrombin complex concentrates contain variable amounts of Factors II and X and may be enriched for Factor VII or contain almost no Factor VII. For the rapid treatment of severe vitamin K deficiency or warfarin overdose, the prothrombin complex concentrates may be very useful; however, for full correction, it

Table 7-2. Cryoprecipitate – Volume 10-15 mL

Coagulation Factor	Per Bag	Half-Life (Hours)
Fibrinogen	150 - 250 mg	100 - 150
Factor VIII	80 - 150 U	12
von Willebrand factor	100 - 150 U	24
Factor XIII	50 - 75 U	150-300

is necessary to use a concentrate enriched for Factor VII. In-vitro activation of the prothrombin complex concentrates yields a product capable of providing hemostasis in patients with antibodies to Factor VIII. Antithrombin concentrates are also available and may have a role in the treatment of bleeding with acquired antithrombin deficiency, such as in DIC. Available coagulation factor concentrates are discussed in detail in Chapter 6.

Hemostatic Agents

Blood components, even with virus inactivation processes, continue to carry real and potential risks, such as virus transmission and allergic reactions. For the management of many hemostatic disorders, the use of a pharmacologic hemostatic agent may either decrease the amount of blood product necessary or obviate their use entirely. The relevant hemostatic agents discussed are desmopressin acetate (DDAVP) (Ferring AB, Malmö, Sweden; distributed by Rhône-Poulenc Rohrer, Collegeville, PA), vitamin K, antifibrinolytic agents, conjugated estrogens, and erythropoietin.

Desmopressin Acetate

Desmopressin acetate (1-deamino-8-D-arginine vasopressin, or DDAVP) is a synthetic derivative of vasopressin (antidiuretic hormone). By a variety of mechanisms, including increasing the plasma levels of Factor VIII and vWF and directly activating

platelets,[5,6] DDAVP improves hemostasis related to platelet dysfunction and disorders of Factor VIII/vWF.[7,8] Repeated administration, however, often leads to a diminishing response (tachyphylaxis).[7] Because of its antidiuretic hormone effects, DDAVP may lead to fluid retention and hyponatremia, especially with repeated use, in the very young or very old, in patients who are also given hypotonic IV fluids, or when free water is not restricted.[7,9] Rarely, this hyponatremia may lead to altered mental function or seizures. Its effects on blood vessel tone may produce either an increase or decrease in the blood pressure, which, in the absence of preexisting hypertension or hypotension, is usually not clinically significant. Other minor but common side effects include facial flushing, nausea, headaches, and abdominal cramping.[8] Thrombosis has been reported after DDAVP administration, but this appears to be an extremely rare event.[10] DDAVP may be given intravenously, subcutaneously, or intranasally.

Vitamin K

Vitamin K is available for oral or parenteral administration and is useful in the prevention and treatment of vitamin K deficiency or oral anticoagulant-related hypocoagulation. While oral vitamin K typically has good bioavailability, its absorption and effect on PT prolongation may be erratic and should not be relied on for the treatment of bleeding related to vitamin K deficiency or oral anticoagulant use. Likewise, subcutaneous or intramuscular vitamin K is not without local adverse effects and does not provide the certainty of correction that is observed with IV administration. Although rapid IV vitamin K administration (eg, 1 mg/minute) has been associated with rare anaphylactic reactions,[11] slower administration (eg, 5 mg over longer than an hour) has not produced these reactions. Accordingly, this author typically administers 1-5 mg at 1 mg per hour by continuous infusion, the dose depending on the individual circumstance. Nonetheless, even when vitamin K is given intravenously, correction of the hemostatic defect usually does not occur for at least 6-8 hours.[12,13] Therefore, for active bleeding or urgent procedures, although vitamin K administration is an important part of the treatment plan, it is insufficient by itself, and the administration of coagulation factors is necessary.

Antifibrinolytic Agents

Antifibrinolytic agents licensed for use in the United States include epsilon aminocaproic acid (EACA) (Amicar, Immunex Corp, Seattle, WA), tranexamic acid, and aprotinin. EACA and tranexamic acid (Cyklokapron, Pharmacia & Upjohn, Kalamazoo, MI) are lysine analogues that inhibit fibrinolysis both by binding to plasminogen, thereby preventing plasminogen from binding to the fibrin clot, where it may become activated to plasmin, and also by binding to plasmin and displacing it from the fibrin clot.[7] Aprotinin (Trasylol, Bayer Corp, West Haven, CT) is a protease inhibitor, that directly inactivates plasmin, thereby preventing fibrinolysis. Each of these agents has been shown to be effective in decreasing blood loss with cardiopulmonary bypass surgery, and they may have a role in other bleeding disorders that involve excessive fibrinolysis. Because clinical data on the use of aprotinin outside cardiopulmonary bypass surgery are lacking, aprotinin is not discussed in this chapter. Common side effects of lysine analogues include gastrointestinal upset, headache, and light-headedness.[7] They should be used with caution in patients with bleeding from the kidney or bladder,

where thrombus formation may lead to ureteral or bladder outlet obstruction. Rarely, rhabdomyolysis may occur.[14] In patients with DIC, the use of antifibrinolytics may lead to unopposed fibrin formation and may aggravate microvascular thrombosis and organ dysfunction.

Conjugated Estrogens

Conjugated estrogens typically administered parenterally in high doses (0.6 mg/kg for 5 days) promote primary hemostasis. Although the exact mechanism remains unknown, potential mechanisms for this include enhanced platelet reactivity, elevations in Factor VIII and vWF, and decreased vascular permeability. In patients with platelet dysfunction, such as those with renal failure or liver disease, estrogen administration usually leads to a shortening of the bleeding time and improved hemostasis. Side effects are uncommon but include fluid retention, hot flashes, and gastrointestinal upset.[15]

Erythropoietin

Erythropoietin is available in a recombinant form of the natural hormone, which stimulates red blood cell production. Erythropoietin can be very effective in correcting anemia associated with decreased erythropoietin, most commonly found in patients with chronic renal failure. The resulting increase in hematocrit leads to improved in-vivo platelet function by assisting in the margination of platelets to the blood vessel wall[16,17] and by directly enhancing platelet function.[18] Erythropoietin therapy in the surgical setting is discussed in Chapter 19, and its nonsurgical use is discussed in Chapter 20.

Acquired Coagulation Disorders

Bleeding in patients with acquired disorders of hemostasis typically involves one or more of the following defects: anemia, coagulation factor deficiency, disseminated intravascular coagulation, excess fibrinolysis, platelet function defect, and thrombocytopenia. Apart from the discussion of acquired hemophilia A and acquired vWD, this list is used here as a menu from which one or more defects are selected for their importance as contributors to each disorder discussed.

Liver Disease

Hemostatic Defects

Patients with significantly impaired hepatic function usually present with a complex bleeding disorder. Depending on such factors as chronicity of the disorder, degree of cholestasis, and nutritional status, each individual patient may have a different pattern of defects and needs to be managed on the basis of this individual pattern. For example, in some patients, vitamin K deficiency plays a major role and simply administering vitamin K is sufficient. Decreased synthesis of multiple coagulation factors, as detected by PT prolongation, is typically present. In other patients, thrombocytopenia and platelet dysfunction may play more important roles. DIC may occur, perhaps related to the decreased clearance of activated coagulation factors, the decreased clearance of tissue-type plasminogen activator, and the decreased synthesis of coagulation and fibrinolysis inhibitors (antithrombin, protein C, protein S, and $\alpha2$-antiplasmin).[19,20]

Laboratory Evaluation

Determination of the complete blood count, PT, and possibly the bleeding time should provide important information about an individual's hemostatic defects. The PT should be sufficient to determine whether a significant decrease in clotting factors is present. Differentiating whether such a decrease is related to vitamin K deficiency or hepatic insufficiency requires reassessment after adequate vitamin K administration.

If the PT is prolonged, determining the fibrinogen level, D-dimer titer, and antithrombin activity help to establish whether DIC is present. Occasionally, quantification of Factor VIII activity may be needed to clarify whether decreased hepatic synthesis of clotting factors or DIC is the primary problem.[19] In DIC, Factor VIII should be decreased or at least decreasing, whereas with hepatic insufficiency, Factor VIII behaves more like an acute phase reactant either primarily or secondary to an increase in vWF and is typically elevated.[21] Similarly, the fibrinogen typically behaves like an acute phase reactant with liver dysfunction and is elevated until the very end stages. In many patients with cirrhosis, the antithrombin level is decreased significantly, and accelerated fibrinogen turnover occurs as evidence of active DIC. This turnover can be normalized by returning the antithrombin level to normal with the administration of antithrombin concentrate.[22]

Primary fibrinolysis also may contribute to excessive bleeding in patients with cirrhosis.[23] This effect is thought to be caused by the impaired clearance of tissue-type plasminogen activator in combination with decreased hepatic synthesis of the primary inhibitor of plasmin, $\alpha2$-antiplasmin.

Most patients with acute or chronic liver disease will manifest some degree of thrombocytopenia,[24] many from splenic sequestration due to portal hypertension. In addition, liver disease may lead to a decrease in thrombopoietin, thereby diminishing the marrow production of platelets, and platelets may also be consumed by DIC.[24]

Platelet function is typically impaired in patients with cirrhosis. The mechanism or mechanisms for this are still the focus of research. Impaired platelet adhesion appears to play an important role in patients with both acute and chronic liver disease[25]; however, increased platelet adhesion has been suggested in patients with acute liver failure.[24]

Treatment

All patients with liver disease and PT prolongation who are bleeding or for whom a surgical procedure is planned should receive vitamin K. Depending on the circumstances, its administration may be oral, subcutaneous, or intravenous. It should not be concluded that a patient's PT prolongation is not caused by vitamin K deficiency until at least 5 mg of vitamin K has been given intravenously.

If vitamin K fails to correct the PT sufficiently in the presence of active bleeding or prior to an urgent invasive procedure and the PT is at least 1.5 times the mean of its normal range (about 18 seconds), FFP may be useful. Lesser degrees of prolongation are probably not responsible for a patient's bleeding problems. Replacement of Factors II, VII, IX, and X can be performed more rapidly with prothrombin complex concentrates than with FFP.[26] Correction of the PT is most effective using Factor VII-enriched prothrombin complex concentrates (ProplexT; Baxter Healthcare Corporation, Glendale, CA).

It should not be overlooked, however, that the prothrombin complex concentrates do not contain either Factor V or Factor XI, both of which usually are decreased significantly in cirrhotic patients. To provide some Factor V and XI correction, Mannucci and colleagues[27] showed that a combination of prothrombin complex concentrates and FFP with Factor VII concentrate was successful in correcting the PT in cirrhotic patients and that no thrombotic complications occurred.

Precipitation of DIC or thrombosis has been a concern with the use of prothrombin complex concentrates in patients with cirrhosis,[28] although many of these reports concern the prothrombin complex con- centrates produced in the 1970s. Currently available prothrombin complex concentrates appear to be less thrombogenic. Moreover, the thrombogenic potential of prothrombin complex concentrates from different manufacturers may vary significantly. The extensive use of two different prothrombin complex concentrates in Scotland in 127 patients with PT prolongation due to cirrhosis was associated with no thrombotic events.[29] The addition of heparin and antithrombin to the prothrombin complex concentrates prior to infusion should greatly reduce this risk further if not eliminate it. (See warfarin therapy section below.)

DDAVP has been shown to shorten the bleeding time in patients with cirrhosis[30-32]; however, the benefit may be short-lived (≤ 4 hours).[33] An increase in plasma levels of vWF and Factor VIII is observed after DDAVP administration to patients with cirrhosis; the increase in vWF may be responsible for the improved bleeding time.[32] This effect on vWF appears to peak at 1 hour after intravenous DDAVP administration and lasts 3-4 hours.[32] As with uremic platelet dysfunction (see below), conjugated estrogens also may improve the bleeding time in patients with cirrhosis.[34] Because of the combination of thrombocytopenia and platelet dysfunction, significant bleeding may occur at platelet counts over 50,000/μL. Patients often require platelet transfusion for active bleeding or prior to invasive procedures if the platelet count is below 50,000/μL.[24] However, trapping of the infused platelets in the enlarged spleen usually will blunt the expected numerical increase in the platelet count in response to platelet transfusion.

The multiple hemostatic defects, in order of frequency and clinical significance, are shown in Table 7-3, with a stepwise approach to their management.

Uremia

Hemostatic Defects

Patients with chronic renal failure typically develop a mild-to-moderate hemorrhagic diathesis, commonly having ecchymoses, epistaxis, and gingival bleeding, as well as gastrointestinal bleeding.[35,36] This has been demonstrated to be related to platelet dysfunction.[37] Multiple mechanisms for this impaired platelet function have been proposed, including an impaired adhesion to endothelium mediated by vWF and glycoprotein Ib[38] and a decrease in platelet-dense granule adenosine diphosphate (ADP) and serotonin.[39] Abnormalities of vWF multimers and decreased platelet vWF may contribute to impaired primary hemostasis in uremic patients.[40] The precise cause or causes for this dysfunction may be related to the interaction of platelets with elevated levels of phenols or urea, other toxins. In addition, the decrease in hematocrit usually seen in patients with chronic renal failure further aggravates in-vivo platelet dysfunction.[36] A direct negative correlation between the hematocrit

Table 7-3. Management of Hemostatic Defects in Liver Disease and a Multistep Approach to Their Treatment*

Hemostatic Defects	Blood Components and Derivatives	Hemostatic Agents
1) Factor deficiency	b) Fresh Frozen Plasma c) Prothrombin complex concentrates	a) Vitamin K
2) Platelet dysfunction	c) Platelets	a) Desmopressin acetate b) Estrogens (conjugated)
3) Thrombocytopenia	Platelets	
4) Disseminated intravascular coagulation	a) Antithrombin concentrate b) Fresh frozen plasma c) Platelets	
5) Anemia	Red Blood Cells	
6) Primary fibrinolysis	b) Cryoprecipitate	a) Epsilon aminocaproic acid/tranexamic acid

*Treatment options are given in preferred order a), b) , and c).

and bleeding time in chronic renal failure patients has been observed.[15,41] The effect of decreased hematocrit on the bleeding time may be related to the rheologic effect of decreased pushing of the platelets to the endothelium[17] and to decreased red cell ADP release with subsequently lesser ADP-induced platelet activation.[16] The levels of clotting factors are usually normal, and elevated levels of fibrinogen, Factor VIII, and vWF are typically present.

Laboratory Evaluation

Although the test for bleeding time has many critics, it remains the most widely used and accepted test of platelet dysfunction in patients with chronic renal failure.[15,42,43] More sophisticated tests of platelet function fail to provide readily available clinically useful information. Determination of the hematocrit is an important part of managing current bleeding and planned invasive procedures, as primary hemostasis is determined in part by the hematocrit.

Treatment

Although the infusion of normal platelets will correct the defect, the correction is usually very transient, as the infused platelets rapidly become dysfunctional in the uremic environment.[36] Fortunately, other interventions have proved effective in improving platelet function, decreasing active bleeding, and preventing excess bleeding with surgical or other interventions in uremic patients. However, platelet transfusion may be helpful in emergencies.

Aggressive dialysis usually improves platelet function but incompletely corrects the hemostatic defect. For major procedures, aggressive dialysis is not sufficient by itself.[35,36] The infusion of cryoprecipitate often promptly shortens the bleeding time and decreases bleeding in many but not all uremic patients.[44] Cryoprecipitate infusion leads to increases in fibrinogen, Factor VIII, and vWF, and its effects may last up to 36 hours.[36] Although the levels of these proteins are increased already, there is some evidence for vWF dysfunction in uremia that might be corrected with cryoprecipitate infusion. However, the unpredictable response to cryoprecipitate and the risk of virus transmission makes pharmacologic agents, such as DDAVP and estrogens, preferrable.

DDAVP has been shown to be a very effective agent in the short-term improvement of hemostasis in uremic patients.[45] The exact mechanism for this is unclear but may include the release of more functional vWF. Some researchers have reported a direct effect on platelets, related to increased serotonin uptake and enhanced dense granule release after DDAVP administration.[46] However, others have reported decreased platelet serotonin following DDAVP.[47] Unfortunately, the effects of DDAVP, which begin within 30 minutes of IV administration, are maximal at approximately 4 hours and in many patients wear off by 6-8 hours. Subcutaneous and intranasal administration of DDAVP have shown efficacy also. The repeated administration of DDAVP may lead to tachyphylaxis[48] and hyponatremia. For cutaneous bleeding in uremic patients, another vasopressin analog, triglycyl-lysine vasopressin, may improve hemostasis even when DDAVP has been ineffective.[49]

Longer-lasting improvement in the bleeding time and hemostasis may be achieved by the administration of high-dose conjugated estrogens. Livio et al[50] showed that daily infusion of 0.6 mg/kg of estrogens shortens the bleeding time and leads to less bleeding. The effect may begin within 12 hours and peaks at 5-7 days, and the improvement in hemostasis may last up to 2 weeks in many patients.[50] A dose of 50 mg of conjugated estrogens given orally also may improve hemostasis, although the duration of improvement in the bleeding time may be much shorter than when the conjugated estrogens are given intravenously.[51] For gastrointestinal bleeding in uremic patients with gastrointestinal

telangiectases, the administration of norethynodrel/mestranol 2.5-5 mg/0.075-0.1 mg has been effective in the treatment for refractory gastrointestinal bleeding; some patients have been treated for up to 28 months.[52] It has been demonstrated recently that estrogens (estradiol -17ß) given at a lower dose via a transdermal patch (50-100 µg/24 hours) also may improve hemostasis over a prolonged period.[53] The precise mechanism of action by which estrogens improve hemostasis in uremic patients is unclear.

The infusion of Red Blood Cells shortens the bleeding time and improves hemostasis in anemic uremic patients when the hematocrit is less than approximately 27%.[16,54] Erythropoietin usually will produce an improvement in the hematocrit in patients with chronic renal failure[55]; it also may enhance platelet function directly and shorten the bleeding time[18] by improving platelet adhesion and aggregation defects in uremic patients.[56] Of course, erythropoietin also may thereby increase the risk of thrombosis, including vascular graft thrombosis, myocardial infarction, and stroke.[57,58] Its effect appears not to be a direct drug effect on the uremic platelets, however, as in-vitro incubation of platelets with erythropoietin does not lead to improved platelet function.[59] The multiple hemostatic defects, in order of frequency and clinical significance, are shown in Table 7-4 with a stepwise approach to their management.

Warfarin Therapy/Vitamin K Deficiency

Hemostatic Defects

Vitamin K deficiency or warfarin administration leads to a decrease in the circulating levels of functional Factors II, VII, IX, and X, and also of the anticoagulants protein C and protein S. The overall effect is to impair hemostasis, such that patients are at risk for bleeding during surgery or invasive procedures and even for spontaneous hemorrhage when vitamin K deficiency is severe or the patient is over-anticoagulated with warfarin. Vitamin K deficiency is relatively common in hospitalized patients. Risk factors for the development of clinically

---

Table 7-4. Management of Hemostatic Defects in Uremia and a Multistep Approach to Their Treatment*

Hemostatic Defect	Blood Components and Derivatives	Hemostatic Agents
1.) Platelet dysfunction	c) Cryoprecipitate	a) DDAVP
	d) Platelets	b) Estrogens (conjugated)
2.) Anemia	b) Red Blood Cells	a) Erythropoietin

*Treatment options are given in preferred order a), b), c), and d).

---

significant vitamin K deficiency include poor diet, malabsorption, antibiotic use, recent surgery, and liver or kidney dysfunction.[13]

Laboratory Evaluation

Determination of the PT with calculation of the international normalized ratio is usually sufficient to determine the degree of coagulopathy related to vitamin K deficiency or oral anticoagulant administration, provided there is no suspicion of additional hemostatic defects.

Treatment

Certainly, the administration of vitamin K plays a role in the management of these patients, but vitamin K may be insufficient by itself, depending on the circumstances. For the vitamin K-deficient patient, options include oral, subcutaneous, or intravenous administration. In the absence of bleeding and with no reason for impaired gastrointestinal absorption, oral administration (eg, 5 mg four times a day for several days) is usually sufficient. If malabsorption exists, subcutaneous administration of 10 mg of vitamin K is usually adequate. If bleeding occurs or if urgent correction is needed, IV administration should lead to more rapid and more certain correction. Very rapid infusion (eg, 5-10 mg given

in less than 5-10 minutes) has been associated with anaphylactic reactions.[11] However, Alperin[13] gave 20-25 mg of vitamin K intravenously over 30 minutes to 42 patients without adverse effects. This author prefers to administer vitamin K intravenously at 1 mg per hour (total dose 1-5 mg) by continuous infusion. Although this approach leads to a slightly slower correction of the PT, it should avoid all anaphylactic reactions. In addition, if immediate surgical intervention is needed or if active bleeding occurs, no quantity or route of vitamin K is going to be effective immediately, and other treatment modalities will be needed.

For immediate reversal of vitamin K deficiency, functional levels of Factors II, VII, IX, and X must be restored. FFP provides this correction, as well as protein C and protein S, but carries the risk of virus transmission and takes time to thaw. Also, if the patient is severely vitamin K deficient or greatly overanticoagulated with warfarin, the large volume of FFP needed—possibly up to 15-20 mL/kg or just over a liter for a 70-kg adult—may become an issue.

The vitamin K-dependent coagulation factors are also available as concentrates (prothrombin complex concentrates). These virus-inactivated blood derivatives were marketed initially for patients with hemophilia B (Factor IX deficiency). Because Factor VII has the shortest half-life of the vitamin K-dependent procoagulant factors, it is essential that a prothrombin complex concentrate be used that contains at least as much Factor VII as the other factors, if not more. Currently, only one product, ProplexT, contains sufficient Factor VII to be useful in this setting; however, the clinical availability of this product has been very limited recently. Prothrombin complex concentrates are rapidly effective in normalizing the PT, but the effect is usually short-lived.[60] However, for life-threatening hemorrhage, prothrombin complex concentrates normalize PT approximately four- to fivefold faster than FFP.[61,62] In high doses and in patients with underlying atherosclerosis or liver disease, these concentrates have been associated with an increased risk of thrombotic complications and DIC.[28,63,64] However, the addition of heparin prior to infusion, about 0.05 U per unit of Factor IX, appears to decrease this complication.[63]

Several prothrombin complex concentrates are available in the United States. Two of these, Konȳne 80 (Bayer Corporation, West Haven, CT) and Profilnine Heat-Treated (Alpha Therapeutics, Los Angeles, CA), contain only 10-20 U of Factor VII per 100 U of Factor IX.[65] By contrast, ProplexT is enriched for Factor VII and contains approximately 400 Units of Factor VII per 100 Units of Factor IX.[65] This author has been using ProplexT for this purpose with rapid correction of the PT and without complications. To avoid the thrombotic complications thought to be related to the small amount (<5%) of activated clotting factors contained in the concentrate, both heparin and antithrombin are added as 0.05-0.1 U per unit of Factor VII prior to infusion. No thrombotic complications have been observed in more than 20 patients treated, and the cost of this combination of prothrombin complex concentrate plus heparin plus antithrombin is less than half the cost of the FFP required to supply the same number of units of Factor VII. In addition, unlike FFP, the concentrates are virus inactivated.

For patients on warfarin, who are either over-anticoagulated or for whom urgent intervention is needed while on therapeutic anticoagulation, several factors must be considered to determine the optimal approach: 1) the strength of the indication for warfarin (ie, can the warfarin be totally reversed without consequence?); 2) the risk of bleeding with the planned procedure or surgery (ie, must the warfarin be stopped or totally reversed, or can the procedure be performed safely with no or only incomplete reversal of anticoagulation?); and 3) the timing of the situation (eg, active bleeding, or emergent or urgent surgery).[66] Depending on the specifics outlined above, options for an individual patient include proceeding without correction of the warfarin, holding the warfarin for several days, and then proceeding when a lesser degree of anti-coagulation exists, or administering a small amount (eg, 0.5-2 mg) of vitamin K intravenously or subcutaneously[67] to lessen the degree of anticoagulation within 6-12 hours. Of note, responses to low-dose vitamin K may be unpredictable.[68,69] Moreover, without additional vitamin K, the PT often will begin to extend again in 2-3 days, necessitating further vitamin K for the treatment of bleeding or for invasive procedures.[70] The administration of FFP or prothrombin complex concentrates will be required if anticoagulation must be reversed immediately.[71]

Disseminated Intravascular Coagulation

Hemostatic Defect

DIC is a complex syndrome of coagulation activation and platelet activation, leading to activation of the fibrinolytic system. Although the consequences of this syndrome initially lead to a hypercoagulable state with thrombotic occlusion of the arterial microvascular system and occasionally larger vessels,[12] in time, a coagulopathy develops with diffuse hemorrhagic consequences.[72] The coagulopathy is multifactorial, involving all hemostatic systems. The concentration of all coagulation factors is decreased by consumption and by degradation by plasmin. Platelets are decreased in number, and their function may be impaired by the action of plasmin and the presence of fibrin(ogen) degradation products. Activation of the fibrinolytic system leads to the degradation of clotting factors, decreased platelet function, and premature dissolution of all thrombi. Patients thus develop bleeding of all types—usually at all sites of invasion, such as IV catheters, endotracheal tubes, etc.

Laboratory Evaluation

Determination of the PT, complete blood count, fibrinogen concentration, and D-dimer titer are usually sufficient to confirm the presence and severity of DIC in a patient with a clinical condition who is expected to be at risk for DIC. Typically, the PT is prolonged with an elevated D-dimer titer, and thrombocytopenia and hypofibrinogenemia are present. Often, however, serial determinations of these laboratory studies are useful to demonstrate a decreasing level of fibrinogen and platelet count, even though their values remain within the normal range. In addition, the determination of the antithrombin level can help support the diagnosis of DIC; a normal or elevated level of antithrombin renders the diagnosis of DIC unlikely.

Treatment

The treatment of bleeding in patients with DIC requires a multistep approach. Most important, the underlying cause for DIC must be identified and treated; otherwise, treatment of the coagulopathy is almost certainly futile. Nonetheless, even with identification and treatment of the underlying disease, it is often necessary to treat abnormalities in the coagulation system to prevent and treat both the thrombotic and hemorrhagic consequences. Simple replacement of depleted coagulation factors with FFP is often unsuccessful in correcting the PT or low fibrinogen in patients with active DIC[12] and may contribute at least theoretically to further microvascular thrombosis.

Because thrombin is the final common denominator in coagulation activation and its thrombotic consequences, its generation and action must be inhibited effectively. Although in many cases of DIC, the coagulation activation shuts off rapidly with treatment of the underlying disease (eg, intrauterine fetal demise with delivery of the fetus), frequently a delay exists prior to shutdown of the

coagulation system activation and its consequences. Therefore, shutting down the coagulation system may be important to achieving a successful outcome. Many clinicians have used heparin or low-molecular-weight heparin in this situation[73]; however, when DIC is active, typically consumption, and perhaps other mechanisms, also have decreased the level of antithrombin, the primary inhibitor of thrombin. Thus, heparin administration is less effective, as it requires antithrombin. In addition, in the patient with acute DIC and active bleeding, the administration of heparin is likely to aggravate the bleeding by interfering with platelet function and increasing vascular permeability. However, in patients with chronic DIC (eg, secondary to malignancy or aortic aneurysms), heparin or low-molecular-weight heparin appears to be effective in controlling the coagulopathy.

Studies of patients with DIC secondary to sepsis have demonstrated that the infusion of antithrombin concentrate leads to significantly more rapid improvement in all coagulation parameters of DIC.[74] These and other studies of patients suggest that this improvement in DIC may be accompanied by an improvement in patient morbidity and mortality.[75] The infusion of antithrombin alone was more effective in shortening the duration of DIC and was associated with less hemorrhage than the infusion of either heparin alone or heparin with antithrombin.[76] Gabexate mesilate, a serine protease inhibitor with antithrombin activity, has shown promise in the treatment of DIC and appears to be associated with less hemorrhage than heparin in acute DIC patients.[77] In obstetric patients with DIC, a study by Maki et al[78] demonstrated improvement in DIC and less bleeding in those patients treated with antithrombin concentrate than in those receiving gabexate mesilate.[78] Likewise, the administration of protein C or activated protein C concentrate may be beneficial in patients with DIC.[79] Both of these concentrates (antithrombin and protein C) have the advantage over heparin of improving the patient's endogenous anticoagulant systems without increasing the risk of hemorrhage. For patients with acute DIC, this author administers antithrombin as a bolus calculated to achieve an antithrombin activity level of at least 140% of normal. The dose is calculated by subtracting the patient's baseline level (eg, 60%) from the target of 140%. Then, the difference is multiplied by the patient's weight in kilograms. Depending on the specific antithrombin concentrate being used, this is divided by 1.4 (Thrombate III, Bayer Corporation) or by 1.0 (ATnativ, Baxter Healthcare Corporation). An antithrombin level is determined 20-30 minutes after the bolus to confirm that the target has been reached. A continuous infusion of antithrombin is then begun at 3-5 U/kg per hour, the rate depending on the severity of DIC. Antithrombin levels are determined every 8-12 hours, and the dose is adjusted to maintain antithrombin activity at or slightly greater than 140%. In most patients, as DIC resolves, the antithrombin infusion rate can be tapered.

Once treatment of the underlying cause of DIC is begun and the prothrombotic process is addressed, as by the administration of antithrombin, it is possible to treat coagulation factor deficiencies and thrombocytopenia effectively with FFP and platelet concentrates without the risk of aggravating the DIC. Parameters for the administration of plasma should be to maintain the PT at less than 1.5 times the mean of the normal range if bleeding occurs or an invasive procedure is planned. If the fibrinogen level is less than 100 mg/dL, fibrinogen can be given via FFP if FFP is being administered already for the treatment of other factor deficiencies or in the form of cryoprecipitate. An increase of 6-7 mg/dL should be expected per bag of cryoprecipitate in a 70-kg adult; however, in the face of ongoing DIC, the recovery and duration of response can be decreased markedly. The platelet count should be greater than 50,000/µL if bleeding occurs or an invasive procedure is planned. For the patient with DIC, probable platelet dysfunction due to fibrin(ogen) degradation products, and other coagulation factor deficiencies, a higher target such as 80,000/µL may be reasonable. Table 7-5 shows the hemostatic defects and a multistep treatment approach for patients with DIC.

Acquired Coagulation Inhibitors

Patients may develop autoantibodies directed against any of the coagulation factors. The patient then develops signs and symptoms similar to those

---

Table 7-5. Management of Hemostatic Defects in Disseminated Intravascular Coagulation and a Multistep Approach to Their Treatment*

Hemostatic Defects	Blood Components and Derivatives	Pharmacologic Agents
1) Disseminated coagulation activation	a) Antithrombin concentrate	b) Heparin
2) Factor deficiencies	a) Fresh Frozen Plasma	
	b) Cryoprecipitate	
3) Thrombocytopenia	Platelets	
4) Platelet dysfunction	Platelets	
5) Anemia	Red Blood Cells	

*Treatment options are given in preferred order a) and b).

in a patient with an inherited deficiency of that factor. Although antibodies against each of the clotting factors have been described, the most commonly occurring antibodies are directed against Factor VIII or vWF. These are the focus of this section.

Acquired Hemophilia A—Factor VIII Autoantibodies

With Factor VIII autoantibodies, a patient with no prior history of bleeding problems, including tolerance of significant operations without excess bleeding, presents with hematomas after relatively minor trauma or manifests marked bleeding after surgery or an invasive procedure. Clinical conditions associated with the development of Factor VIII autoantibodies include postpartum state, connective tissue disorders, and malignancies; however, approximately one-half of cases are idiopathic. Up to one-fifth of patients may die as a result of developing Factor VIII antibody.[80,81]

Laboratory Evaluation

Laboratory evaluation shows an isolated prolongation of the activated partial thromboplastin time, which fails to correct on mixing with normal plasma, indicative of an inhibitor. Assays of clotting factor levels identify an isolated decrease in the level of Factor VIII. It is essential to quantify the amount of antibody in the patient's plasma to determine the optimal approach to the treatment or prevention of bleeding. The method of quantitation developed for the patient with inherited hemophilia A with alloantibodies, called the Bethesda system, is used, although the system performs less precisely for autoantibodies. Basically, the number of inhibitor units is the inverse of the degree of dilution of the patient's plasma that inhibits 50% of the Factor VIII activity in normal plasma. The ability of the patient's antibody to neutralize porcine Factor VIII should be determined simultaneously. On average, these antibodies have about 15% cross-reactivity; however, large interindividual variation exists, and some studies have shown much less (about 2%).[80]

Treatment

The treatment of patients with Factor VIII antibodies requires that two problems be addressed: 1) the elimination of the antibody, and 2) the treatment or prevention of bleeding until the antibody has been eliminated. Obviously, only the most emergent operations should be performed. Any procedures that can be delayed should be, as it might be possible to eradicate the antibody or at least reduce the inhibitor titer.

Patients with low titers of Factor VIII antibody (eg, less than 5 or perhaps even 10 Bethesda U/mL) often can be treated effectively with high doses of Factor VIII. If the inhibitor titer is greater than 10, alternative therapies for the treatment of bleeding need to be sought. If the porcine inhibitor titer is less than 10 Bethesda units, and perhaps even less than 30 U/mL, the administration of porcine Factor VIII is very effective. At least three-fourths of patients achieve hemostatic levels of Factor VIII.[80,82] There are few side effects of porcine Factor VIII, but some patients will develop sufficient titers of antiporcine Factor VIII to render the porcine Factor VIII clinically useless.[82] If the inhibitor titer to both human and porcine Factor VIII is too high, activated or perhaps nonactivated prothrombin complex concentrates should be used to treat bleeding or manage surgical procedures.[83,8] In the near future, another therapeutic agent, recombinant Factor VIIa, should be available. This agent has been shown to be safe and effective in the management of acute bleeding in approximately 75% of inherited and acquired hemophilia A and B patients with inhibitors who have become refractory to all other agents.[85,86] In addition, with very low titers of Factor VIII inhibitor, DDAVP may be helpful in the treatment of minor bleeding or for minor invasive procedures.[87]

While some inhibitors may resolve spontaneously,[88] because the risk of hemorrhage outweighs the risk of the therapies used to try to eliminate the antibody, prompt initiation of immunosuppressive therapy is warranted in most patients.[89] The agents used include prednisone and cyclophosphamide and, less frequently, azathioprine.[89,90] Many patients will respond to high-dose prednisone alone at 1 mg/kg. For patients who fail this therapy, or perhaps those with inhibitor titers greater than 10 Bethesda U/mL, the addition of cyclophosphamide at 2 mg/kg orally each day may increase the remission rate. For patients who are not bleeding, prednisone with or without cyclophosphamide, depending on the inhibitor titer, can be administered and Factor VIII activity levels and Bethesda units determined weekly. Once the inhibitor can no longer be detected and a normal Factor VIII level has been restored, the cyclophosphamide can be discontinued and the prednisone tapered. Some researchers have advocated a more aggressive approach, including the administration of Factor VIII concentrate as a bolus (50-100 U/kg) followed by cycles of cyclophosphamide, vincristine, and prednisone.[91] In a series of 12 patients treated with this regimen, 11 with antibody titers of less than 50 Bethesda U/mL had their inhibitor disappear with three or fewer cycles.[91]

It appears that patients who develop Factor VIII autoantibodies postpartum respond less well to immunosuppression; however, in most patients, the antibody will disappear spontaneously within 2-3 years.[92]

As some inhibitors may return, the patient should be followed with Factor VIII levels for at least 6 months and then be reevaluated subsequently should symptoms return. For patients who fail to respond or who respond incompletely to the above regimens, some researchers have reported responses to intravenous immune globulin. Intravenous immune globulin may reduce the inhibitor titer in one-third to one-half of patients; however, this response is usually transient.[93]

Acquired von Willebrand Disease

Autoantibodies directed against vWF have been reported in a variety of conditions, most commonly with monoclonal gammopathy of unknown significance, but also with lymphoproliferative disorders associated with monoclonal gammopathies, as well as in patients with myeloproliferative disorders.[94] Similar to patients with inherited vWD, patients with acquired vWD manifest mucocutaneous bleeding, including epistaxis, bruising, and prolonged bleeding after cuts and scratches. However, in contrast to patients with inherited vWD, the patient with the acquired disease typically has no personal or family history of a bleeding disorder and often has an identifiable monoclonal gammopathy or a lymphoproliferative disorder, or both.[94,95]

Laboratory Evaluation

Although the activated partial thromboplastin time and bleeding time are typically abnormal in patients with moderate-to-severe acquired vWD, diagnosis rests on identifying the decreased levels of vWF ristocetin cofactor activity and vWF antigen.[94] As a bystander effect, Factor VIII is usually also reduced. The most common mechanism for this disorder is an autoantibody, but, in other patients, adsorption to tumor cells expressing glycoprotein Ib, the receptor for vWF, appears to be etiologic.[94,96] Unfortunately, for most patients with acquired vWD, there is no assay comparable to the Bethesda assay to prove the presence of an antibody and to quantify the antibody concentration.[94] In occasional patients, serial dilutions of the patient's plasma followed by addition to normal plasma and determination of the ristocetin cofactor activity allow a rough gauge of antibody titer; however, for most patients, the antibody is nonneutralizing and does not interfere with the function of the normal vWF in vitro. The quantity of ristocetin cofactor activity, the amount of vWF antigen, and the level of Factor VIII activity, therefore, provide the best information on severity for patient management.

Treatment

For minor bleeding, DDAVP often leads to a brief increase in the levels of Factor VIII and vWF sufficient for hemostasis.[95,97] For the treatment of more significant bleeding or prior to surgery, the provision of vWF is usually necessary. The best currently available products for this include the intermediate-purity Factor VIII concentrates containing both Factor VIII and vWF.[98] These are preferable to cryoprecipitate, which is not virus-inactivated. These components include Humate-P (Behringwerke, Marburg, Germany), Koāte-HP (Bayer Corporation), and Alphanate (Alpha Therapeutics). In clinical studies, these components appear to provide a comparable degree of hemostatic replacement of vWF in patients with inherited vWD. Because the vWF is bound rapidly by antibody and cleared from the circulation, the half-life is shortened and frequent infusions may be necessary. This author administers the intermediate-purity Factor VIII concentrates by continuous infusion with periodic determinations of the vWF ristocetin cofactor activity level. Because the antibody is not directed against Factor VIII, there is typically an accumulation of Factor VIII. If the level of ristocetin cofactor activity is adequate, the Factor VIII is usually much greater, and, therefore, measurement of the Factor VIII levels is unnecessary.

Treatment of the underlying lymphoproliferative disorder (eg, dexamethasone for monoclonal gammopathy of unknown significance) often but not always leads to improvement in the condition.[96] Infusions of intravenous immune globulin are effective in some patients and may increase the yield from intermediate-purity Factor VIII infusions as well, but usually do not lead to any lasting remissions.[99,100] Immunoadsorption or plasmapheresis also can provide an improved response to Factor VIII/vWF infusion in refractory patients.[96] Splenectomy has been reported to induce remissions in some patients.

Conclusion

Acquired disorders of hemostasis are typically multifactorial and present complex therapeutic problems. Systematic laboratory evaluation can assist the physician in determining rational intervention with pharmacologic and biologic treatments. Although this chapter presents guidelines for the therapy of patients with acquired disorders of hemostasis and the supporting rationale, each patient's unique constellation of laboratory abnormalities and clinical signs and symptoms challenges the physician to customize the therapy to the individual patient.

References

1. McVay PA, Toy PTCY. Lack of increased bleeding after paracentesis and thoracentesis in patients with mild coagulation abnormalities. Transfusion 1991;31:164-71.
2. McVay PA, Toy PTCY. Lack of increased bleeding after liver biopsy in patients with mild hemostatic abnormalities. Am J Clin Pathol 1990;94:747-53.
3. Spector I, Corn M, Ticktin HE. Effect of plasma transfusions on the PT and clotting factors in liver disease. N Engl J Med 1966; 275:1032-7.
4. Poon M-C. Cryoprecipitates: Uses and alternatives. Transfus Med Rev 1993;7:180-92.
5. Mannucci PM. Desmopressin (DDAVP) in the treatment of bleeding disorders: The first 20 years. Blood 1997;90:2515-21.
6. Wun T, Paglieroni T, Lachant NA. Physiologic concentrations of arginine vasopressin activate human platelets in vitro. Br J Haematol 1996;92:968-72.
7. Bolan CD, Alving BM. Pharmacologic agents in the management of bleeding disorders. Transfusion 1990;30:541-51.
8. Mannucci PM. Desmopressin: A nontransfusional form of treatment for congenital and acquired bleeding disorders. Blood 1988;72. 1449-55.
9. Weinstein RE, Bona RD, Altman AJ, et al. Severe hyponatremia after repeated intravenous administration of desmopressin. Am J Hematol 1989;32:258-61.
10. Mannucci PM, Lusher JM. Desmopressin and thrombosis (letter). Lancet 1989;2:675-6.
11. Rich EC, Drage CW. Severe complications of intravenous phytonadione therapy. Two cases, with one fatality. Postgrad Med 1982; 72:303-6.
12. Staudinger T, Locker GJ, Frass M. Management of acquired coagulation disorders in

emergency and intensive-care medicine. Semin Thromb Hemost 1996;22:93-104.

13. Alperin JB. Coagulopathy caused by vitamin K deficiency in critically ill, hospitalized patients. JAMA 1987;258:1916-9.

14. Ratnoff OD. Some therapeutic agents influencing hemostasis. In: Colman RW, Hirsh J, Marder VJ, Salzman EW, eds. Hemostasis and thrombosis: Basic principles and clinical practice. 3rd ed. Philadelphia: J.B. Lippincott Company, 1994:1104-33.

15. Eberst ME, Berkowitz LR. Hemostasis in renal disease: Pathophysiology and management. Am J Med 1994;96:168-79.

16. Boneu B, Fernandez F. The role of the hematocrit in bleeding. Transfus Med Rev 1987;1:182-5.

17. Turitto VT, Weiss HJ. Red blood cells: Their dual role in thrombus formation. Science 1980;207:541-3.

18. Cases A, Escolar G, Reverter JC, et al. Recombinant human erythropoietin treatment improves platelet function in uremic patients. Kidney Int 1992;42:668-72.

19. Kelly DA, Summerfield JA. Hemostasis in liver disease. Semin Liver Dis 1987;7:182-91.

20. Verstraete M, Vermylen J, Collen D. Intravascular coagulation in liver disease. Annu Rev Med 1974;25:447-52.

21. Joist JH. Hemostatic abnormalities in liver disease. In: Colman RW, Hirsh J, Marder VJ, Salzman EW, eds. Hemostasis and thrombosis: Basic principles and clinical practice. 3rd ed. Philadelphia: J.B. Lippincott Company, 1994:906-20.

22. Schipper HG, Ten Cate JW. Antithrombin III transfusion in patients with hepatic cirrhosis. Br J Haematol 1982;52:25-33.

23. Francis RB Jr, Feinstein DI. Clinical significance of accelerated fibrinolysis in liver disease. Haemostasis 1984;14:460-5.

24. Pereira SP, Langley PG, Williams CBE. The management of abnormalities of hemostasis in acute liver failure. Semin Liver Dis 1996;16:403-14.

25. Ordinas A, Escolar G, Cirera I, et al. Existence of a platelet-adhesion defect in patients with cirrhosis independent of hematocrit: Studies under flow conditions. Hepatology 1996;24:1137-42.

26. Kooistra T, Van den Berg AP, Emeis JJ, Princen JMG. Modulation of tissue-type plasminogen activator (t-PA) and plasminogen activator inhibitor (PA-I) production by human endothelial cells (EC) and porcine hepatocytes (PH) (abstract). Thromb Haemost 1985;54:171.

27. Mannucci PM, Franchi F, Dioguardi N. Correction of abnormal coagulation in chronic liver disease by combined use of fresh-frozen plasma and prothrombin complex concentrates. Lancet 1976;2:542-5.

28. Menache D. Prothrombin complex concentrates: Clinical use. Ann NY Acad Sci 1981;747-56.

29. Prowse CV, Cash JD. The use of factor IX concentrate in man: A 9-year experience of Scottish concentrates in the South-East of Scotland. Br J Haematol 1981;47:91-104.

30. Mannucci PM, Vicente V, Vianello L, et al. Controlled trial of desmopressin in liver cirrhosis and other conditions associated with a prolonged bleeding time. Blood 1986;67:1148-53.

31. Agnelli G, Parise P, Levi M, et al. Effects of desmopressin on hemostasis in patients with liver cirrhosis. Haemostasis 1995;25:241-7.

32. Burroughs AK, Matthews K, Qadiri M, et al. Desmopressin and bleeding time in patients with cirrhosis. Br Med J 1985;291:1377-81.

33. Cattaneo M, Tenconi PM, Alberca I, et al. Subcutaneous desmopressin (DDAVP) shortens the prolonged bleeding time in patients with liver cirrhosis. Thromb Haemost 1990;64:358-60.

34. Perez EA, Tanaka M, Gandara DR. Conjugated estrogen for platelet dysfunction associated with liver disease (letter). N Engl J Med 1988;318:1543.

35. Couch P, Stumpf JL. Management of uremic bleeding. Clin Pharmacol 1990;9:673-81.

36. Remuzzi G. Bleeding in renal failure. Lancet 1988;1:1205-8.
37. Carvalho AC. Acquired platelet dysfunction in patients with uremia. Hematol Oncol Clin North Am 1990;4:129-43.
38. Escolar G, Cases A, Bastida E, et al. Uremic platelets have a functional defect affecting the interaction of vWF with glycoprotein IIb-IIIa. Blood 1990;76:1336-40.
39. Mezzano D, Tagle R, Panes O, et al. Hemostatic disorder of uremia: The platelet defect, main determinant of the prolonged bleeding time, is correlated with indices of activation of coagulation and fibrinolysis. Thromb Haemost 1996;76:312-21.
40. Gralnick HR, McKeown LP, Williams SB, et al. Plasma and platelet vWF defects in uremia. Am J Med 1988;85:806-10.
41. Small M, Lowe GDO, Cameron E, Forbes CD. Contribution of the haematocrit to the bleeding time. Haemostasis 1983;13:379-84.
42. Jubelirer SJ. Hemostatic abnormalities in renal disease. Am J Kidney Dis 1985;5:219-25.
43. Steiner RW, Coggins C, Carvalho ACA. Bleeding time in uremia: A useful test to assess clinical bleeding. Am J Hematol 1979;7:107-17.
44. Janson PA, Jubelirer SJ, Weinstein MJ, Deykin D. Treatment of the bleeding tendency in uremia with cryoprecipitate. N Engl J Med 1980;303:1318-22.
45. Mannucci PM, Remuzzi G, Pusineri F, et al. Deamino-8-D-arginine vasopressin shortens the bleeding time in uremia. N Engl J Med 1983;308:8-12.
46. Soslau G, Schwartz AB, Putatunda B, et al. Desmopressin-induced improvement in bleeding times in chronic renal failure patients correlates with platelet serotonin uptake and ATP release. Am J Med Sci 1990;300:372-9.
47. Malyszko J, Peitrascek M, Buczko W, Mysliwiec M. Study on mechanisms of a haemostatic effect of 1 deamino-8-D-arginine vaso- pressin (desmopressin) in uraemic patient Folia Haematol 1990;117:319-24.
48. Canavese C, Salomone M, Pacitti A, et al. R duced response of uraemic bleeding time repeated doses of desmopressin (letter). La cet 1985;1:867-8.
49. Garner WL, Rodriguez JL, Thomson PD, al. Control of hemorrhage during renal fa ure with triglycyl-lysine-vasopressin. A Plast Surg 1993;31:78-81.
50. Livio M, Mannucci PM, Viganò G, et al. Co jugated estrogens for the management bleeding associated with renal failure. N En J Med 1986;315:731-5.
51. Shemin D, Elnour M, Amarantes B, et Oral estrogens decrease bleeding time a improve clinical bleeding in patients with nal failure. Am J Med 1990;89:436-40.
52. Bronner MH, Pate MB, Cunningham Marsh WH. Estrogen-progesterone thera for bleeding gastrointestinal telangiectasi in chronic renal failure. Ann Intern M 1986;105:371-4.
53. Sloand JA, Schiff MJ. Beneficial effect of lo dose transdermal estrogen on bleeding tin and clinical bleeding in uremia. Am J Kidn Dis 1995;26:22-6.
54. Fernandez F, Goudable C, Sie P, et al. Lo hematocrit and prolonged bleeding time uraemic patients: Effect of red cell transf sions. Br J Haematol 1985;59:139-48.
55. Moia M, Mannucci PM, Vizzotto L, et al. I provement in the haemostatic defect of ura mia after treatment with recombinant h man erythropoietin. Lancet 1987;2:1227-9
56. Zwaginga JJ, Ijsseldijk MJW, de Groot PG, al. Treatment of uremic anemia with recor binant erythropoietin also reduces the d fects in platelet adhesion and aggregatio caused by uremic plasma. Thromb Haemo 1991;66:638-47.
57. Taylor JE, Belch JJF, McLaren M, et al. Effe of erythropoietin therapy and withdrawal blood coagulation and fibrinolysis in hem dialysis patients. Kidney Int 1993;44:182-9(

58. Tsao C-J, Kao R-H, Cheng T-Y, et al. The effect of recombinant human erythropoietin on hemostatic status in chronic uremic patients. Int J Hematol 1992;55:197-203.

59. El-Shahawy MA, Francis R, Akmal M, Massry SG. Recombinant human erythropoietin shortens the bleeding time and corrects the abnormal platelet aggregation in hemodialysis patients. Clin Nephrol 1994;41:308-11.

60. Taberner DA, Thomson JM, Poller L. Comparison of prothrombin complex concentrate and vitamin K₁ in oral anticoagulant reversal. Br Med J 1976;2:83-5.

61. Fredriksson K, Norrving B, Strömblad L-G. Emergency reversal of anticoagulation after intracerebral hemorrhage. Stroke 1992;23:972-7.

62. Makris M, Greaves M, Phillips WS, et al. Emergency oral anticoagulant reversal: The relative efficacy of infusions of FFP and clotting factor concentrate on correction of the coagulopathy. Thromb Haemost 1997;77:477-80.

63. Lusher JM. Thrombogenicity associated with factor IX complex concentrates. Semin Hematol 1991;28(Suppl 6):3-5.

64. Blatt PM, Lundblad RL, Kingdon HS, et al. Thrombogenic materials in prothrombin complex concentrates. Ann Intern Med 1974;81:766-70.

65. Ginsburg D, Roberts HR, High KA. Hemophilia and von Willebrand disease. In: McArthur JR, Schechter GP, Platt OS, Bajus JL, eds. Hematology—1997. Seattle: University of Washington, 1997:29-45.

66. Kearon C, Hirsh J. Management of anticoagulation before and after elective surgery. N Engl J Med 1997;336:1506-11.

67. Perry DJ, Kimball DB. Low-dose vitamin K for excessively anticoagulated prosthetic valve patients. Mil Med 1982;147:836-7.

68. Shetty HGM, Backhouse G, Bentley DP, Routledge PA. Effective reversal of warfarin-induced excessive anticoagulation with low-dose vitamin K₁. Thromb Haemost 1992;67:13-5.

69. Hirsh J, Poller L. The international normalized ratio. A guide to understanding and correcting its problems. Arch Intern Med 1994;154:282-8.

70. Andersen P, Godal HC. Predictable reduction in anticoagulant activity of warfarin by small amounts of vitamin K. Acta Med Scand 1975;198:269-70.

71. British Committee for Standards in Haematology, Contreras M, Ala FA, et al. Guidelines for the use of FFP. Transfusion Med 1992;2:57-63.

72. Marder VJ, Feinstein DI, Francis CW, Colman RW. Consumptive thrombohemorrhagic disorders. In: Colman RW, Hirsh J, Marder VJ, Salzman EW, eds. Hemostasis and thrombosis: Basic principles and clinical practice. 3rd ed. Philadelphia: J.B. Lippincott Company; 1994:1023-63.

73. Oguma Y, Sakuragawa N, Maki M, et al. Clinical effect of low-molecular-weight heparin (Fragmin) on DIC: A multicenter cooperative study in Japan. Thromb Res 1990;59:37-49.

74. Fourrier F, Chopin C, Huart J-J, et al. Double-blind, placebo-controlled trial of antithrombin III concentrates in septic shock with disseminated intravascular coagulation. Chest 1993;104:882-8.

75. Blauhut B, Necek S, Vinazzer H, Bergmann H. Substitution therapy with an antithrombin III concentrate in shock and DIC. Thromb Res 1982;27:271-8.

76. Vinazzer H. Therapeutic use of antithrombin III in shock and disseminated intravascular coagulation. Semin Thromb Hemost 1989;15:347-52.

77. Umeki S, Adachi M, Watanabe M, et al. Gabexate as a therapy for disseminated intravascular coagulation. Arch Intern Med 1988;148:1409-12.

78. Maki M, Terao T, Ikenoue T, et al. Clinical evaluation of antithrombin III concentrate (BI 6.013) for disseminated intravascular co-

agulation in obstetrics. Well-controlled multicenter trial. Gynecol Obstet Invest 1987; 23:230-40.

79. Okajima K, Imamura H, Koga S, et al. Treatment of patients with disseminated intravascular coagulation by protein C. Am J Hematol 1990;33:277-8.

80. Kessler CM, Ludlam CA. The treatment of acquired factor VIII inhibitors: Worldwide experience with porcine factor VIII concentrate. Semin Hematol 1993;30(Suppl 1):22-7.

81. Green D, Rademaker AW, Briët E. A prospective, randomized trial of prednisone and cyclophosphamide in the treatment of patients with factor VIII autoantibodies. Thromb Haemost 1993;70:753-7.

82. Morrison AE, Ludlam CA, Kessler C. Use of porcine factor VIII in the treatment of patients with acquired hemophilia. Blood 1993; 81:1513-20.

83. Lusher JM. Perspectives on the use of factor IX complex concentrates in the treatment of bleeding in persons with acquired factor VIII induction. Am J Med 1991;91(Suppl 5A): 30S-4S.

84. Negrier C, Goudemand J, Sultan Y, et al. Multicenter retrospective study on the utilization of FEIBA in France in patients with factor VIII and factor IX inhibitors. Thromb Haemost 1997;77:1113-9.

85. Lusher JM. Recombinant factor VIIa (NovoSeven) in the treatment of internal bleeding in patients with factor VIII and IX inhibitors. Haemostasis 1996;26(Suppl 1):124-30.

86. Hay CRM, Negrier C, Ludlam CA. The treatment of bleeding in acquired haemophilia with recombinant factor VIIa: A multicentre study. Thromb Haemost 1997;78:1463-7.

87. Naorose-Abidi SM, Bond LR, Chitolie A, Bevan DH. Desmopressin therapy in patients with acquired factor VIII inhibitors (letter). Lancet 1988;1:366.

88. Lottenberg R, Kentro TB, Kitchens CS. Acquired hemophilia. A natural history study of 16 patients with factor VIII inhibitors receiving little or no therapy. Arch Intern Me 1987;147:1077-81.

89. Söhngen D, Specker C, Bach D, et al. A quired factor VIII inhibitors in nonhem philic patients. Ann Hematol 1997;74:8 93.

90. Shaffer LG, Phillips MD. Successful trea ment of acquired hemophilia with oral in munosuppressive therapy. Ann Intern Me 1997;127:206-9.

91. Lian EC-Y, Larcada AF, Chiu AY-Z. Combin tion immunosuppressive therapy after facto VIII infusion for acquired factor VIII inhit tor. Ann Intern Med 1989;110:774-8.

92. Michiels JJ, Hamulyák K, Nieuwenhuis HI et al. Acquired haemophilia A in wome postpartum: Management of bleeding ep sodes and natural history of the factor VIII i hibitor. Eur J Haematol 1997;59:105-9.

93. Schwartz RS, Gabriel DA, Aledort LM, et a A prospective study of treatment of acquire (autoimmune) factor VIII inhibitors wi high-dose intravenous gammaglobuli Blood 1995;86:797-804.

94. Tefferi A, Nichols WL. Acquired von Will brand disease: Concise review of occu rence, diagnosis, pathogenesis, and trea ment. Am J Med 1997;103:536-40.

95. Jakway JL. Acquired von Willebrand's di ease. Hematol Oncol Clin North Am 199 6:1409-19.

96. Rinder MR, Richard RE, Rinder HM. A quired von Willebrand's disease: A conci review. Am J Hematol 1997;54:139-45.

97. Rodeghiero F, Castaman G, Mannucci PN Clinical indications for desmopress (DDAVP) in congenital and acquired von W lebrand disease. Blood Rev 1991;5:155-61.

98. Rodeghiero F, Castaman G, Meyer D, Ma nucci PM. Replacement therapy with viru inactivated plasma concentrates in von W lebrand disease. Vox Sang 1992;62:193-9

99. van Genderen PJJ, Papatsonis DNM Michiels JJ, et al. High-dose intraveno gammaglobulin therapy for acquired vc

Willebrand disease. Postgrad Med J 1994; 70:916-20.

100. Gross S, Traulle C, Capiod JC, et al. Efficacy of high-dose intravenous gammaglobulin in the management of acquired von Willebrand's disease during orthopedic surgery. Br J Haematol 1992;82:170-1.

In: Mintz PD, ed.
Transfusion Therapy: Clinical Principles and Practice
Bethesda, MD: AABB Press, 1999

8

The Use of Blood Components Prior to Invasive Bedside Procedures: A Critical Appraisal

SUNNY DZIK, MD

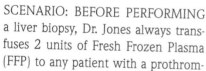 SCENARIO: BEFORE PERFORMING a liver biopsy, Dr. Jones always transfuses 2 units of Fresh Frozen Plasma (FFP) to any patient with a prothrombin time greater than 15 seconds. Dr. Jones will not do a liver biopsy if the platelet count is below 50,000/µL. Comment: *While this approach may not be unusual, little in the medical literature supports the confidence that Dr. Jones places on co-agulation time or platelet count as predictors of bleeding after liver biopsy.*

Scenario: A 1200-gm preterm neonate is given indomethacin to hasten closure of a patent ductus arteriosus. On the second day of life, the infant is suspected of having seizures, and an evaluation reveals an intraventricular hemorrhage. A consultant argues that had a bleeding time been done after the administration of indomethacin, it would have been prolonged and its correction by platelet concentrates would have prevented the bleed. Comment: *This issue has been examined in single- and multicenter studies. The bleeding time did not serve as a guide to identify which infants would develop hemorrhage.*

Scenario: A 60-year-old man in the coronary care unit is recovering from an acute myocardial infarction complicated by left ventricular failure. He has been treated with morphine, aspirin, nitrates, pressors, and afterload-reducing agents, and he has been sustained for 4 days by an intra-aortic counterpulsation balloon pump inserted into his left femoral artery. His balloon pump is about to be removed

Sunny Dzik, MD, Director, Transfusion Medicine, Beth Israel-Deaconess Medical Center, and Assistant Professor of Medicine, Harvard Medical School, Boston, Massachusetts

and his platelet count is 60,000/µL. Platelet concentrates are requested to be given immediately before the balloon pump is removed. Comment: *A better strategy would be to remove the balloon and treat the patient if he demonstrates prolonged bleeding from the wound site. The great majority of patients will not have prolonged bleeding.*

Scenario: A 34-year-old woman with systemic lupus erythematosus is being treated in the medical intensive care unit for suspected sepsis. Her medications include steroids, Plaquenil, broad-spectrum antibiotics, and dopamine. Her platelet count is 30,000/µL, and she requires a central line placement for hemodynamic monitoring and vascular access. The house staff request that the line be placed "under platelet coverage," meaning that it should be inserted while the platelet concentrates are infusing.

The next day, the same woman requires a diagnostic lumbar puncture to evaluate suspected meningitis. The coagulation tests are unchanged. Platelet concentrates are requested again before the procedure because the count is below 50,000/µL. Comment: *There is no evidence that any preprocedure therapy will change the outcome of the central line placement. The concept of "platelet coverage" is probably more fantasy than reality. Literature on the issue of thrombocytopenia and the lumbar puncture is insufficient, and it would be appropriate to honor a request for platelet concentrates before the spinal tap.*

As the above examples illustrate, hemostatic evaluation before a procedure may not correlate with hemorrhage after the procedure. The literature is fairly silent on the value of such testing.[1] Perhaps, the "value" lies in the health-care practitioner's sense of ease if a normal test result is entered into the patient's chart.[2]

Modern medical and surgical therapy rely on a wide variety of invasive bedside procedures. Patients treated in intensive care units are particularly dependent upon such procedures, including advanced cardiovascular monitoring with Swan-Ganz catheters, transbronchial biopsies, endoscopic procedures, invasive radiologic procedures, arterial-venous hemofiltration, dialysis, intra-aortic balloon counterpulsation, and extracorporeal membrane oxygenation. But, while the intensity of bedside invasive procedures has increased, an almost opposite trend has occurred in some surgical specialties, which have shifted from the use of open laparotomy-based procedures to laparoscopic surgical techniques. Thus, the line between minor bedside procedures and more major surgical operative procedures has become less distinct.

Despite these advances, there has been little investigation into the proper preprocedure management of patients with disorders of hemostasis. This is particularly relevant as patients who require multiple invasive procedures are frequently among the most ill in the hospital and often have associated hemostatic disorders resulting from liver disease, multiple medications, nutritional deficiencies, uremia, sepsis, and disseminated intravascular coagulation. Thus, it is not surprising that invasive procedures often must be performed in individuals who have abnormalities of hemostasis documented by laboratory tests. The number of blood components transfused annually in the United States to improve hemostasis before procedures is not reported but is probably considerable. Indeed, it is likely that large numbers of patients are transfused with blood components such as FFP or platelet concentrates before an invasive bedside procedure in order to "treat" abnormalities of hemostasis.

This chapter attempts to identify and critically review the published data concerning the proper hemostatic management of patients undergoing invasive bedside procedures. Three assumptions form the basis for the prophylactic use of blood components before such procedures. One assumption is that abnormal results of commonly used laboratory tests of hemostasis—such as the prothrombin time (PT) and the activated partial thromboplastin time (aPTT)—have *predictive value* to identify patients at risk for bleeding complications during invasive procedures. A second assumption is that blood components administered before procedures are able to correct hemostatic abnormalities. A third assumption is that the correction of hemostatic abnormalities by preprocedure blood components reduces the risk of bleeding at the time of the procedure. Evidence supporting each of these assumptions is reviewed.

Common Laboratory Tests as Predictors of Bleeding

Much of the literature concerning preoperative laboratory tests addresses the predictive value of screening tests performed on a population of patients without known hemostatic defects. Unfortunately, such studies do not specifically address risks for patients with known disorders. However, these studies often include a subgroup of individuals with abnormal hemostasis, whose outcomes may provide useful information. More pertinent are retrospective studies that examine outcomes among a cohort of patients with known abnormalities of hemostasis. Finally, a few prospective studies have investigated outcomes of patients with abnormal hemostasis who undergo procedures.

A basic approach to the analysis of these studies is to define the sensitivity and the predictive value of an abnormal test result. Bleeding is defined as the primary outcome. This may be any form of bleeding (including a simple hematoma) or more substantial bleeding that requires the transfusion of Red Blood Cells. With the use of a simple 2×2 cell, the number of patients with or without an abnormal test result and with or without bleeding can be recorded (see Fig 8-1). According to this approach, the *sensitivity* of any given "cutoff" value for a test of hemostatic function is the percentage of patients with bleeding who also had an abnormal test result. The *predictive value of an abnormal test result* is the percentage of patients with an abnormal test result who bled. Receiver operating characteristics (ROCs) can be used to compare the utility of different tests. With ROC analysis, the cutoff point that defines an abnormal test result is changed throughout the range of values and the corresponding sensitivity and specificity of the test as an indicator of bleeding at each value are determined. The resulting data points are plotted on a standard graph shown in Fig 8-2.

	Bleeding	No bleeding
Abnormal coag	a	b
Normal coag	c	d

Sensitivity = a/(a+c)

Specificity = d/(b+d)

Predictive value of an abnormal test=a/(a+b)

Predictive value of a normal test=d/(c+d)

Figure 8-1. Determining the sensitivity and predictive value of hemostatic tests. After a clinical study defined "bleeding" and the cutoff value for an abnormal test result, the predictive value of that cutoff can be determined as shown.

Bleeding Time

Not so long ago, the template bleeding time was used to predict the risk of bleeding at the time of surgery. Bleeding times were part of the routine

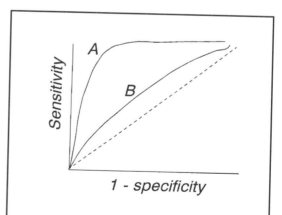

Figure 8-2. Idealized receiver operating curves (ROCs). The sensitivity and (1 − specificity) are plotted for each test over a range of values. The dotted line represents a test with no informative value. The farther away from this line of identity, the more informative the test. The ROC curve of test "A" shows it to be of much greater value than test "B."

preoperative screen done before major surgical procedures, and millions of tests were done yearly in the United States. Patients with prolonged bleeding times were evaluated and might have elective surgery postponed if the prolonged bleeding time was caused by a correctable problem such as aspirin ingestion. Patients facing more urgent surgery would be given platelet concentrate transfusions during surgery as a response to the identified prolonged bleeding time. However, in the late 1980s, a series of papers challenged the view that a prolonged bleeding time was predictive of hemorrhage at surgery. These papers identified that the template bleeding time was originally developed as a method of measuring platelet function and not of predicting bleeding.

In an article by Burns and Lawrence,[3] the clinical utility of a preprocedure bleeding time is questioned. The authors point out numerous technical problems with the reproducibility of the test. Moreover, they note that some studies have found that the skin bleeding time did not correlate with the time of bleeding from other sites. For example, an interesting study of patients taking aspirin noted that the time in which the gastric mucosa bled after biopsy was not affected by aspirin, even though aspirin prolonged the skin bleeding time.[4] This latter study argues against those programs that routinely offer transfusions of platelet concentrates to patients who present with gastrointestinal bleeding and a history of aspirin ingestion. Burns and Lawrence review a number of studies in which the bleeding time was found not to be predictive of the risk of hemorrhage at the time of surgery. These include studies of patients taking aspirin or nonsteroidal anti-inflammatory drugs (NSAIDs), patients with liver disease or myeloproliferative disorders, and patients undergoing cardiac surgery or general surgery.[3] For example, Barber et al[5] studied outcomes among 110 patients with prolonged bleeding times who were identified during the preoperative screening of 1941 patients. Among those 110 patients, there was no correlation between the bleeding time and the estimated blood loss during surgery.

An authoritative review by Lind[6] in 1991 further demonstrates the lack of predictive value of a prolonged bleeding time test. Lind's review of the literature highlights 13 separate reports that question the predictive value of such a test. These studies include a prospective trial by Weksler et al,[7] who administered aspirin to 23 patients the evening before cardiac surgery and documented a prolongation in the bleeding time but found no increase in chest tube drainage or blood transfusion requirements compared with the effects in 26 control subjects. Analogous studies were reported for orthopedic surgery patients taking aspirin[8] and for urologic surgery patients taking ticlopidine.[9]

Nevertheless, studies demonstrate that the bleeding time test is not without any residual merit. In patients with abnormal hemostasis who are undergoing a diagnostic evaluation, the bleeding time can serve to examine the first phase of hemostasis, including platelet adhesion, aggregation, and the formation of a platelet plug. The test remains valuable in the diagnosis and evaluation of patients with von Willebrand's syndrome and platelet storage pool disease.[10] It also can be used to document response to DDAVP (desmopressin) or cryoprecipitate in patients with uremia. The major point of the critical reappraisal of the bleeding time test in the late 1980s was that the test was *not predictive of significant* bleeding at the time of an invasive procedure. Thus, therapeutic maneuvers designed to respond to an abnormal bleeding time are considered not clinically useful. By the mid-1990s, the test dropped from the horizon of preoperative screening tests.

Prothrombin Time; Activated Partial Thromboplastin Time; Platelet Count

Whereas hematologists and surgeons have been quick to drop reliance on the bleeding time as a predictor of hemorrhage and while numerous studies have shown that the PT or aPTT do not serve as useful screening tests for predicting blood loss at surgery, many clinicians continue to make decisions regarding transfusion prior to bedside procedures on the basis of results of the PT, aPTT, and platelet count. While common sense would suggest that patients with thrombocytopenia or elevated coagulation times are at increased risk for bleeding at the time of bedside procedures, there is very little literature to demonstrate a correlation between the degree of abnormality of the laboratory test results and the likelihood of procedure-related hemorrhage. This lack of a strong correlation may relate to the fact that technical mishaps may dominate the cause of procedure-related bleeding, and that the PT and aPTT assays are not able to predict the risk of hemorrhage.

At least four different problems have been found regarding the usefulness of the PT and aPTT. First, the tests are not standardized and not linearly related to the degree of abnormality of hemostasis (see Fig 8-3). Second, reagent sensitivity and reagent stability for the PT and aPTT cause a range of problems with assay performance. As a result, factor levels required to prolong the aPTT can vary from 25-40% of normal.[11] Third, the tests are known to overestimate deficiencies in the upper limb of the cascade and underestimate deficiencies in the lower limb. Fourth, while hemostasis depends on a complex interrelationship between the blood vessel wall, cellular elements of the blood, platelet number and function, fibrin formation, and fibrinolysis, the PT and aPTT examine only fibrin formation in response to an artificial stimulus. Thus, as useful as these assays have been to classify disorders of fibrin formation, they cannot be relied on to reflect with accuracy overall in-vivo hemostasis.

Estimation of the concentration of residual coagulation factors based on the result of the PT or aPTT is certainly inexact. In a clever series of in-vitro mixing-study experiments, Burns et al[12] demonstrated that plasma samples containing 50% activity of a single factor and 100% activity of all other factors (yielding 75% activity of the single deficient factor) had a normal PT and aPTT. However, when two-factor–deficient plasma samples were combined with normal plasma samples such that the resulting mixture contained 75% activity of two coagulation factors and 100% of the rest, the resulting PT and aPTT were prolonged. These results indi-

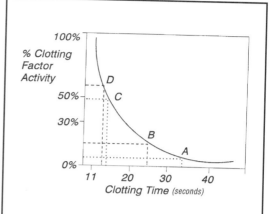

Figure 8-3. General relationship between coagulation time and concentration of coagulation factors. For the patient represented at point "A," a 2-unit Fresh Frozen Plasma (FFP) transfusion that increases the concentration of factors by 10% to point "B" has a dramatic effect on the coagulation time (35-25 seconds). For the patient represented at point "C," a 2-unit FFP transfusion that increases the concentration of factors to point "D" has a trivial impact on the coagulation time (14-13.7 seconds).

cate that prolongations of the PT and aPTT in disorders of coagulation that affect multiple factors (such as hemodilution, liver disease, and therapeutic anticoagulation) represent less of a reduction in factor levels than is generally appreciated or predicted on the basis of widely used information obtained from isolated coagulation deficiencies.

Even in the setting where very minimal blood loss is undesirable, the predictive value of an abnormal hemostatic test result is poor. For example, in a prospective study of 139 patients undergoing cataract extraction, 10.8% of all patients developed hyphemas. Using any abnormality of the PT, aPTT, platelet count, or bleeding time as a predictor of bleeding resulted in an aggregate sensitivity of 30% and a positive predictive value of 18%.[13] For the individual tests, the positive predictive values were as follows: PT was 11%, aPTT was 12%, platelet count was 0%, and bleeding time was 18%.

Very little literature exists to support the notion that transfusing FFP or platelet concentrates to address mild to moderate abnormalities of hemostatic test results will have any impact on the frequency of procedure-related bleeding. When considering the potential value (or lack thereof) of 2 units of FFP administered before a bedside procedure to a patient with an abnormal PT or aPTT, it is essential to review the relationship between the measured coagulation time and the concentration of coagulation factors. An idealized graph of this relationship is shown in Fig 8-3. The relationship is nonlinear. Because the volume of distribution of different coagulation factors varies, the intravascular concentration of different coagulation factors after transfusion ranges from approximately 40-100%. As a result, the transfusion of 2 units of FFP has a variable effect on the residual concentration of clotting factor proteins. As an average estimate in a 70-kg recipient, 2 units of FFP would be expected to increase the concentration of coagulation factors by 10% (5-15%). As shown in Fig 8-3, when the pretransfusion PT is longer than 30 seconds, a 10% increase in coagulation factors will have a dramatic effect on the PT. However, when the pretransfusion PT is below 16 seconds, a 10% increase in coagulation factors will have a trivial impact on the measured PT. This fact is critically important to an understanding of why FFP transfusions given to address mild to moderate prolongation of the PT are probably ineffective.

Other Tests of Hemostasis

Thromboelastography (TEG) is a widely used bedside measure of hemostasis. However, there is no consensus in the literature on its utility as a predictor of bleeding during surgery.[14] In a prospective and controlled trial among coronary bypass patients, Mongan and Hosking[15] report that among 29 individuals with an abnormal TEG-maximal amplitude (TEG-MA) (<50 mm), the 16 patients who received placebo had significantly greater mediastinal chest tube drainage (1352 mL) than the placebo-treated patients with a TEG-MA greater than 50 mm (865 mL). The subgroup with an ab-

normal TEG-MA also received a greater number of transfusions, and those in the subgroup who received desmopressin had less chest tube drainage than those who were not given desmopressin. However, TEG was found to be of no predictive value in a separate study of patients undergoing coronary artery bypass surgery.[16]

HemoSTATUS (Medtronic, Inc, Parker, CO) is a device in which the activated clotting time (ACT) is measured in the presence of platelet activating factor. The platelet-ACT assay was designed to provide additional information on the functional capacity of platelets in hemostasis. In an initial study, the platelet-ACT test was evaluated in 150 patients undergoing cardiac surgery.[17] The test results showed some correlation ($R^2 = 0.65$) with the cumulative chest tube drainage in the first 4 postoperative hours. ROC curves for the platelet-ACT were similar to those for the bleeding time. However, the results of this trial could not be repeated in a subsequent study of the predictive values of the platelet-ACT, the TEG, and routine hemostatic tests performed in 200 patients undergoing cardiopulmonary bypass.[18] ROCs were used to evaluate the performance of the tests to identify more than 200 mL of chest tube blood loss in the first 4 hours in the intensive care unit. Both the platelet-ACT and the TEG-MA measurement correlated only very weakly with 4-hour mediastinal blood loss (platelet-ACT, $R^2 = 0.09$; TEG-MA, $R^2 = 0.1$). ROCs were most favorable for the TEG-MA. There was no correlation between post-protamine platelet-ACT values and the blood transfusion requirement. The performance characteristics of the tests are shown in Table 8-1.

Specific Bedside Procedures

Central Venous Catheter Insertion

Central venous catheters are often inserted in patients who are thrombocytopenic, and this may lead to requests for platelet concentrate transfusions or FFP prior to performing the procedure. Complications of central venous catheter place-

Table 8-1. Test Characteristics for Predicting More Than 200 ML/Hour Chest Tube Blood Loss for 4 Hours

Test	Cutoff value	Sensitivity (%)	Specificity (%)	Positive predictive value (%)	Negative predictive value (%)
PT	15 seconds	67	83	17	96
aPTT	45 seconds	67	76	15	95
Platelet count	100,000/µL	83	66	12	95
Platelet-ACT	70%	67	72	12	95
TEG-MA	44 mm	83	79	23	97

PT = prothrombin time; aPTT = activated partial thromboplastin time; ACT = activated clotting time; TEG-MA = thromboelastography-maximal amplitude.

Positive predictive value is the percentage of patients with a test result more abnormal than the cutoff who bled. Negative predictive value is the percentage of patients with a test result better than the cutoff who did not bleed. Cutoffs were selected to maximize sensitivity and specificity.

ment are unusual and include pneumothorax, air embolus, and bleeding. Most episodes of significant bleeding and hemothorax following subclavian vein catheterization appear to be due to the inadvertent puncture of the subclavian artery in a patient with normal hemostasis rather than to uncontrolled bleeding in a patient with abnormalities.[19]

The need for central venous catheters in patients undergoing orthotopic liver transplantation represents an excellent clinical model with which to explore the relationship between bleeding complications and abnormal preprocedure hemostatic test results. Liver failure patients are a particularly informative population because of the severity and complexity of their abnormalities. Foster et al[20] report results on 202 central venous catheter insertions performed on 40 liver transplant patients with severe hemostatic abnormalities typical of end-stage liver disease. No attempts were made to correct laboratory abnormalities before the procedure. Approximately equal numbers of internal jugular and subclavian insertions were performed. The mean PT activity was 29% of normal

(range=10-39%), the mean aPTT was 92 seconds (range=78-100 seconds), and the mean platelet concentration was 47,000/µL (range=8,000-79,000/µL). Despite these values and the lack of any preprocedure therapy, no serious bleeding complications occurred. One nonhemorrhagic complication that did occur, however, was the inadvertent insertion of the catheter into the subclavian artery. Yet, this paper provides rather striking evidence that central catheter placement by experienced individuals can be performed safely in patients with severe hemostatic defects. In a separate study, Goldfarb and Lebrec[21] report only one hematoma among 1000 attempts at catheterization of the internal jugular vein among patients with significant hemostatic abnormalities undergoing transvenous liver biopsy.

Additional experience with central venous catheter placement in patients with thrombocytopenia or prolongation of the PT and/or aPTT was reported by Doerfler et al.[22] Outcomes were reported among 76 consecutive patients with abnormalities of hemostasis who received 104 central catheters. The patients were ill with a variety of different disorders as seen in intensive care units. Most of the catheter insertions (80%) were subclavian. Seventy-three percent of the patients had platelet counts of less than 100,000/μL. The distribution of insertions was as follows: 22 catheters were placed in patients with platelet counts of 50,000-100,000/μL, 30 catheters were placed in patients with platelet counts of 20,000-50,000/μL, and 11 catheters were placed in patients with platelet counts below 20,000/μL. Thirteen percent of patients had a combination of thrombocytopenia and prolongation of the PT and/or aPTT. These included a patient with a PT of 22.6 seconds, an aPTT above 100 seconds, and a platelet count of 45,000/μL, and a patient with a PT of 15 seconds and a platelet count of 18,000/μL. None of the patients was given transfusions of platelet concentrates or FFP before the procedure to treat the abnormalities of hemostasis; none had serious complications, intrathoracic bleeding, or an unexpected drop in hematocrit. Bleeding occurred in seven individuals and consisted of minor bleeding from the skin suture site in five patients and small (2- to 3-cm), periosteal hematomas of the clavicle in two. All seven patients with these minor bleeding complications had thrombocytopenia ranging from 6,000/μL to 37,000/μL. Yet, most patients with platelet counts in this range did not have even minor bleeding.

Petersen[23] reported results on 516 consecutive patients with internal jugular cannulations performed by anesthesiologists before cardiac surgery. Of these, 252 (49%) were anticoagulated with heparin before surgery, with a target aPTT of 1.5 times control. Central lines were placed within 15 minutes of stopping the heparin, while the patients were still systemically anticoagulated. An observer who was unaware of the anticoagulation status of each patient recorded the presence of an insertion site hematoma. Of the 22 hematomas that occurred, 13 were in anticoagulated patients and 9 were in nonanticoagulated persons. This difference was not significant. No patient's hematoma required drainage or transfusion. There were 22 inadvertent punctures of a carotid artery, 12 in anti-

coagulated patients and 10 in nonanticoagulated patients. Of these 22 arterial punctures, 7 developed hematomas—4 in anticoagulated patients and 3 in nonanticoagulated patients. This large retrospective review found no evidence for hemorrhagic complications of central line placement in anticoagulated patients when performed by an experienced operator.

In 1996, DeLoughery et al[24] reported on an even larger series of patients. They reviewed hemostatic data and bedside transfusion practices on 490 intensive care patients in whom 938 central lines were placed. The study design included adults treated in medical, cardiac, and surgical intensive care units. Most lines were placed in the surgical units, and only 15% were placed in medical patients. Half the lines were radial arterial catheters, 30% were central venous catheters, and 20% were pulmonary artery catheters. At least one hemostatic defect was noted in 388 (41%) line placements, although many of these defects were mild. Patients with more marked hemostatic abnormalities were treated with preprocedure blood components as requested by the clinical staff and not according to any common protocol. Hemostatic tests were not checked after preprocedure treatment to verify any form of correction. For the purpose of the study, the authors developed a hemostatic "score" ranging from 0 (normal) to 15 (worst) to evaluate combinations of laboratory abnormalities. Several patients had marked defects in hemostasis. Forty patients had a PT of 18-24 seconds and nine had a PT of more than 24 seconds. Ninety-four patients had an aPTT of more than 48 seconds, and 65 patients had a platelet count below 50,000/μL; 39 of these patients had counts below 20,000/μL. Thirty patients had a creatinine above 14 mg/dL. For 57 patients, a mean of six blood components was given before the procedure. Bleeding occurred in 16 patients (3%), but 10 of these bleeding incidents involved minor skin oozing at the site of the catheter, which was treated with dressing changes and no transfusions. Three patients developed hematomas at the site of insertion. Two patients (0.4%) developed a hemothorax. One patient had a hemostatic defect score of 9 and the other had a score of only 3. There were too few significant bleeds to correlate with any single laboratory abnormality or with combinations of abnormalities as defined by the hemostatic score. When all forms of bleeding were considered (including minor skin bleeding), the incidence of bleeding was significantly higher on the medical service (9%) than on the surgical (0.6%) or trauma service (1.4%). In addition, a significantly higher proportion of medical patients was given preprocedure transfusions of coagulation factors. While the score was nonpredictive for patients on the surgical service, the risk of any form of bleeding (including minor skin bleeding) on the medical service increased with an increasing score. However, an analysis of multiple cutoff points for abnormal laboratory test results did not reveal any threshold associated with a high predictive value for bleeding.

Several interesting insights emerge from this report. While 41% of the patients demonstrated some form of hemostatic abnormality, preprocedure transfusions were given to only one-third of these patients, and the incidence of bleeding complications in this group was no lower than it was in the other patients. The use of preprocedure transfusions and the incidence of minor bleeding events were far more common on the medical service. The authors interpret their findings to suggest that for many patients, the risk of bleeding relates more directly to the technical skill of the individual doing the line insertion than to the patient's hemostatic status, and that preprocedure transfusions may not reverse that risk.

Other studies have directly documented that the technical skill of the person inserting the catheter appears to be more important than the preprocedure laboratory tests. In one review of more than 700 central line procedures, complication rates were twice as high among inexperienced physicians than among experienced ones.[25]

Liver Biopsy

For a number of reasons, liver biopsy represents an important clinical setting for the evaluation of prophylactic transfusions prior to procedures. First, a large proportion of liver biopsies are done on patients with abnormalities of the PT, aPTT, and platelet count. Second, patients with liver disease are known to have multiple different derangements of hemostasis, including those not measured in routine testing, and therefore represent a "worst case" clinical study group. Third, the procedure is done frequently in a "blind" fashion in that no techniques are used to avoid puncturing large hepatic vessels and no opportunity exists for direct compression of bleeding vessels after the procedure. Fourth, sensitive studies using ultrasound analysis have detected small intrahepatic hematomas in as many as one-quarter of the patients who undergo a liver biopsy.[26] For these reasons, it is not surprising that the guidelines for preprocedure hemostatic values are often more conservative for this procedure than for others. Some programs will not perform closed biopsies on patients with certain locally determined abnormalities of hemostatic screening tests and therefore resort to open biopsy, transvenous biopsy, laparoscopic biopsy,[27] or biopsy followed by gelfoam plugging.[28] Nevertheless, several very informative studies have attempted to identify whether the preprocedure laboratory values can serve as predictors of hemorrhage at the time of liver biopsy.

An early report by Sharma et al[29] raises caution regarding liver biopsies in patients with thrombocytopenia. They studied 87 patients undergoing percutaneous liver biopsy after allogeneic marrow transplantation. Of the three patients who developed intraperitoneal bleeding, two required surgery for ligation of a bleeding vessel. The three patients who bled each had a preprocedure platelet count below 60,000/μL, yet ten additional patients with the same preprocedure platelet count did not bleed (predictive value of 23%). Of interest, two of the three patients who bled were given preprocedure platelet concentrate transfusions to prevent bleeding.

A unique study was reported by Ewe,[30] who performed liver biopsies using a Menghini needle (with 1.8-mm) under direct vision through a laparoscope inserted into the abdomen. After the liver biopsy was taken, the authors measured the number of seconds during which the capsule of the liver was observed to be bleeding into the abdominal cavity; this latter value was referred to as the "liver bleeding time." Two hundred consecutive patients who had a variety of liver ailments including fatty liver, cirrhosis, and metastatic liver disease were studied. No patient carried the diagnosis of primary hepatocellular carcinoma, which is a vascular lesion presumably at greater risk for bleeding. During the study period, no patient was excluded on the basis of preprocedure laboratory test results (PT, platelet count, whole blood clotting time), nor were patients treated with blood components before the procedure. The results showed no correlation between the length of time the liver bled after puncture and the preprocedure laboratory values (see Figs 8-4 and 8-5).[30] Three patients had prolonged bleeding (>15 minutes) after the procedure; these included two patients with a PT of 18.5

seconds (50% activity) and one patient with a PT of 13.5 seconds (100% activity). Platelet counts in these three patients ranged from 50,000 to 150,000/μL. Patients with more markedly prolonged PTs and/or with more markedly depressed platelet counts did not bleed excessively. Multiple logistic regression analysis found no correlation between liver bleeding time and any other variables, including the length of the biopsy cylinder and the underlying disease of the patient.

Lack of evidence for increased bleeding after percutaneous liver biopsy in patients with mild abnormalities of hemostasis was reported by McVay and Toy.[31] These authors reviewed the medical records of 177 patients with a PT or an aPTT at 1.0-1.5 times the midrange normal or with platelet counts of 50,000-100,000/μL. Of these patients, 76 had abnormal PTs, 74 had abnormal aPTTs, 20 had thrombocytopenia, and 7 had incomplete data. Bi-

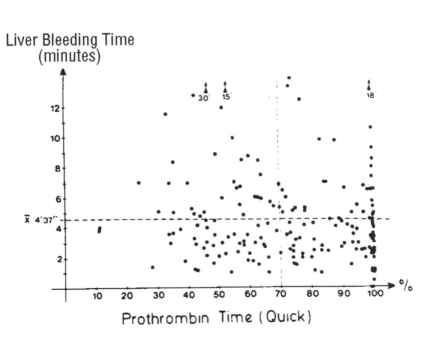

Figure 8-4. Lack of relationship between liver bleeding after biopsy and the preprocedure prothrombin time (PT). The minutes in which the liver was observed to bleed after biopsy are plotted as a function of the percentage of activity of the PT. Used with permission from Ewe.[30]

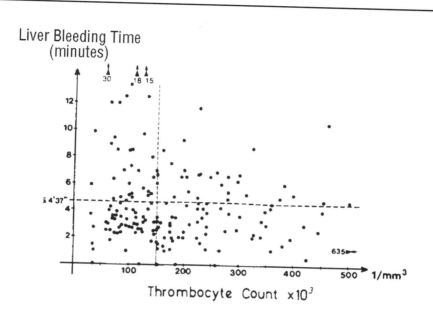

Figure 8-5. Lack of relationship between liver bleeding after biopsy and the preprocedure platelet count. The minutes in which the liver was observed to bleed after biopsy are plotted as a function of the platelet count. Used with permission from Ewe.[30]

opsies were done with either a standard needle (n=155) or a fine needle (n=22). Pre- and postprocedure hemoglobin levels, transfusion records, and review of the medical record were used to identify patients who bled. No patient received FFP or platelet concentrates before the procedure. Procedure-related bleeding was defined as clinical evidence or a 2 g/dL or greater drop in hemoglobin after the procedure. Eight patients (4.5%) bled by these criteria, and 6 (3.4%) were treated with transfusion of Red Blood Cells. Four units of Red Blood Cells were transfused to a 32-year-old woman with a hepatoma, a PT of 13.0 seconds, an aPTT of 38.8 seconds, and a platelet count of 114,000/μL. Six units of Red Blood Cells were transfused to a 65-year-old man with multiple myeloma, a PT of 11.2 seconds, an aPTT of 30.9 seconds, and a platelet count of 16,000/μL. The proportion of patients who bled was not significantly different among those with normal values than among those with mild abnormalities as defined in the study (stated above). When other patient factors were analyzed, the presence of malignancy was seen as an independent risk factor for bleeding complications.

A subsequent report by Caturelli et al[32] evaluated outcomes in patients with more severe abnormalities who underwent percutaneous liver biopsy using a fine needle. The authors report a retrospective study of outcomes among 85 patients with platelet counts below 50,000/μL and/or PTs below 50% of normal activity who received ultrasound-guided fine-needle percutaneous liver biopsies. Each patient received multiple punctures for sampling, and, therefore, the study involved 229 punctures. No patient received any preprocedural FFP or platelet concentrate transfusions; no patient developed signs of bleeding. Abdominal ultrasound studies done within 6 hours of the biopsy showed no evidence of intrahepatic or subcapsular hematoma, no hemoperitoneum, and no he-matomas of the abdominal wall.

Renal Biopsy

Many patients in need of a renal biopsy have acute renal failure and may have the platelet dysfunction associated with uremia. This may be suggested by a long bleeding time, but a normal bleeding time does not ensure normal hemostasis or predict an absence of hemorrhagic complications. The use of DDAVP would seem particularly appropriate as a preprocedure therapy to improve hemostasis, as the drug is known to improve hemostasis in most patients with uremia.

Davis and Chandler[33] studied the predictive value of hemostatic tests prior to biopsy of renal transplants. Bleeding times, PT, aPTT, platelet count, and TEG were performed before allograft bi-opsies in 120 patients. Test results were considered abnormal if they were outside the reference range. Bleeding was defined as a drop of four or more points of the hematocrit or as ultrasound evidence of a perirenal hematoma. Overall, 21% of patients showed evidence of mild bleeding, two showed evidence of hematoma on ultrasound, and none re-quired transfusion for bleeding. Eighty percent of the bleeding patients had normal test results before the biopsy. Of the various tests done, the highest positive predictive value was seen with the angle of the TEG. A weakness of this study is that the number of patients with moderate to severe abnor-malities was very limited. Various other studies have examined the risk of bleeding after kidney bi-opsy and have not found a high predictive value to preprocedure laboratory testing.

Among patients whose renal disease is compli-cated by cirrhosis, there may be even greater con-cern over bleeding risk from a closed renal biopsy. Jouet et al[34] report their experience with 70 pa-tients with cirrhosis and clotting disorders who un-derwent transjugular renal biopsies. Elevated PT was noted in 31 cases (mean=19 seconds; range=12-35 seconds); low platelet count in 19 cases (mean=152,000 µL; range=34,000-420,000/µL); and long bleeding time in 60 cases.

Two patients developed a cervical hematoma re-quiring no additional treatment. Perirenal he-matomas were noted in nine patients; five of these hematomas were clinically insignificant and seen only on ultrasound while the other four were clini-cally significant. Of these four, two were treated with blood transfusions. Four patients had macro-scopic hematuria, one of whom required blood transfusion. This study showed very little hemor-rhagic morbidity at the site of central line insertion. Some patients bled from the renal biopsy site; how-ever, the authors noted that the incidence of bleed-ing complications among these patients with pre-procedure hemostatic abnormalities was no greater than that reported in other series of patients with normal preprocedure evaluation.

Thoracentesis and Paracentesis

Given the low likelihood of any vascular trauma with either of these two bedside procedures, it would not be expected that any form of preproce-dure blood component therapy would be of value. Nevertheless, some physicians may wish to trans-fuse blood components to patients with laboratory abnormalities who are about to undergo bedside thoracentesis. To address this issue, McVay and Toy[35] performed a retrospective review of out-comes in 608 consecutive procedures (391 para-centeses, 207 thoracenteses, and 10 both procedures). The procedures were done in a wide range of hospitalized patients, including those with AIDS, liver cirrhosis, malignancy, renal failure, heart failure, and infection. Pre- and postprocedure hemoglobin levels, transfusion records, and the medical record notes were reviewed to identify pa-tients with bleeding complications. Patients were excluded from the record review if laboratory tests were not obtained or if the patient was actively bleeding. None of the patients was given prophy-lactic FFP infusions before the procedure. The overall frequency of bleeding complications requir-ing red cell transfusions was very low (0.2%). No significant difference was seen in the proportion of procedures with an accompanying hemoglobin de-crease of 2 g/dL or more, or in the average hemoglobin values among patients with a normal PT and/or aPTT compared with those with a prolonged PT and/or aPTT. Nor were any significant differences in hemoglobin changes observed in patients with platelet counts above 100,000/μL compared with those with counts of 50,000-100,000/μL or of 25,000-50,000/μL. Hemoglobin changes among 87 patients with a combined decrease in platelet count and prolongation of the PT or aPTT were no different from those among patients with normal values. Further analysis revealed that a small subgroup of 11 patients with a markedly elevated creatinine (6-14 mg/dL) had a significantly greater (p=0.01) average hemoglobin loss (0.8 g/dL) than the 450 patients with a normal serum creatinine (0.1 g/dL). Only one patient required a red cell transfusion for bleeding associated with the procedure, and this patient had a normal aPTT, platelet count, and creatinine and only a mildly elevated PT (1.3 midrange normal).

Frequently, patients with end-stage liver failure and hemostatic abnormalities are managed with large-volume paracentesis to temporarily address any problems of ascites and volume overload. Webster et al[36] reported a retrospective analysis of 179 outpatients undergoing large-volume paracentesis and reviewed the literature on hemorrhagic complications of large-volume abdominal paracentesis. A total of four patients developed intra-abdominal or abdominal wall bleeding that required a transfusion of red cells. The PTs of the four patients who bled were 14 seconds, 14.5 seconds, 15.2 seconds, and 17 seconds. These values were no different from those found in the 175 patients who did not bleed.

Gastrointestinal Endoscopy and Biopsy

As is widely known to gastroenterologists, most bleeding from the gastrointestinal tract stems from a mucosal lesion or vascular abnormality. Significant gastrointestinal bleeding attributed solely to hemostatic defects is unusual. Nevertheless, transfusions may be requested for patients with abnormal hemostatic test results prior to endoscopic procedures. In some facilities, transfusion of platelet concentrates may be requested to "correct" the platelet defect induced by recent ingestion of aspirin or NSAIDs. The impact of such drugs was addressed in a study by Shiffman et al.[37] Of 694 patients who underwent either upper endoscopy with biopsy or colonoscopy with biopsy or polypectomy, half had recently taken either aspirin or NSAIDs. The incidence of bleeding in this group was compared with that among the half who had not taken either aspirin or NSAIDs. A total of 32 patients bled. Minor bleeding requiring no therapy was more common in the group taking NSAIDs (6%) than among those on no medication (2%). Serious bleeding requiring hospitalization or treatment occurred in four patients who had polypectomies—two taking aspirin or NSAIDs and two not taking medications. Thus, the overall risk of significant gastrointestinal bleeding after endoscopic biopsy was small (<1%), and the risk of serious hemorrhage was not affected by the use of aspirin or NSAIDs.

Epidural Anesthesia; Lumbar Puncture

Because bleeding in the closed space of the subarachnoid or epidural region can produce paraparesis or paraplegia following lumbar puncture, caution should be exercised when doing procedures in patients with hemostatic abnormalities. There are no prospective trials evaluating the risk of spinal hematomas in such patients. The overall incidence of paraparesis or paraplegia following epidural or spinal anesthesia is very low,[38] and most episodes have been attributed to chemical irritation or spinal ischemia rather than to bleeding.[39] Owens et al[38] found 33 cases of spinal hematoma in the literature, most of which involved either thrombocytopenia (range=1000-44,000/μL) or therapeutic anticoagulation.

Waldman et al[40] used a small (25-gauge) needle to administer morphine via a caudal block to 19 thrombocytopenic patients without neurologic complications. The patients' platelet counts were all below 50,000/μL. Rasmus et al[41] reported that none of 14 thrombocytopenic women (platelet counts=15,000-100,000/μL) who received epidural anesthesia at the time of childbirth developed any problems. His review of the literature found no cases of spinal or epidural hematomas in women giving birth. Hew-Wing et al[42] reviewed the literature on the issue of epidurals and thrombocytopenia and could find no case report of a thrombocytopenic patient who developed a hematoma after epidural anesthesia. They did identify a report of eight cases of spinal subdural hematoma among leukemia patients who had received diagnostic lumbar punctures.[43] The authors stated that the belief that epidural anesthesia is contraindicated among patients with fewer than 100,000 platelets/μL has no supporting data.

Rao and El-Etr[44] reported on the incidence of neurologic complications in the setting of low-dose systemic anticoagulation immediately following placement of an epidural catheter in 3164 patients or of a subarachnoid catheter in 847 patients. Patients received spinal anesthesia with a 17-gauge needle prior to systemic low-dose anticoagulation for vascular surgery. The mean heparin dose was 10,500 units per 24 hours. Catheters were left in the spinal space during the operation for 24 hours and after transfer to the recovery care unit; they were then removed while patients were still being treated with heparin. No patients developed peridural hematomas. However, Ruff and Dougherty[45] note five cases of paraplegia among 342 patients who received a diagnostic lumbar puncture and then were given systemic heparin (dose not stated). The literature on lumbar puncture and spinal anesthesia is not sufficient to draw strong conclusions.

Pulmonary Procedures

Special care to provide good hemostasis is prudent when procedures are being done on the oropharynx, trachea, or bronchi, given that excessive bleeding can prove fatal rapidly. A few studies have addressed the potential value of preoperative hemostatic screening prior to tonsillectomy. Kang et al[46] reviewed more than 1000 cases, including 27 children, in whom an abnormality was found in the PT, aPTT, platelet count, or bleeding time. There were 64 episodes of bleeding after the procedure, although most (90%) occurred in patients with normal preoperative hemostatic test results. The sensitivity of any abnormality in results of the four tests was 9%, and the predictive value of an abnormal test result was 22%.

In a recent article, Zwack and Derkay[47] investigated the utility of routine preprocedure PT and aPTT prior to adenotonsillectomy in a large cohort of healthy pediatric patients. Routine hemostatic screening was done among 1750 patients, and selective screening triggered by the patient's history was done in 2624 patients. A total of 38 patients had early or delayed postoperative bleeding that required either a return to the operating room or a delay in discharge. No patient who bled required transfusion. Not surprisingly, the preprocedure hemostatic screening did not predict or correlate with the development of bleeding. While this study documents the lack of predictive value of hemostatic screening prior to adenotonsillectomy in this population, it does not provide primary outcome data on patients undergoing adenotonsillectomy who are known to have abnormal hemostasis.

Kozak and Brath[48] reported on 274 patients undergoing 305 fiberoptic bronchoscopy and biopsy procedures at a tertiary care institution. Prolonged hemostatic studies prior to the procedure are noted in 10% (n=28) of patients. Overall, 35 patients bled, but 32 of these had normal preprocedure hemostatic values. Three patients had severe bleeding and each of them had normal preprocedure test results. The sensitivity of any abnormal hemostatic test result was 8%, and the predictive value of an abnormal test result was 10%. The authors found no utility for prebronchoscopy hemostatic tests. In this study, the number of patients with hemostatic abnormalities was too few to identify low-frequency complications.

Cost-Effectiveness of Prophylactic Components Administered Prior to Bedside Procedures

From the standpoint of blood use and patient exposure to blood components, there is a striking difference between the strategy of *prophylactic use of components* and that of *therapeutic use of components*. For anyone considering these two alternative strategies, it is important to state that there is no evidence in the literature to suggest that a prophylactic strategy is inherently more successful. While the therapeutic transfusion of FFP and platelet concentrates may be of no value in stopping bleeding from a punctured artery (even patients with normal hemostasis will bleed from such local wounds), transfusions given to treat hemostatic abnormalities are expected to be efficacious. The use of a prophylaxis strategy to prevent uncommon bleeding complications requires the transfusion of a large number of patients, the majority of whom would have the same outcome if not transfused.

A comparison of prophylaxis vs therapeutic transfusion strategies for bedside procedures is revealing. For the sake of argument, assume that a typical prophylactic transfusion of 2 units of FFP or 6 units of Platelets is 100% effective in preventing all instances of hemorrhage in patients with a certain degree of hemostatic abnormality—a laboratory value above some threshold. We also can assume that all bleeding complications are exclusively due to hemostatic problems and not to technical mishaps. Under these two assumptions, 200 units of FFP or 600 units of Platelets would be given prophylactically to 100 patients with hemostatic values above the local threshold. This contrasts with a therapeutic transfusion strategy. For example, if each patient has a 5% risk of bleeding in the absence of prophylactic therapy and if the same 200 units of FFP and 600 units of Platelets were distributed to each of the five patients who bleed, then each patient could receive up to 40 units of FFP or up to 120 units of Platelets given therapeutically with equivalent blood usage.

In reality, neither of the above two assumptions is likely to be correct. The extent to which 2 units of FFP or 6 units of Platelets are effective at reversing the risk of bleeding posed by abnormal hemostasis is not known. For the sake of argument, we can assume a 50% success rate. Moreover, the literature amply documents that procedure-related bleeding is not due exclusively to hemostatic ab-

normalities but rather that technical mishaps are the dominant cause of such bleeding episodes. Again, for discussion's sake, we can assume that 80% of all bleeding episodes occurring in patients with abnormal laboratory test results are technical mishaps and that the outcome is not influenced by preprocedure transfusions. Under these two assumptions, the utility of a prophylactic transfusion strategy becomes even less cost-effective compared with that of a therapeutic strategy. The quantity of blood components required to prevent bleeding complications under these latter assumptions is shown in Table 8-2. As shown in the right-hand column of the table, if an equivalent number of components were directed toward a therapeutic strategy, then each patient with a bleeding episode would have access to incredible quantities of therapeutic blood components. The table should be interpreted in light of the studies on central lines among patients undergoing transvenous liver biopsy, which showed a 0.1% risk of bleeding, the studies of thoracentesis and paracentesis in patients with abnormal hemostasis, which showed a 0.2% risk of bleeding, and the studies of liver biopsy patients with abnormal hemostasis, which suggest perhaps a 1.0% risk of bleeding. The literature documents that on the unusual occasions when significant bleeding episodes occur following bedside procedures, the quantity of blood hemorrhaged is replaced by 2-4 units of Red Blood Cells. If viewed from this perspective, a prophylaxis strategy consumes large quantities of blood and exposes large numbers of individuals to transfusion in order to prevent the loss of a small amount of blood.

Recommendations

Prospective, randomized, controlled trials in which patients with similar degrees of abnormal hemostasis are randomly assigned to receive or not receive preprocedure blood components are needed to be able to make firm recommendations on the value of prophylactic transfusions prior to bedside invasive procedures. Given the low incidence of any form of hemorrhagic complications even among patients with known defects, such

Table 8-2. Prophylactic Compared With Therapeutic Blood Component Use

A Risk of bleeding without prophylaxis	B Total no. of bleeders among 10,000 patients	C No. of bleeders owing to technical causes (0.8 of column B)	D No. of bleeders prevented by prophylaxis (0.5 x [B–C])	E No. of patients given prophylactic transfusion without benefit	F No. of therapeutic units available per patient
0.1%	10	8	1	9999	20,000 FFP 60,000 Platelets
1.0%	100	80	10	9990	2000 FFP 6000 Platelets
5.0%	500	400	50	9950	400 FFP 1200 Platelets
10.0%	1000	800	100	9900	200 FFP 600 Platelets

FFP = Fresh Frozen Plasma

studies may need to be multicenter trials in order to accrue a sufficient number of patients to have statistical power. In the absence of such studies, the current literature can serve to suggest some guidelines for the clinical approach to bedside procedures. Some of the published retrospective studies reviewed here include large numbers of patients with documented abnormalities of hemostasis. In particular, the data addressing central venous catheterization would suggest that preprocedure prophylaxis is unlikely to be of any value whatsoever except perhaps in patients with extreme disorders of hemostasis. The literature regarding liver biopsy suggests that most institutions may have developed too conservative a set of guidelines for laboratory parameters prior to this procedure as well. While an important small percentage of patients undergoing liver biopsy bleed and while such bleeding may be severe enough to require surgical intervention, it would appear that the risk of bleeding is more related to the presence of vascular lesions (as found in malignancy) than to laboratory values measured prior to the procedure. Thus, all patients who undergo liver biopsy, including those with normal hemostasis, should be monitored for abdominal pain. Bleeding complications from renal biopsy appear far less often than those from liver biopsy. While the use of DDAVP to improve hemostasis would seem of low risk and of practical value in patients with uremia, a prospective trial of its utility would be welcome. Paracentesis, thoracentesis, or gastrointestinal biopsy appear to be very low-risk procedures, and bleeding complications are not predicted from either laboratory tests or a history of aspirin ingestion. Lumbar space insertions and procedures on the upper airway or bronchi represent events in which excess bleeding may be of greater consequence. There are insufficient data in the literature to promote or disprove the utility of preprocedure blood components for patients with abnormal hemostasis who undergo epidural anesthesia, lumbar punctures, or tracheobronchial procedures. Given the expected predictive value of currently used tests for hemostasis, it is not unreasonable to ignore mild to moderate laboratory abnormalities, nor is it unreasonable to attempt to "correct" moderate to severe defects before such procedures.

When deciding on the clinical approach to a particular patient, clinicians and laboratorians should recognize some of the potent intellectual traps inherent in a prophylactic strategy of blood component use. The decision to transfuse blood components for hemostasis is most defensible when the transfusions are used as a focused therapy for hemorrhage. From the perspective of patient morbidity from transfusion (risk/benefit) as well as of resource usage (cost/benefit), a strategy that uses FFP and platelet concentrates *therapeutically* can justify the aggressive use of blood components to treat bleeding complications. As in the rest of medicine, however, the best decision making is done in the context of the patient's full clinical picture rather than on the basis of laboratory values alone.

References

1. Eika C, Havig O, Godal HC. The value of preoperative haemostatic screening. Scand J Haematol 1978;21:349-54.
2. Suchman AL, Mushlin AI. How well does the activated partial thromboplastin time predict postoperative hemorrhage? JAMA 1986;256:750-3.
3. Burns ER, Lawrence C. Bleeding time: A guide to its diagnostic and clinical utility. Arch Pathol Lab Med 1989;113:1219-24.
4. O'Laughlin JC, Hoftiezer JW, Mahoney JP, Ivey KJ. Does aspirin prolong bleeding from gastric biopsies in man? Gastrointest Endosc 1981;27:1-5.
5. Barber A, Green D, Gailozzo T, Tsao CH. The bleeding time as a preoperative screening test. Am J Med 1985;78:761-4.
6. Lind SE. The bleeding time does not predict surgical bleeding. Blood 1991;77:2547-52.
7. Weksler BB, Pett SB, Alonso D, et al. Differential inhibition by aspirin of vascular and platelet prostaglandin synthesis in atherosclerotic patients. N Engl J Med 1983;308:800-5.

8. Amrein PC, Ellman L, Harris WH. Aspirin induced prolongation of the bleeding time and perioperative blood loss. JAMA 1981;245: 1825-8.

9. Brommer EJ. The effect of ticlopidine upon platelet function, haemorrhage and postoperative thrombosis in patients undergoing suprapubic prostatectomy. J Intern Med Res 1981;9:203-10.

10. Nieuwenhuis HK, Akkerman JW, Sixma JJ. Patients with a prolonged bleeding time and normal aggregation tests may have storage pool deficiency: Studies on one hundred and six patients. Blood 1987;70:620-3.

11. Naghibi F, Yangsook H, Dodds WJ, Lawrence CE. Effects of reagent and instrument on prothrombin times, activated partial thromboplastin times and patient/control ratios. Thromb Haemost 1988;59:455-63.

12. Burns ER, Goldberg SN, Wenz B. Paradoxic effect of multiple mild coagulation factor deficiencies on the prothrombin time and activated partial thromboplastin time. Am J Clin Pathol 1993;100:94-8.

13. Gorman M, Rittersbach GH, Eliason JA, Rosenthal AR. Preoperative prediction of hyphemas. Ophthalmic Surg 1986;17:490-2.

14. Caprini JA, Traverso CI, Walenga JM, et al. Thromboelastography. Semin Thrombst Hemo 1995;21(Suppl 4):1-93.

15. Mongan PD, Hosking MP. The role of desmopressin acetate in patients undergoing coronary artery bypass surgery. Anesthesiology 1992;77:38-46.

16. Dorman H, Spinale FG, Bailey MK, et al. Identification of patients at risk for excessive blood loss during coronary artery bypass surgery: Thromboelastograph versus coagulation screen. Anesth Analg 1993;76:694-700.

17. Despotis GJ, Levine V, Filos K, et al. Evaluation of a new point-of-care test that measures PAF-mediated acceleration of coagulation in cardiac surgical patients. Anesthesiology 1996; 85:1311-25.

18. Ereth MH, Nuttall GA, Klindworth JT, et al. Does the platelet-activated clotting test (HemoSTATUS) predict blood loss and platelet dysfunction associated with cardiopulmonary bypass? Anesth Analg 1997;85:259-64.

19. Vanherweghem JL, Cabolet P, Dhaene M, et al. Complications related to subclavian catheters for hemodialysis. Am J Nephrol 1986;6: 339-43.

20. Foster PF, Moore LR, Sankary HN, et al. Central venous catheterization in patients with coagulopathy. Arch Surg 1992;127:273-5.

21. Goldfarb G, Lebrec D. Percutaneous cannulation of the internal jugular vein in patients with coagulopathies: An experience based on 1,000 attempts. Anesthesiology 1982;56: 321-3.

22. Doerfler ME, Kaufman B, Goldenberg AS. Central venous catheter placement in patients with disorders of hemostasis. Chest 1996;110:185-8.

23. Petersen GA. Does systemic anticoagulation increase the risk of internal jugular vein cannulation? (letter) Anesthesiology 1991;75: 1124.

24. DeLoughery TG, Liebler JM, Simonds V, Goodnight SH. Invasive line placement in critically ill patients: Do hemostatic defects matter? Transfusion 1996;36:827-31.

25. Sznajder JI, Zveibil FR, Bitterman H, et al. Central vein catheterization: Failure and complication rates by three percutaneous approaches. Arch Intern Med 1986;146:259-61.

26. Minuk GY, Sutherland LR, Wiseman DA, et al. Prospective study of the incidence of ultrasound-detected intrahepatic and subcapsular hematomas in patients randomized to 6 or 24 hours of bed rest after percutaneous liver biopsy. Gastroenterology 1987;92:290-3.

27. Iqbal M, Creger RJ, Fox RM, et al. Laparoscopic liver biopsy to evaluate hepatic dysfunction in patients with hematologic malignancies: A useful tool to effect changes in management. Bone Marrow Transplant 1996; 17:655-62.

28. Fandrich CA, Davies RP, Hall PM. Small-gauge gelfoam plug liver biopsy in high-risk

patients: Safety and diagnostic value. Australas Radiol 1996;40:230-4.

29. Sharma S, McDonald GB, Banaji M. The risk of bleeding after percutaneous liver biopsy: Relation to the platelet count. J Clin Gastroenterol 1982;4:451-3.

30. Ewe K. Bleeding after liver biopsy does not correlate with indices of peripheral coagulation. Dig Dis Sci 1981;26:388-93.

31. McVay PA, Toy PTCY. Lack of increased bleeding after liver biopsy in patients with mild hemostatic abnormalities. Am J Clin Pathol 1990;94:747-53.

32. Caturelli E, Squillante MM, Andriulli A, et al. Fine-needle liver biopsy in patients with severely impaired coagulation. Liver 1993;13: 270-3.

33. Davis CL, Chandler WL. Thromboelastography for the prediction of bleeding after transplant renal biopsy. J Am Soc Nephrol 1995;6: 1250-5.

34. Jouet P, Meyrier A, Mal F, et al. Transjugular renal biopsy in the treatment of patients with cirrhosis and renal abnormalities. Hepatology 1996;24:1143-7.

35. McVay PA, Toy PTCY. Lack of increased bleeding after paracentesis and thoracentesis in patients with mild coagulation abnormalities. Transfusion 1991;31:164-71.

36. Webster ST, Brown KL, Luchey MR, Nostrant TT. Hemorrhagic complications of large-volume abdominal paracentesis. Am J Gastroenterol 1996;91:366-8.

37. Shiffman ML, Farrel MT, Yee YS. Risk of bleeding after endoscopic biopsy or polypectomy in patients taking aspirin or other NSAIDs. Gastrointest Endos 1994;40:458-62.

38. Owens EL, Kasten GW, Hessel EA. Spinal subarachnoid hematoma after lumbar puncture and heparinization: A case report, review of the literature, and discussion of anesthetic implications. Anesth Analg 1986;65:1201-7.

39. Kane RE. Neurologic deficits following epidural or spinal anesthesia. Anesth Analg 1981;60:150-61.

40. Waldman SD, Feldstein GS, Waldman JH, et al. Caudal administration of morphine sulfate in anticoagulated and thrombocytopenic patients. Anesth Analg 1987;66:267-8.

41. Rasmus KT, Rottman RL, Kotelko DM, et al. Unrecognized thrombocytopenia in parturients: A retrospective review. Obstet Gynecol 1989;73:943-6.

42. Hew-Wing P, Rolbin SH, Hew E, Amato D. Epidural anaesthesia and thrombocytopenia. Anaesthesia 1989;44:775-7.

43. Edelson RN, Chernik NL, Posner JB. Spinal subdural hematomas complicating lumbar puncture. Occurrence in thrombocytopenic patients. Arch Neurol 1974;31:134-7.

44. Rao TK, El-Etr AA. Anticoagulation following placement of epidural and subarachnoid catheters: An evaluation of neurologic sequelae. Anesthesiology 1981;55:618-20.

45. Ruff RI, Dougherty JH. Complications of lumbar puncture followed by anticoagulation. Stroke 1981;12:879-81.

46. Kang J, Brodsky L, Danziger I, et al. Coagulation profile as a predictor for post-tonsillectomy and adenoidectomy hemorrhage. Int J Pediatr Otorhinolaryngol 1994;28:157-65.

47. Zwack G, Derkay CS. The utility of preoperative hemostatic assessment in adenotonsillectomy. Int J Pediatr Otorhinolaryngol 1997;39: 67-76.

48. Kozak EA, Brath LK. Do "screening" coagulation tests predict bleeding in patients undergoing fiberoptic bronchoscopy with biopsy? Chest 1994;106:703-5.

In: Mintz PD, ed.
Transfusion Therapy: Clinical Principles and Practice
Bethesda, MD: AABB Press, 1999

9

Transfusion in Surgery and Trauma

RICHARD K. SPENCE, MD, FACS; ELAINE K. JETER, MD; AND PAUL D. MINTZ, MD

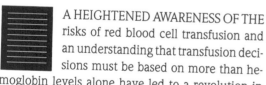

A HEIGHTENED AWARENESS OF THE risks of red blood cell transfusion and an understanding that transfusion decisions must be based on more than hemoglobin levels alone have led to a revolution in surgical transfusion practice. Surgeons have responded to these challenges by reassessing the reasons for transfusion in their patients, increasing the use of autologous blood, and using various approaches to reduce blood loss and transfusion need. Current practice policies recommend that elective transfusion of allogeneic blood be viewed as an outcome to be avoided in surgical patients. Of primary importance is the need for the surgeon to change from a casual approach to allogeneic blood transfusion to one characterized by thoughtful planning. To do this requires both an understanding of the consequences of blood loss anemia in the surgical patient and a structured approach to the transfusion decision.

Physiologic Response to Anemia

Understanding the physiologic response to anemia is essential to making rational transfusion decisions.[1] The heart provides the primary response to acute, surgical anemia by increasing cardiac output through an increase either in heart rate or stroke volume.[2] Because the heart extracts approximately 80% of the oxygen delivered under normal condi-

Richard K. Spence, MD, FACS, Visiting Professor of Surgery, Department of Surgery, State University of New York, Health Sciences Center at Brooklyn, Brooklyn, New York; Elaine K. Jeter, MD, General Pathologist and Transfusion Medicine Physician, Providence Hospital and Clinical Associate Professor, University of South Carolina, Columbia, South Carolina and Clinical Associate Professor, Medical University of South Carolina, Charleston, South Carolina; and Paul D. Mintz, MD, Associate Chair and Professor of Pathology, Professor of Internal Medicine, and Director, Clinical Laboratories and Blood Bank, University of Virginia Health Sciences Center, Charlottesville, Virginia

tions, its ability to increase output is limited by its ability to increase its oxygen consumption. Cardiac oxygen extraction is improved by increasing coronary flow. To do this, the coronary arteries must dilate. In the presence of coronary artery disease, the heart may be unable to provide the work needed to increase total body oxygen delivery without risk to the myocardium. Continued demands on the stressed heart to provide oxygen in the face of anemia may come at the expense of conversion to an anaerobic metabolic state and eventual subendocardial infarction.[3,4] Animal studies of normovolemic hemodilution have shown that the lower limit of cardiac tolerance for anemia lies around 3-5 g/dL.[5,6] Under these conditions, coronary blood flow is shifted from the endocardium to the epicardium, thereby placing subendocardial tissue at an increased risk of ischemia. The addition of an experimental coronary stenosis to this model results in depressed cardiac function at hemoglobin levels of 7-10 g/dL.

Peripheral tissues may also compensate for anemia by increasing oxygen delivery, either by recruiting more capillaries or by increasing blood flow through existing beds. Some tissues, particularly those that are supply-dependent, may compensate by increasing oxygen extraction.[7-9] LASER-Doppler flow studies of the skin, muscle, and splanchnic bed microcirculation suggest that these compensatory mechanisms may be limited and dependent on not only red cell mass but also circulating volume.[10] In the chronically anemic patient, increases in stroke volume and, therefore, in cardiac output are supplemented by increased levels of 2,3-diphosphoglycerate (2,3-DPG). These intracellular changes shift the oxyhemoglobin curve to the right, facilitating oxygen off-load and increasing oxygen delivery.

In most clinical settings, oxygen consumption is relatively independent of hemoglobin level across a wide range of oxygen delivery values because of compensations made in oxygen extraction. As oxygen delivery decreases through a loss of hemoglobin, oxygen extraction should increase from a baseline of 15-25% to maintain a constant oxygen consumption. Any increase in circulating volume

that improves cardiac output will also mathematically improve oxygen delivery regardless of hemoglobin level. However, an improvement in oxygen delivery does not necessarily lead to an increase in oxygen consumption. Wilkerson et al have shown in exchange-transfused baboons that oxygen consumption is maintained down to a hematocrit of 4% if left atrial pressure is held constant.[6] These animals survived by increasing their oxygen extraction ratio significantly. The investigators detected a conversion to anaerobic metabolism at a 10% hematocrit level, which correlated with an oxygen extraction ratio of 50%, suggesting that these two numbers might be useful as transfusion guidelines.

Weiskopf et al induced isovolemic hemodilution in conscious healthy patients prior to anesthesia for surgery and in volunteers not undergoing surgery.[11] Overall, mean hemoglobin concentration was reduced from 13.1 g/dL to 5.0 g/dL. This degree of hemodilution did not increase mean plasma lactate concentration and increased oxygen consumption only slightly (mean = 3.07 mLO$_2$/kg/minute to 3.42 mLO$_2$/kg/minute). These results, along with electrocardiographic monitoring, suggest that at a hemoglobin concentration of 5.0 g/dL in a resting, healthy population, myocardial ischemia would occur infrequently. The authors caution, however, that the results should not be extrapolated to circumstances of increased activity or decreased ability to increase either cardiac output or specific organ or tissue blood flow.

Formulas and relationships useful in evaluating oxygen transport parameters are given in Table 9-1.

Transfusion Decisions in Surgery

Current policies that focus on the use of physiologic transfusion decisions state that blood should be transfused only when there is a documented need to increase oxygen delivery in those patients who are unable to meet demands through normal cardiopulmonary mechanisms.[1,9] This stands to reason because the primary function of Red Blood Cells (RBCs) is to transport oxygen to tissues. Therefore, any red cell transfusion should be physi-

Table 9-1. Oxygen Transport Formulas

Parameter	Formula	Normal Range
Cardiac output (CO)	Stroke volume × heart rate	4-6 L/minute
Arterial oxygen content (CaO_2)	$1.34 \times Hb \times SaO_2 + (0.003 \times PaO_2)$	16-22 mL/dL
Mixed venous oxygen content ($C\bar{v}O_2$)	$1.34 \times Hb \times S\bar{v}O_2 + (0.003 \times P\bar{v}O_2)$	12-17 mL/dL
Oxygen delivery ($\dot{D}O_2$)	$CO \times CaO_2 \times 10$	500-750 mL/minute/m^2
Oxygen consumption ($\dot{V}O_2$)	$CO \times (CaO_2 - C\bar{v}O_2) \times 10$	100-180 mL/minute/m^2
Oxygen extraction ratio	$\dot{V}O_2 / \dot{D}O_2$	0.23 - 0.30

Hb = hemoglobin concentration in g/dL; SaO_2 = arterial oxygen saturation; $S\bar{v}O_2$ = mixed venous oxygen saturation; PaO_2 = arterial oxygen tension; $P\bar{v}O_2$ = mixed venous oxygen tension

ologic; that is, it should provide the additional oxygen delivery needed to correct or protect against the development of tissue hypoxia. Other investigators have rekindled interest in the role of red blood cell transfusion in the correction of hypovolemic anemia and as a mediator of hemostasis.[12]

Most transfusion decisions are made on the basis of isolated hemoglobin and hematocrit values. A National Institutes of Health consensus conference, convened in 1988 to address the topic of perioperative red cell transfusion, focused primarily on the risks of transfusion and the need to modify transfusion practices.[13] It also produced recommendations for a new transfusion trigger that represents an update over the traditional "10/30" rule that had existed for years.[14] The target, or trigger, hemoglobin was lowered to 8 g/dL, and guidelines for transfusion directed attention toward the assessment of clinical need and symptoms rather than at numbers alone. Since then, much has appeared in the literature that has attempted to define further the transfusion trigger.[15-18] Investigators have focused on defining an acceptable hemoglobin level, deriving a trigger from oxygen transport

or metabolic variables, or describing the effect of transfusion in specific clinical settings.

Two concepts form the basis for the use of hemoglobin as a transfusion trigger, the optimal hemoglobin/hematocrit and the minimally acceptable hemoglobin/hematocrit. For many years, they were considered to be one and the same. At the turn of the century, before blood transfusion was possible, surgeons tolerated low hemoglobin levels because there was little one could do to change them. The scientific investigation of blood-oxygen delivery mechanics was in its infancy, transfusion was a very young discipline, and little was known about optimal or minimal hemoglobin levels. By the 1930s, Carrel and Lindberg had demonstrated that isolated organs could survive and grow in an extremely anemic environment, defining the minimally acceptable hemoglobin level for sustained life as approximately 3 g/dL.[18] During the ensuing years, as transfusion became a part of everyday practice, the optimal hemoglobin level was defined clinically. In 1941, less than 10 years after the first blood bank opened, Adams and Lundy recommended that all patients with preoperative hemoglobin levels below 10 g/dL be transfused prior to surgery, basing this decision on their clinical experience and understanding of oxygen transport dynamics.[19] A few years later, Clark et al provided some clinical support for the 10-g/dL level when they proposed that patients with the anemia of "chronic shock" would benefit from preoperative transfusion.[20] The 10-g/dL hemoglobin level, or the 10/30 rule for transfusion, soon became a doctrine that persisted for many years.

Subsequent studies of the role of hematocrit, cardiac function, and oxygen transport have supported 10 g/dL as an optimal level as well. In-vitro rheologic studies of diluted blood pumped through glass tubes at constant pressure showed that oxygen delivery peaks at hematocrit levels of 30% and then declines with progressive hemodilution.[21] Oxygen transport and survival are maximized at hematocrit levels of 30-40% in the experimental animal.[22,23] Czer and Shoemaker determined that an optimal hematocrit of 33% is desirable in critically ill patients, but they emphasized the importance of maintaining adequate volume status over transfusion.[24] Their patients had had acute blood loss from trauma or had undergone emergency surgery. Hemoglobin levels were confounded in their analysis by both the nature of the critical illness and volume replacement. Even so, patients with normal compensatory mechanisms tolerated hematocrit levels as low as 18%. These investigators subsequently demonstrated maintenance of both cardiac output and oxygen consumption in dogs with hematocrit levels as low as 10% as long as volume remained normal.[25]

Several studies designed to establish an optimal hemoglobin level noted that lower levels are tolerated by most patients. Clinical studies give us further information regarding the minimally acceptable hemoglobin level in the form of mortality and morbidity data in anemic surgical patients. Lunn and Elwood described the mortality rate in 1584 surgical patients who received anesthesia.[26] As the hemoglobin level decreased, the mortality increased. However, this study did not assess or control for concurrent medical problems or type of surgical procedure, factors that may have had an effect on survival. Furthermore, mortality rates were not stratified by hemoglobin levels below 10 g/dL, making it impossible to assess the effect of severe anemia on the risk of death. In Rawstron's comparison of 145 patients with preoperative hemoglobin levels of less than 10 g/dL with a group of 412 surgical patients with hemoglobin levels of 10 g/dL or greater, the number of postoperative complications was similar.[27] However, both groups received preoperative transfusion, which may have obscured a difference in operative risk. Outcomes were not stratified for hemoglobin levels below 10 g/dL. Alexiu et al compared the postoperative mortality and morbidity in patients with gastrointestinal bleeding.[28] Sixty-nine transfused patients were compared with 72 patients who were resuscitated with large volumes of dextrose and normal saline. In patients not given blood, the mean preoperative hematocrit was 29% (range = 16-42%), dropping by the second postoperative day to a mean of 23% (range = 10-37%). There was no mortality, and the complication rate was lower than in the transfused group. However, the number of patients with hemoglobin levels below 10 g/dL was not stated, and the presence of potentially confounding medical problems was not included in the analysis. Carson et al have reported the largest retrospective chart study conducted to date of the effect of transfusion on mortality in hopes of defining both the benefits of and the appropriate hemoglobin level for transfusion in the surgical patient.[29] This retrospective study of 8787 consecutive hip fracture patients with a hemoglobin level between 8.0 and 10.0 g/dL was unable to show any effect, either beneficial or adverse, of red cell transfusion on either 30-day or 90-day mortality.

Several studies of anemia and the risk of postoperative morbidity and mortality in Jehovah's Witnesses have been reported.[30,31] Spence et al studied 125 patients undergoing either emergency or elective surgery.[30] The mean preoperative hemoglobin level in those who died was 7.6 g/dL, significantly lower than that in the survivors (11.8 g/dL, p<0.002). The percentage of patients who died with preoperative hemoglobin levels between zero and 6 g/dL was 61.5%; between 6.1 and 8 g/dL,

33.3%; between 8.1 and 10 g/dL, 0%; and greater than 10 g/dL, 7.1%. None of the patients with pre-operative hemoglobin levels greater than 8 g/dL and operative blood loss of less than 500 mL died (upper 95% confidence interval = 5%). However, the study was too small to describe precisely the risk of death in patients with hemoglobin levels between 6 g/dL and 10 g/dL. A subsequent analysis of 113 elective operations in 107 Jehovah's Witness patients showed that mortality was zero with hemoglobin levels as low as 6 g/dL as long as blood loss was kept below 500 mL.[31]

The minimally acceptable hemoglobin in the surgical patient may be that beyond which coronary artery blood flow cannot increase enough to meet myocardial oxygen demands, but this level has yet to be defined in useful clinical terms. In 1990, Robertie and Gravlee recommended accepting a transfusion trigger of 6 g/dL in well-compensated patients with no heart disease and no postoperative complications.[22] A higher trigger—8 g/dL—should be used in patients with stable cardiac disease and when blood loss of approximately 300 mL is expected. Older patients and those with postoperative complications who cannot increase cardiac output to compensate for hemodilution should be transfused when hemoglobin reaches 10 g/dL. In 1997, Hebert and colleagues published the results of two studies addressing the value of transfusion in critically ill patients.[32] A combined retrospective and prospective cohort analysis of 4470 patients admitted to intensive care units with a variety of diagnoses showed that anemia increases the risk of death in critically ill patients and that blood transfusion appears to decrease this risk. However, a concomitant multicenter, randomized, controlled pilot study by the same investigators of two transfusion triggers—one restrictive, 7-9 g/dL; one liberal, 10-12 g/dL—in the treatment of similar patients showed no difference in 30-day and 120-day intensive care unit mortality.[33] Baron's report for the French Consensus Conference on hemodilution in cardiac surgery recommends that a postoperative hematocrit of 25% is acceptable *if* the patient remains asymptomatic. Otherwise, the transfusion decision must include both hematocrit and symptoms.[34]

Because humans tolerate anemia surprisingly well, symptoms and signs caused by decreased red cell mass have limited usefulness as transfusion triggers, especially in the surgical setting.[35] Symptoms of exertional dyspnea do not appear in the otherwise healthy individual until hemoglobin concentration reaches 7 g/dL. Even at this and lower levels, symptoms and signs are variable. Carmel and Shulman reported on the correlation between symptoms and the need for transfusion in 122 medical patients with pernicious anemia.[36] Sixty-two patients with a mean hemoglobin level of 5.5 g/dL were transfused, but only 34 (55%) had symptoms of chest pain, dyspnea at rest, syncope, or lethargy, suggesting an urgent need for additional blood. Muller and colleagues evaluated the use of a 6-g/dL hemoglobin or 20% hematocrit transfusion trigger in 171 patients (100 children, 71 adults).[37] Adults were more likely to demonstrate hemodynamic symptoms at this level of anemia than children, whose predominant symptoms were dyspnea and impaired consciousness. In spite of the severity of the anemia, only 54% of all patients were tachycardic, 32% were hypotensive, 27% had dyspnea, and 35% had impaired levels of consciousness. These symptoms have little usefulness in the postoperative environment.

There have been few clinical studies of the effect of coexisting medical conditions on the ability of the heart to compensate for moderate or severe anemia in surgical patients. In our study of mortality and hemoglobin level in Jehovah's Witnesses, preoperative cardiac disease as defined by the Multifactorial Cardiac Risk Index appeared to worsen outcome.[31] In a smaller study of 47 patients with more severe anemia (mean hemoglobin = 4.6 ± 0.2 g/dL), a history of cardiac, pulmonary, or renal disease had no association with adverse outcome.[38] Two reports of an increased incidence of electrocardiographic evidence of myocardial ischemia in postoperative vascular patients with hematocrits below 29% suggest that patients with cardiac disease may need hemoglobin levels higher than 8 g/dL, although neither report accounts for the presence or severity of underlying heart disease.[39,40] This is corroborated by a retrospective cohort study of 1958 adult Jehovah's Witnesses by Carson and associates.[41] In demonstrating that the nontransfused Jehovah's Witness patient with cardiopulmonary disease is at increased risk of dying as hemoglobin drops below 10 g/dL, this work is the first to provide solid data regarding the relationship between information derived from the history and that derived from the physical examination—that is, symptoms and hemoglobin level.

The above studies show that many patients tolerate a hemoglobin value significantly lower than an optimal level of 10 g/dL. This does not necessarily mean that a *tolerable* hemoglobin level should automatically be considered an *acceptable* level for use as a transfusion trigger in all patients.[42] Conversely, it is unnecessary and potentially risky to transfuse all patients to an optimal hemoglobin of 10 g/dL. The main problem with a hemoglobin-based trigger is its lack of generalizability. Some patients can tolerate very low perioperative hemoglobin levels; others require supranormal values to survive, depending upon diagnosis and clinical condition.

Sepsis and anemia form a particularly lethal combination in the surgical patient, as suggested by a 1990 study, which included 12 septic patients with hemoglobin levels below 5 g/dL, all of whom died.[30] This corroborates the finding of Shoemaker and colleagues that survival is decreased in sepsis when oxygen consumption is compromised, in part because of increased tissue oxygen debt and a resetting of oxygen delivery/consumption interactions.[43] Although their work suggests that transfusing to supranormal hematocrits may be beneficial, transfusion has not always turned the tide in sepsis. It may be that giving additional blood to the compromised, septic patient to improve oxygen delivery cannot alone compensate for the increased tissue oxygen debt.

Other approaches to defining the transfusion trigger in metabolic terms have had limited success. Bihari and Tinker have shown that patients with acute respiratory distress syndrome may have a hidden oxygen debt unrelated to hemoglobin level.[44] They used prostacyclin administration to define oxygen delivery/consumption relationships in hopes of identifying those patients who would benefit from additional oxygen, but this test has not gained widespread use. Spence et al summarized several studies that have been conducted to evaluate the effect of transfusion on oxygen transport in a variety of clinical settings.[45] Pretransfusion oxygen extraction ratios ranged between 24% and 48%, with the highest values seen in patients with cardiogenic shock. The effect of transfusion to a hemoglobin level of 10 g/dL on oxygen extraction ratio was minimal in most patients. The roles of mixed venous oxygen tension and mixed venous oxygen saturation as triggers have yet to be defined. Sowade and colleagues' 1997 study of the role of recombinant human erythropoietin (rHuEPO; Procrit, Ortho Biotech, Raritan, NJ) as an alternative to allogeneic transfusion used the Siggaard-Andersen oxygen status algorithm as an indicator of transfusion need.[46]

Lactate levels are useful correlates of blood loss and injury severity, but they have not been helpful in defining transfusion need.[47] Astiz et al found no correlation between lactate and oxygen delivery in 100 patients with either an acute myocardial infarction or sepsis.[48] Muller and colleagues' analysis of the value of serum lactate measurements as a transfusion trigger in premature infants reached similar conclusions.[49]

We can conclude from the above that the decision to transfuse should be related to the specific patient's needs and condition. Transfusion need should be assessed on a case-by-case basis. This assessment should include a history and physical examination, a review of pertinent laboratory data, consideration of the operation planned and expectant blood loss, and analysis of the risk factors that may contribute to increased morbidity and mortality. The history and physical examination should focus on preexisting diseases or conditions that may increase the risk of blood loss or the need for increased oxygen delivery. The presence of cardiac, pulmonary, and other atherosclerotic disease processes should be assessed and quantified when possible. Surgical patients with coronary artery disease and pulmonary hypoxia will most likely require higher perioperative hemoglobin levels than those with normal hearts and lungs to avoid ischemia and undue cardiac stress. Factors to consider in the surgical transfusion decision are listed in Table 9-2.

Surgical Anemia: Approaches to Treatment

Anemia may present a problem to the surgeon at any time in the perioperative period. Malnourished, iron-deficient patients may present in need of surgery; anemia of blood loss may be an unwanted complication of any surgical procedure. If anemia is discovered during preoperative investigations, the surgeon must decide if the level of anemia and the risk of blood loss from the planned procedure are of enough merit to warrant action. If they are and if surgery can be postponed, the surgeon can use oral iron to correct the anemia. Oral iron therapy should also be used in patients storing autologous blood before surgery and those receiving erythropoietin.[50] If surgery cannot be delayed, if the patient is demonstrably (ie, by laboratory analysis) iron-deficient, or if the level of anemia is severe and life-threatening, the use of IV iron dextran may be considered.[51,52] Because iron dextran may produce anaphylaxis, it should be used according to the dosage instructions issued by its manufacturers.[53] Polysaccharide forms may be better tolerated than dextran preparations.

Table 9-2. Factors to Consider in the Surgical Transfusion Decision

Clinical history
  Cardiopulmonary disease
  Disorder of hemostasis
  Anemia
  Trauma classification
    Mechanism of injury
    Injury severity score
Medications
  Antiplatelet
  Anticoagulants
Clinical symptoms
  Dyspnea on exertion
  Angina
Hemoglobin/hematocrit level
Oxygen delivery/consumption
  Oxygen extraction ratio
  Oxygen partial pressure
  Oxygen saturation
  Serum lactate
  Base deficit
Surgical procedure
  Elective vs emergency
  Laparoscopic vs open
Estimated blood loss
Jehovah's Witness

Allogeneic Blood Use and Risks

The incidence of transfusion-transmitted diseases from allogeneic blood has been reduced by the use of donor history and testing. Allogeneic blood can be made even safer through the use of leukocyte-reduction filters. Leukocyte-reduction filters can limit the number of white blood cells transfused with Red Blood Cells (RBCs), thereby limiting the potential for febrile reactions, exposure to leukocyte-borne viruses such as cytomegalovirus, and the consequences of immunosuppression.[54,55]

Various animal and human studies have demonstrated systemic immunomodulation caused by allogeneic transfusion.[56-59] Both cellular and humoral factors seem to play a role. Macrophage function is altered following allogeneic transfusion, resulting in decreases in migratory capabilities and both eicosanoid and interleukin-2 production. Lymphocyte responses to both antigen and mitogen are suppressed, and suppressor cell activity is increased with concomitant declines in helper:suppressor cell ratios. Both an increased susceptibility to bacterial infection and increased mortality following allogeneic transfusion have been reported, and postsurgical infections may be increased by as much as

30%. Patients transfused during surgery for cancer may have a decreased disease-free interval and shortened survival time. Although these clinical findings are controversial, the surgeon should be aware of the potential risk of transfusion-induced immunosuppression. This potential risk can be decreased either by avoiding allogeneic blood transfusion or by reducing leukocytes with filters when transfusion of allogeneic blood is necessary. Both California and New Jersey require physicians to explain transfusion risks to patients and to offer alternatives. Guidelines for informed consent in surgical transfusion are shown in Table 9-3.

Blood Conservation Strategies

The use of autologous blood is not a new concept to surgeons. This alternative to allogeneic transfusion has been used for several years in orthopedic and cardiac surgery in the form of preoperative autologous donation (PAD) and in urologic procedures in the form of acute normovolemic hemodilution (ANH). PAD is considered a standard of care for elective orthopedic procedures and radical prostatectomy.[60-62]

rHuEPO has been proved to increase red cell mass in patients with anemia caused by both renal failure and chronic disease.[63,64] The drug has also shown usefulness in stimulating erythrocyte production during a course of PAD and is approved for this use in the United States in patients undergoing orthopedic procedures.[65,66] An analysis of the ability of patients scheduled for elective orthopedic procedures to participate in PAD demonstrated that patients at risk for subsequent allogeneic transfusion were those who were anemic at the time of their first autologous blood phlebotomy and those who were required to provide four or more units of blood.[67] Low endogenous erythropoietin levels at the time of the initial encounter have also been shown to prevent completion of a planned collection schedule.[68] To address this problem, Goodnough et al treated a group of nonanemic patients with 600 U/kg of IV rHuEPO twice weekly.[69] When compared with placebo-treated control patients, the rHuEPO patients provided 41% more red cell volume. A subsequent clinical trial of nonanemic patients showed no significant difference in allogeneic blood requirements between rHuEPO-treated (150-180 U/kg three times per

---

Table 9-3. Explanation and Documentation of Informed Consent for Blood Transfusion

1. Explain the blood transfusion procedure.
2. Describe the potential benefits of transfusion.
3. Describe the potential risks of transfusion:
   Transfusion reaction, including fever, chills, shock, heart failure, death
   Hepatitis
   Human immune deficiency virus infection
   Postoperative wound infection
   Other blood-borne infections
4. Describe alternatives to transfusion.
5. Describe the potential risks of no transfusion, including unexpected hemorrhage and the risk of death, with respect to the planned procedure.
6. Answer any questions.
7. Document the above process, including the patient's acceptance or refusal.

week at 4 and 2 weeks before surgery) and untreated patients.[64] However, Biesma et al used rHuEPO therapy to reduce overall exposure to allogeneic blood transfusion when collection was limited to only two units of blood.[70]

Subsequent studies of the impact of rHuEPO on PAD focused on the anemic surgical patient. Mercuriali and European colleagues demonstrated a reduction in allogeneic blood use in orthopedic patients with the use of preoperative rHuEPO and IV iron in a randomized, clinical trial.[71] In a similar US study, allogeneic blood transfusion was required in 31% of placebo-treated patients compared with 20% of rHuEPO-treated patients.[72] Although this difference did not reach statistical significance, the rHuEPO-treated patients did demonstrate the ability to donate more autologous units (4.5 vs 3.0; p <0.001) and to increase their production of red cells (688 vs 353 mL over baseline; p<0.05). These studies have shown that rHuEPO therapy coupled with iron administration can make PAD a successful option for many anemic surgical patients who would otherwise need allogeneic transfusion.

Successful autologous collection before surgery depends on adequate time for donation, a hemoglobin level greater than 11.0 g/dL, the absence of significant patient disease (eg, severe aortic stenosis or active angina) that could render phlebotomy unsafe, the selection of appropriate patients, and both patient and physician cooperation.[73-76] The ideal patient for PAD is one who needs a blood transfusion in the perioperative period and has a window of 2 or more weeks before surgery to donate. PAD blood may be frozen for those patients who need more time. The majority of patients can successfully complete a predonation program without incident. An increased incidence of reactions is associated with donor age under 17 years, weight under 110 lb, female gender, and a history of previous reactions.

Phlebotomy is now being performed in select blood centers with the use of apheresis machines. This process reduces the volume loss associated with standard blood donations. As a consequence, patients can donate more RBCs with less risk of adverse events. This approach makes the process available to more patients but requires additional

logistics and medical expertise, which add to the cost of autologous phlebotomy. The latter is substantial and has caused some to look for other, less expensive alternatives to PAD in the surgical patient.[77]

ANH is the process of removing and temporarily storing blood just before or immediately after the induction of anesthesia and replacing volume losses with either crystalloid or colloid solutions.[76] The removal of one to four units is possible in the patient with a normal hematocrit and results in a postdilutional hematocrit of 20-30%.[21] The advantages of ANH include an improvement in tissue perfusion secondary to decreased viscosity and loss of fewer red cells from bleeding; a major disadvantage is the need for an experienced anesthesiologist or perfusionist. Hemodilution can be performed safely in most patients, with the only contraindications being anemia, which limits the amount of blood that can be removed, and cardiac disease. Monk and colleagues have championed the use of ANH as an alternative to allogeneic blood transfusion in the patient undergoing radical prostatectomy.[78] Their 1995 analysis of rHuEPO therapy as an adjunct to ANH has shown that erythropoietin is effective in both preventing exposure to allogeneic blood and increasing production of RBCs.[79]

Autologous blood may also be obtained through the collection and reinfusion of blood shed in the perioperative period.[80] Intraoperative autotransfusion can be performed with systems that either collect blood directly, anticoagulate it, and reinfuse it through filters or collect the blood, wash it, and reinfuse a concentrated red cell product.[81]

Systems without washing capability collect shed blood via a suction wand or wound drainage catheter. Heparin or citrate-phosphate-dextrose anticoagulant must be added to the collection chamber. The collected blood is then returned to the patient through a filter, which is relied on as the only means of preparing the blood. Filters are capable of removing large debris (eg, bone chips in orthopedic cases) and smaller particulate matter up 260 μ (eg, cellular fragments). Following filtration, the recovered blood contains red cells and platelets suspended in plasma. Unwashed blood may contain vasoactive contaminants, activated clotting factors, fibrin degradation products, and free hemoglobin, all of which can be dangerous. However, unwashed blood appears to be safe if transfusion is limited to small quantities and to appropriate circumstances.

Systems that wash blood and concentrate the red cells have the advantage of providing a cleaner product, free of the contaminants found in unwashed blood. With these systems, blood is collected from the operative field, filtered, anticoagulated, temporarily stored in a reservoir, and then washed for return. The advantage of portability, previously found only with systems that did not wash blood, has been added to washer devices. The machines used are mounted on wheels, allowing easy movement from the operating room to the recovery room or intensive care unit. Smaller washing bowls permit the collection of volumes as small as 100 mL. Collection chambers have been modified to portable, smaller sizes under a "collect first" philosophy. These chambers allow the physician to decide whether it is worthwhile to reinfuse the volume collected, which may have particular applicability for Jehovah's Witness patients. The use of autologous blood and rHuEPO in the surgical setting is also discussed in Chapter 19.

Surgeons are relearning Halstedian principles of gentle tissue handling, anatomic dissection, and minimization of blood loss in all operations. The surgeon should enter the operating room with the goal of preventing as much blood loss as possible by maintaining careful surgical hemostasis.[60] Because transfusion need in surgery is clearly tied to blood loss, reduction of operative blood loss should minimize the need for transfusion; any blood not shed is blood that does not have be replaced. Technical factors and operative approach have a critical effect on blood loss in most procedures.

The success of laparoscopic cholecystectomy has encouraged surgeons to develop similar, alternative approaches to many operations that previously required incision into the chest or abdomen. In many cases, laparoscopic techniques are easier on patients because they produce smaller incisions, lead to more rapid recovery, and result in shorter hospital stays. Laparoscopic techniques in surgery do much to minimize the need for transfusion. The improved visualization of the operative field, coupled with the knowledge that extra care must be taken in dissection through a minimal-access port, has led to a reduction in blood loss from laparoscopic procedures when compared with open techniques.[82-86]

The choice of anesthetic agent and technique may have an effect on surgical blood loss. In this context, Blackwell et al studied the effect of general anesthesia with isoflurane inhalation in 13 patients vs monitored sedation with a continuous IV infusion of propofol in 12 similar patients undergoing endoscopic sinus surgery.[87] Blood loss in the isoflurane group was 251 mL compared with 101 mL in the propofol group (p<0.01).

Locally acting agents that encourage clotting such as fibrin sealants, collagen, and topical thrombin, may be helpful in maintaining hemostasis.[88] Fibrin sealants are discussed in detail in Chapter 10. Antifibrinolytic drugs, such as aprotinin, epsilon aminocaproic acid, desmopressin acetate, and tranexamic acid, may be helpful in reducing blood loss, especially during cardiac surgery.[89] Specific considerations in cardiopulmonary bypass (CPB) surgery are discussed below.

Perioperative rHuEPO has been used in both anemic and nonanemic patients either in anticipation of or following surgical blood loss. Early experience with erythropoietin in Jehovah's Witness patients demonstrated its superiority to hematinics alone in restoring red cell mass following hemorrhage. Atabek et al reported significantly higher hematocrits (19.3% vs 12.5%) after 1 week of rHuEPO in 20 Jehovah's Witnesses with postsurgical, severe anemia (hematocrit <25%) who were compared with a similar group of 20 patients who received only IV iron.[90] Three separate studies of preoperative erythropoietin therapy—two in orthopedic surgery and one in cardiac surgery—have demonstrated the usefulness of rHuEPO in the avoidance of allogeneic blood.[91-93] Considerations in surgical transfusion are summarized in Table 9-4.

Table 9-4. Considerations in Surgical Transfusion

Preoperative
    Antiplatelet/anticoagulant drugs
    Cardiopulmonary status
    Autologous blood collection
    Erythropoietin
    Iron, oral or IV
Intraoperative
    Acute normovolemic hemodilution
    Autotransfusion/cell recovery
    Antifibrinolytics
    Fibrin sealants
    Surgical techniques to reduce blood loss
    Blood substitutes
    Hypotensive/hypothermic anesthesia
    Transfusion trigger
    Leukocyte-reduction filters
Postoperative
    Autotransfusion/cell recovery
    Blood substitutes
    Erythropoietin
    Iron, oral or IV
    Phlebotomy
    Transfusion trigger
    Leukocyte-reduction filters

Considerations in Patients Undergoing Cardiopulmonary Bypass Surgery

Cold Agglutinins

Patients undergoing surgical procedures that require the use of a CPB circuit are typically made hypothermic with a systemic body temperature of 25-32 C. In addition, in almost all such patients, cold cardioplegic solutions are used to prefuse the myocardium to induce asystole during surgery. For certain procedures such as aortic arch reconstruc-

tions and for infants, deep hypothermia is used with systemic temperatures around 18 C. Each of these hypothermic conditions raises concerns when patients are known to have antibodies that agglutinate red cells at such a temperature.

Theoretical concerns include significant intravascular hemolysis and ischemic damage from red cell agglutinates, particularly in the myocardium and cerebral circulations. Although reports of significant complications in this situation are notably rare, they do exist.[94] Still, for clinicians, perfusionists, and transfusion medicine specialists, the patient with a known cold agglutinin scheduled for CPB surgery raises concerns. No studies have definitively related clinical risks to antibody titers or thermal amplitudes, although one report has documented successful surgery in five patients with cold agglutinins with 4 C agglutination titers of less than 1:32.[95] It is, however, possible to make some prudent decisions regarding this clinical circumstance.

Owing to the scarcity of reported problems, it does not seem necessary to perform specialized testing for cold agglutinins in patients scheduled for CPB. An antibody detection test read at room temperature after an immediate spin should detect antibodies that may pose problems. If such a test should detect a red blood cell cold agglutinin, it is reasonable to ascertain whether the antibody reacts at 28 C. If it does, it can be tested for reactivity at successively higher temperatures using 2 C intervals to determine the temperature at which it is no longer reactive or weakly reactive. This information can be provided to the clinicians and perfusionists who then can avoid systemic hypothermia at temperatures at which the antibody is strongly reactive. Although this increases the patient's metabolic rate and oxygen consumption during surgery and requires an increased output from the circuit, such surgery can be performed even normothermically if necessary.

Cardioplegia to induce asystole is typically performed with solutions of electrolytes, and the patient's blood is chilled to approximately 8 C to achieve a myocardial temperature of approximately 10 C. If patients are known to have cold agglutinins, the perfusionist can initially use an all-electrolyte cardioplegic solution at 37 C to flush the heart and can then provide a mixture of autologous blood and electrolyte solution at a temperature above the known thermal amplitude. Alternatively, after a warm flush, pure electrolyte cold flushes have been used, but because back-bleeding is always possible, it seems reasonable to use a cardioplegic solution at a temperature above the known thermal amplitude of the cold agglutinin. The use of warmer cardioplegic solutions increases the myocardium's metabolic rate and thus its need for nutrients. This then requires an increased delivery of cardioplegic solution during surgery. Another alternative is to fibrillate the heart without cardioplegic solution; however, this does not reduce myocardial metabolism to the extent that cardioplegia does.

If agglutination is first noted during an operation, the temperature can be raised immediately, after which a warm retrograde cardioplegic washout by coronary sinus cannulation can be performed.

For those who require deep hypothermia, a retrograde cerebral perfusion with cold autologous blood is typically used. Such a procedure would seem particularly dangerous in patients with cold agglutinins. Preoperative plasmapheresis to remove the cold agglutinin followed by hypothermia above the thermal amplitude of the antibody may be attempted.[96,97] Because cold agglutinins are typically IgM, plasmapheresis would be expected to remove a considerable amount. Alternatively, an attempt could be made to cannulate the arteries emanating from the aortic arch and perfuse each artery normothermically with blood. This adventurous approach adds complexity to the procedure, but for patients from whom a high-titer cold agglutinin cannot be removed by plasmapheresis, it might provide an opportunity to perform what would otherwise be very dangerous surgery.

While the rarity of reports documenting adverse outcomes in patients with cold agglutinins undergoing CPB surgery is reassuring, precautions such as those described above for patients who have cold agglutinins as documented by routine presurgical compatibility testing are prudent, as well as being necessary for patients with symptomatic cold agglutinin disease.

Indications for Transfusion

The hypothermia typically used during CPB reduces oxygen consumption, allowing the patient to tolerate significant isovolemic hemodilution. Helm and Isom have recently proposed indications for red cell transfusion in patients undergoing such surgery.[98] They suggest that a routine preoperative transfusion trigger is a hematocrit lower than 25% in asymptomatic patients weighing more than 80 kg. Smaller patients who experience greater hemodilution while on CPB are typically transfused preoperatively to a hematocrit of 27%. Patients who have continuing myocardial ischemia should be transfused to maintain a hematocrit of approximately 30%. The same guidelines are used for the beginning of the intraoperative period before CPB is initiated. During surgery, the anesthetized patient at typical levels of hypothermia can safely tolerate hematocrits as low as 15%; for patients who are at special risk for reduced cerebral oxygen delivery (eg, those with insulin-dependent diabetes or documented cerebral vascular disease), the hematocrit is maintained at no less than 18% during CPB. As hypothermia ends, these numbers are adjusted to 17% and 20%, respectively, prior to weaning from bypass, and then to 19% and 22%, respectively, in the intraoperative period after bypass is discontinued. During the postoperative period, after recovered blood from the CPB circuit has been reinfused, higher hematocrits are used. In this period, patients are transfused with hematocrits lower than 22% if they are less than 80 years old, and with hematocrits lower than 24% if they are 80 or older. Similar hematocrits are used as triggers during convalescence. Certain patients, however, will benefit from higher hematocrits than those stipulated here. In particular, patients with poor revascularization, low cardiac output, pulmonary dysfunction, or continuing symptoms of atherosclerotic disease may require red cell transfusion at higher hematocrits.

Typically, RBCs are used to provide increased oxygen-carrying capacity. Hemostatic defects may be corrected with specific components. One study, however, concluded that the transfusion of Whole Blood less than 48 hours old was associated with significantly less postoperative blood loss than the transfusion of RBCs, Fresh Frozen Plasma, and platelet concentrates in children under 2 years of age who underwent complex cardiac surgery.[99]

CPB is associated with several hemostatic defects. Decreased coagulation factor levels and fibrinolysis are seen within a few minutes after patients are placed on CPB. Platelet counts typically decline to below $100,000/\mu L$ and remain low during the first few postoperative days, although coagulation factor levels return to normal a few hours after surgery.[100] Decreased platelet reactivity can be documented in response to an in-vivo wound. This "platelet function defect" appears to be not intrinsic to the platelet but due to an unavailability of platelet agonists.[101] Heparin used during CPB may contribute substantially to this, owing to its inhibition of thrombin. Hypothermia may contribute to the thrombocytopenia and increased fibrinolysis.

The laboratory results of hemostasis during and after CPB are not predictive of clinically important hemostatic abnormalities.[100] Thus, the detection of a hemostatic abnormality by laboratory testing should not, in and of itself, be considered a trigger for transfusion. Rather, transfusion should be guided by the patient's clinical condition in association with laboratory studies when feasible. A reasonable guideline in view of the platelet dysfunction in vivo is to maintain a platelet count no lower than $80,000$-$100,000/\mu L$. Certain patients may require higher platelet counts to arrest hemorrhage, and some may tolerate lower counts. One single-donor platelet product provides an appropriate dose for adults, or a pool of five to eight random-donor platelets may be transfused.

As in other surgical settings, it is appropriate in CBP to maintain the prothrombin time (PT) at less than 1.5 times the midpoint of the reference range and to maintain the activated partial thromboplastin time (aPTT) at less than 1.5 times the top of the reference range. A reasonable dose of plasma is one bag per 20 kg of body weight. In this text, "plasma" is used to refer to fresh frozen plasma or pooled solvent/detergent-treated plasma (PLAS+SD, V.I. Technologies, Melville, NY). These products may be used interchangeably and are discussed in Chapter 7. Clinicians should remember that each platelet transfusion will provide 200-300 mL of plasma containing normal or nearly normal levels of coagulation factors.

Cryoprecipitate infusion should be reserved for patients with a documented fibrinogen level of less than 100 mg/dL. One unit per 10 kg is an appropriate dose.

The absence of a statistically significant correlation between laboratory measurements of hemostasis and actual postoperative bleeding suggests that identified laboratory abnormalities should never obscure the possibility that excessive bleeding may be due to an anatomic defect.

Transfusion in Trauma/Massive Transfusion: Overview

At no time in the surgeon's practice is the need for transfusion more apparent than when treating the trauma patient. Both the rapidity and the amount of blood loss and their overall impact on the clinical condition dictate the need for red cell or other component replacement. Patients may be in "shock" clinically without having lost a large number of red cells. Therefore, it is important to determine both the patient's volume and red cell losses. Some patients may require no red cell transfusion; others will require massive transfusion.

Massive transfusion is commonly defined as transfusion approximating or exceeding the patient's blood volume within a 24-hour period.[102] In the adult who weighs 70 kg, this translates to an estimated replacement of 4-5 L of lost blood, or the transfusion of 16-20 units of packed RBCs. A second definition that is suitable for most patients is blood replacement of between 30 and 50% of total blood volume.[103] This definition is more useful in the clinical setting because amounts of blood loss can be tied to clinical signs and symptoms and the development of shock. Trunkey adds further clarification by expressing hemorrhage in terms of rate of blood loss.[104] He defines severe hemorrhage as a rate of blood loss greater than 150 mL per minute, which could lead to the loss of more than one-half of the patient's blood volume within 20 minutes. Although this is relatively easy to recognize from the patient's obvious signs of shock, less severe hemorrhage is more difficult to define on clinical grounds. Blood loss and hemorrhagic shock may be classified as shown in Table 9-5.

While clinical assessment of the patient is the sine qua non in determining the need for transfusion, this should be corroborated with initial laboratory studies. An ABO-Rh type should be performed promptly to provide the patient with type-specific blood. This can be completed in 5-10 minutes and will help preserve the inventory of group O, D-negative RBCs. An initial low hemoglobin in patients with a history of trauma or obvious blood loss (eg, from a gastrointestinal source) should be considered evidence of ongoing blood loss. Those patients whose presenting hemoglobin is consistent with a 40-50% loss of blood volume (6-8 g/dL) should be treated as having massive blood loss.[105] With rapid hemorrhage, the initial hemoglobin and hematocrit may not reflect the degree of blood loss.

Most trauma patients are managed without blood transfusion. Wudel et al at Vanderbilt University found that only 27% of patients admitted to the hospital for trauma over a 5-year period required transfusion.[106] Of these, only 9.6% of the blunt trauma patients required 20 or more units of blood. However, this small percentage contributes a disproportionate share to total deaths following motor vehicle accidents. Frey et al reported that 41% of such deaths are related to uncontrolled hemorrhage.[107] Massive transfusion is needed most commonly in trauma victims, patients with gastrointestinal hemorrhage, or those with ruptured aortic aneurysms.[108-110] It may also follow a variety of elective surgical procedures, especially in those patients with an unexpected congenital or acquired bleeding diathesis.[111,112]

Certain injury patterns in combination with hypotension will prompt the clinician to institute early transfusion. Penetrating injuries of the chest, neck, abdomen, or proximal extremities often lead to ongoing blood loss. Approximately 2% of patients with abdominal injury will present with "ex-

Table 9-5. Classes of Hemorrhage

Class of Hemorrhage	Blood Loss (%TBV)	Heart Rate	Blood Pressure	Tissue Perfusion	Other Clinical Signs	Fluid Therapy
I	<15	Normal or increased	Normal	Normal	None	None
II	15-30	Increased	Normal or decreased	Decreased	Anxiety	1. Crystalloid/colloid 2. Blood +/–
III	30-40	Increased	Decreased	Decreased	Oliguria Confusion	1. Crystalloid/colloid 2. Blood
IV	>40	Increased	Decreased	Decreased	Lethargy Coma	1. Crystalloid/colloid 2. Blood

TBV = Total blood volume

sanguinating hemorrhage."[113] Pelvic fracture associated with severe abdominal injury characteristically causes high blood loss and leads to transfusion.[114]

Overall survival among patients with massive transfusion is between 40 and 60% and correlates with several factors, including age, severe head injury, the duration and magnitude of shock, abdominal trauma as a source of hemorrhage, pelvic fracture, underlying medical conditions particularly of hepatic origin, and nontraumatic surgical emergencies, as well as the number of transfusions given.[115-121] Morbid complications, including multisystem organ failure, increase following massive transfusion in trauma patients.[122]

Two approaches to red cell transfusion may be used in the trauma patient with massive or ongoing hemorrhage: transfusion on the scene and transfusion in the hospital. Transfusion on the scene is rarely done. Proponents of this approach believe that early transfusion offers the theoretical advantage of providing earlier oxygen-carrying capacity through the provision of RBCs as volume replacement.[123,124] This advantage must be weighed, however, against the risks and potential disadvantages, which stem from the following factors:

1. Blood is not the ideal resuscitation fluid. It cannot be infused as rapidly through small-bore IV lines as crystalloid solutions.

2. The ABO group cannot be determined.

3. Because of logistics, group O, D-positive cells are used in most circumstances. This could cause D-negative females of child-bearing potential future problems.

4. The crossmatch cannot be performed. Acute hemolysis may occur in the patient with red blood cell alloantibodies. This may be confusing and/or misdiagnosed in the trauma setting.

In addition, blood transfused on the scene may be lost again before the source of bleeding is identified and controlled. Infusions of large volumes of crystalloid fluids may lead to increased blood pressure, which perpetuates or increases bleeding from open vessels. Major trauma centers now advocate the use of a "scoop-and-run" approach that attempts to minimize blood loss.[125] Trauma victims are moved rapidly from the scene to the trauma center, where the source of bleeding is identified and controlled. Transfusion is given as needed to replace red blood cell losses.

Most transfusions are given on arrival in the hospital emergency department or trauma unit. Group O RBCs can be transfused in life-threatening situations when the blood type is unknown.[126-128] As noted, however, type-specific blood can be provided in 5-10 minutes. Delays may occur in transport and specimen processing, extending the time from blood sampling to transfusion. During blood processing, blood is usually centrifuged, and the RBCs are concentrated and resuspended in an additive solution to extend cell viability and improve flow rates. The transfusion of group O RBCs containing anti-A and anti-B is usually not a significant problem because only small quantities of residual plasma (approximately 20-30 mL) remain in the red cell concentrates resuspended in additive solutions. When the patient's blood type is determined, the patient can be safely switched to his or her own type or to a compatible blood type without concern for hemolysis resulting from the passive transmission of these naturally occurring antibodies. The availability of red blood cell components for emergency transfusion and their immunohematologic risks are presented in Table 9-6.

Care must be taken to follow transfusion protocols in the trauma setting because human error can lead to ABO incompatibility reactions, especially when multiple trauma victims are being treated simultaneously. Errors in patient identification, sample labeling, multiple simultaneous typing procedures, STAT testing, and the urgent nature of the clinical setting all may increase the risk of clerical errors. ABO reactions may be misdiagnosed as coagulopathy due to hypothermia, shock, or hemodilution.

The use of D-positive and D-negative RBCs for transfusion in emergency room/trauma situations varies in different parts of the United States. As a general rule, group O, D-positive red cells should be used in males with penetrating or blunt trauma who have no known history of prior transfusion with D-positive blood. Group O, D-negative blood

Table 9-6. Red Blood Cell (RBC) Component Availability for Emergency Transfusion

Component	Availability	Principal Immunohematologic Risks
Group O RBCs*	0 - 5 minutes	Hemolytic transfusion reaction resulting from patient red blood cell alloantibody (eg, anti-Kell).
ABO-group and Rh-type identical uncrossmatched RBCs or Whole Blood	10 - 15 minutes	Hemolytic transfusion reaction resulting from ABO-incompatible transfusion or other alloantibody present in the patient (eg, anti-Kell).
Crossmatched RBCs or Whole Blood	40 - 60 minutes	Hemolytic transfusion reaction resulting from ABO-incompatible transfusion.

*D-negative for females of child-bearing potential and for others known to have anti-D or to have been exposed to D-positive red blood cells.

is reserved for females of child-bearing potential and for other individuals with known or suspected sensitization to the D antigen. Because only 6% of the population is group O D-negative, many centers do not use this product for all emergency room/trauma center patients. Hemoglobin-derived blood substitutes may provide an answer in the future.[129,130]

Complications of Massive Transfusion

Massive transfusion may be associated with a variety of complications including significant hemostatic and metabolic impairment. Concomitant shock and organ dysfunction (especially hepatic, renal, cardiac, and pulmonary disease) will exacerbate the adverse effects of massive transfusion. Laboratory evaluation can help to ascertain the nature and extent of complications in a particular patient and to guide therapy.

Impaired Hemostasis

Etiology

Impaired hemostasis, a frequent finding in a trauma patient, may be caused by a combination of events, including hypothermia, dilution of platelets and coagulation factors following transfusion, and disseminated intravascular coagulation (DIC). Stored RBCs do not contain functional platelets. Although coagulation factors other than Factors V and VIII are well maintained during refrigerated storage of plasma, RBCs contain only a small volume of plasma and therefore are not a significant source of coagulation factors. In the course of a controlled exchange, approximately 37% of an original blood constituent remains within the circulation following a single blood volume exchange presuming 100% recovery, no ongoing consumption, and no increased introduction into the circulation by synthesis or mobilization.[131] At this level sufficient concentrations of coagulation factor would be present to maintain hemostasis. With an exchange of two blood volumes, intravascular elements would fall to levels of approximately 13%, and an exchange of three blood volumes would result in levels of approximately 5%. Simply on the basis of dilution, hemostatic bleeding would develop at these levels without sufficient replacement.[131-133] In practice, there is considerable variability in the degree of coagulopathy associated with large-volume transfusion.

The presence of DIC is a strong contributor to the development of coagulopathy and thrombocytopenia and also to impaired hemostasis owing to the generation of fibrin degradation products. DIC may aggravate the dilutional coagulopathy.[111,120,134-136] In the setting of massive transfusion, DIC reportedly occurs in 5-30% of trauma patients and is associated with high morbidity and mortality rates.[111,112,116,131,132] Tissue injury and hemolysis with the release of cytokines and tissue thromboplastin into the circulation may cause immediate activation of both the coagulation and fibrinolytic systems, resulting in intense DIC.[137] The degree of DIC is correlated with the intensity and duration of shock. In addition, hypothermia, often present in patients receiving massive transfusions, can impair platelet function and coagulation cascade enzyme reactions.[122,138-140] Associated hepatic and/or renal disease can exacerbate hemostatic dysfunction as well.

Evaluation and Management

Thrombocytopenia is the most common hemostatic abnormality during and after massive transfusion.[141-144] Clinical evidence of thrombocytopenia includes diffuse microvascular bleeding evidenced by oozing from mucosa, wounds, and puncture sites. Although platelets are mobilized from the spleen during blood loss, significant thrombocytopenia develops frequently after 15-20 units of RBCs or Whole Blood are transfused to an adult. There is, however, considerable variability between patient platelet counts and the number of units of blood transfused. Thus, prophylactic platelet transfusions are not indicated in this setting. Rather, if microvascular bleeding occurs, prompt

treatment with platelet transfusion is indicated. Concomitantly, a platelet count should be obtained and should be maintained at a level greater than 80,000-100,000/μL (Table 9-7). Although a platelet count of 50,000-60,000/μL is typically the lower limit for adequate surgical hemostasis, the likelihood of platelet dysfunction resulting from hypothermia and DIC makes it preferable to maintain a higher platelet count. Transfusion of one apheresis platelet concentrate or of five to eight units of pooled random-donor platelets is an appropriate dose. If the platelet count is below 50,000-60,000/μL, it is reasonable to transfuse platelets even if no microvascular bleeding is noted so that posttraumatic and postoperative hemostasis is not impaired. Empiric transfusion of components using a "cookbook" approach without evidence of bleeding should be avoided.

Dilutional coagulopathy can develop when RBCs are used for replacement in massive transfusion. If Whole Blood has been used, it is unusual to see a dilutional coagulopathy. PT and aPTT times may begin to be prolonged as a result of dilution when more than approximately 10 units of RBCs have been transfused. The exact activity levels of clotting factors needed for hemostasis when multiple factor deficiencies coexist are not well defined.[103,117,121] Hiippala, et al found that critical levels of platelets and clotting factors were not reached with blood loss and replacement until more than two estimated blood volumes had been replaced. However, fibrinogen deficits appeared much earlier.[144]

It may be difficult to correlate directly a clinical observation of bleeding with prolongation of the PT and aPTT which are reagent and temperature dependent.[137] Because coagulation testing is routinely performed at 37 C rather than at the patient's actual in-vivo temperature, normal coagulation tests can be obtained even in the presence of clinical evidence of a coagulopathy.[145] Normal test results in this setting suggest that sufficient clotting factors are available for coagulation if normothermia is restored.[146] As for platelets, transfusion by an empiric formula is not indicated. Plasma transfusion is indicated to maintain the PT at less than 1.5 times the

---

Table 9-7. Practice Guidelines for Blood Component Therapy in Surgery and Trauma

Blood Component	Indications	
Platelet concentrates	Massive transfusion Cardiopulmonary bypass surgery Neurologic surgery Ophthalmologic surgery	} Platelet count <80 - 100,000/µL
	Other surgery	Platelet count <60 - 80,000/µL
Plasma (Fresh Frozen or Solvent/ Detergent-Treated)	PT > 1.5 times the midpoint of the reference range and/or aPTT > 1.5 times the top of the reference range	
Cryoprecipitate	Fibrinogen < 100 mg/dL	

PT = prothrombin time; aPTT = activated partial thromboplastin time

---

midpoint of the reference range and the aPTT at less than 1.5 times the top of the reference range (Table 9-7). Plasma infusion at the rate of 1 U/20 kg is a reasonable dose. The fibrinogen concentration should be maintained at greater than 100 mg/dL. Cryoprecipitate (1 U/10 kg) may be used for this purpose. Clinicians should remember that when platelet transfusions are given, approximately 200-300 mL of plasma containing normal or nearly normal levels of coagulation factors is being infused.

The clinician caring for the massively transfused patient should obtain a platelet count, PT, aPTT, and fibrinogen concentration initially and frequently during the course of therapy. The infusion of platelet concentrates, plasma, and cryoprecipitate should be determined by a combination of the results of these assays and the patient's clinical condition. The adherence to specific guidelines can lead to undertransfusion if the decision is based only on laboratory values. Bleeding in trauma patients is often multifactorial and may not correlate directly with laboratory measurements. The location and extent of injuries, duration of shock, responses to resuscitation, and presence of compli-

cating factors such as intracranial bleeding all play a role in the clinical decision to transfuse. In the end, clinical judgment must prevail, even if this results in what appears to be an overuse of components based on laboratory measurements. Recently, the use of fresh Whole Blood when all else fails has been identified as having a potential role in the setting of massive transfusion, although additional studies are needed to confirm this finding.[147]

Citrate Toxicity

Blood components are anticoagulated with sodium citrate. The concentration of citrate in components is listed in Table 9-8. The principal sources of citrate during massive transfusion are platelet concentrates and plasma. Citrate binds divalent cations, including calcium and magnesium. During massive transfusion, the body's ability to excrete and metabolize citrate may be exceeded. This ability may be limited in trauma patients with severe hypotension, hypothermia, hepatic injury, or preexisting hepatic disease. Hypocalcemia and hypomagnesemia may result. Hypocalcemia may manifest

Table 9-8. Citrate Content of Various Anticoagulant-Preservative Formulations

	CPD/CPDA-1	AS-1	AS-3
Grams trisodium citrate ($2H_2O$)	1.656	1.656	2.244
Grams citric acid (H_2O)	0.206	0.206	0.248
Grams citrate per unit	1.261	1.261	1.681
Concentration of citrate per liter (mmol/L)	6.7	6.7	8.9
Concentration of citrate (mg/dL)* in			
Whole Blood	246	206	274
Red Blood Cells (RBCs)	76	54	181
Fresh Frozen Plasma (FFP)	384	384	384
Quantity of citrate (mg)* in			
Whole Blood	1261	1261	1681
RBCs	176	176	596
FFP	843	843	843

CPD = citrate phosphate dextrose; CPDA-1 = citrate phosphate dextrose adenine; AS = additive solution

*Calculated assuming a 450-mL donation, a hematocrit of 41%, and no movement of citrate into cells. For CPD and CPDA-1, calculation assumes the production of RBCs with a hematocrit of 80%; 230 mL of FFP; and 55 mL of Platelets. For AS-1 and AS-3, calculation assumes the production of RBCs with a final hematocrit of 56%; 230 mL of FFP; and 55 mL of Platelets.

Reprinted with permission from Dzik WH, Kirkley SA.[148]

clinically by reduced ventricular function, increased neuromuscular excitability, and arrhythmia including ventricular fibrillation.[149] The electrocardiographic manifestation of hypocalcemia is a prolongation of the QoTc interval. Citrate does not cause levels of calcium to become so low that coagulation is compromised. Hypomagnesemia can also result in neuromuscular excitability and ventricular arrhythmia.

Typically, calcium therapy during massive transfusion is necessary in neonates and patients with hepatic dysfunction. In all massively transfused patients, ionized calcium levels should be used to guide therapy. If levels are below 50% of normal, IV calcium chloride administration is appropriate. If symptoms are not corrected by calcium administration, magnesium levels should be measured.

Each molecule of citrate is metabolized to three molecules of bicarbonate, which can lead to metabolic alkalosis.

Potassium

Potassium leaks from red cells during storage and may accumulate, reaching levels of 7.5 mmol/U.[103] Massive transfusion of units containing increased potassium may lead to transient hyperkalemia, adding to the elevated potassium levels caused by severe shock, renal dysfunction, and muscle necrosis. In most patients, the amount of potassium transfused with RBCs causes little harm because potassium reenters the cells within a few hours after transfusion. Some patients may experience a paradoxical hypokalemia resulting from metabolism of citrate to bicarbonate, with the resultant metabolic alkalosis inducing increased urinary excretion of potassium.[134] The ability to infuse large volumes of stored blood rapidly using high-capacity blood warmers has increased the risk of hyperkalemia in massively transfused patients. Significant hyperkalemia can result in cardiac arrhythmia and reduced myocardial function. Potassium levels must be monitored closely in massively transfused patients.

Red Blood Cell Dysfunction

Erythrocyte 2,3-DPG concentration decreases during storage and drops to less than 10% of the initial level after 10-14 days. The depletion of 2,3-DPG results in a left shift of the hemoglobin-oxygen dissociation curve, which in turn results in increased oxygen affinity and decreased oxygen off-loading from the red cell.[150] For patients with atherosclerotic disease who may not be able to increase myocardial perfusion, the depletion of 2,3-DPG is of concern. Although adverse patient outcomes owing to 2,3-DPG depletion have not been documented, the empiric provision of some blood less than 2 weeks old in older patients or in patients with known atherosclerotic disease who are receiving massive transfusions is a reasonable practice. Alternatively, it may be desirable to maintain a higher hematocrit value (eg, approximately 30%) in such patients.

The stored erythrocyte's deformability may also be limited, restricting its ability to pass through the microcirculation. This capability depends on cellular adenosine triphosphate levels.[151] Up to 25% of transfused erythrocytes may not survive more than a few hours posttransfusion.

Microaggregates

Microaggregates of platelets, leukocytes, and fibrin accumulate in stored RBCs. Many of these particles are not trapped by the standard 170-μ blood filter. Microaggregate filters are available, but there is no convincing evidence that they provide improved pa-tient outcome. These filters may prevent the rapid delivery of blood, so their use is not recommended.

Hypothermia

Blood transfusions can exacerbate the hypothermia already present in patients with major trauma. In turn, the hypothermia can impair hemostasis, reduce the metabolism of citrate, increase hemoglobin oxygen affinity, and reduce myocardial function. The rapid infusion of cold blood centrally could also induce arrhythmia. For these reasons, the warming of blood products and other IV fluids to 37 C with high-flow blood-warming devices approved for this function is appropriate. Insulating the patient's head and extremities and warming the resuscitation room are other measures that may be used.

Dilutional Hypoalbuminemia

If resuscitation is undertaken with RBCs and crystalloid solution, little albumin is being replaced. Although approximately 60% of albumin is normally extravascular, at some point, particularly in patients who may have low albumin concentrations prior to trauma or massive hemorrhage, dilutional albuminemia will result. Clinicians should be mindful of this possibility and measure albumin levels during the course of massive transfusion if albumin solutions are not being used as replacement fluid.

Immune Hemolysis

Incompatible RBCs

ABO-incompatible hemolytic transfusion reactions are the most common cause of acute fatalities from blood transfusion and are related to human error.[152,153] Acute hemolytic reactions caused by naturally occurring alloantibodies (anti-A or anti-B) lead to complement activation, red cell lysis, and liberation of free hemoglobin.[154] These events may result in acute renal failure, DIC, and death. A hemolytic reaction in a critically injured or massively transfused patient may be overlooked. The clinical findings of hemoglobinuria, hypotension, fever, and microvascular hemorrhage may be attributed to traumatic injury.

Passive Antibody

Uncrossmatched group O RBCs are often used for emergency transfusion. The small amount of plasma in these components does not pose a problem for the recipient regardless of the patient's blood group. Furthermore, once the patient's own blood group has been determined, it is safe to switch the blood group of the infused red cells to that of the recipient without concern for the small amount of passive antibody that has been infused with the group O RBCs. This will conserve the supply of group O units.

Conclusion

Blood transfusion is an essential element of surgical and trauma therapy. Clinicians must be guided by the patient's clinical status and laboratory results in determining when, what, and how much to transfuse. The use of large quantities of blood components brings additional risks to patients already compromised by surgery and/or serious injury.

References

1. Greenburg AG. Pathophysiology of anemia. Am J Med 1996;101(2A):7-11S.
2. Ostgaard G. Perioperative and postoperative normovolemic anemia. Physiological compensation, monitoring and risk evaluation. Tidsskr Nor Laegeforen 1996;116:57-60.
3. Buckberg G, Brazier J. Coronary blood flow and cardiac function during hemodilution. Bibl Haematol 1974;41:173-89.
4. Doak GJ, Hall RI. Does hemoglobin concentration affect perioperative myocardial lactate flux in patients undergoing coronary artery bypass surgery? Anesth Analg 1995; 80:910-6.
5. Geha AS, Baue AE. Graded coronary stenosis and coronary flow during acute normovolemic anemia. World J Surg 1978;2:645-51.
6. Wilkerson DK, Rosen AL, Sehgal LR, et al. Limits of cardiac compensation in anemic baboons. Surgery 1988:103:665-70.
7. Tuman KJ. Tissue oxygen delivery: The physiology of anemia. Anesthesiol Clin North Am 1990;9:451-69.
8. Kleen M, Habler O, Hutter J, et al. Effects of hemodilution on splanchnic perfusion and hepatorenal function, I: Splanchnic perfusion. Eur J Med Res 1997;2:413-8.
9. Guidelines for red blood cell and plasma transfusion for adults and children. Report of the Expert Working Group. Can Med Assoc J 1997;156 (11 Suppl):S5-6.
10. Erni D, Banic A, Wheatley AM, Sigurdsson GH. Haemorrhage during anaesthesia and surgery: Continuous measurement of microcirculatory blood flow in the kidney, liver, skin and skeletal muscle. Eur J Anaesthesiol 1995;12:423-9.
11. Weiskopf RB, Viele MK, Feiner J, et al. Human cardiovascular and metabolic response to acute, severe isovolemic anemia. JAMA 1998;279:217-21.
12. Valeri CR, Crowley JP, Loscalzo J. The red blood cell transfusion trigger: Has the sin of commission now become the sin of omission? Transfusion 1998;38:602-10.
13. Office of Medical Applications and Research, National Institutes of Health. Perioperative red blood cell transfusion. JAMA 1988;260: 2700-3.
14. Adams RC, Lundy JS. Anesthesia in cases of poor surgical risk. Some suggestions for decreasing the risk. Surg Gynecol Obstet 1942; 74:1011-9.
15. Wedgewood JJ, Thomas JG. Peri-operative haemoglobin: An overview of current opinion regarding the acceptable level of haemoglobin in the peri-operative period. Eur J Anaesthesiol 1996;13:316-24.

16. Lundsgaard-Hansen P. Safe hemoglobin or hematocrit levels in surgical patients. World J Surg 1996;20:1182-8.

17. Stehling L, Simon TL. The red cell transfusion trigger. Physiology and clinical studies. Arch Pathol Lab Med 1994;118:429-34.

18. Lou S, Low TC. Perioperative transfusion strategies: A national survey among anaesthetists. Ann Acad Med Singapore 1997;26:193-9.

19. Diamond LK. A history of blood transfusion. In: Wintrobe MM, ed. Blood, pure and eloquent: A story of discovery, of people, and of ideas. New York: McGraw-Hill 1980:659-83.

20. Clark JH, Nelson W, Lyons C, et al. Chronic shock: The problem of reduced blood volume in the chronically ill patient. Ann Surg 1947;125:618-20.

21. Stehling L, Zauder HL. Acute normovolemic hemodilution. Transfusion 1991:31;857-68.

22. Robertie PG, Gravlee GP. Safe limits of hemodilution and recommendations for erythrocyte transfusion. Int Anesthesiol Clin 1990:28:197-204.

23. Chapler CK, Cain SM. The physiologic reserve in oxygen carrying capacity: Studies in experimental hemodilution. Can J Physiol Pharmacol 1986;64:7-12.

24. Czer LSC, Shoemaker WC. Optimal hematocrit value in critically ill postoperative patients. Surg Gynecol Obstet 1978;147:363-8.

25. Schwarz S, Frantz RA, Shoemaker WC. Sequential hemodynamic and oxygen transport responses in hypovolemia, anemia, and hypoxia. Am J Physiol 1981;241: (Heart Circ Physiol 10): HH64-72.

26. Lunn JN, Elwood PC. Anemia and surgery. Br Med J 1970;3:71-3.

27. Rawstron ER. Anemia and surgery. A retrospective clinical study. Aust N Z J Surg 1970;39:425-32.

28. Alexiu O, Mircea N, Balaban M, et al. Gastrointestinal hemorrhage from peptic ulcer. An evaluation of bloodless transfusion and early surgery. Anaesthesia 1975;30:609-15.

29. Carson JL, Duff A, Berlin JA, et al. Perioperative blood transfusion and postoperative mortality. JAMA 1998;279:199-205.

30. Spence RK, Carson JA, Poses R, et al. Elective surgery without transfusion: Influence of preoperative hemoglobin level and blood loss on mortality. Am J Surg 1990;59:320-4.

31. Carson JA, Spence RK, Poses R, et al. Severity of anemia and operative mortality and morbidity. Lancet 1988;2:727-9.

32. Hebert PC, Wells GA, Tweedale M, et al. Does transfusion practice affect mortality in critically ill patients? Am J Respir Crit Care Med 1997;155:1618-23.

33. Hebert PC, Wells GA, Marshall JC, et al. Transfusion requirements in critical care. A pilot study. JAMA 1995;273:1439-44.

34. Baron JF. Which lower value of haematocrit or haemoglobin concentration should guide the transfusion of red blood cell concentrates during and after extracorporeal circulation? Ann Fr Anesth Reanim 1995;14(Suppl 1):21-7.

35. Linman JW. Physiologic and pathophysiologic effects of anemia. N Engl J Med 1968;279:812-8.

36. Carmel R, Shulman IA. Blood transfusion in medically treatable chronic anemia. Pernicious anemia as a model for transfusion overuse. Arch Pathol Lab Med 1989;113:995-7.

37. Muller G, N'tita I, Nyst M, et al. Application of blood transfusion guidelines in a major hospital of Kinshasa, Zaire (letter). AIDS 1992;6:431-2.

38. Spence RK, Costabile JP, Young GS, et al. Is hemoglobin level alone a reliable predictor of outcome in the severely anemic patient? Am J Surg 1992;58:92-5.

39. Nelson AH, Fleisher LA, Rosenbaum SH. The relationship between postoperative anemia and cardiac morbidity in high risk vascular patients in the ICU (abstract). Crit Care Med 1992;20(Suppl):S71.

40. Christopherson R, Frank S, Norris E, et al. Low postoperative hematocrit is associated

with cardiac ischemia in high-risk patients (abstract). Anesthesiology 1991;75(3A): A100.

41. Carson JA, Duff A, Poses R, et al. Effect of anemia and cardiovascular disease on surgical mortality and morbidity. Lancet 1996; 348:1055-60.

42. Lum G. Should the transfusion trigger and the hemoglobin low critical limit be identical? Ann Clin Lab Sci 1997;27:130-4.

43. Shoemaker WC, Appel PL, Kram HB. Tissue oxygen debt as determinant of lethal and non-lethal postoperative organ failure. Crit Care Med 1988;16:1117-20.

44. Bihari DJ, Tinker J. The therapeutic value of prostaglandins in multiple organ failure associated with sepsis. Intensive Care Med 1988; 15:2-7.

45. Spence RK, Cernaianu AC, Carson J, Del Rossi AJ. Transfusion and surgery. Curr Probl Surg 1993;30:1101-80.

46. Sowade O, Gross J, Sowade B, et al. Evaluation of oxygen availability with oxygen status algorithm in patients undergoing open heart surgery treated with epoietin beta. J Lab Clin Med 1997;127:97-105.

47. Bannon MP, O'Neill CM, Martin M, et al. Central venous oxygen saturation, arterial base deficit, and lactate concentration in trauma patients. Am J Surg 1995;61:738-45.

48. Astiz ME, Rackow EC, Falk JL, et al. Oxygen delivery and consumption in patients with hyperdynamic septic shock. Crit Care Med 1987;15:26-8.

49. Muller JC, Schwarz U, Schaible TF, et al. Do cardiac output and serum lactate levels indicate blood transfusion requirements in the anemia of prematurity? Intensive Care Med 1996;22:472-6.

50. Van Wyck DB. Iron management during recombinant human erythropoietin therapy. Am J Kidney Dis 1989;14(2 Suppl 1):9-13.

51. Tasaki T, Ohto H, Noguchi M, et al. Iron and erythropoietin measurement in autologous blood donors with anemia: Implications for management. Transfusion 1994;34:337-43.

52. Weisbach V, Eckstein R. Iron homeostasis in preoperative autologous blood donation. Infusionsther Transfusionsmed 1996;23(3): 161-70.

53. Ashby EC. Total dose iron-dextran infusions in general surgery. Lancet 1967;2:807-9.

54. Popovsky MA. Quality of blood components filtered before storage and at the beside: Implications for transfusion practice. Transfusion 1996;36:470-4 .

55. Higgins VL. Leukocyte-reduced blood components: Patient benefits and practical applications. Oncol Nurs Forum 1996;23:659-67.

56. Bradley J. The blood transfusion effect: Experimental aspects. Immunol Lett 1991;29: 127-32.

57. Klein HG. Immunologic aspects of blood transfusion. Semin Oncol 1994;21(2 Suppl 3):16-20.

58. Triulzi D, Blumberg N, Heal J. Association of transfusion with postoperative bacterial infection. Crit Rev Clin Lab Sci 1990;28:95-107.

59. Blumberg N, Heal J. Transfusion-induced immunomodulation and its possible role in cancer recurrence and perioperative bacterial infection. Yale J Biol Med 1990;63:429-33.

60. Spence RK for the Blood Management Practice Guidelines Conference. Surgical red blood cell transfusion practice policies. Am J Surg 1995;170(6A Suppl):3-15S.

61. Goodnough LT, Grishaber JE, Birkmeyer JD, et al. Efficacy and cost-effectiveness of autologous blood predeposit in patients undergoing radical prostatectomy procedures. Urology 1994;44:226-31.

62. Sculco TP. Blood management in orthopedic surgery. Am J Surg 1995;170(6A Suppl):60-3S.

63. Nissenson AR. Erythropoietin treatment in peritoneal dialysis patients. Perit Dial Int 1994;14(Suppl 3):S63-9.

64. Spivak JL. Recombinant human erythropoietin and the anemia of cancer (editorial). Blood 1994;84:997-1004.

65. Goodnough LT, Price TH, Friedman KD, et al. A Phase III trial of recombinant human erythropoietin therapy in nonanemic orthopedic patients subjected to aggressive removal of blood for autologous use: Dose, response, toxicity, and efficacy. Transfusion 1994;34:66-71.

66. Beris P, Mermillod B, Levy G, et al. Recombinant human erythropoietin as adjuvant treatment for autologous blood donation. A prospective study. Vox Sang 1993;65:212-8.

67. Goodnough LT, Vizmeg A, Robecks R, et al. Prevalence and classification of anemia in elective orthopedic surgery patients: Implications for blood conservation program. Vox Sang 1992;63:90-5.

68. Goodnough LT, Brittenham G. Limitations of the erythropoietic response to serial phlebotomy: Implications for autologous blood donor programs. J Lab Clin Med 1990;115:28-35.

69. Goodnough LT, Rudick S, Price TH, et al. Increased collection of autologous blood preoperatively with recombinant human erythropoietin therapy. N Engl J Med 1989;321:1163-7.

70. Biesma DH, Marx JJ, Kraaijenhagen RJ, et al. Lower homologous blood requirement in autologous blood donors after treatment with recombinant human erythropoietin. Lancet 1994;344:367-70.

71. Mercuriali F, Zanella A, Barosi G, et al. Use of erythropoietin to increase the volume of autologous blood donated by orthopedic patients. Transfusion 1993;33:55-9.

72. Price TH, Goodnough LT, Vogler WR, et al. Improving the efficacy of autologous blood donation with low hematocrit: A randomized, double-blind, controlled trial of recombinant human erythropoietin. Am J Med 1996;101(Suppl 2A):22-7S.

73. Healy JC, Frankforter SA, Graves BK, et al. Preoperative autologous blood donation in total-hip arthroplasty. A cost-effectiveness analysis. Arch Pathol Lab Med 1994;118:465-70.

74. Britton L, Eastlund D, Dziuban S, et al. Predonated autologous blood use in elective cardiac surgery. Ann Thorac Surg 1989;47:529-32.

75. Spiess BD. Pro: Autologous blood should be available for elective cardiac surgery. J Cardiothorac Vasc Anesth 1994;8:231-7.

76. D'Ambra MN, Kaplan DK. Alternatives to allogeneic blood use in surgery: Acute normovolemic hemodilution and preoperative autologous donation. Am J Surg 1995;170:6A(Suppl):49-52S.

77. Goodnough LT, Monk TG, Brecher ME. Autologous blood procurement in the surgical setting: Lessons learned in the last 10 years. Vox Sang 1996;71:133-41.

78. Monk TG, Goodnough LT, Birkmeyer JD, et al. Acute normovolemic hemodilution is a cost-effective alternative to preoperative autologous donation in patients undergoing radical retropubic prostatectomy. Transfusion 1995;35:559-65.

79. Monk TG, Goodnough LT, Andriole GL, et al. Preoperative recombinant human erythropoietin therapy enhances the efficacy of acute normovolemic hemodilution. Anesth Analg 1995;80:S230.

80. Williamson KR, Taswell HF. Intraoperative blood salvage: A review. Transfusion 1991;31:662-75.

81. Giordano GF, Giordano DM, Wallace BA, et al. An analysis of 9918 consecutive perioperative autotransfusions. Surg Gynecol Obstet 1993;176:103-10.

82. Senagore AJ, Luchtefeld MA, Mackeigan JM, Mazier WP. Open colectomy versus laparoscopic colectomy: Are there differences? Am J Surg 1993;59:549-54.

83. Go H, Takeda M, Takahashi H, et al. Laparoscopic adrenalectomy for primary aldosteronism: A new operative method. J Laparoendosc Surg 1993;3:455-9.

84. Suzuki K, Kageyama S, Ueda D, et al. Laparoscopic adrenalectomy: Clinical experience with 12 cases. J Urol 1993;150:1099-102.

85. Vietz PF, Ahn TS. A new approach to hysterectomy without colpotomy: Pelviscopic in-

trafascial hysterectomy. Am J Obstet Gynecol 1994;170:609-13.

86. Arbogast JD, Welch RA, Riza ED, et al. Laparoscopically assisted vaginal hysterectomy appears to be an alternative to total abdominal hysterectomy. J Laparoendosc Surg 1994;4:185-90.

87. Blackwell KE, Ross DA, Kapur P, Calcaterra TC. Propofol for maintenance of general anesthesia: A technique to limit blood loss during endoscopic sinus surgery. Am J Otolaryngol 1993;14:262-6.

88. Kram H, Nathan R, Stafford F, et al. Fibrin glue achieves hemostasis in patients with coagulation disorders. Arch Surg 1989;124:384-8.

89. Rosengart TK. Pharmacologic approaches to coagulation (aprotinin, epsilon amino caproic acid, DDVP, tranexamic acid therapy). In: Krieger KH, Isom OW, eds. Blood conservation in cardiac surgery. New York: Springer-Verlag, 1998:381-95.

90. Atabek U, Alvarez R, Pello MJ, et al. Erythropoietin accelerates hematocrit recovery in post-surgical anemia. Am J Surg 1994;61:74-7.

91. Canadian Orthopedic Perioperative Erythropoietin Study Group. Effectiveness of perioperative recombinant human erythropoietin in elective hip replacement. Lancet 1993;341:1227-32.

92. Faris P. Use of recombinant human erythropoietin in the perioperative period of orthopedic surgery. Am J Med Suppl 1996;101 (2A):28-32.

93. D'Ambra MN, Lunch KE, Bocaggno J, et al. Effect of perioperative administration of recombinant human erythropoietin in CABG patients(abstract). Anesthesiology 1992;77:A159.

94. Wertlake PT, McGinniss MH, Schmidt PJ. Cold antibody and persistent intravascular hemolysis after surgery under hypothermia. Transfusion 1969;9:70-3.

95. Moore RA, Geller EA, Mathews ES, et al. The effect of hypothermic cardiopulmonary bypass on patients with low-titer, nonspecific cold agglutinins. Ann Thorac Surg 1984;37:233-8.

96. Klein HG, Kalz IL, McIntosh CL, et al. Surgical hypothermia in a patient with a cold agglutinin: Management by plasma exchange. Transfusion 1980;20:354-7.

97. Paccagnella A, Simini G, Nieri A, et al. Cardiopulmonary bypass and cold agglutinin (letter). J Thorac Cardiovasc Surg 1988;95:543.

98. Helm RE, Isom OW. Indications for red cell transfusion. In: Krieger KH, Isom OW, eds. Blood conservation in cardiac surgery. New York: Springer-Verlag, 1998:397-438.

99. Manno CS, Hedberg KW, Kim HC, et al. Comparison of the hemostatic effects of fresh whole blood, stored whole blood, and components after open heart surgery in children. Blood 1991;77:930-6.

100. Gelb AB, Roth RI, Levin J, et al. Changes in blood coagulation during and following cardiopulmonary bypass. Am J Clin Pathol 1996;106:87-99.

101. Kestin AS, Valeri CR, Khuri SF, et al. The platelet function defect of cardiopulmonary bypass. Blood 1993;82:107-17.

102. Vengelen-Tyler V, ed. Technical manual. 12th ed. Bethesda, MD: American Association of Blood Banks, 1993:345.

103. Ross S, Jeter E. Massive transfusion. In: Petz LD, Swisher SN, Kleinman S, et al, eds. Clinical practice of transfusion medicine. 3rd ed. New York: Churchill-Livingstone, 1995:563-79.

104. Trunkey D. Trauma. Sci Am 1983;249:28-30.

105. Knottenbelt J. Low initial hemoglobin levels in trauma patients: An important indicator of ongoing hemorrhage. J Trauma 1991;31:1396-9.

106. Wudel J, Morris J, Yates K, et al. Massive transfusion: Outcome in blunt trauma patients. J Trauma 1991;31:1-7.

107. Frey C, Huelke D, Gikas P. Resuscitation and survival in motor vehicle accidents. J Trauma 1969;9:292-8.

108. Yavorski R, Wong R, Maydonovitch C, et al. Analysis of 3,294 cases of upper gastrointestinal bleeding in military medical facilities. Am J Gastroenterol 1995;90:568-73.

109. Harrigan C, Lucas C, Ledgerwood A, Mammen E. Primary hemostasis after massive transfusion for injury. Surgery 1985;98:836-40.

110. Phillips T, Soulier G, Wilson R. Outcome of massive transfusion exceeding two blood volumes in trauma and emergency surgery. J Trauma 1987;27:903-8.

111. Wilson R, Mammen E, Walt E. Eight years of experience with massive blood transfusion. J Trauma 1971;11:275-8.

112. Rutledge R, Sheldon G, Collins M. Massive transfusion. Crit Care Clin 1986;2:791-83.

113. Olsen W. Quantitative peritoneal lavage in blunt abdominal trauma. Arch Surg 1972; 104:536-9.

114. Mucha P, Welch T. Hemorrhage in major pelvic fractures. Surg Clin North Am 1988; 68:757-80.

115. Sawyer P, Harrison C. Massive transfusion in adults. Vox Sang 1990;58:199-202.

116. Kivioja A, Myllynen P, Rokkanen P. Survival after massive transfusions exceeding four blood volumes in patients with blunt injuries. Am J Surg 1991;57:398-402.

117. Harvey M, Greenfield T, Sugrue M, Rosenfeld D. Massive blood transfusion in a tertiary referral hospital. Clinical outcomes and hemostatic complications. Med J Aust 1995; 163:356-9.

118. Harrigan C, Lucas C, Ledgerwood A. The effect of hemorrhagic shock on the clotting cascade in injured patients. J Trauma 1989;29: 1416-20.

119. Mitchell KJ, Moncure KE, Onyeije C, et al. Evaluation of massive volume replacement in the penetrating trauma patient. J Natl Med Assoc 1994;86:926-9.

120. Canizaro P, Possa M. Management of massive hemorrhage associated with abdominal trauma. Surg Clin North Am 1990;70:621-5.

121. Faringer P, Mullins R, Johnson R, Trunkey D. Blood component supplementation during massive transfusion of AS-1 red cells in trauma patients. J Trauma 1993;34:481-6.

122. Samama CM. Traumatic emergencies and hemostasis. Can J Anesthesiol 1995;43: 479-82.

123. Schmidt P. Use of Rh positive blood in emergency situations. Surg Gynecol Obstet 1988; 167:229-33.

124. Schwab C, Shayne J, Turner J. Immediate trauma resuscitation with type O uncrossmatched blood: A two-year prospective experience. J Trauma 1986;26:897-902.

125. Bickell WH, Wall MJ Jr, Pepe PE, et al. Immediate versus delayed fluid resuscitation for hypotensive patients with penetrating torso injuries. N Engl J Med 1994;331: 1105-9.

126. Janvier G, Fialon P, Guinier MC, et al. Strategy of erythrocyte transfusion and plasma use in traumatic emergencies. Can J Anaesthesiol 1994;42:643-9.

127. Audibert G. Indications of blood components and outcome of transfusion practices in hemorrhage of multiple trauma. Can J Anaesthesiol 1994;42:391-4.

128. Gervin A, Fischer R. Resuscitation of trauma patients with type-specific uncrossmatched blood. J Trauma 1984;24:327-31.

129. Gervin A. Transfusion, autotransfusion, and blood substitutes. In: Moore E, Mattox K, Feliciano D, eds. Trauma. 2nd ed. Norwalk, CT.: Appleton and Lange, 1991:165-73.

130. Bowersox JC, Hess JR. Trauma and military applications of blood substitutes. Artif Cells Blood Substit Immobil Biotechnol 1994;22: 145-57.

131. Counts R, Haisch C, Simon T, et al. Hemostasis in massively transfused trauma patients. Ann Surg 1979;190:91-6.

132. Humphries JE. Transfusion therapy in acquired coagulopathies. Hematol Oncol Clin North Am 1994;8:1181-201.

133. Murray DJ, Pennell BJ, Weinstein SL, Olsen JD. Packed red cells in acute blood loss: Dilutional coagulopathy as a cause of surgical bleeding. Anesth Analg 1995;80:336-42.

134. Collins J. Problems associated with the massive transfusion of stored blood. Surgery 1974; 75:274-8.

135. Lucas C, Ledgerwood A. Clinical significance of altered coagulation test after massive transfusions for trauma. Am J Surg 1981;47:125-9.

136. Hewson J, Neame P, Kumar N, et al. Coagulopathy related to dilution and hypotension during massive transfusion. Crit Care Med 1985;13:387-92.

137. Bick R. Disseminated intravascular coagulation and related syndromes: A clinical review. Semin Thromb Hemost 1988;14:299-305.

138. Schmied H, Kurz A, Sessler DI, et al. Mild hypothermia increases blood loss and transfusion requirements during total hip arthroplasty. Lancet 1996;347:289-92.

139. Nathan HJ, Polis T. The management of temperature during hypothermic cardiopulmonary bypass, II: Effect of prolonged hypothermia. Can J Anaesthesiol 1995;42:672-6.

140. Valeri C, Cassidy G, Khuri S, et al. Hypothermia-induced reversible platelet dysfunction. Ann Surg 1987;205:175-80.

141. Harke H, Rahman S. Haemostatic disorders in massive transfusion. Bibl Haematol 1980; 46:179-83.

142. Noe D, Graham S, Luff R, Sohmer P. Platelet counts during rapid massive transfusion. Transfusion 1982;22:392-6.

143. Mannucci P, Federici A, Sirchia G. Hemostasis testing during massive blood replacement. Vox Sang 1982;42:113-8.

144. Hiippala ST, Myllyla GJ, Vahtera EM. Hemostatic factors and replacement of major blood loss with plasma-poor red cell concentrates. Anesth Analg 1995;81:360-5.

145. Rohrer MJ. Effect of hypothermia on the coagulation cascade. Crit Care Med 1992;20: 1402-8.

146. Nicholls MD, Whyte G. Red cell, plasma and albumin transfusion decision triggers. Anaesth Intensive Care 1993;21:156-62.

147. Erber WN, Tan J, Grey D, Lown JA. Use of unrefrigerated fresh whole blood in massive transfusion. Med J Aust 1996;165:11-3.

148. Dzik WH, Kirkley SA. Citrate toxicity during massive blood transfusion. Transfus Med Rev 1988;2:76-94.

149. Bunker J. Metabolic Effects of blood transfusions. Anesthesiology 1966;27:446-50.

150. Valeri C, Gray A, Cassidy G, et al. The 24-hour post-transfusion survival, oxygen transport function, and residual hemolysis of human outdated-rejuvenated red cell concentrate after washing and storage at 4 degrees C for 24 to 72 hours. Transfusion 1984;24: 323-8.

151. Wolfe L. The membrane and lesions of storage in preserved red cells. Transfusion 1985; 25:185-9.

152. Sazama K. Reports of 355 transfusion-associated deaths: 1976 through 1985. Transfusion 1990;30:583-8.

153. Gloe D. Common reactions to transfusions. Heart Lung 1991;20:506-12.

154. Seyfried H, Walewska I. Immune hemolytic transfusion reactions. World J Surg 1987; 11:25-9.

In: Mintz PD, ed.
Transfusion Therapy: Clinical Principles and Practice
Bethesda, MD: AABB Press, 1999

10

Clinical Uses of Fibrin Sealant

WILLIAM D. SPOTNITZ, MD, AND ROSANNE L. WELKER, PhD

 FIBRIN SEALANT HAS GROWN IN importance and use in the past 25 years. Its use in an extensive range of surgical procedures has been described in a large body of literature. This chapter reviews the more recent clinical uses of fibrin sealant, paying particular attention to hemostatic, tissue sealing, and drug carrier applications. It also discusses potential complications associated with fibrin sealant use, as well as developing methods for improving its safety. To emphasize the scientific rigor of this field, this chapter uses the term *fibrin sealant* rather than *fibrin glue* to describe this class of tissue adhesives. It also describes fibrin sealants made in local blood banks, as opposed to commercial or investigational fibrin sealants, as *blood-bank produced* instead of the unfortunate and derogatory term *homemade*, which has gained some widespread use.

Fibrin sealant, a surgical tissue adhesive composed primarily of fibrinogen and thrombin, mimics the final stage of the natural clotting mechanism. The process by which fibrinogen and thrombin combine in the presence of Factor XIII and calcium chloride to form fibrin sealant has been well described in the literature.[1-3] Fibrin sealant is biodegradable by the process of fibrinolysis and consequently may be combined with antifibrinolytic agents,[4] such as epsilon aminocaproic acid (Amicar, Immunex Corp, Seattle, WA), tranexamic acid (Cyklokapron, Pharmacia & Upjohn, Kalamazoo, MI), or aprotinin (Trasylol, Bayer Corp, West Haven, CT), to reduce intrinsic and extrinsic degradation.

William D. Spotnitz, MD, Professor, Department of Surgery, and Director, Tissue Adhesive Center, University of Virginia Health System, Charlottesville, Virginia; and Rosanne L. Welker, PhD, Academic Instructor, Division of Technology, Culture and Communication, School of Engineering and Applied Sciences, University of Virginia; and Publications Coordinator, Tissue Adhesive Center, University of Virginia Health System, Charlottesville, Virginia

Fibrin sealant has been used for three general purposes: to achieve hemostasis, to seal tissues, and to provide a delivery system for other biologic agents (see Fig 10-1). As a hemostatic agent, fibrin sealant can help surgeons address a variety of clotting disorders.

This effect is particularly important for anticoagulated patients undergoing cardiovascular procedures. Depending on the particular surgical site, the fibrin sealant is applied using one of several techniques that keep the fibrinogen and thrombin separate, mixing only upon the site of application. For larger surface areas with slow bleeding, a spray technique is used.[5] For suture lines, a light spray technique or syringes with blunt-nose cannulas are used. Cellulose sponge (Gelfoam; Upjohn Laboratories, Kalamazoo, MI) or collagen fleece (Avitene Nonwoven Web; Alcon Laboratories, Fort Worth, TX) may enhance the hemostatic effects at sites of heavier, localized bleeding. For very localized sites, such as the bronchial tree or a femoral arteriotomy, the fibrin sealant can be delivered through a catheter system.[6-8] Surgeons must remember, however, that fibrin sealant cannot substitute for meticulous surgical technique and cannot stop bleeding when traditional surgical methods such as sutures are required.

Fibrin sealant has been available commercially in Europe, Canada, and Japan. Until recently, however, the US Food and Drug Administration (FDA) had not approved fibrin sealant for the market because of concerns about possible viral disease transmission. Compassionate use guidelines have allowed some uses of fibrin sealant, and investigational fibrin sealants are now being tested on a large scale in the United States for possible FDA approval. In May, 1998, the FDA approved one fibrin sealant commercial preparation for use as an adjunct to hemostatis in cardiopulmonary bypass surgery, for the sealing of anastomoses in the closure of temporary colostomies, for the treatment of spleen injuries, and as an adjunct to surgical methods of hemostasis. This product is manufactured by Österreichisches Institut Für Haemoderivate GMBH (Vienna, Austria) and distributed by Baxter Healthcare Corporation (Hyland Division, Glendale, CA) under the brand name Tisseel and by Haemacure Corporation (Quebec, Canada) under the brand name Hemaseel.

At the University of Virginia, fibrin sealant is produced in the blood bank by combining commercial bovine thrombin with either single donor or autologous fibrinogen concentrates.[9] In general, higher fibrinogen concentrations increase the mechanical strength of the sealant and higher concentrations of thrombin increase the speed of polymerization; however, excessively high concentrations of either component can be disadvantageous.[10,11] The fibrinogen concentration used at the University of Virginia is 30-40 mg/mL and provides adequate

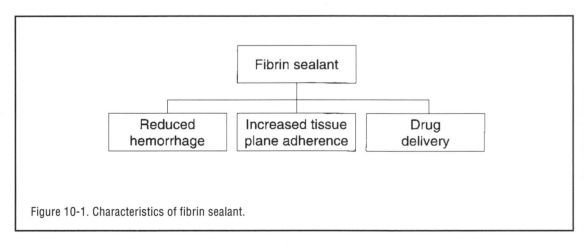

Figure 10-1. Characteristics of fibrin sealant.

clinical strength, while the thrombin concentration is relatively high (1000 N.I.H. units/mL), which causes the sealant to activate rapidly. The most common methods for separating fibrinogen from Whole Blood or Fresh Frozen Plasma include cryoprecipitation and various forms of chemical precipitation using ammonium sulfate,[12] polyethylene glycol,[13] or ethanol,[14] as well as the varying of centrifuge speeds and anticoagulants.[15] However, cryoprecipitation remains the gold standard.[16,17] Because using fresh plasma to produce fibrinogen results in a significant waste of unstable clotting factors, the University of Virginia's blood bank processes stored plasma using a cryoprecipitation method.[9]

Fibrin sealant has proved its value in a number of different surgical specialties, including cardiovascular, thoracic, vascular, oncologic, plastic, neurologic, ophthalmologic, orthopedic, trauma, head and neck, gynecologic, urologic, gastrointestinal, minimally invasive, and dental surgery. Its use in each of these areas, as well as its drug-delivery capabilities and its potential complications, is discussed below with attention to the more recent literature. At the University of Virginia, fibrin sealant has been used since 1985 in more than 3000 patients for a variety of surgical applications constituting about 5% of all operations each year. In more than 90% of these uses, the surgeons have judged

the fibrin sealant effective and have not had to re-operate.[18] No increase in surgical infection rates has been noted in these patients.

Fibrin Sealant in Cardiovascular Surgery

Achieving hemostasis after cardiovascular surgery represents a principal challenge in cardiovascular surgery, not only because complex suturing can produce additional bleeding but also because patients are frequently anticoagulated, which compromises their own hemostatic mechanisms (see Fig 10-2). Numerous animal and human studies suggest that fibrin sealant is a very effective adjunct to cardiovascular surgery. In fact, cardiovascular surgeons remain the primary users of fibrin tissue adhesives. One review of clinical studies of fibrin sealant in cardiothoracic surgery noted that through 1995, none of the 24 published clinical studies had demonstrated a deleterious effect from the use of fibrin sealant.[19] At the University of Virginia, thoracic and cardiovascular surgical procedures account for the majority of fibrin sealant uses. It has been used successfully there to seal complex suture lines, vascular conduits, cannulation sites, and vascular anastomoses (see Figs 10-3 and 10-4). It has controlled diffuse mediastinal bleeding and reduced transfusion requirements sig-

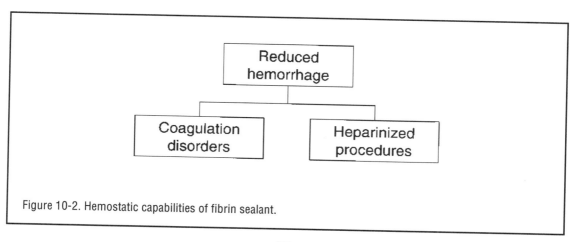

Figure 10-2. Hemostatic capabilities of fibrin sealant.

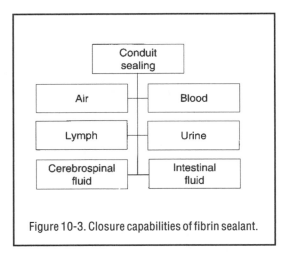

Figure 10-3. Closure capabilities of fibrin sealant.

may prove advantageous for reoperations because it seems to inhibit the formation of intrapericardial adhesions; however this use remains controversial.[23]

Fibrin sealant applied topically along arterial suture lines has been shown to (p < 0.014) reduce time to hemostasis significantly.[24,25] Researchers have studied such use for fully heparinized patients undergoing carotid endarterectomy with a polytetrafluoroethylene (PTFE) patch,[24] arterial bypass surgery with a PTFE bypass graft,[25] and aortic aneurysm repair with a woven Dacron graft.[25,26] In animal studies, fibrin sealant has sealed atrial rupture in a porcine model[27] and plugged femoral arteriotomy sites after cardiac catheterization in canine models successfully.[7,8]

Investigators have reported the effective use of fibrin sealant to treat Teflon patches for mitral valve replacement under the challenging condition of irregular and massive calcification.[28] Free-wall left-ventricular rupture has been repaired successfully with a pericardial patch reinforced with fibrin sealant.[29] For such procedures, fibrin sealant's hemostatic and biodegradable qualities are crucial. Rein-

nificantly.[20] Some researchers have described the effective use of an antibiotic-fibrin sealant mixture both to achieve hemostasis at the time of median sternotomy and to prevent postoperative wound infection complications.[21] Fibrin sealant alone has been used to stop pericardial leakage and preserve systemic pulmonary shunts.[22] Fibrin sealant even

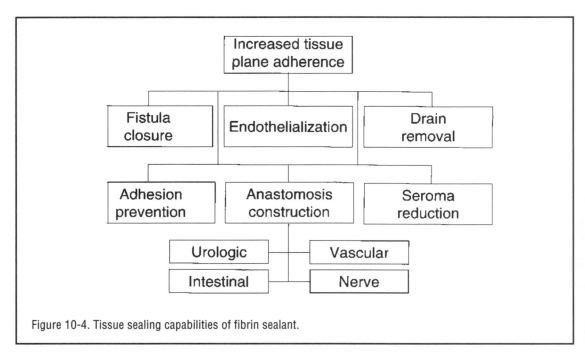

Figure 10-4. Tissue sealing capabilities of fibrin sealant.

forcing patch closure with fibrin sealant also appears to reduce the number and the size of residual ventricular septal defects.[30]

Fibrin sealant combined with endothelial cell growth factor not only assists in the adherence of muscle flap to the myocardium in cardiomyoplasty, but also can promote angiogenesis.[31] In that application, the fibrin sealant seems to imitate the extracellular matrix for endothelial cells, supporting their growth.[31] Site-specific angiogenesis (see Fig 10-5) can also be enhanced with the application of fibrin sealant seeded with angiogenic growth factor alpha–endothelial cell growth factor.[32]

Fibrin Sealant in Thoracic Surgery

Because of its changes in volume and surface areas, the lung surface represents a challenge to fibrin sealant use. The changes in size often cause the weaker fibrin sealant-to-tissue bond, as opposed to the stronger internal sealant-to-sealant bond, to break. Thus, the sealant may become detached from the lung surface when pulmonary ventilation occurs, changing the lung surface area.

However, several researchers have detailed successful methods for closing bronchopleural fistulas with fibrin sealants.[33-39] Recently, investigators have used fibrin sealant in high-risk patients to seal not only small proximal bronchopleural fistula, but also the muscle flap cavity to avoid pulmonary resection and thoracoplasty.[40] Closing bronchopleural fistula with fibrin sealant applied through a fiber-optic flexible bronchoscope, which enables better visualization and, hence, more precise application of the fibrin sealant, can prevent more invasive surgery,[6] as well as the trauma and hospital cost associated with more invasive procedures.

Methods for applying fibrin sealant to minimize air leakage and pleural drainage have also been frequently detailed.[33,41-43] In animal studies, the application of fibrin sealant has brought about hemostasis and stopped air leaks more effectively than the application of cryoprecipitate or topical collagen.[44,45] In a clinical study, the application of fibrin sealant following pulmonary resection reduced both leakage and hospital stay.[46] Other researchers have used fibrin sealant to reinforce suture lines after thoracotomy or resection.[47] Although these authors did not note a significant reduction in leak-

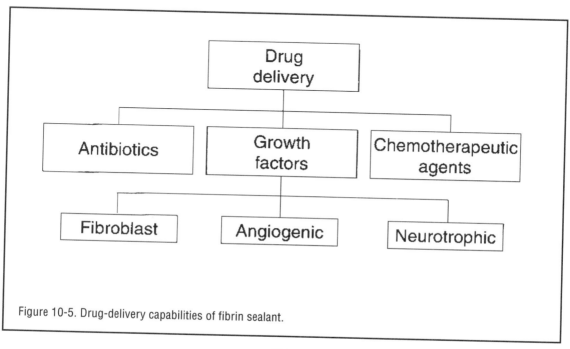

Figure 10-5. Drug-delivery capabilities of fibrin sealant.

age, they found the adhesive conferred other benefits, such as the reinforcement of suture lines and the closure of nonsuturable sites.

When used in clinical trials on lobectomy and pneumonectomy, fibrin sealant both reduced leakage and produced greater airway pressure tolerance.[42] In a 1977, randomized, clinical study of postthoracotomy alveolar air leaks, however, investigators found no statistically significant advantage to spraying fibrin sealant on the lung surface before closure.[48] This study focused on those patients for whom all conventional methods of treating persistent, moderate-to-severe alveolar air leak had failed, with the authors noting that previous studies were not randomized and used a heterogeneous group of surgical procedures. The authors concluded that fibrin sealant appears unable to manage such severe air leaks. The study, however, used a very small volume of fibrin sealant (5 mL), which was allowed to set for only 2 minutes before ventilation resumed, and investigators did not apply fibrin sealant prophylactically.

Other studies have noted significant advantages to using fibrin sealant during pulmonary procedures.[44-46,49,50] In thorascopic procedures, it has been used successfully to seal pneumothorax.[51,52] A case even has been reported of its successful use in resolving pneumothorax in an infant.[53]

Fibrin Sealant in Vascular Surgery

In addition to the routine use of fibrin sealant to augment hemostasis in vascular procedures, investigators report that coating expanded PTFE grafts with fibrin sealant used as a carrier for fibroblast growth factor type I and heparin enhances endothelialization in animal models.[54-58] Other studies by the same investigators suggest that this technique may decrease platelet deposition and early graft thrombogenicity.[59,60]

Fibrin sealant also has a role as a carrier in the design of bioprostheses to maximize the patency and function of engineered blood vessels.[61] Researchers have performed in-vitro and in-vivo experiments to determine how different substrates influence the process of endothelialization. By developing appropriate delivery systems, these researchers hope to manipulate the biologic response to various substrates in order to encourage or inhibit tissue growth, as required.[56-58,62] Fibrin sealant, because it is bioresorbable, appears to be an excellent candidate for the delivery of substrates such as heparin and growth factors (see Fig 10-5).[61]

In microvascular surgery, researchers using rat models have developed a telescoping anastomotic technique with fibrin sealant treatment. This method appears to secure the inserted vessel better and to reduce aneurysmal dilation of vein grafts.[63] In a subsequent study by the same researchers, the fibrin sealant method achieved a statistically higher patency rate ($p < 0.05$) than did the same telescoping technique used without fibrin sealant.[64] Other investigators also have reported that using fibrin sealant as an adjunct to end-to-side anastomosis achieves patency results comparable to those for suture techniques but provides the advantages of a simpler method, better hemostasis, and less tissue trauma.[65] In the anastomosis of very small vessels, a novel technique has been developed using disolvable stents made of mono-, di-, and triglycerides, with fibrin sealant treated anastomosis.[66] As compared with suture methods, this method is faster and easier and it achieves better short-term patency rates, but it is associated with lower long-term patency rates because of aneurysm formation. The authors of this study speculate that increasing the long-term strength of the fibrin sealant by increasing its Factor XIII concentration may alleviate this problem.[66] Other researchers suggest that negatively charged fibrin sealant may provide additional strength and may reduce rates of microvascular anastomotic thrombosis.[67]

Fibrin Sealant in Oncologic Surgery

Both animal and human studies have demonstrated the effective use of fibrin sealant to reduce serous drainage and seroma formation (see Fig 10-4) following axillary dissection in the treatment of breast cancer.[68-71] In addition, as discussed below, fibrin sealant can be used to deliver chemotherapeutic agents.

In a randomized, prospective, clinical study of axillary dissection, researchers at the University of Virginia used autologous fibrin sealant to reduce serous drainage significantly and allow earlier drain removal.[70] Control and treatment groups underwent identical surgical procedures by a single surgeon who was unaware of their status until the axillary dissection. After achieving hemostasis with sutures and electrocautery, the treatment group had fibrin sealant sprayed over suture lines, exposed axilla, and the chest wall. Both groups then had the skin flaps closed immediately with sutures. On every postoperative day, mean cumulative drainage volumes were reduced significantly in the fibrin sealant group (p <0.002), which allowed the axillary drains to be removed 3 days earlier. The authors of that study note that the fibrin sealant may allow for drainless surgery when this procedure is complicated by seroma formation. They also note that a rapidly clotting sealant and immediate wound closure are essential to the success of this method.[70]

A subsequent study of 40 patients undergoing axillary lymphadenectomy found that the application of a small volume (4 mL) of fibrin sealant followed by rapid wound closure reduced lymphatic drainage significantly.[72] That study was part of a multicenter, prospective, Phase II, FDA trial. Some controversy remains over the ability of fibrin sealant to reduce drainage, however, as another study did not find that the application of a commercial fibrin sealant after breast surgery reduced either serous drainage or the formation of cysts and fistula to a statistically significant degree.[73] The divergent findings in these studies may result from the different surgical techniques employed. Specifically, the best results occur with a technique of rapid wound closure immediately following fibrin sealant application in order to seal tissues and eliminate spaces where seroma fluid could accumulate.

Fibrin Sealant in Plastic Surgery

At the University of Virginia, plastic surgery is the third, most frequent, surgical specialty using fibrin sealant. It is a particularly effective hemostatic agent following burn debridement,[74] and it also appears to enhance the initial adherence and long-term viability of skin grafts. In a study of the effect of fibrin sealant on wound drainage using a rabbit model, autologous fibrin sealant applied to skin flaps over the parotid inhibited seroma and hematoma formation.[75] The ability of fibrin tissue adhesives to seal potential cavities may shorten hospital stays and help eliminate the need for drains (see Fig 10-4).

In a study of patients undergoing face lifts, drains were eliminated successfully for the fibrin sealant-treated group, and there were statistically significant reductions in major hematoma formation (p < 0.03) and in the edema and ecchymosis rate (p < 0.006).[76] In animal models for mastectomy[68] and for radical neck dissection,[77] fibrin sealant reduced seroma formation by enhancing tissue apposition and adherence as well as by reducing lymphatic leakage.

Fibrin Sealant in Neurosurgery

At the University of Virginia, neurosurgery is the second most frequent user of fibrin sealant. The tissue-sealing effects of fibrin sealant are particularly useful here because of the inability of cerebrospinal fluid (CSF) to form clots. Fibrin sealant can provide a watertight seal (see Fig 10-3), so adding antifibrinolytic agents to the sealant may be particularly useful in this nonclotting environment. Fibrin sealant has been used effectively to reduce CSF leakage at the time of dural closure.[78] It also has been used to augment closure of CSF fistulas during reoperative procedures.[78] Investigators have described a successful technique using fibrin sealant during the microscopic surgical repair of CSF rhinorrhea.[79] Researchers have also reported the successful use of fibrin sealant to close an intranasal meningoencephalocele, with no postoperative CSF leakage.[80]

Some invasive surgical procedures may be avoided altogether by using computerized, tomography-guided application of fibrin sealant to seal CSF leaks.[81] One study, however, reported no decrease in CSF leak following the application of fibrin sealant during acoustic neuroma surgery.[82] These authors conclude that fibrin sealant affords no advantage, yet they do not note the thrombin concentration of the adhesive they made, and they claim that the fibrinogen concentration of their sealant is comparable to that of commercial formulations. In a study of 31 patients undergoing lateral suboccipital craniectomy, surgeons used a mixture of allogeneic fibrin sealant and autologous bone chips to induce osteoregeneration of the occipital bone.[83] The authors of that study report satisfactory regeneration in 81% of the patients and nearly complete regeneration in 45%, and they suggest that adding a growth factor to the fibrin sealant might produce even better results.[83]

A case has been reported, however, of the postsurgical development of a spinal arachnoid cyst that researchers speculate may have been caused in part by the fibrin sealant used to reconstruct the suboccipital bone defect.[84] These authors speculate that the bone filler and fibrin sealant may have blocked CSF flow, leading to the cyst formation.

Animal studies have demonstrated the safety and usefulness of using fibrin sealant in intradural procedures. Such studies are important for demonstrating the feasibility of using fibrin sealant as a vehicle for the delivery of chemotherapeutics and other drugs to the brain tissue (see Fig 10-5). Researchers have reported that applying fibrin sealant to parenchymal tissue in rats increases mononuclear cell numbers and promotes angiogenesis at the wound site significantly. This study did not provide any evidence of significant detrimental effects on neuronal or glial cells.[85] Yet, another study, which also used a rat model, demonstrated that fibrin sealant is an excellent delivery system for glial cell line-derived neurotrophic factor into central nervous system tissues, permitting prolonged delivery.[86]

Several studies using rat models have been published on the use of fibrin sealant to assist spinal cord and nerve repair (see Fig 10-4). One experiment used fibrin sealant with compressive wiring of the posterior spinal processes to effect regeneration of 5-HT nerve fibers following complete spinal cord transection.[87] The authors of that experiment speculate that the adhesive provided a bridge supporting the growth of the nerve fibers. Fibrin sealant and compressive wiring also have been shown to assist in the repair of complete spinal cord gaps bridged with nerve grafts.[88] In a model for hand surgery, fibrin sealant was used to repair peripheral nerve transection with results comparable to those of microsuture technique.[89] This success, as the author of the study points out, contradicts earlier notions that the fibrin sealant method would cause more anastomotic failures, yet the application remains controversial.

Fibrin Sealant in Ophthalmologic Surgery

Commercial fibrin sealant has been used successfully to close conjunctival wounds after trabeculectomy.[90] In a study of six patients, the fibrin sealant provided a watertight seal and did not interfere with healing, and the authors note the promise of this application given the disadvantages of using sutures at the conjunctiva. Other researchers have also reported less early postoperative tissue trauma and patient discomfort when conjunctival wounds are closed with fibrin sealant rather than sutures.[91] Using small amounts of fibrin sealant as an adjunct to vitrectomy and gas tamponade decreases procedural time and appears to improve anatomic and functional results.[92]

In a study of scleral tunnel laceration repairs using a rabbit model, closure with sutureless self-sealing methods was compared with closure with cyanoacrylate adhesive or fibrin sealant.[93] These investigators found that the fibrin sealant method produces results comparable to the sutureless method and causes significantly less tissue trauma than does the cyanoacrylate method. They suggest that fibrin sealant may be an excellent adjunct to the sutureless method by providing additional tensile strength to the wound and by enhancing collagen fiber formation and crosslinking to promote healing across the wound. Investigators using a rabbit model also have used fibrin sealant successfully to reattach extraocular muscles,[94] a method that is particularly effective for larger muscle recessions (≥ 6 mm). The authors of that study conclude that fibrin sealant is safer than traditional suturing methods because of the statistically significant decrease in endophthalmitis seen ($p = 0.013$).

Fibrin Sealant in Orthopedic Surgery

In orthopedic surgery, fibrin sealant has been used as an effective adjunct to implant fixation,[95] spinal fusion,[96,97] fracture fixation,[98-103] bone graft filling,[104-108] bone induction,[109-113] repair of tendon and articular defects,[114-124] and increased fibroblast ingrowth.[125] Fibrin sealant also has been used successfully with bone fragments to reduce CSF leakage and reconstruct the mastoid bone following the transpetrosal-presigmoid approach in seven patients.[126] Its use to achieve rapid hemostasis during orthopedic procedures is particularly important. It may allow for forms of anticoagulation to be used during such procedures to help avoid deep vein thrombosis, pulmonary embolism, and death.[127,128] The use of fibrin sealant alone as a means of enhancing osteoinduction is controversial, however, with literature from 1991 and 1992[110-113] documenting a positive effect only when the sealant was combined with growth factors.[109] A review of musculoskeletal applications notes that the low inherent tensile strength of fibrin sealant often demands the adjunct use of other supporting materials.[16]

Fibrin Sealant in Trauma Surgery

A 1998 review of fibrin sealant applications in the management of trauma patients noted that this adhesive may be the best adjunctive hemostatic agent for parenchymal injuries of abdominal solid organs.[129] Both animal and human studies support the use of fibrin sealant to control bleeding at traumatic injuries, an application particularly important for injuries to the liver or spleen.[130,131] The use of this hemostatic agent may allow for splenorrhaphy instead of splenectomy, thereby preventing future infection by encapsulated organisms, particularly pneumococcus, and preserving the patient's immune responses. Fibrin sealant also can be an ap-

propriate adjunct to transplant preservation techniques. Researchers studying renal allograft rupture found that fibrin sealant with collagen foam can reduce hemorrhage and aid graft preservation if rejection can be reduced.[132] The authors of that study note that the fibrin sealant method, as compared with suturing methods, reduces tissue manipulation and trauma and thus promotes transplant preservation. As an adjunct to liver resection, preoperative embolization using fibrin sealant on portions scheduled for removal stimulates hypertrophy of the nonembolized sections, thus enhancing overall postresection liver function.[133]

Researchers have begun developing applications for fibrin sealant that are appropriate for mass casualty situations and severe crushing injuries of the extremities.[129,134] These developments include fibrin sealant-treated pressure dressings, which significantly reduced blood loss and supported mean arterial pressure in a pig study.[135] Such dressings would be advantageous in emergent care for massive extremity wounds and other soft tissue injuries.[129,134,135]

Fibrin Sealant in Head and Neck Surgery

Achieving hemostasis after tonsillectomy with fibrin sealant rather than diathermy has been reported to reduce postoperative pain significantly ($p < 0.05$), as measured by interincisor distance and a visual linear analog scale.[136] During parotidectomy closure, fibrin sealant permits the elimination of drains and may reduce the risk of facial paralysis by reducing the formation of hematoma; it also may reduce the risk of salivary fistula formation.[137] A canine model suggests that applying fibrin sealant treated with fibroblast growth factors in tandem with omental wrapping may enhance the revascularization of tracheal autografts.[138] In a study using autologous fibrin sealant during endoscopic sinus surgery, the adhesive eliminated the need for packing and improved healing with decreased scarring, as compared with control sides for the same patients.[139]

Fibrin sealant has been used successfully to assist reconstruction of the ossicular chain to treat conductive hearing loss.[140] One study, which compared a commercial fibrin sealant with an autologous fibrin sealant made from the precipitation of fibrinogen produced from an ethanol/freezing method, demonstrated no adverse tissue reactions to either adhesive, even when injected directly into rat auricles.[141] That study did note, however, the superior bonding strength of the commercial adhesive. European studies report the effective repair of labyrinthine fistulae using a mixture of fibrin sealant and bone filler to promote osteogenesis.[142] For the treatment of atrophic rhinitis, mixing a bone filler cement of hydroxyapatite granules and calcium triphosphate with fibrin sealant allows for more accurate molding and placement of the implant and reduces the volume of nasal fossae.[143] However, a 1997 review of otologic and neurotologic uses of fibrin sealant noted that excessively thick application may result in impaired healing, pseudopolyps, granulomas, and fibromas.[144]

Fibrin Sealant in Gynecologic and Urologic Surgery

A review of fibrin sealant applications in reproductive surgery notes that thus far the adhesive has been demonstrated to be successful in animal models, but no controlled clinical trials support human use.[145] Oviduct anastomosis using autologous fibrin sealant has been achieved in rabbit models with patency rates comparable to those for microsuture techniques and with statistically significant (p < 0.001) shortened operating time.[146] Similarly, researchers using fibrin sealant in a rat model of vasoepididymostomy reported patency rates comparable to those for microsuture techniques and a simplified procedure.[147] Investigators comparing the formation of adhesions after using various wound repair methods found that using fibrin sealant or a commercial antiadhesive barrier as an adjunct to suturing with prolene, compared with using catgut sutures, reduced significantly the rate of adhesion formation (p < 0.0001) following reproductive pelvic surgery in rats.[148]

The effects of fibrin sealant on adhesion prevention and peritoneal healing—issues of concern following both laparoscopic procedures and more invasive pelvic surgery—have been investigated. Researchers using an atraumatic microsurgical technique found that using fibrin sealant did reduce the formation of adhesions (although not to a statistically significant degree) and was associated with satisfactory healing, showing no evidence of inflammation.[149] Other investigators, using a rabbit model of reproductive surgery, compared fibrin sealant with a nonsuture method and found no significant difference in the rate of adhesion formation or in the reproductive outcome.[150] A group of researchers has developed a reproducible rat model for investigating the effects of various antiadhesive agents on peritoneal adhesion formation.[151] Having compared fibrin sealant and Ringer's lactate solution, dextran 70, modified carboxymethylcellulose, an absorbable knitted cellulose material, silicone elastomer film, and expanded PTFE membrane, the authors found that fibrin sealant demonstrated some success in decreasing the rate of peritoneal adhesions, performing second only to the carboxymethylcellulose method. They noted the advantages of fibrin sealant's biodegradability and noninflammatory qualities.

Commercial fibrin sealant has been used instead of sutures to achieve endoscopic colposuspension in women with stress urinary incontinence.[152] While long-term effects are not known yet, this sutureless method appears to provide comparable results with less tissue trauma.

Animal studies on laparoscopic ureterotomy have reported better results using fibrin sealant as compared with laser weld and mechanical suturing; in particular, the fibrin sealant method prevented leakage best, producing significantly higher flow rates than found in the control group.[153] In a study comparing different methods for achieving tissue approximation during laparoscopic pelviureteric anastomoses in a pig model, fibrin sealant effected patent anastomoses with a simpler technique, shorter procedural time, and better histologic results than suture, gelatin/resorcin/for-maldehyde glue, and laser tissue welding methods.[154] In a 1997 clinical study on humans, fibrin sealant proved to be an effective adjunct to laparoscopic pyeloplasty by significantly shortening the procedure time ($p < 0.001$) and reducing postoperative pain ($p < 0.0015$).[155] In an earlier study of fibrin sealant in laparoscopic uretal reanastomosis using a pig model, however, researchers reported an increased rate of fibrosis and inflammation as compared with suture methods.[156] The authors of that study speculate that the use of a cross species-derived fibrin sealant, composed of bovine thrombin and an unidentified fibrinogen source, may have contributed to the inflammatory response.

Fibrin Sealant in Gastrointestinal Surgery

Researchers have developed a sutureless technique using a sliding, absorbable, intraluminal, nontoxic stent with fibrin sealant to treat gastrointestinal anastomosis with excellent results.[157] This improved method causes minimal tissue damage and faster healing than suture methods. However, the use of fibrin sealant to close colonic anastomoses has met with controversial results.[158-160] Such use requires caution at the moment and further investigation.

Studies have reported the successful use of fibrin sealant to repair perforated peptic ulcers.[161-163] In a clinical study of 100 patients with comparable, perforated, peptic ulcers, researchers compared three treatment methods: standard laparotomy with omental patch repair, laparoscopic suture patch repair, and laparoscopic fibrin sealant repair.[162] Both laparoscopic procedures required significantly longer operating times but resulted in less pain and tissue trauma than laparotomy. The authors of that study note that the fibrin sealant closure method was much easier to perform than the suture patch method, and they suggest that the fibrin sealant can be used to reinforce patch placement.[162] In a 1997 randomized clinical study of 854 patients with bleeding peptic ulcers, researchers found that repeated endoscopic injections of fibrin

sealant worked significantly better than a single endoscopic injection of polidocanol to manage recurrent bleeding.[163]

Fibrin Sealant for Preventing or Closing Fistulas

It is reported that sealing suture lines with fibrin sealant, as compared with using sutures alone, results in a significantly lower rate of postoperative fistula formation ($p = 0.04$), after pancreatectomy.[164] Some researchers have published case studies in which the application of fibrin sealant, followed by octreotide treatment, resolved post-transplant pancreatic fistulas.[165]

Several studies document the successful use of fibrin sealant instead of sutures to seal fistulas (see Fig 10-4). In a small, randomized trial, investigators reported the successful use of fibrin glue to close low-output enterocutaneous fistulas, with a significantly faster healing time ($p < 0.01$).[166] Other researchers, in a study of 15 patients, found that the application of fibrin sealant is an effective method for closing persistent perineal fistulas.[167] In that study, the first application of fibrin sealant closed the fistula completely in the majority of patients. The authors stress the importance of antibiotic treatment prior to fibrin sealant application in order to reduce the population of bacteria capable of lysing the adhesive and the need to repeat the treatment more than once to ensure long-term success. In a case report detailing the effective use of fibrin sealant to seal a contaminated fistula with vesicointestinal communication, investigators again emphasized the need to pretreat the area with antibiotics.[168] Another study using autologous fibrin sealant to close rectovaginal and anorectal fistulas also pretreated with antibiotics and reported favorable results.[169] The authors noted that although the fistulas did not heal completely in the patients with Crohn's disease and with human immunodeficiency virus (HIV), those patients did report significantly less drainage.

Researchers have developed a fistuloscopic method for delivering fibrin sealant to the site of enterocutaneous fistulas.[170] This technique offers an effective alternative to long-term conservative management and invasive surgical procedures. Those who reported this development discourage the use of pressure to apply the fibrin sealant, noting the risk of air embolism.[170] Investigators have detailed the endoscopic application of fibrin sealant to close upper gastrointestinal fistulas in four patients.[171] The authors of that report also noted the advantage of this less invasive procedure. A case study also has been published in which surgeons reported the successful use of fibrin sealant to close a kidney transplant-ureteral fistula; the adhesive itself forms a clot to occlude the fistula in the short term and promotes local fibroblastic tissue growth for long-term occlusion.[172] In another case, surgeons used fibrin sealant to eliminate a prostatic-urethral-cutaneous fistula.[173]

Fibrin Sealant in Minimally Invasive Surgery

Fibrin sealant is an excellent adjunct to minimally invasive procedures, with or without video assistance, as it often affords simpler, shorter operations with less tissue trauma and pain to the patient. As more surgeons develop less invasive surgical procedures, such as minimally invasive coronary artery bypass grafting,[174] fibrin sealant may prove to be an important adjunct to procedures that decrease hospital stays and costs. In a review of forehead endoscopic procedures in 206 patients, researchers at one institution report that fibrin sealant-based procedures, as compared with bicoronal approaches, provided stable fixation as well as multidirectional displacement, with minimal complications.[175] There also has been increased attention to endoscopic procedures in head and neck surgery,[176] including transnasal repairs of CSF leaks.[177] The need for less invasive gynecologic procedures has been recognized also,[178] and fibrin sealant could augment them. Finally, in a recent prospective study comparing open cholecystectomy and laparoscopic cholecystectomy in cirrhotic patients, researchers report that the minimally invasive procedure resulted in significantly less bleeding ($p < 0.05$), significantly less hospital time ($p < 0.01$), and no

blood transfusion requirements.[179] The authors that study find laparoscopic cholecystectomy to the procedure of choice for cirrhotic patients, a ptient population for whom cholecystectomy usally is discouraged. While the above studies did n incorporate fibrin sealant into their methods, t surgical adhesive is potentially valuable in mai minimally invasive procedures because of its ea of use and biodegradability.

A thoracoscopic technique has been describ that uses fibrin sealant to treat large emphysem tous bullae.[180] The authors of that study point o the advantages of this less traumatic method for p tients with advanced lung disease, who may poor candidates for more invasive surgery. F searchers also have used a percutaneous transth racic method with fibrin sealant to close airspac after pulmonary resection, again avoiding more i vasive reoperation.[181]

Fibrin Sealant in Dental Surgery

A body of literature has developed exploring t use of fibrin sealant in dental surgery, particula in patients with hemophilia and other coagu pathies (see Fig 10-2). Some studies have report that fibrin sealant does not provide a statistica significant advantage over nonfibrin sealant met ods for treating gingival recession defects moderate-to-severe periodontitis.[182,183] An earl study, however, did show a statistically significa advantage to using fibrin sealant as an adjunct treating gingival recession.[184] Other researchers, cusing on patients with coagulopathies such as h mophilia, have reported that autologous fibr sealant, in combination with tranexamic swis and-swallow rinses and sutures, decreased blee ing associated with tooth extraction sign cantly.[185,186]

Other Surgical Uses of Fibrin Sealar

Fibrin sealant is well suited to the delivery of dru and biologics to wound sites and injured tissue (s Fig 10-5) because 1) it can be applied in a si specific manner, 2) it can be composed of only h man components to reduce immunogenicity, 3) it does not interfere with natural healing mechanisms, and 4) it is biodegradable over time in the tissue.[187] Antifibrinolytics added to the sealant can slow its rate of resorption and, hence, extend its release of biologically active agents.[4] Several research teams have developed methods for seeding fibrin sealants with antibiotics and have explored the mechanisms of drug release, and the time of release, from the sealant.[187,188] In particular, fibrin sealant has been studied for its ability to carry antibiotics, chemotherapeutics, osteoinducers, growth factors, and antiproliferative agents.[189]

Native or cultured skin grafts can be destroyed by microbial contamination. Theoretically, site-specific application of fibrin sealant carrying antibacterial agents may counteract such contamination and, thus, promote engraftment. One in-vitro study found a short-term, drug-delivery effect for burn wounds but suggested that higher fibrinogen concentrations might lengthen the effect.190

Investigators also have used fibrin sealants to administer epidermal growth factors continuously to a wound site. One group of researchers, using a murine model, has developed a novel method of suspending growth factors in the fibrin sealant that then is applied to the wound site.[191] These investigators note that this technique may help to develop novel gene therapies for chronic wounds.[191]

Chemotherapy can also take advantage of fibrin sealant. Fibrin sealant has been shown to work effectively as a local drug carrier. In one rat study, doxorubicin was delivered successfully to a malignant AH60C tumor using a commercial fibrin sealant, with sodium alginate to prolong the release of the doxorubicin.[192] Another study suggests that fibrin sealant can deliver chemotherapeutic agents successfully and effectively to osteosarcomas in rats.[193]

Fibrin sealant also has proved to be an excellent surgical adjunct for patients with hemostatic disorders during procedures such as circumcision, hip and knee replacement, open-heart surgery, pseudotumor resection, and hemophilic bone cysts.[145,194] Such use of fibrin sealant has reduced blood losses, Factor VIII requirements, and overall inpatient time by permitting multiple procedures.[145,194,195]

Potential Complications

The use of fibrin sealant is associated with several potential complications. The transmission of blood-borne disease remains a primary concern, with one case of HIV transmission apparently associated with fibrin sealant having been reported recently.[196] Viral elimination methods, including solvent/detergent treatment,[197] ultrafiltration,[3] and dry-heat inactivation,[198] have been developed to remove viruses such as hepatitis and HIV from pooled-plasma sources. The fibrin sealant recently approved by the FDA employs cryoprecipitation and washing, freeze-drying, and vapor-heating processes to reduce viral contamination. Autologous methods should also eliminate blood-borne disease transmission for patients, although clinical personnel remain at risk and should use meticulous techniques to protect themselves and avoid introducing exogenous contamination.[199,200] Emergency procedures require nonautologous methods. Virus-inactivated, pooled- plasma products should be useful in this setting. Alternatively, infectious disease-screened, single-donor fibrinogen concentrate could be used. Despite the theoretical risk of blood-borne disease transmission, in more than 12 years of fibrin sealant use at the University of Virginia, there have been no reports of such an occurrence.

Allergic reaction to the bovine thrombin used in most blood bank-produced fibrin sealants is another risk associated with fibrin sealant use. Reports of complications resulting from bovine thrombin exist; these include anaphylaxis, abnormal Factor V antibodies, hypotension, and other coagulopathies.[201-206] Using a human or recombinant rather than a bovine thrombin source can eliminate this adverse reaction. The fibrin sealant recently approved by the FDA uses human thrombin, although it also employs a bovine-derived antifibrinolytic. In 1997, some investigators reported on in-vitro studies that were conducted on a sealant using batroxobin instead of thrombin.[207]

A method for producing an entirely autologous fibrin sealant has been described.[199] In this method, the autologous plasma is treated with biotinylated batroxobin to produce an acid-soluble fibrin polymer, which then is isolated. The remaining biotinylated batroxobin is extracted. The fibrin polymerizes as it is brought to a neutral pH. The process requires only a small volume of blood from the patient and can be completed in 30 minutes. The resulting fibrin sealant has been tested in heparinized animal models and reportedly demonstrates good hemostatic effects.

When applied to an already contaminated site, fibrin sealant can be associated with an increased risk of infection by providing a growth medium of proteins. At the University of Virginia, the infection rates associated with fibrin sealant use remain a low 1.4% for superficial infections and 0.7% for major wound infections.[208] Combining antibiotics with the fibrin sealant may prove to be an advantageous method for reducing and treating infection.[187,189]

Finally, fibrin sealant use may result in clotting at undesirable locations, such as chest tubes. Fibrin sealant or thrombin alone may be injected into the arterial system, causing dangerous embolization or intravascular coagulation. Meticulous surgical and application techniques as well as experience with fibrin sealant should minimize the incidence of such complications.

Conclusion

Fibrin sealant has been used effectively in a wide variety of surgical procedures, with new applications being developed continuously. Given its hemostatic, tissue sealing, and carrier capabilities, it should continue to hold significant advantages for surgeons. The recent FDA approval of a fibrin sealant should encourage the commercial and clinical development of additional safe and effective commercial fibrin sealants in the United States. Such commercial products, approved by the FDA, would be expected to reduce the risks of many blood-borne diseases by reducing the use of single-donor, nonautologous, untreated plasma. They might also reduce the risks of anaphylaxis, hypotension, and coagulopathy by using human or recombinant instead of bovine thrombin. Finally, such safer commercial fibrin sealants would have marked applications in emergency procedures that do not lend themselves to autologous donation methods for producing fibrin sealant; for nonemergency situations, however, autologous fibrinogen concentrates may continue to have a therapeutic role. Antivirus treatments, such as nanofiltration and pasteurization, exist for pooled plasma but may not eradicate infectious agents completely.[3] Although virus inactivation of pooled plasma by solvent/detergent treatment alone,[197] for example, prevents the risk of transmitting lipid-coated viruses, other infectious agents, both known and unknown, are still potentially transmissible. Fibrin sealant appears to be a significant adjunct to meticulous surgical technique, potentially providing faster, safer, and more effective patient care.

References

1. Sierra DH. Fibrin sealant adhesive systems: A review of their chemistry, material properties, and clinical applications. J Biomater Appl 1993;7:309-52.
2. Brennan M. Fibrin glue. Blood Rev 1991;5:240-4.
3. Radosevich M, Goubran HA, Burnouf T. Fibrin sealant: Scientific rationale, production methods, properties, and current clinical use. Vox Sang 1997;72:133-43.
4. Pipan CM, Glasheen WP, Matthew TL, et al. The effects of antifibrinolytic agents on the life span of fibrin sealant. J Surg Res 1992;53:402-7.
5. Baker JW, Spotnitz WD, Nolan SP. A technique for spray application of fibrin glue during cardiac operations. Ann Thorac Surg 1987;43:564-5.
6. Glover W, Chavis TV, Danial TM, et al. Fibrin glue application via the flexible fiberoptic bronchoscope: Closure of bronchopleural fistulas. J Thorac Cardiovasc Surg 1987;9:470-2.
7. Ismail S, Combs MJ, Goodman NC, et al. Reduction of femoral arterial bleeding post catheterization using percutaneous applic

tion of fibrin sealant. Cathet Cardiovasc Diagn 1995;34:88-95.

8. Falstrom JK, Goodman NC, Ates G, et al. Reduction of femoral artery bleeding post catheterization using fibrin enhanced collagen sealant. Cathet Cardiovasc Diagn 1997;41: 79-84.

9. Spotnitz WD, Mintz PD, Avery N, et al. Fibrin glue from stored human plasma: An inexpensive and efficient method for local blood bank preparation. Am Surg 1987;53: 460-4.

10. Siedentop KH, Park JJ, Sanchez B. An autologous fibrin tissue adhesive with greater bonding strength. Arch Otolaryngol Head Neck Surg 1995;121:769-72.

11. Sanders RP, Goodman NC, Amiss LR Jr, et al. Effect of fibrinogen and thrombin concentrations on mastectomy seroma prevention. J Surg Res 1996;61:65-70.

12. Park MS, Cha CL. Biochemical aspects of autologous fibrin glue derived from ammonium sulfate precipitation. Laryngoscope 1993;103:193-6.

13. Epstein GH, Weisman RA, Zwillenberg S, Schreiber AD. A new autologous fibrinogen-based adhesive for otologic surgery. Ann Otol Rhinol Laryngol 1986;95:40-5.

14. Kjaergard HK, Weis-Fogh US, Sorensen H, et al. A simple method of preparation of autologous fibrin glue by means of ethanol. Surg Gynecol Obstet 1992;175:72-3.

15. DePalma L, Criss VR, Luban NLC. The preparation of fibrinogen concentrate for use as fibrin glue by four different methods. Transfusion 1993;33:717-20.

16. Silver FH, Wang M-C, Pins GD. Preparation and use of fibrin glue in surgery. Biomaterials 1995;16:891-903.

17. Silver FH, Wang M-C, Pins GD. Preparation of fibrin glue: A study of chemical and physical methods. J Appl Biomater 1995;6:175-83.

18. Spotnitz WD. Fibrin sealant in the United States: Clinical use at the University of Virginia. Thromb Haemost 1995;74:482-5.

19. Kjaergard HK, Fairbrother JE. Controlled clinical studies of fibrin sealant in cardiothoracic surgery—A review. Eur J Cardiothorac Surg 1996;10:727-33.

20. Spotnitz WD, Dalton MS, Baker JW, Nolan SP. Reduction of perioperative hemorrhage by anterior mediastinal spray application of fibrin glue during cardiac operations. Ann Thorac Surg 1987;44:529-31.

21. Watanabe G, Misaki T, Kotoh K. Microfibrillar collagen (Avitene) and antibiotic-containing fibrin glue after median sternotomy. J Card Surg 1997;12:110-1.

22. García-Guereta L, Burgueros M, Borches D, et al. Cardiac tamponade after a systemic-pulmonary shunt complicated by serous leakage. Ann Thorac Surg 1997;63:248-50.

23. Boris WJ, Gu J, McGrath LB. Effectiveness of fibrin glue in the reduction of postoperative intrapericardial adhesions. J Invest Surg 1996; 9:327-33.

24. Milne AA, Murphy WG, Reading SJ, Ruckley CV. Fibrin sealant reduces suture line bleeding during carotid endarterectomy: A randomized trial. Eur J Vasc Endovasc Surg 1995;10:91-4.

25. Milne AA, Murphy WG, Reading SJ, Ruckley CV. A randomized trial of fibrin sealant in peripheral vascular surgery. Vox Sang 1996;70: 210-2.

26. Meisner H, Struck E, Schmidt-Habelmann P, Sebening F. Fibrin sealant application: Clinical experience. Thorac Cardiovasc Surg 1982;30:232-3.

27. Kjaergard HK, Axelsen P, Weis-Fogh US. Repair of experimental atrial rupture with fibrin glue. Injury 1995;26:147-9.

28. Ruvolo G, Speziala G, Voci P, Marino B. "Patch-glue" annular reconstruction for mitral valve replacement in severely calcified mitral annulus. Ann Thorac Surg 1997;63: 570-1.

29. Hvass U, Chatel D, Frikha I, et al. Left ventricular free wall rupture: Long-term results with pericardial patch and fibrin glue repair. Eur J Cardiothorac Surg 1995;9:75-6.

30. Von Segesser LK, Fasnacht MS, Vogt PR, et al. Prevention of residual ventricular septal defects with fibrin sealant. Ann Thorac Surg 1995;60:511-6.

31. Chekanov V, Nikolaychik V, Tchekanov G. The use of biologic glue for better adhesion between the skeletal muscle flap and the myocardium and for increasing capillary ingrowth. J Thorac Cardiovasc Surg 1996;111:678-9.

32. Fasol R, Schumacher B, Schlaudraff K, et al. Experimental use of a modified fibrin glue to induce site-directed angiogenesis from the aorta to the heart. J Thorac Cardiovasc Surg 1994;107:1432-9.

33. Bayfield MS, Spotnitz WD. Fibrin sealant in thoracic surgery: Pulmonary applications, including management of bronchopleural fistula. Chest Surg Clin N Am 1996;6:567-83.

34. Matthew TL, Spotnitz WD, Daniel TM, et al. Closure of small bronchopleural fistulas using fibrin sealant through the flexible fiberoptic bronchoscope. Chest(Suppl)1988;94:77.

35. York EL, Lewall DB, Hirji M, et al. Endoscopic diagnosis and treatment of postoperative bronchopleural fistula. Chest 1990;97:1390-2.

36. Regel G, Sturm JA, Neumann C, et al. Occlusion of bronchopleural fistula after lung injury—A new treatment by bronchoscopy. J Trauma 1989;29:223-6.

37. McManigle JE, Fletcher GL, Tenholder MF. Bronchoscopy in the management of bronchopleural fistula. Chest 1990;97:1235-8.

38. Salmon CJ, Pon RB, Westcott JL. Endobronchial vascular occlusion coils for control of a large parenchymal bronchopleural fistula. Chest 1990;98:233-4.

39. Yasuda Y, Mori A, Kato H, et al. Intrathoracic fibrin glue for postoperative pleuropulmonary fistula. Ann Thorac Surg 1991;51:242-4.

40. Francel TJ, Lee GW, Mackinnon SE, Patterson GA. Treatment of long-standing thoracostoma and bronchopleural fistula without pulmonary resection in high risk patients. Plast Reconstr Surg 1997;99:1046-53.

41. Matar AF, Hill JG, Duncan W, et al. Use of biological glue to control pulmonary air leaks. Thorax 1990;45:670-4.

42. Mouritzen C, Dromer M, Keinecke HO. The effect of fibrin glue to seal bronchial and alveolar leakages after pulmonary resections and decortications. Eur J Cardiothorac Surg 1993;7:75-80.

43. Turk R, Weidringer JW, Hartel W, et al. Closure of lung leaks by fibrin gluing: Experimental investigations and clinical experiences. Thorac Cardiovasc Surg 1983;31:185-6.

44. DeRisis D, Cohen H, Takita H, et al. Hemostasis in experimental pulmonary injury. J Surg Oncol 1982;19:208-10.

45. McCarthy PM, Trastek VF, Bell DG, et al. The effectiveness of fibrin glue sealant in reducing experimental pulmonary air leak. Ann Thorac Surg 1988;45:203-5.

46. Fleischer, AJ, Evans KG, Nelems B, et al. Effect of routine fibrin glue use on the duration of air leaks after lobectomy. Ann Thorac Surg 1990;49:133-4.

47. Thetter O. Fibrin adhesive and its application in thoracic surgery. Thorac Cardiovasc Surg 1981;29:290-2.

48. Wong K, Goldstraw P. Effect of fibrin glue in the reduction of postthoracotomy alveolar air leak. Ann Thorac Surg 1997;64:979-81.

49. Vincent JG, Van DE, Wal HJ, et al. Postponing the limits: Multiple and repeated pulmonary metastasectomy by parenchymal-sparing electrocautery incision. Helv Chir Acta 1990;57:295-300.

50. Uyama T, Monden Y, Harada K, et al. Drainage of giant bulla with balloon catheter using chemical irritant and fibrin glue. Chest 1988;94:1289-90.

51. Hansen MK, Kruse-Anderson S, Watt-Boolsen S, et al. Spontaneous pneumothorax and fibrin glue sealant during thoracoscopy. Eur J Cardiothorac Surg 1989;3:512-4.

52. Hauck H, Bull PG, Pridun N. Complicated pneumothrax: Short- and long-term results

of endoscopic fibrin pleurodesis. World J Surg 1991;15:146-50.

53. Kuint J, Lubin D, Martinowitz U, Linder N. Fibrin glue treatment for recurrent pneumothorax in a premature infant. Am J Perinatol 1996;13:245-7.

54. Zarge JI, Huang P, Husak V, et al. Fibrin glue containing fibroblast growth factor 1 and heparin with autologous endothelial cells reduces intimal hyperplasia in a canine carotid artery balloon injury model. J Vasc Surg 1997; 25:840-8.

55. Gray JL, Kang SS, Zenni GC, et al. FGF-1 affixation stimulates ePTFE endothelialization without intimal hyperplasia. J Surg Res 1994; 57:596-612.

56. Kang SS, Gosselin C, Ren D, Greisler HP. Selective stimulation of endothelial cell proliferation with inhibition of smooth muscle cell proliferation by fibroblast growth factor-1 plus heparin delivered from fibrin glue suspensions. Surgery 1995;118:280-7.

57. Gosselin C, Ren D, Ellinger J, Greisler HP. In vivo platelet deposition on polytatrefluoroethylene coated with fibrin glue containing fibroblast factor 1 and heparin in a canine model. Am J Surg 1995;170:126-30.

58. Gosselin C, Vorp DA, Warty V, et al. ePTFE coating with fibrin glue, FGF-1, and heparin: Effect on retention of seeded endothelial cells. J Surg Res 1996;60:327-32.

59. Zarge JI, Gosselin C, Huang P, Greisler HP. Platelet deposition on ePTFE grafts coated with fibrin glue with or without FGF-1 and heparin. J Surg Res 1997;67:4-8.

60. Zarge JI, Husak V, Huang P, Greisler HP. Fibrin glue containing fibroblast growth factors type I and heparin decreases platelet deposition. Am J Surg 1997;174:188-92.

61. Greisler HP, Gosselin C, Ren D, et al. Biointeractive polymers and tissue engineered blood vessels. Biomaterials 1996;17:329-36.

62. Weatherford DA, Sackman JE, Reddick TT, et al. Vascular endothelial growth factor and heparin in a biologic glue promote human aortic endothelial cell proliferation with aor-

tic smooth muscle cell inhibition. Surgery 1996;120:433-9.

63. Saitoh S, Nakatsuchi Y. Long-term results of vein grafts interposed in arterial defects using the telescoping anastomotic technique and fibrin glue. J Hand Surg [Br] 1996;21B:47-52.

64. Saitoh S, Nakatsuchi Y. Telescoping and glue technique in vein grafts for arterial defects. Plast Reconstr Surg 1995;96:1401-8.

65. Padubidri AN, Browne E, Kononov A. Fibrin glue-assisted end-to-side anastomosis of rat femoral vessels: Comparison with conventional suture method. Ann Plast Surg 1996; 37:41-7.

66. Moskovitz MJ, Bass L, Zhang L, Siebert JW. Microvascular anastomoses utilizing new intravascular stents. Ann Plast Surg 1994;32: 612-8.

67. Dowbak GM, Rohrich RJ, Robinson JB Jr, Peden E. Effectiveness of a new non-thrombogenic bio-adhesive in microvascular anastomoses. J Reconstr Microsurg 1994;10: 383-6.

68. Lindsey WH, Masterson T, Spotnitz WD, et al. Seroma prevention using fibrin glue in a rat mastectomy model. Arch Surg 1990; 125:305-7.

69. Lindsey WH, Becker DG, Hoare JR, et al. Comparison of topical fibrin glue, fibrinogen, and thrombin in preventing seroma formation in a rat model. Laryngoscope 1995;105: 241-3.

70. Moore MM, Nguyen DHD, Spotnitz WD. Fibrin sealant reduces serous drainage and allows for earlier drain removal after axillary dissection: A randomized prospective trial. Am Surg 1997;63:97-102.

71. Kulber DA, Bacilious N, Peters ED, et al. The use of fibrin sealant in the prevention of seromas. Plast Reconstr Surg 1997;99:842-9.

72. Moore MM, Burak WE, Nelson E, et al. Fibrin sealant reduces the amount and duration of fluid drainage after axillary lymphadenectomy. Am Coll Surg 1997;48:866-7.

73. Medl M, Mayerhofer K, Peters-Engl C, et al. The application of fibrin glue after axillary lymphadenectomy in the surgical treatment of human breast cancer. Anticancer Res 1995; 15:2843-6.

74. Stuart JD, Kenney JG, Spotnitz WD, et al. Application of single donor fibrin glue to burns. J Burn Care Rehabil 1988;9:619-22.

75. Bold EL, Wanamaker JR, Zins JE, Lavertu P. The use of fibrin glue in the healing of skin flaps. Am J Otolaryngol 1996;17:27-30.

76. Marchac D, Sandor G. Face lifts and sprayed fibrin glue: An outcome analysis of 200 patients. Br J Plast Surg 1994;47:306-9.

77. Lindsey WH, Spotnitz WD, Llaneras MR, et al. Seroma prevention using fibrin glue during modified neck dissection in a rat model. Am J Surg 1988;156:310-3.

78. Shaffrey CI, Spotnitz WD, Shaffrey ME, Jane JA. Neurosurgical applications of fibrin glue: Augmentation of dural closure in 134 patients. Neurosurgery 1990;26:207-10.

79. Yoon JH, Lee JG, Kim SH, Park IY. Microscopical surgical management of cerebrospinal fluid rhinorrhea with free grafts. Rhinology 1995;33:208-11.

80. Khan MA, Salahuddin I. Intranasal meningoencephalocele and the use of fibrin glue. Ear Nose Throat J 1997;76:464-7.

81. Patel MR, Louie W, Rachlin J. Postoperative cerebrospinal fluid leaks of the lumbosacral spine: Management with percutaneous fibrin glue. AJNR: Am J Neuroradiol 1996;17:495-500.

82. Lebowitz RA, Hoffman RA, Roland JT, Cohen NL. Autologous fibrin sealant in the prevention of cerebrospinal fluid leak following acoustic neuroma surgery. Am J Otol 1995;16:172-4.

83. Sawamura Y, Terasaka S, Ishii N, et al. Osteoregenerative lateral suboccipital craniectomy using fibrin glue. Acta Neurochir (Wien) 1997;139:446-52.

84. Taguchi Y, Suzuki R, Okada M, Sekino H. Spinal arachnoid cyst developing after surgical treatment of a ruptured vertebral artery aneurysm: A possible complication of topical use of fibrin glue. J Neurosurg 1996;84:526-9.

85. Muhammad AKMG, Yoshimine T, Maruno M, et al. Topical application of fibrin adhesive in the rat brain: Effects on different cellular elements of the wound. Neurol Res 1997;19:84-8.

86. Cheng H, Hoffer B, Strömberg I, et al. The effect of glial cell line-derived neurotrophic factor in fibrin glue on developing dopamine neurons. Exp Brain Res 1995;104:199-206.

87. Cheng H, Olson L. A new surgical technique that allows proximodistal regeneration of 5-HT fibers after complete transection of the rat spinal cord. Exp Neurol 1995;136:149-61.

88. Cheng H, Cao Y, Olson L. Spinal cord repair in adult paraplegic rats: Partial restoration of hind limb function. Science 1996;273:510-3.

89. Povlsen B. A new fibrin seal: Functional evaluation of sensory regeneration following primary repair of peripheral nerves. J Hand Surg (Br) 1994;19B:250-4.

90. O'Sullivan F, Dalton R, Rostron CK. Fibrin glue: An alternative method of wound closure in glaucoma surgery. J Glaucoma 1996;5:367-70.

91. Biedner B, Rosenthal G. Conjunctival closure in strabismus surgery: Vicryl versus fibrin glue. Ophthalmic Surg Lasers 1996;27:967.

92. Tilanus MAD, Deutman AF. Full-thickness macular holes treated with vitrectomy and tissue glue. Int Ophthalmol 1995;18:355-8.

93. Kim JC, Bassage SD, Kempski MH, et al. Evaluation of tissue adhesives in closure of scleral tunnel incisions. J Cataract Refract Surg 1995;21:320-5.

94. Spierer A, Barequet I, Rosner M, et al. Reattachment of extraocular muscles using fibrin glue in a rabbit model. Invest Ophthalmol Vis Sci 1997;38:543-6.

95. Hetherington VJ, Park JB, Park SH, et al. Effects of fibrin sealant on the fixation of po-

rous titanium and pyrolitic carbon implants. J Foot Surg 1989;28:145-50.

96. Ono K, Shikata J, Shimizu K, Yamamuro T. Bone-fibrin mixture in spinal surgery. Clin Orthop 1992;275:133-9.

97. Vaquero J, Arias A, Oya S, et al. Effect of fibrin glue on postlaminectomy scar formation. Acta Neurochir 1993;120:159-63.

98. Angermann P, Riegels-Nielsen P. Fibrin fixation of osteochondral talar fracture. Acta Ortho Scand 1990;61:551-3.

99. Arce AA, Garin DM, Garcia VM, Jansana JP. Treatment of radial head fractures using a fibrin adhesive seal. J Bone Joint Surg Br 1995; 77:422-4.

00. Havranek P, Hajkova H. Fibrin glue osteosynthesis of epiphyseal injuries in children. Acta Univ Carol (Med) 1989;35:255-64.

01. Marchac D, Renier D. Fibrin glue in craniofacial surgery. J Craniofac Surg 1990;1:32-4.

02. Scapinelli R. Treatment of fractures of the humeral capitulum using fibrin sealant. Acta Orthop Trauma Surg 1990;109:235-7.

03. Visuri T, Kuusela T. Fixation of large osteochondral fractures of the patella with fibrin adhesive system. Am J Sports Med 1989;17: 842-5.

04. Hotz G. Alveolar ridge augmentation with hydroxylopatite using fibrin sealant for fixation. Int J Oral Maxillofac Surg 1991;20: 204-7.

05. Oberg S, Kahnberg KE. Combined use of hydroxy-apatite and Tisseel in experimental bone defects in the rabbit. Swed Dent J 1993;17:147-53.

06. Ono K, Yamamuro T, Nakamura T. Apatite-wollastonite containing glass ceramic granule-fibrin mixture as a bone graft filler: Use with low granular deposits. J Biomed Mater Res 1990;24:11-20.

07. Shen WJ, Chung KC, Wang GW, et al. Demineralized bone matrix in the stabilization of porous-coated implants in bone defects in rabbits. Clin Orthop 1993;293:346-52.

108. Wittkampf ARM. Fibrin glue as cement for HA-granules. J Craniomaxillofac Surg 1989; 17:179-81.

109. Arnaud E, Wybier M, de Vernejoul MC. Potentiation of transforming growth factor (TGF-β1) by natural coral and fibrin in a rabbit cranioplasty model. Calcif Tissue Int 1994; 54:493-8.

110. Pinholt EM, Solheim E, Bang G, Sudmann E. Bone induction by composites of bioresorbable carriers and demineralized bone in rats. J Oral Maxillofac Surg 1992;50:1300-4.

111. Schwarz N, Redl H, Zeng L, et al. Early osteoinduction in rats is not altered by fibrin sealant. Clin Orthop 1993;293:353-9.

112. Vachon AM, McIlwraith CW, Keeley FW. Biochemical study of repair of induced osteochondral defects of the distal portion of the radial carpal bone in horses by use of periosteal autografts. Am J Vet Res 1991;52: 328-32.

113. Vachon AM, McIlwraith CW, Trotter GW, et al. Morphologic study of induced osteochondral defects of the distal portion of the radial carpal bone in horses by use of a glued periosteal graft. Am J Vet Res 1991;52:317-27.

114. Hashimoto J, Kurosaka M, Yoshiya S, Hirohata K. Meniscal repair using fibrin sealant and endothelial cell growth factor. Am J Sports Med 1992;20:537-41.

115. Homminga GN, Bulstra SK, Bouwmeester PSM, van der Linden AJ. Perichondrial grafting for cartilage lesions of the knee. J Bone Joint Surg Br 1990;72:1003-7.

116. Homminga GN, van der Linden TJ, Terwindt-Rouwenhorst EAW, Drukker J. Repair of articular defects by perichondrial grafts. Acta Orthop Scand 1989;60:326-9.

117. Ishimura M, Tamai S, Fujisawa Y. Arthroscopic meniscal repair with fibrin glue. J Arthroscopy 1991;7:177-81.

118. Lusardi DA, Cain JE. The effect of fibrin sealant on the strength of tendon repair of full thickness tendon lacerations in the rabbit Achilles tendon. J Foot Ankle Surg 1994;33: 443-7.

119. Nabeshima Y, Kurosaka M, Yoshiya S, Mizuno K. Effect of fibrin glue and endothelial growth factor on the early healing response of the transplanted allogenic meniscus. A pilot study. Knee Surg Sports Traumatol Arthrosc 1995;3:34-8.

120. Niedermann B, Boe S, Lauritzen J, Rubak JM. Glued periosteal grafts in the knee. Acta Orthop Scand 1985;56:457-60.

121. Redaelli C, Niederhauser U, Carrel T, et al. Rupture of the Achilles tendon: Fibrin gluing or suture. Chirurg 1992;63:572-6.

122. Tsai CL, Liu TK, Liu CN, Lim AC. Meniscal repair with autogenous periosteum and fibrin adhesive system. Chin Med J 1992;49:170-6.

123. Widenfalk B, Engkvist O, Ohlsen L, Segerstrom K. Perichondrial arthroplasty using fibrin glue and early mobilization. Scand J Plast Reconstr Surg 1986;20:251-8.

124. Wong TY, Jin YT, Laskin DM. Autologous pericranial graft resurfacing after high condylectomy and discectomy of the temporomandibular joint in rabbits. J Oral Maxillofac Surg 1996;54:747-52.

125. Schlag G, Redl H. Fibrin sealant in orthopedic surgery. Clin Orthop 1988;227:269-85.

126. Tokora K, Chiba Y, Murai M, et al. Cosmetic reconstruction after mastoidectomy for the transpetrosal-presigmoid approach. Neurosurgery 1996;39:186-7.

127. Curtin W, Wang G-J, Goodman N, et al. Reduction of bleeding using cryo-based fibrin sealant in a canine anticoagulated knee arthroplasty model. Am Coll Surg 1997;48:558-60.

128. Tredwell SJ, Sawatzky B. The use of fibrin sealant to reduce blood loss during Cotrel-Dubousset instrumentation for idiopathic scoliosis. Spine 1990;15:913-5.

129. Ochsner MG. Fibrin solutions to control hemorrhage in the trauma patient. J Long-Term Effects Med Implants 1998;8:161-73.

130. Ishitani MB, McGahren ED, Sibley DA, et al. Laparoscopically applied fibrin glue in experimental liver trauma. J Pediatr Surg 1989; 24:867-71.

131. Uranüs S, Mischinger H-J, Pfeifer J, et al. Hemostatic methods for the management of spleen and liver injuries. World J Surg 1996; 20:1107-12.

132. Heimbach D, Miersch WD, Buszello H, et al. Is the transplant-preserving management of renal allograft rupture justified? Br J Urol 1995;75:729-32.

133. Nagino M, Nimura Y, Kamiya J, et al. Selective percutaneous transhepatic embolization of the portal vein in preparation for extensive liver resection: The ipsilateral approach. Radiology 1996;200:559-63.

134. Holcomb JB, Pusateri AE, Hess JR, et al. Implications of new dry fibrin sealant technology for trauma surgery. Surg Clin North Am 1997;77:943-52.

135. Larson MJ, Bowersox JC, Lim RC, Hess JR. Efficacy of a fibrin hemostatic bandage in controlling hemorrhage from experimental arterial injuries. Arch Surg 1995;130:420-2.

136. Moralee SJ, Carney AS, Cash MP, Murray JAM. The effect of fibrin sealant haemostasis on post-operative pain in tonsillectomy. Clin Otolaryngol 1994;19:526-8.

137. Depondt J, Koka VN, Nasser T, et al. Use of fibrin glue in parotidectomy closure. Laryngoscope 1996;106:784-7.

138. Nakanishi R, Nagaya N, Yoshimatsu T, et al. Optimal dose of basic fibroblast growth factor for long-segment orthotopic tracheal autografts. J Thorac Cardiovasc Surg 1997; 113:26-36.

139. Gleich LL, Rebeiz EE, Pankratov M, Shapshay SM. Autologous fibrin tissue adhesive in endoscopic sinus surgery. Otolaryngol Head Neck Surg 1995;112:238-41.

140. Minatogawa T, Iritani H, Ishida K, Node M. Allograft stapes surgery for conductive hearing loss in patients with ossicular chain anomalies. Eur Arch Otorhinolaryngol 1996; 253:283-6.

141. Siedentop KH, Chung SE, Park JJ, et al. Evaluation of pooled fibrin sealant for ear surgery. Am J Otol 1997;18:660-4.

142. Vanclooster C, Debruyne F, Vantrappen GR, et al. Labyrinthine fistulae: A retrospective analysis. Acta Otorhinolaryngol Belg 1997; 51:119-21.

143. Bertrand B, Doyen A, Eloy P. Triosite implants and fibrin glue in the treatment of atrophic rhinitis: Technique and results. Laryngoscope 1996;106:652-7.

144. Selesnick S, Mouwafak A-R. Adhesives in otology and neurotology. Am J Otolaryngol 1997;18:81-9.

145. Martinowitz U, Saltz R. Fibrin sealant. Curr Opin Haematol 1996;3:395-402.

146. Rajaram S, Rusia U, Agarwal S, Agarwal N. Autologous fibrin adhesive in experimental tubal anastomosis. Int J Fertil Menopausal Stud 1996;41:458-61.

147. Shekarriz BM, Thomas AJ Jr, Sabanegh E, et al. Fibrin-glue assisted vasoepididymostomy: A comparison to standard end-to-end microsurgical vasoepididymostomy in the rat model. J Urol 1997;158:1602-5.

148. Myinbayev OA, Rubliva KJ. Use of chemiluminescent method for evaluation of postoperative adhesion formation after reproductive pelvic surgery: An experimental study. Am J Reprod Immunol 1996;36:238-41.

149. Evrard VAC, DeBellis A, Boeckx W, Brosens IA. Peritoneal healing after fibrin glue application: A comparative study in a rat model. Hum Reprod 1996;11:1877-80.

150. Marana R, Muzii L, Catalano GF, et al. Use of fibrin sealant for reproductive surgery: A randomized study in a rabbit model. Gynecol Obstet Invest 1996;41:199-202.

151. Harris ES, Morgan RF, Rodeheaver GT. Analysis of the kinetics of peritoneal adhesion formation in the rat and evaluation of potential antiadhesive agents. Surgery 1995; 117:663-9.

152. Kiilholma P, Haarala M, Polvi H, et al. Sutureless endoscopic colposuspension with fibrin sealant. Techniques Urol 1996;1:81-3.

153. Wolf JS Jr, Soble JJ, Nakada SY, et al. Comparison of fibrin glue, laser weld, and mechanical suturing device for the laparoscopic closure of ureterotomy in a porcine model. J Urol 1997;157:1487-92.

154. Eden CG, Coptcoat MJ. Assessment of alternative tissue approximation techniques for laparoscopy. Br J Urol 1996;78:234-42.

155. Eden CG, Sultana SR, Murray KHA, Carruthers RK. Extraperitoneal laparoscopic dismembered fibrin-glued pyeloplasty: Medium-term results. Br J Urol 1997;80:382-9.

156. McKay TC, Albala DM, Gehrin BE, Castelli M. Laparoscopic ureteral reanastomosis using fibrin glue. J Urol 1994;152:1637-40.

157. Detweiler MB, Verbo A, Kobos JW, et al. A sliding, absorbable, reinforced ring and an axially driven stent placement device for sutureless fibrin glue gastrointestinal anastomosis. J Invest Surg 1996;9:495-504.

158. Byrne DJ, Hardy J, Wood RAB, et al. Adverse influence of fibrin sealant on the healing of high-risk sutured colonic anastomoses. J R Coll Surg Edinb 1992;37:394-8.

159. van der Ham AC, Kort WJ, Weijma IM, et al. Effect of fibrin sealant on the integrity of colonic anastomoses in rats with faecal peritonitis. Eur J Surg 1993;159:425-32.

160. Valleix D, Descottes B. Pregluing of circular instrumental anastomoses. Surg Gynecol Obstet 1990;170:161-2.

161. Berg PL, Barina W, Born P. Endoscopic injection of fibrin glue in peptic ulcer hemorrhage: A pilot study. Endoscopy 1994;26: 528-30.

162. Lau WY, Leung KL, Zhu XL, et al. Laparoscopic repair of perforated peptic ulcer. Br J Surg 1995;82:814-6.

163. Rutgeerts P, Rauws E, Wara P, et al. Randomized trial of single and repeated fibrin glue compared with injection of polidocanol in treatment of bleeding peptic ulcer. Lancet 1997;350:692-6.

164. Suzuki Y, Kuroda Y, Morita A, et al. Fibrin glue sealing for the prevention of pancreatic

fistulas following distal pancreatectomy. Arch Surg 1995;130:952-5.

165. Wadström J, Gannedahl G, Wahlberg J, Frödin L. Persistent pancreatic fistula after pancreas transplantation treated with fibrin glue and octreotide. Transplant Proc 1995;27:3491-2.

166. Hwang TL, Chen MF. Randomized trial of fibrin tissue glue for low output enterocutaneous fistula. Br J Surg 1996;83:112.

167. Hjortrup A, Moesgaard F, Kjaergard J. Fibrin adhesive in the treatment of perineal fistulas. Dis Colon Rectum 1991;34:752-4.

168. Moesgaard F, Hoffmann S, Nielsen R. Successful fibrin seal closure of a contaminated fistula. Acta Chir Scand 1989;155:427-8.

169. Abel ME, Chiu YSY, Russell TR, et al. Autologous fibrin glue in the treatment of rectovaginal and complex fistulas. Dis Colon Rectum 1993;36:447-9.

170. Lange V, Meyer G, Wenk H, Schildberg FW. Fistuloscopy—An adjuvant technique for sealing gastrointestinal fistulae. Surg Endosc 1990;4:212-6.

171. Cellier C, Landi B, Faye A, et al. Upper gastrointestinal tract fistulae: Endoscopic obliteration with fibrin sealant. Gastrointest Endosc 1996;44:731-3.

172. Tsurusaki T, Sakai H, Nishikido M, et al. Occlusion therapy for an intractable transplant-uretal fistula using fibrin glue. J Urol 1996;155:1698.

173. Felipetto R, Vigano L, Cecchi M, et al. Use of fibrin sealant in the treatment of prostatic cutaneous fistula in a case of pseudomonas prostatitis. Int Urol Nephrol 1995;27:563-5.

174. King RC, Reece TB, Shockey KS, et al. Minimally invasive coronary artery bypass grafting decreases hospital stay and cost. Ann Surg 1997;225:805-9.

175. Marchac D, Ascherman J, Arnaud E. Fibrin glue fixation in forehead endoscopy: Evaluation of our experience with 206 cases. Plast Reconstr Surg 1997;100:704-14.

176. Cravello L, Demontgolfier R, Dercole C, et al. Endoscopic surgery—The end of classic surgery. Eur J Obstet Gynecol Reprod Bio 1997;75:103-6.

177. Wormald PJ, McDonogh M. "Bath-plug" technique for the endoscopic management of cerebrospinal fluid leaks. J Laryngol Oto 1997;111:1042-6.

178. Gates EA. New surgical procedures: Can ou patients benefit while we learn? Am J Obstet Gynecol 1997;176:1293-8.

179. Yerdel MA, Koksoy C, Aras N, et al. Laparoscopic versus open cholecystectomy in cirrhotic patients—A prospective study. Sur Laparosc Endosc 1997;7:483-6.

180. Hillerdal G, Gustafsson G, Wegenius G, et al. Large emphysematous bullae: Successful treatment with thoracoscopic technique using fibrin glue in poor-risk patients. Chest 1995;107:1450-3.

181. Samuels LE, Shaw PM, Blaum LC. Percutaneous technique for management of persistent airspace with prolonged air leak using fibrin glue. Chest 1996;109:1653-5.

182. Trombelli L, Scabbia A, Wikesjö UM, Calura G. Fibrin glue application in conjunction with tetracycline root conditioning and coronally positioned flap procedure in the treatment of human gingival recession defects. Clin Periodontol 1996;23:861-7.

183. Trombelli L, Scabbia A, Scapoli C, Calura G Clinical effect of tetracycline demineralization and fibrin-fibronectin sealing system application on healing response following flap debridement surgery. J Periodontol 1996;67 688-93.

184. Trombelli L, Schincaglia GP, Zangari F, et al. Effects of tetracycline HCl conditioning and fibrin-fibronectin system application in the treatment of buccal gingival recession with guided tissue regeneration. J Periodonto 1995;66:313-20.

185. Rakocz M, Mazar A, Varon D, et al. Dental extractions in patients with bleeding disorders. Oral Surg Oral Med Oral Pathol 1993 75:280-2.

186. Rakocz M, Lavie G, Martinowitz U. Glanzmann's thrombasthenia: The use of autolo

gous fibrin glue in tooth extractions. ASDC: J Dent Child 1995;62:129-31.

187. Singh MP, Brady R Jr., Drohan W, MacPhee MJ. Sustained release of antibiotics from fibrin sealant. In: Sierra D, Saltz R, eds. Surgical adhesives and sealants: Current technology and applications. Lancaster, PA: Technomic, 1996:121-33.

188. Greco F, DePalma L, Spagnolo N. Fibrin-antibiotic mixtures: An in vitro study assessing the possibility of using a biologic carrier for local drug delivery. J Biomed Mater Res 1991;25:39-51.

189. MacPhee MJ, Singh MP, Brady R Jr, et al. Fibrin sealant: A versatile delivery vehicle for drugs and biologics. In: Sierra D, Saltz R, eds. Surgical adhesives and sealants: Current technology and applications. Lancaster, PA: Technomic, 1996:109-20.

190. Boyce ST, Holder IA, Supp AP, et al. Delivery and release of antimicrobial drugs released from human fibrin sealant. J Burn Care Rehabil 1994;15:251-5.

191. Rosenthal FM, Cao L, Tanczos E, et al. Paracrine stimulation of keratinocytes in vitro and continuous delivery of epidermal growth factor to wounds in vivo by genetically modified fibroblasts transfected with a novel chimeric construct. In Vivo 1997;11:201-8.

192. Kitazawa H, Sata H, Adachi I, et al. Microdialysis assessment of fibrin glue containing sodium alginate for local delivery of doxorubicin in tumor-bearing rats. Biol Pharm Bull 1997;20:278-81.

193. Miura S, Mii Y, Miyauchi Y, et al. Efficacy of slow-releasing anticancer drug delivery systems on transplantable osteosarcomas in rats. Jpn J Clin Oncol 1995;25:61-71.

194. Martinowitz U, Schulman S, Horoszowski H, Heim M. Role of fibrin sealants in surgical procedures on patients with hemostatic disorders. Clin Orthop 1996;328:65-75.

195. Horoszowski H, Heim M, Schulman S, et al. Multiple joint procedures in a single operative session on hemophilic patients. Clin Orthop 1996;328:60-4.

196. Wilson SM, Pell P, Donegan EA. HIV-1 transmission following the use of cryoprecipitated fibrinogen as gel/adhesive (abstract). Transfusion(Suppl)1991;31:51S.

197. Horowitz B, Prince AM, Hammon J. Viral safety of solvent/detergent-treated blood products. Blood Coagul Fibrinolysis 1994; 5:S21-8.

198. Cierniewski CS, Pluskota E, Cieslak M, et al. Antigenic properties of fibrinogen component of Hemaseel™ HMN subjected to antiviral severe dry heat treatment. Thromb Res 1996;82:349-59.

199. Cederholm-Williams SA. Therapeutic use of fibrin—A new class of fibrin sealant with minimal risks. Ukr Biokhim Zh 1996;68:34-6.

200. Gammon R, Avery N, Mintz P. Fibrin sealant: An evaluation of methods of production and the role of the blood bank. J Long-Term Effects Med Implants 1998;8:103-16.

201. Nichols WL, Daniels TM, Fisher PK, et al. Antibodies to bovine thrombin and coagulation Factor V associated with surgical use of topical bovine thrombin or fibrin "glue": A frequent finding (abstract). Blood 1993;82:59a.

202. Berruyer SI, Amiral J, French P, et al. Immunization by bovine thrombin used with fibrin glue during cardiovascular operations: Development of thrombin and Factor V inhibitors. J Thorac Cardiovasc Surg 1993;105:892-7.

203. Rapaport SI, Zivelin A, Minow RA, et al. Clinical significance of antibodies to bovine and human thrombin and Factor V after surgical use of bovine thrombin. Am J Clin Pathol 1992;97:84-91.

204. Kachuger MS, Eide TR, Manecke GR, et al. The hemodynamic effects of topical fibrin during cardiac operations. J Cardiothorac Anesth 1989;3:745-7.

205. Muntean W, Zenz W, Finding K, et al. Inhibitor to Factor V after exposure to fibrin sealant during cardiac surgery in a two-year-old child. Acta Paediatr 1994;83:84-7.

206. Israels SJ, Israels ED. Development of antibodies to bovine and human Factor V in two children after exposure to topical bovine

thrombin. Am J Pediatr Hematol Oncol 1994; 16:249-54.

207. Dascombe WH, Dumanian G, Hong C, et al. Application of thrombin based fibrin glue and non-thrombin based batroxobin glue on intact human blood vessels: Evidence of transmural thrombin activity. Thromb Haemost 1997;78:947-51.

208. Matthew TL, Spotnitz WD, Kron IL, et al. Four years experience with fibrin sealant in thoracic and cardiovascular surgery. Ann Thorac Surg 1990;50:40-4.

In: Mintz PD, ed.
Transfusion Therapy: Clinical Principles and Practice
Bethesda, MD: AABB Press, 1999

11

Transfusion Practice in Solid Organ Transplantation

GLENN RAMSEY, MD, AND PAUL D. MINTZ, MD

ORGAN TRANSPLANTATION IS A routine procedure at many medical centers, but probably only a few aspects of blood banking support can be considered established practice. This chapter discusses preoperative and perioperative transfusions in organ transplantation patients and posttransplantation red blood cell antibodies emanating from graft lymphocytes.

The best-accepted practices are accurate donor and recipient ABO grouping, blood ordering schedules, the use of autologous blood in many patients, and cytomegalovirus (CMV)-reduced-risk transfusions in selected patients. Two aspects of transfusion support are generally agreed upon: avoidance of intentional pretransplantation transfusions and the close monitoring of hemostasis, to varying de-

grees, during liver transplantation. Also noted are some areas in which more information is desirable: leukocyte reduction, blood irradiation, aprotinin usage, and the effect of donor leukocyte microchimerism on graft survival. Finally, recipient hemolysis resulting from the synthesis of anti-A and/or anti-B by donor lymphocytes is discussed and issues regarding the transfusion of the recipient who is D-negative or who has RBC alloantibodies are considered.

Best-Accepted Practices

ABO Grouping

Organ transplants must be ABO-compatible in standard practice because of the powerful comple-

Glenn Ramsey, MD, Co-Director, Blood Bank, Northwestern Memorial Hospital, and Associate Professor of Pathology, Northwestern University, Chicago, Illinois, and Paul D. Mintz, MD, Associate Chair and Professor of Pathology, Professor of Internal Medicine, and Director, Clinical Laboratories and Blood Bank, University of Virginia Health Sciences Center, Charlottesville, Virginia

ment-fixing effect of ABO antibodies on endothelial cells. Therefore, accurate ABO grouping of donors and recipients is required.

When a trauma victim receives large amounts of uncrossmatched group O Red Blood Cells (RBCs) before a blood bank sample is obtained, ambiguity in typing may result. If the trauma is fatal, the blood bank might not be aware of subsequent organ donation from the victim. Accordingly, caution should be used in assigning a blood group in this circumstance. If there is significant doubt, it may be best to report the blood type as unknown so that an organ procurement agency can review this with the blood bank.

Blood Ordering Schedules

As for other surgical procedures, each transfusion service can establish blood ordering schedules for organ transplantation. Table 11-1 shows typical crossmatch orders for each organ, based on recent

Table 11-1. Red Blood Cell (RBC) Crossmatching for Organ Transplants

Organ	Typical RBC Crossmatch Order (in units)
Liver, adult	10-20 (varies with risk)
Liver, pediatric	5-10 (varies with size)
Heart	4-6
Heart-lung	4-6
Lung, single	2
Lung (sequential double)	6
Kidney	0-2
Pancreas	0-2

studies.[1-3] Predictions of blood use in liver transplant patients are inexact, and there is always the chance of a major hemorrhage, but the initial number of crossmatches can be tailored to the patient's risk. Some adults, such as those with hepatoma or metabolic disease, come to transplantation with good hepatic and hemostatic function, and crossmatching 10 units is adequate at the beginning. Orders for pediatric liver recipients are adjusted for size; three to five units are appropriate for neonates.

Use of Autologous Blood

Intraoperative red cell recovery is usually used in adult liver transplantation. Often, one-third to one-half of the total RBCs used is from intraoperative recovery. This can be crucial support in massively transfused patients. Blood recovery can also be worthwhile in complicated heart transplant patients with previous surgery or other reasons for bleeding.

Preoperative autologous blood donations can be made in several settings by prospective patients. A small subset of liver transplant patients, such as those with amyloidosis or other metabolic diseases, has fairly well-preserved hematologic function. When the hematocrit and clotting factors are sufficient, RBCs and plasma can be frozen in advance. After careful evaluation, some heart and lung transplant patients can tolerate RBC donations.

Because of organ shortages, some pediatric liver transplantation programs are harvesting left lobes from parents or other family members for small patients. These donors can donate blood in advance and/or can undergo hemodilution before the procedure. Living related kidney donors usually do not need blood.

Cytomegalovirus-Reduced-Risk Transfusions

In the 1991 survey of 25 North American transplantation centers conducted by Danielson et al,[4] a substantial percentage of centers provided CMV-seronegative cellular blood components to both seropositive and seronegative recipients. This was true of most heart, lung, and pediatric liver transplantation programs and of some kidney and adult liver programs. However, the publication did not comment on the impact of the organ donor's CMV status.

More recently, in 1997, the American Association of Blood Banks (AABB) issued a bulletin on the prevention of transfusion-transmitted CMV.[5] The document includes a discussion of whether CMV-seropositive organ transplant recipients should receive CMV-reduced-risk blood. On the basis of available evidence, the document concludes that "the additional clinical benefit from CMV-reduced-risk blood in this setting is expected to be marginal." Even in CMV-*seronegative* patients receiving CMV-seronegative livers and CMV-untested blood components, CMV infection rates are low (8-10%). To date, the transmission of a second strain of CMV by transfusion has not been documented. Therefore, the AABB bulletin concludes that CMV-reduced-risk blood is indicated in CMV-seronegative recipients of organs from CMV-seronegative donors (barring massive transfusion need) but is not indicated in CMV-seropositive patients or in recipients of organs from CMV-seropositive donors. The issue of CMV prevention by leukocyte-reduced blood components is considered in Chapter 16.

Transfusion Support

Pretransplantation Transfusions

Twenty-five years ago, Opelz et al[6] reported that pretransplantation blood transfusions were associated with improved cadaver renal graft survival. Transfusions from prospective living kidney donors became a common practice to induce tolerance (at least among those recipients who did not become sensitized to their potential donor). Some studies showed that transfusions were beneficial mainly if the donor and recipient shared one HLA-DR antigen. However, leukocytes in blood components were thought to mediate this immunosuppressive effect, as evidenced by the fact that frozen-thawed RBC transfusions did not improve graft survival.

All of this has passed largely from the scene, and today's general practice is not to transfuse organ transplant candidates intentionally. Improved immunosuppression by cyclosporine and tacrolimus (FK506) has neutralized much of the beneficial effect. In addition, increased concern about transfusion-transmitted infections has dampened enthusiasm for this approach. In the 1990s, the use of erythropoietin has greatly reduced the need for transfusions in renal failure. The use of erythropoietin in the nonsurgical setting is discussed in Chapter 19.

However, in 1997, Opelz and colleagues[7] published a reexamination of the issue in cadaver kidney recipients. Beginning in 1987, they conducted a multicenter randomized prospective trial in which patients received either three unselected routine RBC units or none, before transplantation. The 205 transfusion recipients had significantly better 1-year (90% vs 82%) and 5-year (79% vs 70%) graft survivals compared with the 218 nontransfused patients. In multivariate analysis, transfusions were beneficial independent of other factors, such as HLA matching, HLA antibodies, disease, age, or gender.

Also in 1997, Koneru et al[8] retrospectively analyzed the transfusion history of 121 liver recipients. Transfusion 90 days or more before the transplantation was independently associated with fewer severe or recurrent rejection episodes (18% of patients), compared with the proportion of episodes among those who had not been transfused (42% of patients). However, graft and patient survival were not different.

Thus, the book is not yet closed on the transfusion effect. As discussed below, the related concept of microchimerism is also under active investigation. Yet, the growing trend of leukocyte reduction might negate this beneficial effect as well, if and when it is present. As the infection risks of transfusions recede in coming years, further investigations of the immunologic effects of transfusions will continue.

Liver Transplantation Hemostasis

In liver transplantation, transfusion and hemostasis therapy is usually guided by close laboratory monitoring. The patient's condition and clotting function often change rapidly during surgery. In conjunction with clinical observations of bleeding, the hematocrit, platelet count, prothrombin time, activated partial thromboplastin time, and the fibrinogen level are the basic parameters for guiding blood component therapy.

To guide transfusions and other hemostatic measures, many programs augment routine testing with thromboelastography (TEG).[9-10] This is a test done in the operating suite to visualize in-vitro whole blood clotting. The time until clotting starts is slowed by low coagulation factor levels and by heparin or heparin-like substances released from the donor liver when it is unclamped. Low platelet or fibrinogen levels impede the rate of clot formation and its strength, as reflected by the angle and amplitude of the TEG tracing. These effects usually can be detected within 30 minutes after sampling, a turnaround time comparable to maximally "stat" laboratory testing.

TEG testing is better than other laboratory tests in two ways. First, fibrinolysis, a well-known complication that may develop during or near the anhepatic phase, can be detected within 20-60 minutes, much faster than by other methods such as euglobulin lysis (up to 2 hours). Second, drugs can be added to the TEG blood sample to assess their effects in the patient. The antifibrinolytic agent epsilon-aminocaproic acid and the heparin-inactivating drug protamine can be previewed in the TEG before use.

The pathophysiology, evaluation, and treatment of the hemostatic defects present in patients with hepatic dysfunction are discussed in detail in Chapter 7.

Areas of Interest

HLA alloimmunization against donor antigens impairs graft survival in kidney and heart transplant recipients. Therefore, logic would suggest that the leukocyte reduction of cellular blood components may be useful in patients with renal and cardiac problems who might be future transplantation candidates. On the other hand, leukocyte reduction might negate any graft-protective effect conferred by prior transfusions. As leukocyte-reduced components become more widely available, further study of this question will be useful.

Most centers do not irradiate blood components routinely for organ transplant patients. In the survey by Danielson et al,[4] only one of 25 centers routinely used gamma-irradiated blood components. However, there are a few reports of transfusion-associated graft-vs-host disease in these patients.[11] Additional analyses of any future cases would be important for the field. The irradiation of blood components to prevent graft-vs-host disease is discussed in Chapter 17.

Aprotinin, a bovine lung protein that inhibits fibrinolysis and may prevent platelet dysfunction during cardiac bypass, is licensed in the United States for reducing blood transfusions in cardiac surgery. Numerous liver transplantation centers in Europe report impressive reductions in blood use when aprotinin is given intraoperatively. Aprotinin also has shown promise in reducing blood loss in heart and lung transplant recipients. However, in liver transplant recipients, tipping the scales too far toward clotting might lead to hepatic arterial thrombosis and graft loss. Consensus on the use of aprotinin has not been reached yet.

Donor leukocyte microchimerism is under active investigation as a mechanism to improve graft survival. Starzl and colleagues[12] propose that the long-term presence of donor leukocytes may lead to tolerance of the graft. They are conducting trials of infusions of cadaver marrow stem cells at the time of liver, kidney, and heart transplantation. This is reminiscent of the proposed tolerizing effect of prior transfusions discussed previously. Thus far, reductions in rejection episodes have been seen, but graft survival is generally similar to that among control subjects.

Immunohematologic Considerations

Antibodies From Graft Lymphocytes

In 1964, Starzl et al[13] suggested that ABO-mismatched liver allografts could result in recipient red blood cell hemolysis. Subsequently, this type of graft-vs-host reaction has been reported following liver,[14-18] kidney,[19-22] pancreas,[23,24] spleen,[25] heart,[26,27] and heart-lung[24,26-29] transplantation. The reactions may arise after what often are called "ABO-unmatched" or "minor-mismatched" transplants (ie, group O allografts transplanted to non-group-O patients, or non-group-AB allografts transplanted to group AB patients). The reactions are caused by the synthesis of anti-A and/or anti-B by donor lymphocytes that accompany the transplanted organ. This clinical problem also has been seen following hematopoietic progenitor cell transplantation as discussed in Chapter 12. While the majority of cases of immune hemolysis resulting from antibody synthesized by passenger lymphocytes involve anti-A or anti-B, several reports of anti-D arising from transplanted kidneys, livers, and lungs have been reported.[30-38] Most, but not all,[33,35] of these reports noted anti-D in the donor prior to transplantation.

In a review of this phenomenon, Ramsey[39] reported that the frequency of ABO antibodies and hemolysis following minor-mismatched allograft transplantation was 17 and 9%, respectively, in kidney transplant recipients; 40 and 29%, respectively, in liver transplant patients; and 70% for both in heart-lung transplant recipients. There was no effect on the likelihood of hemolysis occurring in relation to age, race, or gender of the donor or the recipient, of cadaver vs living kidney donors, or of the recipient's A_2 or secretor status.[39] The frequency of passenger-lymphocyte-induced hemolysis is increased in patients taking cyclosporine compared with earlier immunosuppressive treatments.[39] The ABO antibodies are typically IgG, have appeared 7-10 days after allotransplantation, and have persisted for approximately 1 month. IgG allotyping of the implicated antibodies has provided firm evidence that the antibodies are of donor origin. Many patients have required transfusions for this self-limited process, and a number of cases of hemolysis-induced acute renal failure have been reported.[19,20,22,23,40] One death has been noted owing to complications of hemolysis.[40] In particularly fulminant cases, RBC or plasma exchange has been performed.[19,40]

When minor ABO-incompatible allografts are transplanted, the frequency and severity of recipient hemolysis increase with the lymphoid content of the transplanted organs. In these settings, several of transfusion strategies are possible. In kidney and heart transplant recipients, transfusion support is usually modest and the likelihood of hemolysis is relatively low. Thus, it is appropriate to provide transfusions of the recipient's ABO group and to switch to donor ABO group only if incompatible crossmatches are noted. In liver and heart-lung transplant recipients, the likelihood of severe hemolysis is significantly higher, so alternative strategies should be considered. Possibilities include 1) transfusing exclusively donor group RBCs from the beginning of surgery; 2) transfusing recipient group RBCs at the beginning of surgery but switching to donor group RBCs for the final part of surgery and for subsequent postoperative transfusions; 3) transfusing recipient group RBCs, but performing postoperative direct antiglobulin tests on specimens received for compatibility testing and switching to donor ABO group RBCs if the direct antiglobulin test results become positive owing to anti-A and/or anti-B; or 4) transfusing recipient group RBCs until incompatibility is noted in a crossmatch. Although there is no standardized approach in this regard, the first option seems overly conservative and potentially wasteful, particularly because most of these situations will involve group O solid organ allografts, which would lead to a reduction of the group O blood supply. However, any of the other options represents reasonable practice. We have elected to wait for incompatible crossmatches before switching to donor group RBCs for transfusion.

The D-Negative Recipient

Solid organ allograft recipients who are D negative and do not have anti-D may pose special challenges for the clinician and transfusion service. Because pregnancy may occur after organ allografting, most clinicians would attempt to provide D-negative RBCs to females with childbearing potential. If D-positive platelets are transfused, the provision of Rh

Immune Globulin to prevent alloimmunization to red blood cells contaminating the platelet concentrates is appropriate.

It is reasonable to provide D-negative RBCs to all D-negative patients undergoing solid organ transplantation in order to avoid sensitization to D, given that some of these patients will require prolonged postoperative transfusion and a few may require a second transplant. However, a relatively low rate of D immunization from incompatible transfusions during transplantation procedures has been reported, perhaps owing to the postoperative immunosuppression of these patients. In one series, none of 16 liver or heart allograft recipients who were transfused with D-positive RBCs was reported to make anti-D.[41] To conserve the supply of D-negative blood, some programs have elected to transfuse D-positive RBCs to D-negative males and D-negative females who are not with childbearing potential, provided that these patients have no anti-D detected before transfusion.[42] Some programs also have restricted the amount of D-negative blood provided to females with childbearing potential to an arbitrary number of units (eg, 10).[42] If D-negative patients are transfused with D-positive RBCs, it is necessary to consider when to begin providing D-negative RBCs. A reasonable approach is to do so after the second or third postoperative day if transfusions are still needed. This protects the patient from an exacerbation of immune hemolysis in case an anamnestic response to anti-D is forthcoming.

The Recipient With Red Blood Cell Alloantibodies

Patients who require liver allografts and who have circulating red blood cells alloantibodies often pose a special challenge because they may be expected to require large quantities of blood. In such patients, the preferable practice is to obtain a sufficient quantity of antigen-negative red cells to provide for the patient's anticipated needs during and after surgery. A second approach, which would be most feasible for patients with low titers of anti-

bodies (eg, less than 1:8) or could be used if an insufficient number of antigen-negative units were available, would be to reserve a specified number of antigen-negative units for use at the beginning and again at the end of surgery. If an antibody detection test is demonstrated to be nonreactive during surgery owing to the washout of the alloantibody as a result of blood loss, antigen-positive immediate-spin crossmatch-compatible units could be used. At the end of surgery, the final six units that are transfused should be antigen-negative to prevent postoperative hemolysis as alloantibody is resynthesized or reenters the intravascular space from the extravascular fluid.[42] In one series of seven evaluable patients managed in this fashion, five had no hemolysis and two had delayed immune hemolysis, although one of these two had an underlying hemolytic anemia (paroxysmal nocturnal hemoglobinuria).[43] An additional strategy would be to use preoperative plasmapheresis to remove clinically significant low-titer antibodies. However, because IgG is predominantly extravascular, this approach, while possibly successful, may prove inefficacious. Further issues in massive transfusion are discussed in Chapter 9.

Posttransplantation Red Blood Cell Alloantibodies of Recipient Origin

RBC alloantibodies of recipient origin have been reported after solid organ transplantation despite the intensive immunosuppressive therapy provided to these patients.[44,45] In one report,[44] 9% of liver transplant recipients developed new red blood cell alloantibodies of host origin. Jacobs et al[45] noted the simultaneous development of a delayed hemolytic transfusion reaction owing to a recipient anti-E and the appearance of anti-A from passenger lymphocytes.

Allograft Donor Infectious Disease Testing

Viruses present in donor organ allografts may be transmitted to the recipient. Cases of human immunodeficiency virus-type 1 (HIV-1) transmission by kidney,[46-49] heart,[48,50] liver,[46,51] pancreas,[48] bone,[49,52] and skin[53] allografts from HIV-1-infected donors have been reported. Most of these reports document the infection of recipients before HIV-1 antibody screening of organ and tissue donors was implemented in 1985. Other reports have documented HIV-1 transmission by organ and tissue donors who were in the window period of HIV-1 infection before the presence of detectable antibody was noted[54] or in urgent transplantation before the donor's reactive test result for HIV-1 antibody was available.[51]

One case of HIV-1 transmission is of particular importance with respect to transfusion medicine.[55] In this report, HIV-1 was transmitted to a patient who had received a cadaveric renal transplant from a donor who had received massive blood transfusions prior to death. A specimen obtained from the donor drawn immediately posttransfusion was negative for HIV-1 antibody. On the basis of this test, a kidney was harvested for transplantation. After transplantation, donor blood samples that had been collected before any transfusions were given were analyzed and found to be HIV-1 antibody-positive, as were blood samples obtained 12 hours after the donor received his transfusions. This latter sample was positive presumably because extravascular fluid with antibody had entered the intravascular space. The recipient of this donor's kidney was infected with HIV-1. This case is instructive with regard to the need to test donor blood for infectious disease markers, either prior to the transfusion of blood components, if possible, or, if pretransfusion specimens are not available, as close to the time of organ harvesting as possible.

In July 1997, the US Food and Drug Administration issued a guidance document regarding the screening and testing of donors of human tissue intended for transplantation. This document may be found on the World Wide Web at http://www.fda.gov/cber/gdlns/tissue2.txt. This guidance document states that all donors of human tissue intended for transplantation should be tested and found to be negative for antibodies to HIV-1, HIV-2, and hepatitis C virus, as well as for hepatitis B surface antigen. HIV antigen testing is not included as a requirement.

The document includes a flowchart for determining if a donor specimen is suitable for infectious disease testing. This flowchart stipulates that if the donor has received more than 2 L of blood or colloid within the previous 48 hours, or 2 L of crystalloid within the previous 1 hour, or 2 L of a combination of the above, an algorithm should be applied. This algorithm stipulates that if the amount of colloid infused within the previous 48 hours plus the amount of crystalloid infused in the previous 1 hour exceed one plasma volume, or if the amount of blood transfused in the previous 48 hours plus the amount of colloid infused in the previous 48 hours plus the amount of crystalloid infused in the previous 1 hour exceed one blood volume, then a specimen should not be used for infectious disease testing and the prospective donor should be rejected. The document also stipulates that if the prospective donor is less than 12 years old and no pretransfusion/infusion sample is available, the algorithm should be applied if the donor received any transfusion or infusion of fluids.

The guidance document also addresses viral marker test performance, donor behavioral history screening, and methods of ascertaining clinical and physical evidence of HIV and hepatitis infections.

Solid Organ Donation

There is a continuing shortage of organs available for transplantation. At present, organ procurement and distribution associations have undertaken the principal responsibility for public education regarding organ donation. Because blood donors may be more willing to serve as organ donors than nonblood donors,[56] it is logical for community blood services to play an active role in public education regarding the need for organ donation.

References

1. Ramsey G, Sherman LA. The new age of organic blood banking. Transfusion 1998;38: 9-11.

2. Sherman LA, Ramsey G. Solid organ transplantation. In: Rossi EC, Simon TL, Moss GS, Gould SA, eds. Principles of transfusion medicine. 2nd ed. Baltimore: Williams and Wilkins, 1996:635-40.

3. Triulzi DJ, Griffith BP. Blood usage in lung transplantation. Transfusion 1998;38:12-5.

4. Danielson CFM, Filo RS, O'Donnell JA, McCarthy LJ. Institutional variation in hemotherapy for solid organ transplantation. Transfusion 1996;36:263-7.

5. Leukocyte reduction for the prevention of transfusion-transmitted cytomegalovirus (TT-CMV). Association Bulletin #97-2. Bethesda, MD: American Association of Blood Banks, 1997.

6. Opelz G, Mickey MR, Sengar DPS, Terasaki PI. Effect of blood transfusions on subsequent kidney transplants. Transplant Proc 1973;5:253-9.

7. Opelz G, Vanrenterghem Y, Kirste G, et al. Prospective evaluation of pretransplant blood transfusions in cadaver kidney transplants. Transplantation 1997;63:964-7.

8. Koneru B, Harrison D, Rizwan M, et al. Blood transfusions in liver recipients: A conundrum or a clear benefit in the cyclosporine/tacrolimus era? Transplantation 1997;63:1587-90.

9. Kang Y. Thromboelastography in liver transplantation. Semin Thromb Hemost 1995;21 (Suppl 4):34-44.

10. Kang Y. Coagulation and liver transplantation: Current concepts. Liver Transplant Surg 1997; 3:465-7.

11. Wisecarver JL, Cattral MS, Langnas AN, et al. Transfusion-induced graft-versus-host disease after liver transplantation. Documentation using polymerase chain reaction with HLA-DR sequence-specific primers. Transplantation 1994;58:269-71.

12. Starzl TE, Demetris AJ, Murase N, et al. The future of transplantation: With particular reference to chimerism and xenotransplantation. Transplant Proc 1997;29:19-27.

13. Starzl TE, Marchioro TL, Huntley RT, et al. Experimental and clinical homotransplantation of the liver. Ann N Y Acad Sci 1964;120:739-65.

14. Ramsey G, Nusbacher J, Starzl TE, Lindsay GD. Isohemagglutinins of graft origin after ABO-unmatched liver transplantation. N Engl J Med 1984;311:1167-70.

15. Dzik WH, Jenkins RL. Renal failure from ABO hemolysis due to anti-A of graft origin following liver transplantation (abstract). Transfusion 1987;27:550.

16. Ramsey G, Cornell FW, Hahn LF, et al. Red cell antibody problems in 1000 liver transplants. Transfusion 1989;29:396-400.

17. Brecher ME, Moore SB, Reisner RK, et al. Delayed hemolysis resulting from anti-A, after liver transplantation. Am J Clin Pathol 1989; 91:232-5.

18. Bracey AW. Anti-A of donor lymphocyte origin in three recipients of organs from the same donor. Vox Sang 1987;53:181-3.

19. Lundgren G, Asaba H, Bergström J, et al. Fulminating anti-A autoimmune hemolysis with anuria in a renal transplant recipient: A therapeutic role of plasma exchange. Clin Nephrol 1981;16:211-4.

20. Mangal AK, Growe GH, Sinclair M, et al. Acquired hemolytic anemia due to "auto"-anti-A or "auto"-anti-B induced by group O homograft in renal transplant recipients. Transfusion 1984;24:201-5.

21. Mangal AK, Logan D, Sinclair M, Stillwell G. Protection against hemolysis in ABO mismatched renal transplantation. Transfusion 1984;24:363-4.

22. Nyberg G, Sandberg L, Rydberg L, et al. ABO autoimmune hemolytic anemia in a renal transplant patient treated with cyclosporin. A case report. Transplantation 1984;37:529-30.

23. Swanson JL, Sastamoinen RM, Steeper TA, Sebring ES. Gm allotyping to determine the origin of red cell antibodies in recipients of solid organ transplants. Vox Sang 1987;52:75-8.

24. Albrechtsen D, Solheim BG, Flatmark A, et al. Autoimmune hemolytic anemia in cyclospor-

ine-treated organ allograft recipients. Transplant Proc 1988;20:959-62.

25. Salamon DJ, Ramsey G, Nusbacher J, et al. Anti-A production by a group O spleen transplanted to a group A recipient. Vox Sang 1985;48:309-12.

26. Solheim BG, Albrechtsen DA, Berg KJ, et al. Hemolytic anemia in cyclosporine-treated recipients of kidney or heart grafts from donors with minor incompatibility for ABO antigens. Transplant Proc 1987;19:4236-8.

27. Solheim BG, Albrechtsen D, Egeland T, et al. Auto-antibodies against erythrocytes in transplant patients produced by donor lymphocytes. Transplant Proc 1987;19:4520-1.

28. Hunt BJ, Amin S, Yacoub M, et al. Immune hemolysis after minor ABO-mismatched heart-lung transplants. Transplant Proc 1987; 19:4600.

29. Hunt BJ, Yacoub M, Amin S, et al. Induction of red blood cell destruction by graft-derived antibodies after minor ABO-mismatched heart and lung transplantation. Transplantation 1988;46:246-9.

30. Kenwright MG, Sangster JM, Sachs JA. Development of RhD antibodies after kidney transplantation. Br Med J 1976;2:151-2.

31. Ramsey G, Israel L, Lindsay GD, et al. Anti-Rh₀(D) in two Rh-positive patients receiving kidney grafts from an Rh-immunized donor. Transplantation 1986;41:67-9.

32. Swanson J, Sebring E, Sastamoinen R, Chopek M. Gm allotyping to determine the origin of the anti-D causing hemolytic anemia in a kidney transplant recipient. Vox Sang 1987;52:228-30.

33. Flesland O, Solheim BG, Bergan A. Humeral graft versus host reaction with anti-D production. 1990 Joint Congress of the American Association of Blood Banks and the International Society of Blood Transfusion Book of Abstracts. Arlington, VA: American Asscociation of Blood Banks, 1990:34.

34. Calhoun B, Pothiawala M, Musa G, Baron B. Indicators of clinically significant red cell antibodies produced by sensitized lymphocytes in liver transplant patients. Immunohematology 1991;7:37-9.

35. Schwartz D, Götzinger P. Immune-haemolytic anaemia (IHA) after solid organ transplantation due to rhesus antibodies of donor origin: Report of 5 cases. Beitr Infusionsther 1992; 30:367-9.

36. Knoop C, Andrien M, Antoine M, et al. Severe hemolysis due to a donor anti-D antibody after heart-lung transplantation: Association with lung and blood chimerism. Am Rev Respir Dis 1993;148:504-6.

37. Lee JH, Mintz PD. Graft versus host anti-Rh₀(D) following minor Rh-incompatible orthotopic liver transplantation. Am J Hematol 1993;44:168-71.

38. Saba NF, Sweeney JD, Penn LC, et al. Anti-D in a D-positive renal transplant patient. Transfusion 1997;37:321-4.

39. Ramsey G. Red cell antibodies arising from solid organ transplantation. Transfusion 1991;31:76-86.

40. Minakuchi J, Toma H, Takahashi K, Ota K. Autoanti-A and -B antibody induced by ABO unmatched blood group kidney allograft. Transplant Proc 1985;17:2297-300.

41. Ramsey G, Hahn LF, Cornell FW, et al. Low rate of rhesus immunization from Rh-incompatible blood transfusions during liver and heart transplant surgery. Transplantation 1989;47:993-5.

42. Dzik WH. Solid organ transplantation. In: Petz LD, Swisher SN, Kleinman S, et al, eds. Clinical practice of transfusion medicine. New York: Churchill Livingstone Inc, 1996: 783-806.

43. Ramsey G, Cornell FW, Hahn LF, et al. Incompatible blood transfusions in liver transplant patients with significant red cell alloantibodies. Transplant Proc 1989;21:3531.

44. Blomqvist BI, Wikman A, Shanwell A, Eleborg L. Erythrocyte antibodies in liver transplantation: Experiences from Huddinge University Hospital. Transplant Proc 1991;23: 1944-5.

45. Jacobs LB, Shirey RS, Ness PM. Hemolysis due to the simultaneous occurrence of passenger lymphocyte syndrome and a delayed hemolytic transfusion reaction in a liver transplant patient. Arch Pathol Lab Med 1996; 120:684-6.

46. Human immunodeficiency virus infection transmitted from an organ donor screened for HIV antibody—North Carolina. Morb Mortal Wkly Rep 1987;36:306-8.

47. Kumar P, Pearson JE, Martin DH, et al. Transmission of human immunodeficiency virus by transplantation of a renal allograft, with development of the acquired immunodeficiency syndrome. Ann Intern Med 1987;106:244-5.

48. Erice A, Rhame FS, Heussner RC, et al. Human immunodeficiency virus infection in patients with solid-organ transplants: Report of five cases and review. Rev Infect Dis 1991;13: 537-47.

49. Simonds RJ, Holmberg SC, Hurwitz RL, et al. Transmission of human immunodeficiency virus type 1 from a seronegative organ and tissue donor. N Engl J Med 1992;326:726-32.

50. Dummer JS, Erb S, Breinig MK, et al. Infection with human immunodeficiency virus in the Pittsburgh transplant population: A study of 583 donors and 1043 recipients, 1981–1986. Transplantation 1989;47:134-40.

51. Samuel D, Castaing D, Adam R, et al. Fatal acute HIV infection with aplastic anaemia, transmitted by liver graft. Lancet 1988;1: 1221-2.

52. Transmission of HIV through bone transplantation: Case report and public health recommendations. Morb Mortal Wkly Rep 1988; 37:597-9.

53. Clarke JA. HIV transmission and skin grafts (letter). Lancet 1987;1:983.

54. Quarto M, Germinario C, Fontana A, Barbuti S. HIV transmission through kidney transplantation from a living related donor (letter). N Engl J Med 1989;320:1754.

55. Bowen PA, Lobel SA, Caruana RJ, et al. Transmission of human immunodeficiency virus (HIV) by transplantation: Clinical aspects and time course analysis of viral antigenemia and antibody production. Ann Intern Med 1988; 108:46-8.

56. Szuflad P, DeSantis D, Dzik W. Attitudes toward solid organ donation: Blood donors vs non-blood donors (abstract). Transfusion 1993;33:93S.

In: Mintz PD, ed.
Transfusion Therapy: Clinical Principles and Practice
Bethesda, MD: AABB Press, 1999

12

Transfusion Therapy in Hematopoietic Stem Cell Transplantation

RICHARD C. FRIEDBERG, MD, PhD

 RECENT TECHNOLOGIC ADVANCES in the capability to ablate endogenous marrow and repopulate with exogenous stem cells have generated novel transfusion support problems. The term "bone marrow" transplantation has been correctly superseded by "hematopoietic stem cell," "stem cell," or "progenitor cell" transplantation. Regardless of the descriptive term used, however, the procedure introduces unique considerations that differentiate transfusion support for stem cell transplant recipients from that for more traditional oncology patients.[1,2]

Historically, blood groups were considered a static characteristic for a given individual, much like a fingerprint. The "forward grouping" identi-

fied ABO antigens and the "reverse grouping" identified ABO antibodies (isohemagglutinins). In this paradigm, each blood group had specific rules for ABO antigens and antibodies that were present. With stem cell transplantation, however, an individual's blood group may be dynamic. Classic ABO markers—antigens expressed and antibodies present—may change at different times. Moreover, the waxing and waning of donor (novel) and recipient (previous) ABO markers can follow complex kinetics. Patients in the midst of the transplantation and engraftment process may switch among the various combinations of none, one, or two of the traditional blood groups during different phases of the treatment. In fact, because different cell lines and components engraft at different times and have

Richard C. Friedberg, MD, PhD, Associate Professor of Pathology, Associate Head, Transfusion Medicine, and Associate Medical Director, Blood Bank, Division of Laboratory Medicine, Department of Pathology, University of Alabama at Birmingham, and Chief, Pathology and Laboratory Medicine Service, Birmingham Veterans Affairs Medical Center, Birmingham, Alabama

different half-lives, a dynamic, though often transient, chimera is possible. Many of the standard transfusion protocols have had to be reconsidered. The advent of marrow ablation and successful repopulation with genetically distinct totipotent stem cells as standard therapies have altered the transfusion landscape radically. To bridge the hematopoietic gap adequately between marrow ablation and stable engraftment, the transfusion support team must consider independently the donor-recipient relationship, forward grouping, and reverse grouping, as well as additional considerations such as cytomegalovirus (CMV) serostatus, filtration, and irradiation at each step of the transplantation process.

Transfusion therapy for the patient undergoing stem cell transplantation can vary depending on the relationship between donor and recipient. The donor source may be autologous, syngeneic, or allogeneic. Autologous transplants are more correctly described as "replants" or "rescues" because the transplanted material is genetically identical (unless modified ex vivo). Syngeneic transplantation is an option for patients with a healthy monozygotic (identical) twin. By definition, monozygotic twins are identical for all 23 pairs of chromosomes; therefore, they have the same HLA genes on the short arm of chromosome 6 (ie, they are HLA-identical) as well as the same ABH glycosyltransferases encoded on the distal end of the long arm of chromosome 9 (ie, they are ABO-identical). In contrast, nonmonozygotic twins are not necessarily HLA-identical and are ABO-identical only if the independently segregating chromosome 9 also matches. Conceptually, syngeneic transplantation falls midway between autologous and allogeneic transplantation, having the advantage of being HLA- and ABO-identical with minimal risk of graft-vs-host disease (GVHD). Allogeneic transplantation introduces additional potential complications with greater degrees of incompatibility. For example, donor-recipient blood group pairings can be identical, major incompatible, minor incompatible, or both major and minor incompatible. Related allogeneic transplantation is ideally HLA-matched and has significant degrees of

matching for non-HLA genes (eg, ABO) due to consanguinity. In contrast, unrelated donors are (usually) HLA-matched, which indicates genetic agreement of only select HLA loci. The remainder of the genome, including the ABO loci, is typically quite disparate. Thus, there exists a spectrum of compatibility dependent on the donor-recipient relationship, which directly affects the transfusion support protocols for stem cell transplant recipients.

Provision of Blood Products

Transplantation Phases

From the transfusion point of view, the transplantation process can be divided into three phases: 1) pretransplant, 2) peritransplant, and 3) posttransplant. During the pretransplant phase, the stem cell transplant candidate is much like any other oncology patient in terms of component selection and support, except for the roles played by familial donations and the gamma irradiation of blood components transfused to patients who are candidates for autologous hematopoietic stem cell harvesting. Family members should be avoided as blood donors to prevent alloimmunization against minor histocompatibility and "private" antigens. Such alloimmunization could theoretically make a future related transplantation less likely to be successful.

The peritransplant period begins once the transplantation has begun—that is, at the point of myeloablation—and continues until both engraftment and the patient have stabilized. The actual transplantation itself may require little, if any, blood bank activity. For the blood bank to ascertain its capability to support the patient until engraftment has stabilized, identification of the myeloablation and transplantation phase is critical. Whereas these steps are discrete points in time, engraftment is a gradual and continuous process. It is usually detected through the identification of some novel donor stem cell-derived marker found in the recipient. Patients in the midst of the transplantation and engraftment process may even switch among the various combinations of none, one, or two blood groups during different phases of treatment. In fact, different cell lines and components engraft at different times and have different half-lives, thereby creating a dynamic chimera. Moreover, immune reconstitution biology and kinetics depend on the stem cell source and the relationship between donor and recipient.[3] Therefore, the transfusion support team must consider the antigen (forward grouping) and antibody (reverse grouping) status independently.

The initial phase of posttransplantation hematopoietic reconstitution depends on committed progenitors. The quantity of committed progenitors infused will vary with the total CD34[+] cell count, component source (marrow vs. peripheral blood), and preharvest use of hematopoietic stem cell growth factors. Generally, initial recovery is evident within 2 weeks. Sustained hematopoiesis, which depends on self-repopulating progenitor cells and/or totipotent stem cells, is usually evident within 3-5 weeks. The reconstitution of immune functions differs temporally from that of other hematopoietic elements.[3] The first population of cells to reappear is CD5[+] B cells. Even with physical return, however, T-cell and B-cell functions in the immediate posttransplant phase are typically abnormal and variable. Normal total peripheral cell counts are reached within 3 months, but white blood cell (WBC) subsets are often irregular for much longer. Donor-specific antigens, isohemagglutinins or other antibodies, restriction fragment length polymorphism, or cytogenetic analysis may be useful in allogeneic transplantation to determine engraftment.

Determining engraftment does not establish that the original (recipient) hematopoietic lineages have been fully replaced, given that stable chimeras are not uncommon. Therefore, the loss of some recipient marker should also be identified. Logically, engraftment is difficult to prove with autologous transplantation, unless a marker gene is inserted ex vivo. As Gale and Butturini have noted, "No dose of chemotherapy or total body [ir]radiation, within the limit which can be given without irreversibly damaging non-hematopoietic tissues, completely eliminates endogenous hematopoietic

stem cells. Consequently, recovery of hematopoiesis after high doses of drugs and [ir]radiation and transplantation is not unequivocal evidence that hematopoietic cells in the graft were responsible for recovery."[4] Detection of engraftment is usually the first sign that the transplantation process is proceeding into the posttransplant phase. This phase is noteworthy for hematologic and systemic instability, which resolves as the patient recovers from the effects of treatment regimens that would be lethal if the hematopoietic stem cells were not protected ex vivo. Blood cell consumption often outdistances the recovering marrow's generation capability, and exogenous support is typically required. The point at which external hematologic support is no longer required is difficult to estimate a priori. In some patients, certain cell lines fail to engraft, and these patients can remain dependent on external support indefinitely.

Red Blood Cells

Blood product support during autologous transplantation is not markedly different from routine blood product support of the patient with malignancy, except that, in the prior circumstance, all cellular products should be gamma irradiated to prevent GVHD, and CMV-seronegative patients should receive CMV-reduced-risk cellular blood components. Red Blood Cells (RBCs) should be ABO-identical; if this is not possible, the introduction of foreign isohemagglutinin should be minimized.

In addition to the same routine difficulties in providing support to autologous transplant patients, allogeneic transplant recipients introduce novel and significant problems for transfusion medicine personnel. Each allogeneic transplantation needs to be assessed from the points of view of cell lines involved, antigens expressed, and antibodies present at the various stages of engraftment. ABO-identical allogeneic stem cell transplantation require blood product support similar to that for autologous transplantation. Issues regarding CMV are discussed below and in Chapter 16.

One of the most challenging considerations in the peritransplant period is the support for ABO-mismatched allogeneic transplantations,[5] which depends on whether the transplantation introduces a novel ABO antigen (major incompatible), a novel ABO antibody (isohemagglutinin, minor incompatible), or both novel ABO antigen and antibody (both major and minor incompatible). The breakdown into these groupings is critical to an understanding of the required support at the various stages of engraftment. ABO-mismatched recipients are also in particular danger if engraftment is not accompanied by complete ablation of the recipient hematopoietic lineages: a stable chimera may produce both antigen-bearing red cells and the corresponding antibody-producing lymphocytes, with potential for severe ongoing hemolytic sequelae. Such situations are also occasionally seen complicating ABO-mismatched liver transplantation, in which passenger donor lymphocytes can transiently engraft.[6]

Major incompatible (ABO-mismatch) transplantation involves the introduction of a foreign ABO antigen, ie, a group O recipient of a transplant from a group A, B, or AB donor (Table 12-1). In each of these cases, the recipient has a preformed circulating isohemagglutinin targeting the emerging ABO antigen on the engrafting donor stem cells. Initial concerns should center on the possibility of a severe hemolytic transfusion reaction during the stem cell infusion due to contaminating donor red cells. Therefore, the pretransplant ex-vivo stem cell processing should include red blood cell depletion. Later concerns include graft rejection or delayed engraftment. Although the myeloablative therapy theoretically destroys isohemagglutinin-producing lymphocytes, the residual recipient IgG isohemagglutinins will continue to circulate with a half-life of approximately 3 weeks. As the engrafting marrow produces erythrocytes bearing the donor ABO antigen, the direct antiglobulin test (DAT) may show positive results, and intravascular hemolysis, although rare, can become significant. Therefore, physicians providing blood product support for major incompatible transplantation must consider both donor ABO antigen and recipient isohemagglutinin. RBCs should be of the recipient (original) ABO group and washed free of antidonor isohemagglutinin until the DAT results become negative and the antidonor isohemagglutinin is no longer

Table 12-1. Transfusion Support Beginning at Myeloablation for Major ABO-Incompatible Hematopoietic Stem Cell Transplantation

Recipient	Donor	Washed RBCs*	Platelets: First Choice	Platelets: Second Choice	Platelets: Third Choice	Platelets: Fourth Choice	Fresh Frozen Plasma
O	A	O	A	AB	B, O	-	A, AB
O	B	O	B	AB	A, O	-	B, AB
A	AB	A	AB	A	B	O	AB
B	AB	B	AB	B	A	O	AB
O	AB	O	AB	A, B	O	-	AB

*Until the direct antiglobulin test is negative and antidonor isohemagglutinin is no longer detectable; thereafter, transfuse donor ABO group.

detectable. Plasma components should be of the donor ABO group. Inventory concerns may necessitate the transfusion of ABO-incompatible plasma products (eg, Fresh Frozen Plasma [FFP] and platelet concentrates), which may not necessarily lead to acute complications; nevertheless, plasma compatibility should be maintained whenever possible (see Table 12-1).

Minor incompatible (ABO-mismatched) transplantation involves the introduction of foreign isohemagglutinin—for example, a group AB recipient from a group O, A, or B donor; a group A recipient from a group O donor; or a group B recipient from a group O donor (Table 12-2). In each of these cases, the recipient has preexisting red cell antigens that will be targets for the donor isohemagglutinins in the stem cell preparation as well as those produced in vivo following lymphocyte engraftment. Initial concerns regard the possibility of an acute hemolytic transfusion reaction during the transplantation due to donor isohemagglutinins. Therefore, stem cell processing should include plasma depletion (washing) to avoid the transfusion of incompatible plasma. With engraftment, the DAT results may become positive because residual recipient

RBCs will continue to circulate with a lifespan dependent on the extent of bleeding, laboratory testing, and natural destruction. Therefore, physicians providing blood product support must consider both donor (antirecipient) isohemagglutinins and recipient ABO antigens. RBCs should be of the donor ABO group and should be washed to remove antirecipient isohemagglutinin until original erythrocytes are no longer detectable. Plasma components should be of the recipient ABO group until original erythrocytes are no longer detectable (see Table 12-2).

The final ABO-mismatched allogeneic transplantation category is combined major and minor incompatible, in which both foreign antigens and isohemagglutinins are introduced—for example, a group B recipient of group A stem cells or a group A recipient of group B stem cells (Table 12-3). The generation of novel antigen and antibody, as well as the loss of recipient antigen and antibody, occurs at different stages of the process. Initial concerns are similarly detailed for both the major and minor incompatible transplantation, and, therefore, stem cell processing should include both red cell depletion and plasma depletion to minimize the possibil-

Table 12-2. Transfusion Support Beginning at Myeloablation for Minor ABO-Incompatible Hematopoietic Stem Cell Transplantation

Recipient	Donor	Washed RBCs*	Platelets: First Choice[†]	Platelets: Second Choice	Platelets: Third Choice	Platelets: Fourth Choice	Fresh Frozen Plasma[†]
A	O	O	A	AB	B, O	-	A, AB
B	O	O	B	AB	A, O	-	B, AB
AB	O	O	AB	A, B	O	-	AB
AB	A	A	AB	A	B	O	AB
AB	B	B	AB	B	A	O	AB

*Wash until recipient erythrocytes are no longer detectable.
[†]Until recipient erythrocytes are no longer detectable; thereafter, transfuse donor ABO group.

Table 12-3. Transfusion Support Beginning at Myeloablation for Combined Major and Minor ABO-Incompatible Hematopoietic Stem Cell Transplantation

Recipient	Donor	Washed RBCs*	Platelets: First Choice[†]	Platelets: Second Choice[‡]	Platelets: Third Choice	Fresh Frozen Plasma[†]
A	B	O	AB	A, B	O	AB
B	A	O	AB	B, A	O	AB

*Until direct antiglobulin test is negative and antidonor isohemagglutinin is no longer detectable; thereafter, transfuse donor ABO group.

[†]Until recipient erythrocytes are no longer detectable; thereafter, transfuse donor ABO group.

[‡]Selection is dependent on red cells circulating in patient.

ity of an acute hemolytic transfusion reaction. Physicians providing blood product support must consider both donor and recipient isohemagglutinins and ABO antigens. RBCs should be washed group O products (ie, no A or B antigen) until the DAT results become negative and the original antidonor isohemagglutinin is no longer detectable. Ideally, plasma components should be group AB (ie, no A or B antibody) until original red cells are no longer detectable. Again, inventory concerns may necessitate the transfusion of non-AB plasma products containing undesired isohemagglutinins; nonetheless, plasma compatibility should be maintained if at all reasonably possible.

Given the tremendous variation in red cell genotypes, all allogeneic transplantations can be assumed to introduce a new alloantigen, lymphocytes capable of generating a new alloantibody, or both. Novel (donor-derived) antigens are a problem only if the recipient has the corresponding antibody a priori, in which case RBC transfusion support needs to use antigen-negative cells until the antibody is not detectable. The time to loss of detectable antibody will typically depend on the immunoglobulin's half-life: about 21-23 days for most IgG, about 7 days for IgG3, and about 5 days for IgM. A novel donor antigen should not elicit the corresponding antibody because the recipient's lymphocytes are also of donor origin and will not produce the corresponding antibody. Donor-derived antibodies against red cell antigens may be a problem because the original red cells can survive long enough for lymphocyte engraftment and antibody production. However, this should be a significant problem only if the donor has been sensitized to the antigen prior to stem cell harvest. In general, mismatches of red cell antigens that do not have naturally occurring antibodies should be treated in much the same manner as they are in regular blood banking: if the patient becomes sensitized (ie, develops a positive indirect antiglobulin test), antigen-negative RBC transfusion support should be provided.

For example, consider an Rh-mismatched transplantation. Unlike ABO alloantibodies, anti-D alloantibodies are not "naturally occurring," so a D-positive recipient of a D-negative stem cell product is not necessarily receiving foreign antigen or antibody unless, of course, the donor has a preexisting anti-D secondary to a previous exposure (eg, pregnancy).[7] The recipient will ultimately produce D-negative red cells, yet he or she has a significant likelihood of developing a de novo anti-D after transplantation because residual circulating red cells can stimulate anti-D production. Of note is that the lymphocytes that produce the anti-D must be of donor origin. In the opposite situation, a D-negative recipient of a D-positive stem cell product is unlikely to develop an anti-D de novo since the only lymphocytes capable of producing anti-D should be destroyed by the myeloablative therapy. A preexisting anti-D should be treated like an ordinary isohemagglutinin, with antigen-negative RBC transfusion support until the antibody is no longer detectable. D-negative patients receiving D-positive platelets may benefit from intravenous Rh Immune Globulin administration.[8] Mismatches of other red cell antigens that do not have naturally occurring antibodies should be treated as for other patients: if the patient becomes sensitized (ie, develops a detectable antibody), antigen-negative RBC support should be provided.

Posttransplantation blood product support follows the same indications as routine oncologic blood product support, with the particular consideration being that the safe point to stop gamma irradiation of blood products is unknown. Therefore, many practitioners routinely request irradiated products for the life of the patient. With the increasing population of stem cell transplant survivors, currently unforeseen long-term complications will certainly become apparent.

Detailed indications for RBC transfusion have been discussed elsewhere.[9,10] In general, anemia, decreased red cell mass (hematocrit $<\sim$21-27%, hemoglobin $<\sim$7-9 g/dL), and active bleeding with hypotension and tachycardia are considered appropriate indications. There are no data, however, to support the promotion of wound healing, decreased risk of infection, improved general well-being, or earlier discharge from hospital.[11] The so-called transfusion trigger, or minimum hematocrit, is not well defined. Generally, a hematocrit of less than 5% is lethal to most animals, while a hematocrit of less than 12% is commonly associated with neurologic symptoms in humans. However, animals studied on 100% F_IO_2 can carry enough dioxygen in plasma alone to support minimal resting me-

tabolism. Obviously, patient clinical conditions are highly variable. A 1988 National Institutes of Health consensus conference on perioperative blood transfusion suggested that patients with a hemoglobin concentration below 7 g/dL generally require RBC transfusion. The report notes that "healing is not compromised by normovolemic anemia unless it is extreme. There is no support for transfusion to a certain hemoglobin level or hematocrit to promote wound healing. Likewise, there is no clear evidence that anemia increases the incidence or severity of postoperative infections."[10]

Platelet Concentrates

Whereas the indications for RBC or FFP transfusion are familiar to many medical practitioners, the appropriate indications for platelet transfusion are less well known. The principal indication is severe thrombocytopenia or thrombocytopathy.[12-18] The transfusion platelet count of 20,000-30,000/μL has been a commonly accepted threshold, although without factual basis.[17] Recent studies have validated lower transfusion thresholds with significant reductions in platelet consumption and associated risks.[15,19-22] Generally, if the platelet count is less than about 5000/μL, prophylactic transfusion is appropriate. If it is less than about 10,000/μL, platelet transfusion is reasonable if the patient is febrile or hemorrhagic. Rebulla and colleagues[21] demonstrated in a 1997 study that the risk of major bleeding during induction chemotherapy in patients with acute myeloid leukemia (or when the body temperature exceeds 38 C, active bleeding is present, or invasive procedures are needed) is similar with transfusion thresholds of 20,000/μL and 10,000/μL. The use of the lower threshold reduced platelet use by 21.5%.[21] For stem cell transplantation patients in particular, the rate of reduction in the platelet count may be more significant than the specific count at a given point in time.[23] Considerations should include that platelet transfusion will not limit gross active bleeding and that trace erythrocytes may induce red cell alloimmunization.[8,24] Whenever possible, the plasma in platelet concentrates should be compatible with recipient RBCs (see tables). The selection of pooled platelet concentrates as opposed to those collected by apheresis often depends on availability, although optimal selection based on ABO grouping and CMV status is often easier with apheresis platelets; however, these considerations must be balanced against availability and cost concerns. Hospital costs for apheresis platelets and pooled random-donor platelet concentrates vary markedly across the United States, with the cost per dose of apheresis platelets vs pooled platelets ranging anywhere from approximately equivalent to twice as expensive.[25] The concept that apheresis platelets result in lower rates of alloimmunization than pooled platelets has not been supported by data, at least not when all blood products are leukocyte reduced.[26] Issues regarding CMV are discussed below and in Chapter 16.

Occasionally, however, the posttransfusion survival of donor platelets is insufficient to provide the adequate levels perceived as necessary for prophylaxis against hemorrhage, and additional platelet doses do not significantly increase the circulating platelet count. This refractoriness to platelet transfusion has challenged and frustrated many clinicians and investigators. Appropriate evaluation of refractory states must take into account the facts that 1) a "dose" of platelets, as opposed to a specific quantity, is variable; 2) interindividual intravascular volume varies markedly; and 3) platelet counts may be less accurate at very low concentrations. Platelet refractoriness can be the net result of a variety of independent and coincident factors[25,27] (eg, disseminated intravascular coagulation, splenomegaly, fever), although the presence or absence of any of these factors does not necessarily equate with refractoriness. In fact, for individual patients, the clinical conditions known to be associated with refractoriness may or may not do so, and the significance of each condition cannot be predicted a priori.[27]

Patients can be refractory to platelet transfusion for any one or more of a variety of unrelated reasons, and alloimmunization is but one aspect of the problem. The distinction between refractoriness and alloimmunization is important because, unlike refractoriness based on a clinical condition, true alloimmunization can often be circumvented by the appropriate selection of platelet concentrates.[27,28] For example, platelet crossmatching is of benefit only when antibody-mediated clearance is the cause of the refractoriness; it does not help in circumventing alloimmunization when refractoriness is due to a clinical condition. Indeed, the effective management of clinically important refractoriness requires identification of the significant causative etiologic factors in each patient.[27] Causes can be multiple and cannot be considered mutually exclusive. Platelet refractoriness might be less of a problem if platelets were transfused only when clinically necessary instead of for prophylaxis based on oft-stated but poorly justified numerical criteria.[14,15,17] Of 13 recent studies of platelet refractoriness that specifically mentioned a threshold for prophylactic platelet transfusion, only two[21,29] used $10,000/\mu L$, one[30] used $10,000\text{-}20,000/\mu L$, one[31] used $15,000\text{-}20,000/\mu L$, and nine[32-40] used platelet transfusion triggers equal to or greater than $20,000/\mu L$. Heddle and Blajchman note that "there have not been any formal studies that validate the correlation of bleeding with either platelet refractoriness to allogeneic platelet transfusions or the presence of HLA-alloantibodies in a patient's serum."[41] Many stable oncology patients maintain platelet counts below $20,000/\mu L$ without either significant bleeding or adequate posttransfusion increments.[15,20,21,23] If these patients do not need to be transfused with platelets, the problem of refractoriness for them may be moot. Indeed, given that a majority of platelet concentrates is transfused for prophylaxis, a large part of the platelet refractoriness problem may be an attempt to treat a number rather than a clinical condition.[42,43] Platelet transfusion therapy is discussed in detail in Chapter 4.

Fresh Frozen Plasma

For major-mismatched ABO-incompatible transplantation, plasma components should be of the donor ABO group. Inventory concerns may necessitate the transfusion of ABO-incompatible plasma products (and platelet concentrates), which may not necessarily lead to acute complications; nevertheless, plasma compatibility should be maintained whenever possible. For minor-mismatched ABO-incompatible transplantation, plasma components should be of the recipient ABO group until original recipient red cells are no longer detectable. For both major- and minor-mismatched ABO-incompatible transplantation, plasma components should be group AB (ie, no A or B antibody) until recipient red cells are no longer detectable. Again, inventory concerns may necessitate the transfusion of ABO-incompatible plasma products containing undesired isohemagglutinins, but plasma compatibility should be maintained if at all reasonably possible. Detailed indications for FFP transfusion are discussed in chapters 7 and 8 and elsewhere.[44,45] According to the National Institutes of Health consensus conference on FFP, "There is no justification for the use of FFP as a volume expander or as a nutritional source."[45] CMV is not known to be transmissible by FFP, and CMV serostatus of the component is not taken into account when this product is transfused.

Modifications to Blood Components

CMV-Reduced-Risk Cellular Components

Transplantation patients are vulnerable to CMV primarily because of the immunosuppressive treatment regimens used to improve allograft survival. CMV-seronegative recipients who become infected with CMV while immunocompromised are at the greatest risk of developing the disease. CMV infection can be primary, a superinfection with a second strain, or a reactivation of latent disease. The virus can be acquired either from the community or iatrogenically from blood products or the allograft itself. Stem cell transplant recipients are at particular risk because of their profound immunosuppression and the fact that the leukocytes that harbor the virus are themselves part and parcel of the transplantation. Although the donor and recipient may not be restricted on the basis of CMV serostatus, the blood products transfused to support the recipient can be specifically selected, when appropriate, to minimize CMV transmission. Those stem cell transplantation patients who are at significant risk of acquiring transfusion-transmitted CMV should receive blood products that carry a reduced risk of CMV.

The relative risk for CMV among transplantation patients is stratified according to the serostatus of the donor and recipient. Seronegative recipients of seronegative transplants are at significant risk of transfusion-transmitted CMV infection because of the combination of severe immunocompromise along with the lack of protective CMV antibodies. On the other hand, seropositive recipients of seropositive transplants are not necessarily at significant risk of transfusion-transmitted CMV infection as these patients may be expected to have CMV antibody both before and after the transplantation. Superinfection has been reported from allografts but not from blood products. Seronegative recipients of seropositive transplants inherently receive a transplantation product that may carry the CMV virion but also receive the lymphocytes capable of producing protective IgG antibodies. Therefore, these patients are at greatest risk *prior to* the engraftment of donor lymphocytes and the consequent production of CMV antibody. On the other hand, seropositive recipients of seronegative transplants are at the greatest risk of CMV infection at any time after myeloablation because they harbor the virus yet lose the controlling antibody. A 1997 American Association of Blood Banks (AABB) Ad Hoc Committee on Prevention of CMV Transmission concluded in an Association Bulletin that CMV-seronegative patients who receive allogeneic hematopoietic stem cell transplantation should receive CMV-reduced-risk blood products, regardless of the donors' serostatus.[46] The Committee also recommended that CMV-seronegative patients undergoing autologous hematopoietic stem cell transplantation should receive CMV-reduced-risk cellular blood components.[46]

The definition of CMV-reduced-risk components is in an evolutionary state.[47-49] Traditionally, CMV-seronegative products have been provided for this purpose. With CMV seroprevalence ranging from 50 to 85% across the United States, many areas cannot supply sufficient seronegative products to meet the demand. Also, seronegative products can theoretically transmit CMV as a result of false-negative screening results, subdetectable antibody titers, transient viremia in seropositive patients quenching detectable antibody, and window-period infections. Untested or seropositive products with fewer than 5×10^6 WBCs, including frozen-deglycerolized RBCs and acellular products such as FFP and cryoprecipitate AHF, are considered to pose a reduced risk of CMV because the CMV virion is known to be highly associated with WBCs.[49-52] RBCs and platelet concentrates, however, must be adequately leukocyte reduced. Leukocyte reduction technology has been steadily improving with controlled filtration through specifically designed filters. More recently, platelet collection systems modified to minimize leukocyte content at collection have become available and provide CMV-reduced-risk apheresis concentrates. If, however, all cellular blood products transfused to stem cell transplantation recipients are adequately leukocyte reduced, the issue of using only seronegative products for at-risk patients becomes irrelevant. The AABB Bulletin concludes that either leukocyte-reduced or CMV-seronegative RBCs and platelet concentrates may be used as CMV-reduced-risk components.[47] Reduced-risk CMV blood components are discussed in greater detail in Chapter 16.

Leukocyte Reduction

Leukocyte reduction to remove most of the WBCs in RBCs and platelets can be performed by a number of methods. Older methods such as hydroxyethyl starch sedimentation, inverted differential centrifugation, and saline washing achieved 80-90% leukocyte reduction, with approximately 5-20% red cell loss in time-consuming, open-system processes. More recent methods use filtration over polyester fibers chemically coated to increase the specificity of leukocyte adsorption and trapping.[53-57] Currently available filters remove approximately 4 logs (99.99%) of leukocytes. The enumeration of residual leukocytes requires specialized techniques.[58]

Leukocyte reduction is intended to minimize conditions mediated at least in part by cotransfused WBCs, including HLA alloimmunization, febrile transfusion reactions, some transfusion-transmissible viral and bacterial diseases (eg, CMV, human T-cell lymphotropic virus I and II, *Yersinia enterocolitica*), and transfusion-associated immunomodulation.[26,34,36,41,50,52,53,59-71] However, typical leukocyte reduction techniques are not reliable or efficient enough yet to prevent transfusion-associated GVHD. More recent arguments center on the relative value of the timing of leukocyte reduction: at collection (prestorage), in the laboratory, or at the bedside (poststorage).[62,72-77] At present, to prevent alloimmunization, the timing of leukocyte reduction has not been proved to be significant. However, fewer febrile reactions are observed with prestorage leukocyte reduction because this prevents cytokines from accumulating during storage.

Overall, the literature is not definitive yet regarding the cost-benefit analysis of universal leukocyte reduction. Controlled studies are inconclusive or subject to numerous confounding issues. For example, most efficacy studies evaluating the role of leukocyte reduction for preventing alloimmunization vary markedly in both the breadth and depth of confounding factors: 1) definitions of alloimmunization, refractoriness, and leukocyte reduction; 2) quality control of leukocyte-reduced products, including counting methods and timing concerns; and 3) consistency of evaluation for significant clinical and historical factors such as disease, treatment regimen, previous transfusions, or pregnancy.[36,41,43] These inherent difficulties in evaluating potential studies may partly explain the broad range of published conclusions. More recent studies, such as the large-scale Trial to Reduce Alloimmunization to Platelets (TRAP), have more clearly established the value of leukocyte reduction (and ultraviolet [UV] irradiation) in the prevention of alloimmunization.[26] The TRAP study demonstrated that both leukocyte reduction by filtration and UV-B irradiation were equally effective in prevening alloantibody-mediated refractoriness to platelet transfusion during chemotherapy for acute myeloid leukemia. Nevertheless, lymphocytotoxic antibody did develop in 19% of the 36 patients with no prior alloantigen exposure who received treated transfusions in accord with all study guidelines. Thus, leukocyte reduction is not a foolproof method of preventing alloimmunization. The overall conclusion from the published literature is that it does reduce the primary development of Class I HLA alloantibodies but has no proven role in limiting anamnestic responses or nonalloimmune refractoriness. The literature regarding transfusion-associated immunomodulation is even more diverse.[72] Nonetheless, the apparent benefits of leukocyte reduction warrant its routine use among aggressively transfused patients, including all stem cell transplantation recipients, in whom HLA alloimmunization would result in significant complications. To be fully effective, however, leukocyte reduction must be used throughout the preparative, myeloablation, and maintenance regimens. Leukocyte reduction is discussed in greater detail in chapter 16.

Gamma Irradiation

Generally, the indications for gamma irradiation are limited to both immunocompromised and non-immunocompromised patients who are receiving cellular components (RBCs, Whole Blood, granulocyte concentrates, platelet concentrates, and fresh plasma) and are at risk for transfusion-associated GVHD.[78-82] The required central dose of 2500 cGy inhibits lymphocyte proliferation, thereby preventing transfusion-associated GVHD.[83] Gamma irradiation induces cellular damage via the formation of hydroxyl and/or superoxide radicals, typically from radiolysis of water. These free radicals lead to tertiary structural changes, such as polymerization of long-chain fatty acids, disruption of peptide bonds, and generation of the disulfide bridge linking juxtaposed thiol groups. Gamma irradiation does not reduce immunogenicity, presumably because it has no effect on the expression of the costimulatory signal (cf, UV irradiation). At typical doses, granulocytes retain normal antibacterial and

chemotactic functions while red cells suffer reversible membrane damage. Leukocyte antigens, other cellular antigens, and passenger viruses remain largely unaffected, and reactions against these antigens are not diminished. Gamma irradiation is discussed in greater detail in Chapter 17.

The question of gamma irradiation to prevent lymphocyte engraftment is slightly different for the stem cell transplantation recipient than for the routine oncology patient. Passenger lymphocytes in randomly selected blood products can engraft and proliferate just as readily in myeloablated recipients as can the specifically selected stem-cell–enriched products. In patients who have not yet undergone myeloablation, transfused lymphocytes may transiently engraft just as they do in other patients. Lymphocytes that do engraft should be cleared by the myeloablative therapy. The crucial difference is that any transient engraftment of lymphocytes prior to stem cell collection may be protected ex vivo from postcollection myeloablation. Therefore, independent of the criteria for gamma irradiation for oncology patients, blood products that may leave lymphocytes circulating at the time of a future stem cell collection should be gamma irradiated prior to transfusion. Thus, it is prudent to irradiate cellular blood components for any patient who is anticipated to undergo a stem cell collection.

Ultraviolet Irradiation

UV involves wavelengths from 200 to 400 nm. UV-A (320-400 nm) has the greatest transmission through standard blood bag plastics and biologic effects predominantly limited to the concurrent presence of photosensitizing agents. UV-A is used to crosslink DNA in conjunction with psoralen derivatives (eg, 8-methoxypsoralen) in therapies such as PUVA (psoralen plus UV-A) or photopheresis. UV-B (280-320 nm) appears to induce the loss or inactivation of HLA Class II antigen expression on lymphocytes and may also induce the loss of ICAM-1 from antigen-presenting cells.[84] UV-B appears to prevent transfusion-associated GVHD and alloimmunization and may be useful for purging marrow of alloreactive T lymphocytes prior to transplantation. UV-C (200-280 nm) has the greatest biologic activity of the UV spectrum but is highly toxic, even at relatively low energies.

The use of UV irradiation to prevent transfusion-associated GVHD and alloimmunization is still experimental, and data are still variable.[85-90] Confounding the efficacy question are the formidable practical and technical problems that remain because plasma, hemoglobin, and plastic absorb UV photons, which results in a photon path length through standard blood products of only a few millimeters. Animals transfused with UV-irradiated blood have lower rates of alloimmunization, yet still can mount normal immune responses to microbial antigens.[91] More recent studies, such as the large-scale TRAP, have supported the value of UV irradiation (and leukocyte reduction) in the prevention of alloimmunization.[26]

Volume Reduction

Volume reduction is accomplished by centrifugation to concentrate cellular components and is indicated only for patients who are extremely sensitive to volume overload. RBCs without additive solutions (eg, CPD or CPDA-1) are relatively concentrated already (hematocrit of 75-80%). The volume reduction of platelet concentrates by centrifugation inherently results in some platelet activation and in the concomitant loss of storage-induced platelet-derived procoagulant microparticles as well as of whole platelets. Also, the actual quantity of platelets in a unit can vary by a factor of two. The value of additional concentration must be weighed against selecting a smaller or more concentrated unit.

Washed Products

Washing cellular products removes plasma proteins, antibodies, and electrolytes. In addition, most WBCs (~90%) and platelets (20-90%) are cleared from washed RBCs, depending on the centrifugation speed and the number of washes. Washing platelets does not remove leukocytes because only constituents lighter than what is retained are removed. The indications for washed products in

the general population are generally limited to s[...] vere allergic responses to infused plasma not co[...] trollable with antihistamines. In the stem ce[...] transplantation population, however, washe[...] products are used most commonly during the pe[...] transplantation phase when the RBC products ar[...] plasma products desired are not of the same bloc[...] group. For example, a group O recipient of a grou[...] A stem cell product will need to be supported wi[...] group O cells washed free of anti-A and group A [...] AB plasma products (see tables). Washed produc[...] have traditionally been required for patients wi[...] paroxysmal nocturnal hemoglobinuria, but eve[...] this has been questioned.[92] Washing platelet conce[...] trates may also significantly affect the quality of t[...] remaining platelets, as well as lead to the loss of pr[...] coagulant microparticles.[93] If necessary, washin[...] should be done with an ACD-saline solution [...] Washing platelet concentrates prior to filtration m[...] result in an extreme reduction in platelet quantity.[...] platelets must be washed and leukocyte-reduced, [...] is preferable to filter before washing. Filtration aft[...] washing has resulted in platelet yields as low as 12[...] of the initial count.[95]

Conclusion

Clinicians caring for patients who are undergoin[...] hematopoietic stem cell transplantation must [...] mindful of many transfusion-related issues. T[...] fact that many patients change blood groups rais[...] particular challenges for the blood bank and clir[...] cal team. The ability to provide blood componen[...] with significantly reduced risk for alloimmuniz[...] tion, CMV transmission, transfusion reactions, ar[...] GVHD has afforded opportunities for improved p[...] tient care.

References

1. McCullough J. The role of the blood bank [...] transplantation. Arch Pathol Lab Med 199[...] 115:1195-200.
2. Anderson KC. The role of the blood bank [...] hematopoietic stem cell transplantatio[...] Transfusion 1992;32:272-85.

3. Lenarsky C. Immune recovery after bone marrow transplantation. Curr Opin Hematol 1995;2:409-12.

4. Gale RP, Butturini A. Transplants of blood-derived hematopoietic cells. Bone Marrow Transplant 1990;5(Suppl 1):2-4.

5. Lasky LC, Warkentin PI, Kersey JH, et al. Hemotherapy in patients undergoing blood group incompatible bone marrow transplantation. Transfusion 1983;23:277-85.

6. Ramsey G, Nusbacher J, Starzl TE, Lindsay GD. Isohemagglutinins of graft origin after ABO-unmatched liver transplantation. N Engl J Med 1984;311:1167-70.

7. Heim MU, Schleuning M, Eckstein R, et al. Rh antibodies against the pretransplant red cells following incompatible bone marrow transplantation. Transfusion 1988;28:272-5.

8. Heim MU, Bock M, Kolb HJ, et al. Intravenous anti-D gammaglobulin for the prevention of rhesus isoimmunization caused by platelet transfusions in patients with malignant diseases. Vox Sang 1992;62:165-8.

9. Welch HG, Meehan KR, Goodnough LT. Prudent strategies for elective red blood cell transfusion. Ann Intern Med 1992;116:393-402.

10. National Institutes of Health Consensus Conference. Perioperative red cell transfusion. JAMA 1988;260:2700-3.

11. Kim DM, Brecher ME, Estes TJ, Morrey BF. Relationship of hemoglobin level and duration of hospitalization after total hip arthroplasty: Implications for the transfusion target. Mayo Clin Proc 1993;68:37-41.

12. Baer MR, Bloomfield CD. Controversies in transfusion medicine. Prophylactic platelet transfusion therapy: Pro. Transfusion 1992;32:377-80.

13. Schiffer CA. Prophylactic platelet transfusion. Transfusion 1992;32:295-8.

14. Patten E. Controversies in transfusion medicine. Prophylactic platelet transfusion revisited after 25 years: Con. Transfusion 1992;32:381-5.

15. Gmur J, Burger J, Schanz U, et al. Safety of stringent prophylactic platelet transfusion policy for patients with acute leukemia. Lancet 1991;338:1223-6.

16. Belt RJ, Leite C, Haas CD, Stephens RL. Incidence of hemorrhagic complications in patients with cancer. JAMA 1978;239:2571-4.

17. Beutler E. Platelet transfusions: The 20,000/µL trigger. Blood 1993;81:1411-3.

18. National Institutes of Health Consensus Conference. Platelet transfusion therapy. JAMA 1987;257:1777-80.

19. Morrow JF, Braine HG, Kickler TS, et al. Septic reactions to platelet transfusions. JAMA 1991;266:555-8.

20. Solomon J, Bofenkamp T, Fahey JL, et al. Platelet prophylaxis in acute non-lymphoblastic leukemia (letter). Lancet 1978;1:267.

21. Rebulla P, Finazzi G, Marangoni F, et al. The threshold for prophylactic platelet transfusions in adults with acute myeloid leukemia. N Engl J Med 1997;337:1870-5.

22. Kruskall MS. The perils of platelet transfusion (editorial). N Engl J Med 1997;337:1914-5.

23. Del Rosario MLU, Kao KJ. Determination of the rate of reduction in platelet counts in recipients of hematopoietic stem and progenitor cell transplant: Clinical implications for platelet transfusion therapy. Transfusion 1997;37:1163-8.

24. McLeod BC, Piehl MR, Sassetti RJ. Alloimmunization to RhD by platelet transfusions in autologous bone marrow transplant recipients. Vox Sang 1990;59:185-9.

25. Friedberg RC. Clinical and laboratory factors underlying refractoriness to platelet transfusions. J Clin Apheresis 1996;11:143-8.

26. Trial to Reduce Alloimmunization to Platelets Study Group. Leukocyte reduction and ultraviolet B irradiation of platelets to prevent alloimmunization and refractoriness to platelet transfusions. N Engl J Med 1997;337:1861-9.

27. Friedberg RC, Donnelly SF, Boyd JC, et al. Clinical and blood bank factors in the management of platelet refractoriness and alloimmunization. Blood 1993;81:3428-34.

28. Friedberg RC, Donnelly SF, Mintz PD. Independent roles for platelet crossmatching and HLA in the selection of platelets for alloimmunized patients. Transfusion 1994;34:215-20.

29. Novotny VMJ, van Doorn R, Witvliet MD, et al. Occurrence of allogeneic HLA and non-HLA antibodies after transfusion of prestorage filtered platelets and red blood cells: A prospective study. Blood 1995;85:1736-41.

30. Sintnicolaas K, van Marwijk Kooy M, van Prooijen HC, et al. Leukocyte depletion of random single-donor platelet transfusions does not prevent secondary human leukocyte antigen-alloimmunization and refractoriness: A randomized prospective study. Blood 1995;85:824-8.

31. Klingemann HG, Self S, Banaji M, et al. Refractoriness to random donor platelet transfusions in patients with aplastic anaemia: A multivariate analysis of data from 264 cases. Br J Haematol 1987;66:115-21.

32. Bishop JF, McGrath KM, Wolf MM, et al. Clinical factors influencing the efficacy of pooled platelet transfusions. Blood 1988;71:383-7.

33. Oksanen K, Kekomaki R, Ruutu T, et al. Prevention of alloimmunization in patients with acute leukemia by use of white cell-reduced blood components—a randomized trial. Transfusion 1991;31:588-94.

34. van Marwijk Kooy M, van Prooijen HC, Moes M, et al. Use of leukocyte-depleted platelet concentrates for the prevention of refractoriness and primary HLA alloimmunization: A prospective, randomized trial. Blood 1991;77:201-5.

35. Sniecinski I, O'Donnell MR, Nowicki B, Hill LR. Prevention of refractoriness and HLA-alloimmunization using filtered blood products. Blood 1988;71:1402-17.

36. Andreu G, Dewailly J, Leberre C, et al. Prevention of HLA immunization with leukocyte-poor packed red cells and platelet concentrates prepared by filtration. Blood 1988;72:964-9.

37. Williamson LM, Wimperis JZ, Williamson P, et al. Bedside filtration of blood products in the prevention of HLA alloimmunization—a prospective randomized study. Blood 1994;83:3028-35.

38. Doughty DA, Murphy MF, Metcalfe P, et al. Relative importance of immune and non-immune causes of platelet refractoriness. Vox Sang 1994;66:200-5.

39. Oksanen K. Leukocyte-depleted blood components prevent platelet refractoriness in patients with acute myeloid leukemia. Eur J Haematol 1994;53:100-7.

40. Bishop JF, Matthews JP, McGrath K, et al. Factors influencing 20-hour increments after platelet transfusion. Transfusion 1991;31:392-6.

41. Heddle NM, Blajchman MA. The leukodepletion of cellular blood products in the prevention of HLA-alloimmunization and refractoriness to allogeneic platelet transfusions. Blood 1995;85:603-6.

42. Pisciotto PT, Benson K, Hume H, et al. Prophylactic versus therapeutic platelet transfusion practices in hematology and/or oncology patients. Transfusion 1995;35:498-502.

43. Friedberg RC, Mintz PD. Causes of refractoriness to platelet transfusion. Curr Opin Hematol 1995;2:193-8.

44. Braunstein AH, Oberman HA. Transfusion of plasma components. Transfusion 1984;24:281-6.

45. National Institutes of Health Consensus Conference. Fresh frozen plasma. Indications and risks. JAMA 1985;253:551-3.

46. Leukocyte reduction for the prevention of transfusion-transmitted cytomegalovirus (TT-CMV). Association Bulletin 97-2. Bethesda, MD: American Association of Blood Banks Bulletin, 1997.

47. Miller WJ, McCullough JJ, Balfour HH, et al. Prevention of cytomegalovirus infection following bone marrow transplantation: A randomized trial of blood product screening. Bone Marrow Transplant 1991;7:227-34.

48. Hillyer CD, Emmens RK, Zago-Novaretti M, Berkman EM. Methods for the reduction of transfusion-transmitted cytomegalovirus infection: Filtration versus the use of seronega-

tive donor units. Transfusion 1994;34:929-34.

49. Przepiorka D, Leparc GF, Werch J, Lichtiger B. Prevention of transfusion-associated cytomegalovirus infection. Practice parameter. AJCP 1996;106:163-9.

50. De Witte T, Schattenberg A, Van Dijk BA, et al. Prevention of primary cytomegalovirus infection after allogeneic bone marrow transplantation by using leukocyte-poor random blood products from cytomegalovirus-unscreened blood-bank donors. Transplantation 1990;50:964-8.

51. Bowden RA, Slichter SJ, Ayers M, et al. A comparison of filtered leukocyte-reduced and cytomegalovirus (CMV) seronegative blood products for the prevention of transfusion-associated CMV infection after marrow transplant. Blood 1995;86:3598-603.

52. van Prooijen HC, Visser JJ, van Oostendorp WR, et al. Prevention of primary transfusion-associated cytomegalovirus infection in bone marrow transplant recipients by the removal of white cells from blood components with high-affinity filters. Br J Haematol 1994;87:144-7.

53. Lichtiger B, Leparc GF. Leukocyte-poor blood components: Issues and indications. Crit Rev Clin Lab Sci 1991;28:387-403.

54. Steneker I, Biewenga J. Histologic and immunohistochemical studies on the preparation of white cell-poor red cell concentrates: The filtration process using three different polyester filters. Transfusion 1991;31:40-6.

55. Kickler TS, Bell W, Drew H, Pall D. Depletion of white cells from platelet concentrates with a new adsorption filter. Transfusion 1989;29:411-4.

56. Ciavarella D, Snyder EL. Clinical use of blood transfusion devices. Transfus Med Rev 1988;2:95-111.

57. Steneker I, Prins HK, Florie M, et al. Mechanisms of white cell reduction in red cell concentrates by filtration: The effect of the cellular composition of the red cell concentrates. Transfusion 1993;33:42-50.

58. Rawal BD, Schwadron R, Busch MP, et al. Evaluation of leukocyte removal filters modeled by use of HIV-infected cells and DNA amplification. Blood 1990;76:2159-61.

59. Lane TA, Anderson KC, Goodnough LT, et al. Leukocyte reduction in blood component therapy. Ann Intern Med 1992;117:151-62.

60. Kim DM, Brecher ME, Bland LA, et al. Prestorage removal of Yersinia enterocolitica from red cells with white cell-reduction filters. Transfusion 1992;32:658-62.

61. Andreu G. Role of leukocyte depletion in the prevention of transfusion- induced cytomegalovirus infection. Semin Hematol 1991;28:26-31.

62. Andreu G. Early leukocyte depletion of cellular blood components reduces red blood cell and platelet storage lesions. Semin Hematol 1991;28:22-5.

63. Meryman HT. Transfusion-induced alloimmunization and immunosuppression and the effects of leukocyte depletion. Transfus Med Rev 1989;3:180-93.

64. Bowden RA, Slichter SJ, Sayers MH, et al. Use of leukocyte-depleted platelets and cytomegalovirus-seronegative red blood cells for prevention of primary cytomegalovirus infection after marrow transplant. Blood 1991;78:246-50.

65. Sirchia G, Rebulla P, Mascaretti L, et al. The clinical importance of leukocyte depletion in regular erythrocyte transfusions. Vox Sang 1986;51(Suppl 1):2-8.

66. Rebulla P, Bertolini F, Parravicini A, Sirchia G. Leukocyte-poor blood components: A purer and safer transfusion product for recipients? Transfus Med Rev 1991;4:19-23.

67. Wenz B. Clinical and laboratory precautions that reduce the adverse reactions, alloimmunization, infectivity, and possible immunomodulation associated with homologous transfusions. Transfus Med Rev 1990;4:3-7.

68. Oksanen K, Elonen E, Finnish Leukemia Group. Impact of leucocyte-depleted blood components on the haematological recovery

and prognosis of patients with acute myeloid leukemia. Br J Haematol 1993;84:639-47.

69. Heddle NM. The efficacy of leukodepletion to improve platelet transfusion response: A critical appraisal of clinical studies. Transfus Med Rev 1994;8:15-28.

70. Shimizu T, Uchigiri C, Mizuno S, et al. Adsorption of anaphylatoxins and platelet-specific proteins by filtration of platelet concentrates with a polyester leukocyte reduction filter. Vox Sang 1994;66:161-5.

71. Blumberg N, Heal JM. Immunomodulation by blood transfusion: An evolving scientific and clinical challenge. Am J Med 1996;101:299-308.

72. Wenz B, Ciavarella D, Freundlich L. Effect of prestorage white cell reduction on bacterial growth in platelet concentrates. Transfusion 1993;33:520-3.

73. Blajchman MA, Bardossy L, Carmen RA, et al. An animal model of allogeneic donor platelet refractoriness: The effect of the time of leukodepletion. Blood 1992;79:1371-5.

74. Brecher ME, Pineda AA, Torloni AS, et al. Prestorage leukocyte depletion: Effect on leukocyte and platelet metabolites, erythrocyte lysis, metabolism, and in vivo survival. Semin Hematol 1991;28:3-9.

75. Humbert JR, Fermin CD, Winsor EL. Early damage to granulocytes during storage. Semin Hematol 1991;28:10-3.

76. Heal JM, Cohen HJ. Do white cells in stored blood components reduce the likelihood of posttransfusion bacterial sepsis? Transfusion 1991;31:581-3.

77. Popovsky MA. Quality of blood components filtered before storage and at the bedside: Implications for transfusion practice. Transfusion 1996;36:470-4.

78. Leitman SF, Holland PV. Irradiation of blood products. Indications and guidelines. Transfusion 1985;25:293-300.

79. Linden JV, Pisciotto PT. Transfusion-associated graft-versus-host disease and blood irradiation. Transfus Med Rev 1992;6:116-23.

80. Greenbaum BH. Transfusion-associated graft-versus-host disease: Historical perspec-

tives, incidence, and current use of irradiated blood products. J Clin Oncol 1991;9:1889-902.

81. Pritchard SL, Rogers PCJ. Rationale and recommendations for the irradiation of blood products. Crit Rev Oncol Hematol 1987;7:115-24.

82. Prdzepiorka D, Leparc GF, Stovall MA, et al. Use of irradiated blood components. Practice parameter. Am J Clin Pathol 1996;106:6-11.

83. Moroff G, Leitman SF, Luban NLC. Principles of blood irradiation, dose validation, and quality control. Transfusion 1997;37:1084-92.

84. Deeg HJ, Sigaroudinia M. Ultraviolet B-induced loss of HLA Class II antigen expression on lymphocytes is dose, time, and locus dependent. Exp Hematol 1990;18:916-9.

85. Tandy NP, Pamphilon DH. Platelet transfusions irradiated with ultraviolet-B light may have a role in reducing recipient alloimmunization. Blood Coagul Fibrinolysis 1991;2:383-8.

86. Grana NH, Kao KJ. Use of 8-methoxypsoralen and ultraviolet-A pretreated platelet concentrates to prevent alloimmunization against Class I major histocompatibility antigens. Blood 1991;77:2530-7.

87. Lindahl-Kiessling K, Safwenberg J. Inability of UV-irradiated lymphocytes to stimulate allogeneic cells in mixed lymphocyte culture. Int Arch Allergy Immunol 1971;41:670-8.

88. Andreu G, Boccaccio C, Klaren J, et al. The role of UV radiation in the prevention of human leukocyte antigen alloimmunization. Transfus Med Rev 1992;6:212-24.

89. Grijzenhout MA, Aarts-Riemens MI, de Gruijl FR, et al. UVB irradiation of human platelet concentrates does not prevent HLA alloimmunization in recipients. Blood 1994;84:3524-31.

90. Blundell EL, Pamphilon DH, Menitove JE, et al. A prospective, randomized study of the use of platelet concentrates irradiated with ultraviolet-B light in patients with hematologic malignancy. Transfusion 1996;36:296-302.

91. Deeg HJ, Graham TC, Gerhard Miller L, et al. Prevention of transfusion-induced graft-

versus-host disease in dogs by ultraviolet irradiation. Blood 1989;74:2592-5.

92. Brecher ME, Taswell HF. Paroxysmal nocturnal hemoglobinuria and the transfusion of washed red cells. A myth revisited. Transfusion 1989;29:681-5.

93. Tans G, Rosing R, Christella M, et al. Comparison of anticoagulant and procoagulant activities of stimulated platelet and platelet-derived microparticles. Blood 1991;77:2641-8.

94. Pineda AA, Zylstra VW, Clare DE, et al. Viability and functional integrity of washed platelets. Transfusion 1989;29:524-7.

95. Bredehoeft SJ, Campbell ML. Impact of modification sequence on platelet yield in preparation of small volume platelet products (abstract). Transfusion 1993;33:6S.

In: Mintz PD, ed.
Transfusion Therapy: Clinical Principles and Practice
Bethesda, MD: AABB Press, 1999

13

Mononuclear Cell Transfusion: Immunotherapy Using Allogeneic Donor-Derived Lymphocytes

JONG-HOON LEE, MD, AND HARVEY G. KLEIN, MD

THE AVAILABILITY OF INCREAS-ingly sophisticated blood collection and storage systems has improved the ability to maintain adequate tissue oxygenation or to achieve hemostasis in patients requiring transfusion support. In addition to providing these critical supportive functions more effectively through red blood cell, platelet, and plasma transfusions, scientific and technical advances have provided the basis for preparing cell concentrates to be used clinically as a form of immunotherapy. Although the terms transfusion ther-apy and transfusion support have been used interchangeably in the past, transfusion medicine of the future will likely distinguish clearly between these terms. Lymphocyte transfusions may prove to be useful in the adoptive transfer of donor immunity (adoptive immunotherapy) to treat solid tumors, leukemia, human immunodeficiency virus (HIV) infection, and a variety of other immune-related disorders.

The therapeutic potential of lymphocytes remains an area of active investigation. Although clinical experience to date has not been extensive,

Jong-Hoon Lee, MD, Chief, Blood and Plasma Branch, Division of Blood Applications, Office of Blood Research and Review, Center for Biologics Evaluation and Research, Food and Drug Administration, Rockville, Maryland, and Harvey G. Klein, MD, Chief, Department of Transfusion Medicine, Warren G. Magnuson Clinical Center, National Institutes of Health, Bethesda, Maryland

The views of the authors represent scientific opinion and should not be construed as opinion or policy of the United States Food and Drug Administration or of the National Institutes of Health.

lymphocyte transfusion has been successful enough in treating chronic myelogenous leukemia (CML) recurring after an allogeneic hematopoietic transplantation to merit consideration as one of the standard clinical therapies for selected patients. In this clinical setting, the transfusion of allogeneic lymphocytes derived from the original hematopoietic progenitor cell donor—so-called donor- derived lymphocytes (DDLs)—may be considered investigational primarily from the standpoint of the number of cells and conditions of cell administration. Other considerations, while intriguing, should be confined to controlled, investigational protocols.

The Graft-vs-Leukemia Effect

Data from recent studies in animal models[1,2] have been consistent with the initial observation by Barnes and Loutit[3] in 1957 that transplanted marrow may have activity against residual leukemia. An analysis of the clinical marrow transplantation experience provides indirect evidence of an antileukemic activity in humans—now commonly referred to as the graft-vs-leukemia (GVL) effect—particularly in patients with CML, including: 1) leukemic relapse rates correlate inversely with rates of graft-vs-host disease (GVHD),[4-7] 2) leukemic relapse rates correlate with the degree of T-cell depletion in the hematopoietic graft,[5,8-11] and 3) spontaneous disease remission has been associated with flares of GVHD.[12-14] Furthermore, leukemias appear to recur more often after a syngeneic than after an allogeneic marrow transplant.[5] In 1990, Kolb et al[15] first provided direct clinical evidence for the GVL effect: the transfusion of DDLs in conjunction with the administration of interferon alpha (IFN-α) induced cytogenetic remission in three patients with CML in relapse following allogeneic marrow transplantation.

Donor-Derived Lymphocytes in Relapsed Chronic-Phase Chronic Myelogenous Leukemia

The initial clinical evidence for GVL activity has been confirmed through numerous independent studies.[16-25] The experiences of both the European Group for Blood and Marrow Transplantation, which involved 135 patients (75 evaluable with CML) at 27 transplant centers,[26] and the 25 North American marrow transplantation programs, which involved 140 patients (55 evaluable with CML),[27] are presented in Table 13-1. The studies collectively show that, in relapsed chronic-phase CML, the transfusion of allogeneic DDLs induces clinical remission at a rate approaching 80%, and molecular remission (ie, the inability to detect bcr-abl mRNA transcript using polymerase chain reaction) may be achieved in nearly all patients entering clinical remission.[26,27] In these early studies, infusion of small numbers of lymphocytes (10^7) usually sufficed, and cells collected by leukapheresis were often aliquoted and stored for repeated treatment. The host's circulation, which often contains a mixture of both donor and host cells during chronic-phase relapse, typically converts to cells of only donor origin, and the cells with the Philadelphia chromosome disappear. The time to remission ranges from 1 to 9 months, with an approximate mean of 3 months.[20,26,27] The efficacy of DDL transfusion therapy in relapsed chronic-phase CML appears durable: the probability of such a patient remaining in remission at 3 years after therapy approaches 90% (89.6% at 2 years[27] and 87% at 3 years[26]). Observation continues to determine the mean duration of remission.

Disease Activity and Response Rate

Among the many clinical variables analyzed thus far, a few are emerging as predictors of a positive outcome. As might be expected, a low level of disease activity and early intervention with DDLs (within 2 years of transplantation) may further improve the already impressive results observed in relapsed chronic-phase CML.[26-28] Response rates for a select group of patients receiving prompt DDL therapy after the early detection of relapse (cytogenetic or molecular) approach 100%. However, future clinical trials should define the overall clinical effectiveness of such an aggressive approach. Despite the anticipated high response rate, early DDL inter-

Table 13-1. The North American[27] and European[26] Experiences with Donor-Derived Lymphocyte Transfusion as Adoptive Immunotherapy of Leukemias in Relapse Following Allogeneic Marrow Transplantation

Relapsed Leukemia	No. of Patients			Remission Rate (%)		
	NA	E	NA&E	NA	E	NA&E
Chronic myelogenous leukemia in chronic-phase relapse	37	67	104	76	79	78
Chronic myelogenous leukemia in accelerated-phase relapse	18	8	26	28	13	23
Acute myelogenous leukemia	39	17	56	15	29	20
Acute lymphocytic leukemia	11	12	23	18	0	9

NA = North American experience; E = European experience.

The original marrow grafts (and subsequently, donor-derived lymphocytes) were harvested from related donors (typically from an HLA-identical sibling) in 92% of all patients (range=87% in ALL to 96% in AML, both in the North American experience).

vention may not be clinically justified if patients suffer substantial therapy-related morbidity and mortality, and if the natural history of nonhematologic relapse proves to be relatively mild and indolent.

Adverse Effects

The major adverse effects of DDL therapy are the clinical manifestations of transfusion-associated GVHD. The severity of GVHD seen in up to 80% of cases has been milder than might be expected, given the large number of allogeneic T cells transfused. The pattern of organ involvement is comparable to that seen after marrow transplantation. There is, however, a suggestion of less skin involvement, perhaps owing to the absence of a toxic conditioning regimen.[20,22-24,26] Myelosuppression, which occurs in as many as 50% of the patients (including those with transient isolated leukopenia), appears to result from insufficient donor-derived hematopoietic reserve or from the destruction of residual host hematopoiesis prior to donor engraftment. Myelosuppression has been reversed by transfusing additional donor-derived hemato-poietic progenitor cells without additional patient conditioning.[29,30] Transfusing these cells instead of DDLs from the outset, however, may not prevent myelosuppression,[31] possibly because the lymphocytes typically transfused several weeks prior to the progenitor cell support serve as a cellular form of a necessary conditioning regimen.

In the post-marrow transplantation setting, transfusion-associated GVHD appears to be a less fearful consequence of allogeneic lymphocytes than in the conventional transfusion setting, because donor-derived hematopoietic progenitor cells are often available to initiate marrow rescue. Nevertheless, GVHD, including marrow aplasia, accounts for much of the mortality seen in approximately one-fourth of the patients receiving DDLs.[16-24,26,27]

Separating Graft-vs-Leukemia Effect From Graft-vs-Host Disease

As might be expected from the early reports about the GVL effect, GVHD occurring after DDL transfusion correlates highly with antileukemic response.[26,27] Studies at the molecular, cellular, and clinical levels, however, suggest that the GVL effect and GVHD may be overlapping but distinct, clinically separable phenomena.[30-41] As the recognized mediators and effectors of GVHD, T cells and T-cell subsets have already received much investigative attention. Selective CD8 T-cell depletion appears to be more effective than pan-T-cell depletion in preserving the GVL effect.[8,10,17,32,33,39,42]

In a study reported in 1995, Pan et al[43] also demonstrated that, at least in the murine model, the peripheral circulation may be enriched in type 2 helper T cells through the administration of granulocyte colony-stimulating factor (G-CSF). If applicable to humans, the enrichment of type 2 helper T cells in the peripheral circulation as a result of G-CSF mobilization at least partially explains the relatively mild and less frequent occurrence of GVHD when peripheral blood cells rather than marrow progenitor cells are used to effect hematopoietic reconstitution. The possible applicability to humans suggests the targeting of CD4 T-cell subsets through donor G-CSF stimulation to minimize GVHD without compromising the antileukemic effect of DDLs.

In addition to T cells and T-cell subsets, natural killer (NK) cells may also prove important in the pathophysiology of the GVL effect.[19,35-40,44-48] NK cells cultured in interleukin-2 (IL-2) for 1 week develop cytolytic activity against acute myelogenous leukemia (AML) blasts. The major histocompatibility complex (MHC) nonrestricted T cells derived from the same NK cell donor, however, were ineffective under equivalent conditions. Against normal marrow progenitor cells, the IL-2-activated NK cells showed little cytolytic activity, whereas the T cells were effective in cell lysis and the inhibition of colony formation.

The congenital absence (or depletion) of NK cells in animal models increases the susceptibility to leukemias, which may be reversed by activating or adoptively transferring NK cells.[44-46] Clinical observations are consistent with these findings; subjects with defective NK cell function or low NK cell activity appear to be more susceptible to cancer, particularly to hematologic malignancies.[47] Although IL-2 increases the number of circulating NK cells and may be effective in the treatment of leukemias,[48] cytokine toxicity[49,50] and the concern for acutely exacerbating GVHD after allogeneic marrow transplantation[48,51] have limited its use in conjunction with DDLs. IL-2, however, may prove to be an important tool in separating the GVL effect from GVHD. Its use as a low-dose continuous infusion in conjunction with T-cell depletion has been suggested to be effective in controlling GVHD while retaining the GVL effect.[32,52,53]

Adjunctive Interferon-α and Cell Dose

As reported in the studies to date, patients who received IFN-α in addition to DDLs showed no higher response rate than patients treated with DDL transfusion alone. Despite the anticipated antiproliferative effect on leukemic cells, the upregulation of histocompatibility molecules, and the consequent enhancement of cell-mediated immunity, the coadministration of IFN-α appears not to augment significantly the GVL effect delivered by DDLs.[26,27] As with the adjunctive use of IFN-α, the lymphocyte dose does not correlate with the antileukemic response: nucleated cell doses that differ by more than 30-fold (0.34 to 12.3×10^8 cells/kg) appear to be equally effective.[15-24] Prospective, controlled, randomized clinical trials are necessary to better define the role of adjunctive IFN-α and the dose of lymphocytes for a given patient. Although clinically well justified and apparently logical, the practice of reserving adjunctive IFN-α and larger cell doses for patients with more advanced disease introduces a significant subject selection bias into an uncontrolled trial.

The wide range of response times (1-9 months) after DDL transfusion therapy complicates the recognition of clinically significant variables that affect the separation of GVL effect from GVHD. The selective depletion of T-cell subsets,[32,39] the adjunctive use of cytokines including IFN-α and IL-2,[21,23] the alteration of the cell dose and the transfusion schedule,[22,54] and the manipulation of DDLs to control the cell life span after transfusion[55,56] all continue to receive clinical attention in the attempt to separate the GVL effect from GVHD.

Cytokines have not been administered to a donor in a deliberate attempt to control the cell composition of DDLs. Donor cytokine stimulation before cell collection may complement subsequent laboratory cell processing of the collected DDLs in efforts to optimize the safety and efficacy of the DDL component. In transplantation using circulating hematopoietic progenitor cells (HPCs), donor cytokine stimulation to mobilize progenitors from the marrow compartment into the peripheral circulation has been essential to collecting an effective progenitor cell component.[57] As with donor cytokine stimulation, the potential to increase the specificity and cytotoxicity of DDLs against tumor cells by culturing them in the presence of recipient-derived leukemic cells in vitro has not been explored extensively to date. Given the diversity of tumor antigens and the broad range in immunogenicity, a patient-specific approach to the preparation of DDLs (tumor-activated DDLs) may prove effective in separating the antileukemic activity from GVHD. The use of tumor-activated lymphocytes has enhanced the effectiveness of adoptive immunotherapy in solid cancers, particularly in advanced melanomas (see tumor-infiltrating lymphocytes [TILs] below).[49,58-60]

The Experience in Epstein-Barr Virus-Related Lymphoproliferative Disorders

The clinical experience with Epstein-Barr virus-related lymphoproliferative disorders (EBV-LPDs) occurring after marrow transplantation illustrates the potential to separate the GVL effect from GVHD, even if the two phenomena result from inseparable pathogenetic mechanisms. This experience further suggests the possibility of controlling other viral complications associated with marrow transplantation. The incidence of EBV-LPD occurring in T-cell-depleted allogeneic marrow transplant recipients has been estimated to be 6-12%[61] and may prove higher with accumulating clinical experience.[62] The secondary lymphomas occurring in this clinical setting respond readily to the transfusion of DDLs at a dose approximately 1 log lower than that typically used for activity against the primary leukemic disease. In the limited number of studies to date, sustained clinical remissions have been achieved with only mild GVHD, and patients have often required no additional maintenance therapy.[61,63,64]

In 1997, Bonini et al[55] described a complex but powerful strategy involving the genetic modification of DDLs to separate the GVL effect from GVHD; it entails taking advantage of the different clinical time courses associated with the GVL effect and GVHD. In a patient with an aggressive EBV-induced B-cell lymphoma of donor origin as a complication of T-cell-depleted, HLA-identical sibling marrow transplantation, the transfusion of DDLs (1.5×10^6 lymphocytes/kg) transduced with a construct containing the thymidine kinase gene resulted in a prompt remission of the disease within 2 weeks. A marker gene allowed the circulating donor cells to be tracked as they increased to 13.4% of the total circulating mononuclear cells (MNCs). The patient's acute GVHD occurring at 4 weeks (2 weeks after complete remission was achieved) responded dramatically to the intravenous administration of ganciclovir (two doses of 10 mg/kg), and the number of circulating DDLs also promptly decreased.[55] Despite the technical demands and safety concerns, the use of gene-modified DDLs represents one innovative therapeutic model that might prove effective even if the GVL effect and GVHD result from inseparable common pathogenetic mechanisms. The potential of gene-modified DDLs as a standard therapy against GVHD is being explored in the laboratory[56,65] and in the clinic.[55,66,67]

The activity of DDLs against EBV-LPD that occurs as a complication of using a T-cell-depleted hematopoietic allograft may not be relevant to the potential for GVL activity against the primary disease for which the transplantation was performed, or against EBV-LPD had that been the primary disease. The molecular mechanisms and the cellular interactions involved with DDL-induced antitumor activity have not been sufficiently defined to allow a prediction about the GVL effect against the primary disease in the setting of DDL-responsive secondary EBV-LPDs. If significantly less frequent recurrence of the primary disease and longer patient survival in patients with DDL-responsive EBV-LPDs are documented, this therapy may represent a broadly targeted antitumor effect. Because EBV-LPD is a tumor resulting from infection by a transforming virus, the insight into the mechanisms of antitumor activity in this disease may be applicable to the adoptive immunotherapy of other viral diseases, including hepatitis[68] and HIV.[69-79]

The Donor-Derived Lymphocyte Component

Beyond reporting the total cell dose used for an entire course of DDL transfusion therapy, the studies to date have not routinely described the specific characteristics of the DDL blood component. Typically, a target cell dose of 5×10^8 MNCs/kg (range=2-8×10^8 MNCs/kg) are collected from the original HLA-matched sibling donor using an automated blood cell separator in three (range=1-12) procedures over a period of 1 week (range=1 day to 4 months). The design of the cell collection schedule and the choice of instrumentation to be used are often influenced by practical considerations, including donor availability, adequacy of the donor's venous access, and the operator's hemapheresis skills. Between 1 and 2×10^8 MNCs/kg containing 50-60% T cells may be collected at each 3-hour leukapheresis procedure. The resulting DDL components are typically transfused without further laboratory manipulation (or after T-cell depletion to minimize GVHD) and without storage.

For patients with relapsed CML who respond to DDL transfusion, the pattern of responses to date suggests that: 1) clinical remission is not seen within the first month after the initial DDL transfusion, 2) the probability of achieving remission is approximately 30% by 2 months, 3) the probability increases thereafter by 20% per month over the next 3 months, and 4) nearly all responses are seen within 8 months.[27] These observations, based on a limited number of 33 successful patients, invite future confirmation.

The high incidence of GVHD observed in up to 80% of patients receiving unmodified DDLs may be minimized to as low as 30% by using T-cell-depleted components, but this would be achieved at the expense of increasing the risk for treatment failure.[26,27] Although a detailed description of the manufacturing process has not been a focus of clinical attention for the newly emerging cellular blood component, the increasing use of DDLs to treat chronic-phase CML in relapse after allogeneic marrow transplantation should lead to a better characterization of the many variables that may affect the safety and efficacy of this treatment in the near future. The current efforts to separate the GVL effect from GVHD target a major issue that is only one of many important investigative areas for identifying the relevant product variables subject to eventual standardization.

Advanced-Phase Chronic Myelogenous Leukemia and Other Hematologic Malignancies

DDL transfusion therapy has been much more effective in the chronic phase of CML than in its advanced phases or in other leukemias.[20-24,26,27,80] Antigenically less differentiated, more rapidly proliferating cells in the accelerated phases of CML or in acute leukemias have been more resistant to control through the adoptive transfer of cellular immunity. A composite clinical response of approximately 25% in the transformed phases of the disease contrasts sharply with the threefold higher response rate in chronic-phase relapse. The responses in accelerated CML have also been less durable. In many patients, the specific forms of disease relapse have paralleled the original disease stage at transplantation, and the form of CML relapse appears to be a meaningful predictor of response to DDL therapy. It has also been suggested that with rapidly proliferating disease, male recipients of lymphocytes from female donors may respond more favorably than individuals receiving DDL therapy under other donor-recipient gender combinations.[81]

Response rates in hematologic malignancies other than CML have been comparable to those in accelerated-phase CML. An analysis of the collective response rate of approximately 20% in 103 patients with a variety of disorders[26,27] has been complicated by many clinical variables, including the role of chemotherapy typically administered 1 week prior to the lymphocyte transfusion. To date, DDL transfusion therapy has been attempted in AML, acute lymphocytic leukemia, multiple myeloma, non-Hodgkin's lymphoma, Hodgkin's disease, myelodysplastic syndrome, polycythemia vera, juvenile CML, and chronic lymphocytic leukemia.[26,27] Myeloid diseases, including myelodysplastic syndromes, appear to respond more favorably than lymphoid leukemias; in acute lymphocytic leukemia, complete remission has been seen in only two of 23 evaluable patients (9%) in comparison with the approximately 20% response rate in 56 patients with AML.[26,27] Despite its lymphoid origin, multiple myeloma may respond to DDL therapy at a rate comparable to that of AML, and a T-cell dose of greater than 1×10^8/kg has been suggested as being predictive of a clinical graft-vs-myeloma response.[82-84] As expected, favorable clinical predictors of GVL effect in acute leukemias include the development of GVHD after DDL transfusion and a long duration of remission following initial marrow transplantation. A few reports have suggested that IFN-α, which appears not to affect the response rate in CML, may be more effective in acute leukemias.[26,53,85] Among other diseases treated to date, DDL immunotherapy has been successful in treating myelodysplastic syndrome and polycythemia vera,[24,26,27,85] but no responses have been reported in non-Hodgkin's lymphoma, Hodgkin's disease, juvenile CML, or chronic lymphocytic leukemia.

Solid Cancers and Other Immune-Related Disorders

Besides leukemias, the adoptive transfer of donor immunity through lymphocyte transfusion has been under investigation to treat a variety of disorders in which immune dysfunction plays an important pathogenetic role. In fact, adoptive immunotherapy as a therapeutic concept arose with the observation of the lymphokine-activated killer (LAK) phenomenon in 1980,[86] well before the report by Kolb et al[15] in 1990 about DDLs and relapsed CML, in which a heterogeneous population of MHC nonrestricted lymphocytes gain the ability to lyse tumor cells under the influence of IL-2. Coculturing lymphocytes and tumor cells in IL-2 results in the generation of MHC Class I-restricted T cells with a more potent and specific antitumor activity—the TILs—now also referred to as tumor-derived activated cells, or TDAC.[87] These lymphocyte-based cancer therapies require significant ex-vivo cell manipulation, have been limited largely to the autologous setting, and depend critically on the influence of IL-2 used either during ex-vivo cell culture (LAK cells and TILs) or in conjunction with cell transfusion (LAK cells). LAK cells and TILs continue to receive investigative attention on the basis of observed clinical response rates of up to 40% in selected patients with advanced malignancies,[49,50,58-60,87] as does lymphocyte transfusion in general in treating many immune-related disorders including HIV,[69-79] cancer,[49-51,58-60,87] and autoimmune disorders.[88-92] Innovative approaches for preparing specific DDL populations ex vivo by using antigen-pulsed dendritic cell stimulation are moving from the research laboratory to the clinic.[93] DDL transfusion as defined in this chapter represents only one of many developing lymphocyte-based therapies that has shown particular promise in managing patients with relapsed chronic-phase CML following allogeneic marrow transplantation.

The Regulatory Perspective

Adequate doses of DDLs may be collected using instrumentation and operating procedures that closely resemble those used in a standard apheresis volunteer platelet donation. Few adverse donor effects have been associated with the lymphocytapheresis procedures; mild citrate toxicity is expected in about one-third of the donors. As in any cytapheresis procedure, the purity and cell yield of the DDL component depend on donor variables (peripheral lymphocyte count, hematocrit, adequacy of venous access), instrument characteristics (efficiency of cell interface detection and cell separation), and operator variables (volume of processed blood, venous flow rate, operational skill). The degree of ex-vivo component processing and cell manipulation required depends on the extent to which control over the GVL effect and GVHD is attempted. Cryopreserving the lymphocyte component may allow flexibility in designing the optimal transfusion schedule.

Although these product manufacturing issues have received little regulatory attention with respect to the DDL component, the collection, laboratory processing, storage, and final preparation of DDLs for patient transfusion should be performed in accordance with current good manufacturing practice (cGMP) regulations as defined by the Center for Biologics Evaluation and Research (CBER) of the Food and Drug Administration (FDA), and may be subject to the agency's Investigational New Drug Application (IND) requirements especially when expanded or genetically modified.[94,95] In many marrow transplantation centers, the functions associated with component manufacturing are performed or coordinated by blood bank laboratories as the arm of the hospital service that has traditionally provided blood cell-based therapeutic products under stringent regulatory oversight, both internal and external to the institution.

Blood MNCs have received much investigative attention as a new class of blood components, of which circulating HPCs are being used almost routinely in many marrow transplantation centers. While blood MNCs have not been formally regulated beyond adherence to cGMP regulations, more specific regulations may be promulgated in the future. Vigorously debated questions as to when, by whom, how, and to what extent the manufacture of circulating HPCs should be regulated may be resolved within the next few years.

Circulating Hematopoietic Progenitor Cells

Driven by the increasing clinical use of circulating HPCs, the FDA has taken the lead in formulating a regulatory strategy toward these cells under intense scrutiny by both the transfusion and the transplantation communities. Further evolution of the regulatory strategy is anticipated before final rules may be established. It is difficult to predict if and when blood MNCs will be regulated in a manner analogous to the more traditional blood components such as Whole Blood, Red Blood Cells, Platelets, Plasma, and Cryoprecipitated Anti-Hemophilic Factor. The regulation of these traditional components has been changing as well, because of: 1) the record of product safety over the past decade, 2) the public pressure to reduce the reporting burden on the regulated industry, resulting in CBER's Changes to be Reported and Blood Reinvention initiatives, and 3) CBER's effort to harmonize its operation with that of the Center for Drug Evaluation and Research under the Biologics License Application initiative. In-depth analyses of these transitional CBER initiatives in regulating the conventional blood components and their effect on shaping the regulation of newly emerging blood components are beyond the scope of this discussion. However, a closer look at the evolution of the current regulatory approach toward circulating HPCs may provide insight as to how novel blood components, including DDLs, may be regulated in the future.

Public Workshops About Circulating Hematopoietic Progenitor Cells

The FDA sponsored two public workshops, both in conjunction with the National Heart, Lung, and

Blood Institute of the National Institutes of Health. The primary objective of these workshops was the exchange and collection of scientific information relevant to the quality control procedures applicable to the manufacture of umbilical cord (December 1995) and peripheral blood (February 1996) HPCs intended for use in marrow reconstitution. At each workshop, the agency's respective regulatory proposal was distributed as a draft guidance document in which specific requirements for filing an IND were outlined. Well over 500 letters were received from the public in response to the workshops and the draft proposals, the overwhelming majority of which urged CBER to follow the formal rule-making process subject to an obligatory consideration of all public comments. In clear recognition of the public perception that the IND regulatory mechanism applicable to a typical new biologic drug under development is not well suited for the regulation of circulating HPCs, with which there has already been a considerable amount of clinical experience, the FDA proposed a new regulatory strategy. This strategy is targeted more broadly at biologic products having new clinical applications as a result of rapidly advancing technologies, including circulating HPCs. As before, a public meeting held in March 1997 allowed direct participation by interested public sectors and focused attention on the agency's document, "Proposed Approach to Regulation of Cellular and Tissue-Based Products" (tissue proposal), issued on February 28, 1997.

The New Regulatory Proposal: Circulating Hematopoietic Progenitor Cells as Tissue

Under the authority of the Public Health Service Act and the Federal Food, Drug, and Cosmetic Act, the new tissue proposal underscores three basic requirements common to the manufacturing of biologic products. The two general requirements—to avoid collecting, as the starting material tissues that may transmit infectious diseases; and to ensure that subsequent laboratory procedures do not introduce contaminants or unduly compromise the quality of the final product—are applicable to the manufacture of all cellular and tissue-based products. However, the third requirement—to demonstrate clinical safety and efficacy under an IND—applies only to products that: 1) have been more than minimally manipulated in the laboratory in a way that alters the inherent biologic characteristics of the original cells or tissues, 2) are intended to be used for purposes other than the inherent biologic functions of its cells or tissues, 3) result from combining the original material with nontissue components, or 4) have systemic effects. The complementary terms "more than minimally manipulated" and "minimally manipulated" focus on biologic function at the cellular level; the simple selection of a cell subpopulation is considered minimal manipulation, whereas cytokine or genetic manipulation result in a product considered to be more than minimally manipulated by the agency subject to IND requirements.

Specific Guidelines for Circulating Hematopoietic Progenitor Cells and Applicability to Donor-Derived Lymphocytes

In addition to these general guidelines, the new tissue proposal also outlines guidelines specific to circulating HPCs that distinguish the product's autologous or related allogeneic (first-degree blood relation) uses from its unrelated allogeneic use. Despite (at least) the expected systemic effects of circulating HPCs, a clinical demonstration of product safety and efficacy is *not* required for *autologous* or *related allogeneic* uses, provided that the circulating HPC product *is not* more than minimally manipulated, *is* intended to be used for hematopoietic support, and *does not* contain nontissue material. Even for unrelated allogeneic use, the requirement to demonstrate product safety and efficacy applies if, and only after, CBER does not establish specific product standards by the year 2001, 3 years after the issuance of the January 20, 1998 *Federal Register* notice[96] in which the agency calls for data to support product standards for unrelated allogeneic circulating HPCs. When successfully developed, CBER plans to use the standards directly in evaluating licensure applications in lieu of reviewing clinical safety and efficacy data collected under an IND. Sufficient public support of the agency's February 28, 1997, tissue proposal should lead to its solidification as legally binding regulations under the rule-making process. Mature lymphocytes are not specifically addressed in the new tissue proposal; as such blood establishments engaging in the manufacture of DDLs are well advised to register with CBER, adhere to cGMP regulations in component manufacturing, and consult CBER about IND filing requirements as part of the ongoing dialogue between the FDA and the regulated industry that shapes the agency's thinking.

References

1. Truitt RL, LeFever AV, Shich CC-Y, et al. Graft-vs-leukemia effect. In: Burakoff SJ, Deeg HJ, Ferrara J, Atkinson K, eds. Graft-vs-host disease: Immunology, pathophysiology, and treatment. New York: Marcel Dekker, 1990: 177-81.

2. Kloosterman TC, Tielmans MJ, Martens AC, et al. Quantitative studies on graft-versus-leukemia after allogeneic bone marrow transplantation in rat models for acute myelocytic and lymphocytic leukemia. Bone Marrow Transplant 1994;14:15-9.

3. Barnes DHW, Loutit JF. Treatment of murine leukaemia with X-rays and homologous bone marrow. Br J Haematol 1957;3:241-52.

4. Gale RP, Butturini A. How do transplants cure chronic myelogenous leukemia (editorial)? Bone Marrow Transplant 1992;9:83-5.

5. Horowitz MM, Gale RP, Sondel PM, et al. Graft-versus-leukemia reactions after bone marrow transplantation. Blood 1990;75: 555-62.

6. Weiden PL, Flournoy N, Sanders JE, et al. Anti-leukemic effect of graft-versus-host disease contributes to improved survival after allogeneic marrow transplantation. Transplant Proc 1981;13:248-51.

7. Weiden PL, Sullivan K, Flournoy N, et al. The Seattle Marrow Transplant Team: Antileuke-mic effect of chronic graft-versus-host disease. Contribution to improved survival after allogeneic marrow transplantation. N Engl J Med 1981;304:1529-31.

8. Goldman JM, Gale RP, Horowitz MM, et al. Bone marrow transplantation for chronic myelogenous leukemia in chronic phase. Increased risk for relapse associated with T-cell depletion. Ann Intern Med 1988;108:806-7.

9. Apperley JF, Mauro FR, Goldman JM, et al. Bone marrow transplantation for chronic myeloid leukaemia in first chronic phase: Importance of a graft-versus-leukaemia effect. Br J Haematol 1988;69:239-45.

10. Marmont A, Horowitz MM, Gale RP, et al. T-cell depletion of HLA-identical transplants in leukemia. Blood 1991;78:2120-30.

11. Offit K, Burns JP, Cunningham I, et al. Cytogenetic analysis of chimerism and leukemia relapse in chronic myelogenous leukemia patients after T cell-depleted bone marrow transplantation. Blood 1990;75:1346-55.

12. Odom LF, August CS, Githen JH, et al. Remission of relapsed leukaemia during graft-versus-host reaction. Lancet 1978;2:537-40.

13. Higano CS, Brixey M, Bryant EM, et al. Durable complete remission of acute nonlymphocytic leukemia associated with discontinuation of immunosuppression following relapse after allogeneic bone marrow transplantation. A case report of a probable graft-versus-leukemia effect. Transplantation 1990;50: 175-7.

14. Collins RH, Rogers ZR, Bennett M, et al. Hematologic relapse of chronic myelogenous leukemia following allogeneic bone marrow transplantation: Apparent graft-versus-leukemia effect following abrupt discontinuation of immunosuppression. Bone Marrow Transplant 1990;10:391-5.

15. Kolb HJ, Mittermueller J, Clemm C, et al. Donor leukocyte transfusions for treatment of recurrent chronic myelogenous leukemia in marrow transplant patients. Blood 1990;76:2462-5.

16. Bar BM, Schattenberg A, Mensink EJ, et al. Donor leukocyte infusions for chronic mye-

loid leukemia after allogeneic bone marrow transplantation. J Clin Oncol 1993;11:513-9.

17. Drobyski WR, Keever CA, Roth MS, et al. Salvage immunotherapy using donor leukocyte infusions as treatment for relapsed chronic myelogenous leukemia after allogeneic bone marrow transplantation: Efficacy and toxicity of a defined T-cell dose. Blood 1993;82:2310-8.

18. Helg C, Roux E, Beris P, et al. Adoptive immunotherapy for recurrent CML after BMT. Bone Marrow Transplant 1993;12:125-9.

19. Jiang YZ, Cullis JO, Kanfer EJ, et al. T cell and NK cell mediated graft-versus-leukaemia reactivity following donor buffy coat transfusion to treat relapse after marrow transplantation for chronic myeloid leukaemia. Bone Marrow Transplant 1993;11:133-8.

20. Porter DL, Roth MS, McGarigle C, et al. Induction of graft-versus-host disease as immunotherapy for relapsed chronic myeloid leukemia. N Engl J Med 1994;330:100-6.

21. Slavin S, Ackerstein A, Weiss L, et al. Immunotherapy of minimal residual disease by immunocompetent lymphocytes and their activation by cytokines. Cancer Invest 1992;10:221-7.

22. Johnson BD, Drobyski WR, Truitt RL. Delayed infusion of normal donor cells after MHC-matched bone marrow transplantation provides an antileukemia reaction without graft-versus-host disease. Bone Marrow Transplant 1993;11:329-36.

23. Hertenstein B, Wiesneth M, Novotny I, et al. Interferon-alpha and donor buffy coat transfusions for treatment of relapsed chronic myeloid leukemia after allogeneic bone marrow transplantation. Transplantation 1993;56:1114-8.

24. Collins RH, Pineiro LA, Nemunaitis JJ, et al. Transfusion of donor buffy coat cells in the treatment of persistent or recurrent malignancy after allogeneic bone marrow transplantation. Transfusion 1995;35:898-9.

25. Sullivan KM, Storb R, Buckner CD, et al. Graft-versus-host disease as adoptive immunotherapy in patients with advanced hematological neoplasms. N Engl J Med 1994;320:100-4.

26. Kolb HJ, Schattenberg A, Goldman JM, et al. Graft-versus-leukemia effect of donor lymphocyte transfusions in marrow grafted patients. Blood 1995;86:2041-50.

27. Collins RH, Shpilberg O, Drobyski WR, et al. Donor leukocyte infusions in 140 patients with relapsed malignancy after allogeneic bone marrow transplantation. J Clin Oncol 1997;15:433-44.

28. van Rhee F, Lin F, Cullis JO, et al. Relapse of chronic myeloid leukemia after allogeneic bone marrow transplant: The case for giving donor leukocyte transfusions before the onset of hematologic relapse. Blood 1994;83:3377-83.

29. Keil F, Haas O, Fritsch G, et al. Donor leukocyte infusion for leukemic relapse after allogeneic marrow transplantation: Lack of residual donor hematopoiesis predicts aplasia. Blood 1997;89:3113-7.

30. Keil F, Kalhs P, Haas OA, et al. Graft failure after donor leucocyte infusion in relapsed chronic myeloid leukaemia: Successful treatment with cyclophosphamide and antithymocyte globulin followed by peripheral blood stem cell infusion. Br J Haematol 1996;94:120-2.

31. Flowers M, Sullivan KM, Martin P, et al. Use of peripheral blood stem cells for immune therapy (abstract). Blood 1995;86(Suppl 1):564a.

32. Weiss L, Lubin I, Factorowich I, et al. Effective GVL effects independent of GVHD after T cell-depleted allogeneic bone marrow transplantation in a murine model of B cell leukemia/lymphoma. J Immunol 1994;153:2562-7.

33. Glass B, Uharek L, Gassmann W, et al. Graft-versus-leukemia activity after bone marrow transplantation does not require graft-versus-host disease. Ann Hematol 1992;64:255-9.

34. Bortin MM, Rimm AA, Saltzstein EC, Rodey GE. Graft versus leukemia, III: Apparent inde-

pendent antihost and antileukemia activity of transplanted immunocompetent cells. Transplantation 1973;16:182-8.

35. Lotzova E. Interleukin-2 generated killer cells, their characterization and role in cancer therapy. Cancer Bull 1987;39:30-8.

36. Lotzova E, McCredie KB, Muesse L, et al. Natural killer cells in man: Their possible involvement in leukemia and bone marrow transplantation. In: Baum SJ, Ledney GD, eds. Experimental hematology today. New York: Springer-Verlag, 1979:207-13.

37. Lotzova E, Savary CA, Keating MJ. Leukemia diseased patients exhibit multiple defects in natural killer cell lytic machinery. Exp Hematol 1983;10:83-95.

38. Schirrmacher V, Beckhove P, Kruger A, et al. Effective immune rejection of advanced metastasized cancer. Int J Oncol 1995; 6:505-7.

39. Rocha M, Umansky V, Lee K, et al. Differences between graft-versus-leukemia and graft-versus-host reactivity, I: Interaction of donor immune T cells with tumor and/or host cells. Blood 1997;89:2189-202.

40. Lotzova E. Role of interleukin-2 activated MHC-nonrestricted lymphocytes in antileukemia activity and therapy. Leuk Lymphoma 1992;7:15-28.

41. Johnson BD, Hanke CA, Truitt RL. The graft-versus-leukemia effect of post-transplant donor leukocyte infusion. Leuk Lymphoma 1996;23:1-9.

42. Giralt S, Hester J, Huh Y, et al. CD8-depleted donor lymphocyte infusion as treatment for relapsed chronic myelogenous leukemia after allogeneic bone marrow transplantation. Blood 1995;86:4337-43.

43. Pan L, Delmonte J, Jalonen CK, Ferrara JLM. Pretreatment of donor mice with granulocyte colony-stimulating factor polarizes donor T lymphocytes toward type-2 cytokine production and reduces severity of experimental graft-versus-host disease. Blood 1995;86:4422-9.

44. Warner J, Dennert F. In vivo function of a cloned cell line with NK activity: Effects on bone marrow transplants, tumor development and metastases. Nature 1982;300:31-4.

45. Kasai M, Yoneda T, Habu S, et al. In vivo effect of anti-sialo GM-1 antibody on natural killer activity. Nature 1981;291:334-5.

46. Kiessling R, Klein E, Wigzell H. Natural killer cells in the mouse, I: Cytotoxic cells with specificity for mouse Moloney leukemia cells. Specificity and distribution according to genotype. Eur J Immunol 1975;5:112-7.

47. Abo T, Roder JC, Abo W, et al. Natural killer (HNK-1+) cells in Chédiak-Higashi patients are present in normal numbers but are abnormal in function and morphology. J Clin Invest 1982;70:193-7.

48. Robertson MJ, Ritz J. Biology and clinical relevance of human natural killer cells. Blood 1990;76:2421-38.

49. Dutcher JP, Creekmore S, Weiss GR, et al. A phase II study of interleukin-2 and lymphokine-activated killer cells in patients with metastatic malignant melanoma. J Clin Oncol 1989;7:477-85.

50. Rosenberg SA, Yang JC, Topalian SL, et al. Treatment of 283 consecutive patients with metastatic melanoma or renal cell cancer using high-dose bolus interleukin 2. JAMA 1994;271:907-13.

51. Kohler PC, Hank JA, Exten R, et al. Clinical response of a patient with diffuse histiocytic lymphoma to adoptive chemoimmunotherapy using cyclophosphamide and alloactivated haploidentical lymphocytes. A case report and phase I trial. Cancer 1985;55:552-60.

52. Soiffer RJ, Murray C, Gonin R, Ritz J. Effect of low-dose interleukin-2 on disease relapse after T-cell-depleted allogeneic bone marrow transplantation. Blood 1994;84:964-71.

53. Slavin S, Naparstek E, Nagler A, et al. Allogeneic cell therapy with donor peripheral blood cells and recombinant human interleukin-2 to treat leukemia relapse after allogeneic bone marrow transplantation. Blood 1996;87:2195-204.

54. Mackinnon S, Papadopoulos B, Carabasi MH, et al. Adoptive immunotherapy evaluating escalating doses of donor leukocytes for relapse of chronic myeloid leukemia after bone marrow transplantation: Separation of graft-versus-leukemia responses from graft-versus-host disease. Blood 1995;86:1261-8.

55. Bonini C, Ferrari G, Verzeletti S, et al. HSV-TK gene transfer into donor lymphocytes for control of allogeneic graft-versus-leukemia. Science 1997;276:1719-24.

56. Tiberghien P, Reynolds CW, Keller J, et al. Ganciclovir treatment of herpes simplex thymidine kinase-transduced primary T lymphocytes: An approach for specific in vivo T-cells depletion after bone marrow transplantation. Blood 1994;84:1333-41.

57. Weaver CH, Buckner CD, Longin K, et al. Syngeneic transplantation with peripheral blood mononuclear cells collected after the administration of recombinant human granulocyte colony-stimulating factor. Blood 1993; 82:1981-4.

58. Fisher RI, Coltman CA, Doroshow JH, et al. Metastatic renal cancer treated with interleukin-2 and lymphokine-activated killer cells. Ann Intern Med 1988;108:518-23.

59. Berendt MJ, North RJ. T-cell-mediated suppression of anti-tumor immunity: An explanation for progressive growth of an immunogenic tumor. J Exp Med 1980;151:69-80.

60. Greenberg PD, Cheever MA. Treatment of disseminated leukemia with cyclophosphamide and immune cells: Tumor immunity reflects long-term persistence of tumor-specific donor T cells. J Immunol 1984;133:3401-7.

61. Papadopoulos EB, Ladanyi M, Emanuel D, et al. Infusions of donor leukocytes to treat Epstein-Barr virus-associated lymphoproliferative disorders after allogeneic bone marrow transplantation. N Engl J Med 1994;330: 1185-91.

62. Shapiro RS, McClain K, Frizzera G, et al. Epstein-Barr virus associated B cell lymphoproliferative disorders following bone marrow transplantation. Blood 1988;71:1234-43.

63. Heslop HE, Brenner MK, Rooney CM. Donor T cells as therapy for EBV lymphoproliferation post bone marrow transplantation. N Engl J Med 1994;331:679-80.

64. Caldas C, Ambinder R. Epstein-Barr virus and bone marrow transplantation. Curr Opin Oncol 1995;7:102-6.

65. Munshi NC, Govindarajan R, Drake R, et al. Thymidine kinase (TK) gene-transduced human lymphocytes can be highly purified, remain fully functional, and are killed efficiently with ganciclovir. Blood 1997;89:1334-40.

66. Rooney CM, Smith CA, Ng CYC, et al. Use of gene-modified virus-specific T lymphocytes to control Epstein-Barr virus-related lymphoproliferation. Lancet 1995;345:9-13.

67. Bordignon C, Bonini C, Verzeletti S, et al. Transfer of the HSV-tk gene into donor peripheral blood lymphocytes for in vivo modulation of donor anti-tumor immunity after allogeneic bone marrow transplantation. Hum Gene Ther 1995;6:813-7.

68. Shouval D, Ilan Y. Immunization against hepatitis B through adoptive transfer of immunity. Intervirology 1995;38:41-6.

69. Davis KC, Hayward A, Ozturk G, Kohler PF. Lymphocyte transfusion in a case of acquired immunodeficiency syndrome. Lancet 1983; 1:599-600.

70. Klein HG. Apheresis, immunoreconstitution and AIDS. Ther Plasmapheresis 1993;12: 21-3.

71. Lane HC, Zunich KM, Wilson W, et al. Syngeneic bone marrow transplantation and adoptive transfer of peripheral blood lymphocytes in human immunodeficiency virus (HIV) infection. Ann Intern Med 1990;113:512-9.

72. Walker CM, Moody DH, Stites DP, Levy JA. CD8+ lymphocytes can control HIV infection in vitro by suppressing virus replication. Science 1986;234:1563-6.

73. Wiviott LD, Walker CM, Levy JA. CD8+ lymphocytes suppress HIV production by autologous CD4+ cells without eliminating the in-

fected cells from culture. Cell Immunol 1990; 128:628-34.

74. Walker CM, Levy JA. A diffusible lymphokine produced by CD8+ T lymphocytes suppresses HIV replication. Immunology 1989;66:628-30.

75. Pantaleo G, De Maria A, Koenig S, et al. CD8+ T lymphocytes of patients with AIDS maintain normal broad cytolytic function despite the loss of human immunodeficiency virus-specific cytotoxicity. Proc Natl Acad Sci U S A 1990;87:4818-22.

76. Plata F, Autran B, Martins LP, et al. AIDS virus-specific cytotoxic T lymphocytes in lung disorders. Nature 1987;328:348-51.

77. Whiteside TL, Elder EM, Moody D, et al. Generation and characterization of ex vivo propagated autologous CD8+ cells used for adoptive immunotherapy of patients infected with human immunodeficiency virus. Blood 1993; 81:2085-92.

78. Ho M, Armstrong J, McMahon D, et al. A phase I study of adoptive transfer of autologous CD8+ T lymphocytes in patients with acquired immunodeficiency syndrome (AIDS)-related complex or AIDS. Blood 1993; 81:2093-101.

79. Lieberman J, Skolnik PR, Parkerson GR, et al. Safety of autologous ex vivo-expanded human immunodeficiency virus (HIV)-specific cytotoxic T-lymphocyte infusion in HIV-infected patients. Blood 1997;90:2196-206.

80. Szer J, Grigg AP, Phillips GL, Sheridan WP. Donor leucocyte infusions after chemotherapy for patients relapsing with acute leukaemia following allogeneic BMT. Bone Marrow Transplant 1993;11:109-11.

81. Goulmy E, Termijteelen A, Bradley BA, Van Rood JJ. Y-antigen killing by T cells of women is restricted by HLA. Nature 1977;266:544-5.

82. Lokhorst HM, Schattenberg A, Cornelissen JJ, et al. Donor leukocyte infusions are effective in relapsed multiple myeloma after allogeneic bone marrow transplantation. Blood 1997; 90:4206-11.

83. Verdonck LF, Lokhorst HM, Dekker AW, et al. Graft-versus-myeloma effect in two cases. Lancet 1996;347:800-1.

84. Tricot G, Vesole DH, Jagannath S, et al. Graft-versus-myeloma effect: Proof of principle. Blood 1996;87:1196-8.

85. Porter DL, Roth MS, Lee SJ, et al. Adoptive immunotherapy with donor mononuclear cell infusions to treat relapse of acute leukemia or myelodysplasia after allogeneic bone marrow transplantation. Bone Marrow Transplant 1996;18:975-80.

86. Lotze MT, Line BR, Mathisen DJ, et al. The in vivo distribution of autologous human and murine lymphoid cells grown in T-cell growth factor (TCGF): Implications for the adoptive immunotherapy of tumors. J Immunol 1980; 125:1487-93.

87. Oldham RK, Lewko WM, Good RW, Sharp E. Cancer biotherapy with interferon, interleukin-2 and tumor-derived activated cells (TDAC). In Vivo 1994;8:653-64.

88. Bux J, Westphal E, de Sousa F, et al. Alloimmune neonatal neutropenia is a potential side effect of immunization with leukocytes in women with recurrent spontaneous abortions. J Reprod Immunol 1992;22:299-302.

89. Smith JB, Cowchock FS, Lata JA, Hankinson BT. The number of cells used for immunotherapy of repeated spontaneous abortion influences pregnancy outcome. Reprod Immunol 1992;22:217-24.

90. Pozzilli P, Ghirlanda G, Manna G, et al. White cells transfusion in recent onset type 1 diabetes. Diabetes Res 1986;3:273-6.

91. Krug J, Verlohren H-J, Bierwolf B, et al. Lymphocyte transfusion in recent onset type I diabetes mellitus—a one-year follow-up of cell-mediated anti-islet cytotoxicity and C-peptide secretion. J Autoimmun 1990;3:601-9.

92. Cavanaugh J, Chopek M, Binimelis J, et al. Buffy coat transfusions in early type 1 diabetes. Diabetes 1987;36:1089-93.

93. Shurin MR. Dendritic cells presenting tumor antigen. Cancer Immunol Immunother 1996; 43:158-64.

94. Food and Drug Administration. Department of Health and Human Services. Application of current statutory authorities to human somatic cell therapy products and gene therapy products. Fed Regist 1993;58:53248-51.

95. Kessler DA, Siegel JP, Noguchi PD, et al. Regulation of somatic-cell therapy and gene therapy by the Food and Drug Administration. N Engl J Med 1993;329:1169-73.

96. Food and Drug Administration. Department of Health and Human Services. Request for proposed standards for unrelated allogeneic peripheral and placental/umbilical cord blood hematopoietic stem/progenitor cell products; Request for comments. Fed Regist 1998;63:2985-8.

In: Mintz PD, ed.
Transfusion Therapy: Clinical Principles and Practice
Bethesda, MD: AABB Press, 1999

14

Immune Globulin Therapy

E. RICHARD STIEHM, MD

 IMMUNOGLOBULIN THERAPY IS used to 1) provide immunoglobulin for patients with antibody deficiency (eg, agammaglobulinemia); 2) provide temporary (passive) immunity to a susceptible subject following exposure to an infection, toxin, or drug (eg, rabies); 3) inhibit inflammation or immune activation in immunoregulatory disorders (eg, Kawasaki syndrome); 4) prevent specific antibody production in certain patients (eg, an Rh-negative mother); and 5) treat certain infectious diseases (eg, parvovirus B19).[1]

Three types of preparations are used in immunoglobulin therapy: 1) standard human immune serum globulin for general use, which is available in two forms—intramuscular immune globulin (IG) and intravenous immune globulin (IVIG); 2) special high-titered IGs and IVIGs with a known antibody content for specific illnesses; and 3) animal serums and antitoxins. These are listed in Table 14-1.

Whole blood, plasma, or serum can also be used in passive immunization.

Immunoglobulin treatment is not always effective, its duration is short and variable (1-6 weeks), and undesirable reactions may occur, especially if the product is not of human origin. The special high-titered IG and IVIG are identical to regular IG and IVIG except that the former are derived from patients hyperimmunized or convalescing from a specific infection and the antibody content to the specific antigen is assayed; thus, they are useful in several disorders in which IG or IVIG is of little or no value.

Animal Sera and Antitoxins

In certain clinical situations in which immunoglobulin therapy is indicated (eg, diphtheria, snake and spider bites, digitalis overdose), only animal sera are available. Such sera are derived from the

E. Richard Stiehm, MD, Professor and Chief, Division of Immunology, UCLA Children's Hospital, Los Angeles, California

Table 14-1. Antibody Preparations Available for Passive Immunity in the United States

Product	Abbreviations or Brand Names	Principal Use
STANDARD HUMAN IMMUNE SERUM GLOBULINS	HISG, Gammaglobulin	
Intravenous immune globulin	IVIG, IGIV	Treatment of antibody deficiency, immune thrombo-cytopenic purpura (ITP), Kawasaki syndrome, other immunoregulatory and inflammatory diseases
Intramuscular immune globulin	IG	Treatment of antibody deficiency, prevention of measles, hepatitis A
SPECIAL HUMAN IMMUNE SERUM GLOBULINS*		
Hepatitis B (IM)	HBIG	Prevention of hepatitis B
Varicella zoster (IM)	VZIG	Modification or prevention of chicken pox
Rabies (IM)	RIG	Prevention of rabies
Tetanus (IM)	TIG	Prevention or treatment of tetanus
Vaccinia (IM)	VIG	Prevention or treatment of smallpox, vaccinia
Western equine encephalitis (WEE) (IM)†	WEE-IG	Prevention, after laboratory accident with WEE virus
Rh₀ (D) Immune Globulin (IM)	RhIG	Prevention of sensitization to the D antigen
Rh₀ (D) Immune Globulin (IV)	WinRho SD	Treatment of ITP
Cytomegalovirus (CMV) (IV)	CytoGam	Prevention and treatment of cytomegalovirus (CMV) infection
Respiratory syncytial virus (RSV) (IV)	RespiGam	Prevention of RSV infection

Table 14-1. Antibody Preparations Available for Passive Immunity in the United States (continued)

Product	Abbreviations or Brand Names	Principal Use
ANIMAL SERA AND ANTITOXINS		
Tetanus antitoxin (equine)	TAT	Prevention or treatment of tetanus (when TIG is unavailable)
Diphtheria antitoxin (equine)	DAT	Treatment of diphtheria
Botulism antitoxin (equine)		Treatment of botulism
Latrodectus mactans antivenin (equine)		Treatment of black widow spider bites
Crotalidae polyvalent antivenin (equine)		Treatment of most snake bites
Micrurus fulvius antivenin (equine)		Treatment of coral snake bites
Digoxin immune Fab fragments (ovine)		Digoxin or digitoxin overdose
Anti-CD3 monoclonal antibody (murine)	Muromonab-CD3	Immunosuppression
Anti-interleukin-2 (IL-2) receptor (CD25) monoclonal antibody (humanized murine)	Zenapak-Dadizamab	Immunosuppression
Anti-CD-20 monoclonal antibody (humanized murine)	Rituxan-Rituximab	Treatment of lymphoma
Lymphocyte immune globulin, antithymocyte globulin (equine)	ATG, Atgam	Immunosuppression

* IM=intramuscular; IV=intravenous.

† Available from the US Centers for Disease Control.

serum of immunized animals, usually horses (equine). Because these sera are foreign proteins, a significant risk is associated with their use. Thus, they should be administered only when specifically indicated, after sensitivity tests, and by a physician prepared to deal with a hypersensitivity reaction. A careful history must be taken before an animal serum is injected. Inquiry must be made about asthma, hay fever, urticaria, and previous injections of animal sera. Patients with a history of asthma, allergic rhinitis, or other allergic symptoms on exposure to horses may be dangerously sensitive to the corresponding serum and should receive it only with the utmost caution.

Sensitivity Tests for Animal Serum

A scratch, prick, or puncture skin test, followed by an intradermal skin test, should always be performed before any injection of animal serum, whether or not the patient has had the serum previously. A scratch, prick, or puncture test is performed by applying a drop of 1:100 dilution in saline of the serum to the site of a superficial scratch, prick, or puncture on the volar aspect of the forearm and observing it for 20 minutes. A positive control (histamine phosphate 0.1%) and a negative control (saline) should also be applied. A positive reaction consists of erythema or wheal formation at least 3 mm greater in diameter than that produced by the control. (It should be noted that prior use of antihistaminics may render these test results negative.) If the scratch, prick, or puncture test result is negative, an intradermal test is performed by injecting 0.1 mL of a 1:100 saline dilution. The reaction is read after 10-30 minutes and is positive if a wheal appears that is again at least 3 mm greater than that produced by the control. In persons with a history of allergy, the initial test dose is reduced to 0.05 mL of a 1:1000 dilution. Again, positive (histamine phosphate 0.01%) and negative control tests should be performed.

Although intradermal skin tests have resulted in fatalities, the scratch, prick, or puncture tests have not. Accordingly, a skin test should never be performed (nor a serum injected) unless a syringe containing 1 mL of 1:1000 epinephrine is within immediate reach. Skin tests can indicate the probability of sensitivity. However, a negative skin test result is not an absolute guarantee of the absence of sensitivity. Therefore, either a specific history of allergy or a positive skin test with horse serum is sufficient reason for special caution. A positive history of sensitivity to horse dander indicates the need for extreme caution.

Administration of Animal Serum

If the history and sensitivity test results are negative, the indicated dose of serum may be given intramuscularly (IM) with epinephrine at hand. The patient should be watched closely for an hour for an adverse reaction. Intravenous (IV) injection may be indicated if a high concentration of circulating antibody is required rapidly, as in severe tetanus or diphtheria. In such instances, a preliminary dose of 0.5 mL of serum should be diluted in 10 mL of either physiologic saline or 5% glucose solution. This preparation should be given intravenously over 5 minutes, and the patient should be watched for 30 minutes for reactions. If no reaction occurs, the remainder of the serum, diluted 1:20, may be given at a rate not to exceed 1 mL per minute.

If the skin test result is positive or there is a history of allergy to animal serum, the need for the serum is unquestioned, and provided epinephrine is at hand, a procedure commonly called desensitization can be undertaken. Desensitization, which should be performed by trained personnel with the necessary emergency equipment and drugs immediately available, consists of periodic (at 15-minute intervals) injection or infusion of progressively larger doses of the serum, starting at a very low dose, until tolerance is achieved. Schedules for IV and intradermal-subcutaneous-IV desensitization are available.[2] However, it is unlikely that any significant desensitization will occur. This procedure merely results in establishing temporary tolerance to the serum. The administration of sera after desensitization must be continuous; protection after desensitization is lost rapidly.

Hypersensitivity Reactions to Animal Serum

Hypersensitivity reactions to animal serum may be of the following four general types: 1) anaphylactic reactions consisting of urticaria, dyspnea, cyanosis, shock, and unconsciousness occurring seconds to minutes after an injection; 2) acute febrile reactions consisting of moderate or severe hyperpyrexia within 2 hours after an injection; 3) serum sickness reactions consisting of urticaria, arthritis, adenopathy, and fever occurring hours to days after an injection, depending on the dose and the presence or degree of prior sensitization (serum sickness occurs within hours to a few days after the second injection and within 7-12 days after the first injection); and 4) delayed reactions of varying nature, including peripheral (serum) neuritis.

Intramuscular Immune Globulin

Pharmacology

Human IG is prepared by the fractionation of pooled human serum by the Cohn alcohol fractionation procedure (from which it derives its alternative name of Cohn Fraction II). The fractionation procedure removes most other serum proteins, hepatitis viruses, and human immunodeficiency viruses (HIV-1 and HIV-2), thus providing a safe product for IM injection. It is reconstituted as a sterile 16.5% solution (165 mg/mL) containing thimerosal as a preservative, and it contains a wide spectrum of antibodies to viral and bacterial antigens. IG is 95% IgG, with trace quantities of IgM and IgA and other serum proteins. IgM and IgA are therapeutically insignificant because of their short half-lives (<7 days) and their low concentrations.

IG is approved for IM or subcutaneous use only; IV injection of IG is contraindicated. IG aggregates in vitro to complexes of high molecular weight [9.55 to 40 Svedberg units(s)], which are strongly anticomplementary. Such aggregates are probably responsible for some of the occasional systemic reactions seen to IG. The incidence of these reactions is increased if the recipient had received IG previously or if IG is inadvertently given intravenously.

Intramuscular Immunoglobulin in Antibody Immunodeficiencies

The usual dose of IG for antibody immunodeficiency is 100 mg/kg per month, about equivalent to 0.7 mL/kg per month of the commercially available 16.5% (165 mg/mL) product. A double or triple dose is given at the onset of therapy, usually at 1- to 2-day intervals. The maximum dosage should not exceed 20 or 30 mL per week after the initial loading doses. Few studies evaluating the optimal dosage are available; however, the Medical Research Council Working Party found that 25 mg/kg per week (100 mg/kg/month) was equivalent therapeutically to 50 mg/kg per week, but that 10 mg/kg per week was inadequate.[3]

Injections of IG are given initially at monthly intervals. If the patient continues to have infection or if a characteristic symptom (such as cough, conjunctivitis, diarrhea, arthralgia, or purulent nasal discharge) recurs at the end of the injection period, the interval between doses usually is decreased to 3 or 2 weeks.

Intramuscular IG should be given at multiple sites to avoid injecting more than 5 mL (or 10 mL in a large adult) at any one site. The buttocks are the preferred sites, but the thighs can also be used. Tenderness, sterile abscesses, fibrosis, and sciatic nerve injury may result from these injections. The danger of sciatic nerve injury is especially great in the small, malnourished infant with inadequate muscle and fat in the gluteal regions. IG should not be given to patients with severe thrombocytopenia because of the risk of hematoma and infection.

An intramuscular injection of 100 mg/kg of IG usually raises the IG serum level by 100 mg/dL after 2-4 days. Thus, a recent IG injection usually does not obscure the diagnosis of hypogammaglobulinemia.[4]

Intramuscular Immunoglobulin in Measles and Hepatitis A Prophylaxis

High-titered IGs are not available for measles, hepatitis A, poliomyelitis, or rubella exposures, but regular IG has antibody to these viruses and can be used in susceptible subjects following exposure. The protective doses of IG in these conditions, which vary considerably, are given elsewhere[1] and in the package inserts. Prophylaxis for poliomyelitis and rubella is rarely indicated.

Adverse Effects of Intramuscular Immunoglobulin

Although IG is one of the safest biologic products available, rare anaphylactic reactions to IM injections have been reported, particularly in patients requiring repeat injections. The Medical Research Council Working Party noted such reactions in 33 of 175 patients (19%) treated over a 10-year period.[3] Symptoms included anxiety, nausea, vomiting, malaise, flushing, facial swelling, cyanosis, and loss of consciousness. In all, there were 85 reactions to about 40,000 injections. In eight patients, the injections were stopped as a result of these adverse effects, and one death was recorded. Reactions occurred at any stage of treatment and were unrelated to any particular IG lot number or its anticomplementary activity. Should anaphylactic reactions occur, immediate treatment with epinephrine and antihistamines is indicated. Often, these reactions can be minimized with a pretreatment similar to that used in IVIG therapy (see below).

Immunoglobulin injections or infusions may inhibit antibody responses to vaccine antigens, such as measles or varicella. Siber et al[5] recommend an interval between IVIG or IG therapy and vaccine administration of 3 months for immunoglobulin doses below 40 mg/kg, 6 months for doses of 40-80 mg/kg, 8 months for doses of 80-400 mg/kg, and 12 months for large doses (1-2 g/kg).

Late side effects to IG injections are uncommon; however, some patients develop fibrosis of the buttocks or localized subcutaneous atrophy at the site of repeated injections. Repeated injections of IG may also cause elevated mercury levels as a result of the thimerosal preservative. One patient developed symptoms of acrodynia (mercury toxicity) as a result of such therapy.[6]

Slow Subcutaneous Intramuscular or Intravenous Immunoglobulin

As an alternative to IM injections, IG can be given to immunodeficient patients by slow (0.05-0.2 mL/kg per hour) subcutaneous injections. These injections, which can be self-administered into the abdominal wall with the use of a battery-operated pump, are well tolerated and enable patients to receive higher quantities of IG to maintain higher serum IgG levels. This approach is used in several European countries because of the high cost of IVIG. The usual dose is 100 mg/kg per week. This route has been used successfully in immunodeficient patients who have had anaphylactic reactions to IVIG or poor venous access.[7] Gardulf et al[8] shortened the administration time of subcutaneous IG by using a rate of 10 mL per hour with only minimal adverse reactions. UCLA Children's Hospital has used IVIG preparations (10-12%) because IVIG contains no mercury preservative and IM preparations in the United States contain thimerosal.[7]

High-Titered Immune Globulin

High-titered human IGs for IM use are available for the prevention of certain infectious diseases, notably hepatitis B, varicella, rabies, and tetanus, and as an immunosuppressive agent for D-negative individuals exposed to D-positive erythrocytes (see Table 14-1). The indications and doses for each of these products vary considerably and are available elsewhere and in the package inserts.[1]

Three high-titered human IVIGs are also available: cytomegalovirus (CMV)-IVIG, respiratory syncytial virus (RSV)-IVIG, and Rh$_o$ (D)-IVIG (Tables 14-1 and 14-2). CMV-IVIG (CytoGam; MedImmune, Gaithersburg, MD) is used in the posttransplantation period to prevent CMV infection or treat ongoing CMV infection (along with antivirals).[9] RSV-IVIG (RespiGam; MedImmune) is used in high-risk infants (owing, eg, to premature delivery, bronchopulmonary dysplasia, chronic heart and/or lung disease) of less than 2 years, to prevent RSV infection.[10] Rh$_o$ (D)-IVIG (WinRho SD, Cangene, Winnipeg, Canada) is used in the treatment

Table 14-2. Intravenous Immune Globulin (IVIG) Preparations in the United States

Trade Name	Generic	Manufacturer
Standard IVIGs		
Gamimune-N	IVIG	Bayer
Sandoglobulin	IVIG	Sandoz (Novartis)
Gammagard SD	IVIG	Baxter
Polygam SD	IVIG	American Red Cross
Iveegam	IVIG	Immuno-US
Gammar P	IVIG	Centeon
Venoglobulin S	IVIG	Alpha Therapeutics
High-Titered IVIGs		
CytoGam	CMV-IVIG	MedImmune
RespiGam	RSV-IVIG	MedImmune
WinRho SD	RhIG-IVIG	Cangene

of immune thrombocytopenia (ITP) in D-positive individuals.[11] The anti-D coats the erythrocytes, which in turn cause an Fc receptor blockade, thus decreasing the clearance of antibody-coated platelets. Several studies indicate that such therapy is at least as effective as high-dose IVIG therapy in treating ITP.[12]

Intravenous Immune Globulin

IVIG is treated human immune serum globulin that has been rendered free of large-molecular-weight complexes and is thus safe for IV infusion. Several methods to treat Cohn Fraction II have been used to eliminate these complexes: treatment with proteolytic enzymes, ultracentrifugation, reduction of sulfhydryl bonds followed by alkylation, and incubation at low pH. Solvent/detergent treatment or pasteurization is also now used to ensure virus inactivation. Although these additional procedures increase its cost, IVIG has several advantages over intramuscular IG, including that: 1) larger quantities of immunoglobulin (Ig)G can be given, 2) high levels of serum IgG can be achieved rapidly, 3) pain-

ful IM injections are avoided, 4) tissue pooling and local proteolysis are avoided, and 5) self-administration is possible.

The first IVIG produced in the United States in 1981 was Gamimune (Cutter Laboratories, now Bayer Corp, West Haven, CT), a reduced and alkylated 5% solution containing 10% maltose. The second IVIG product was prepared by acidification and treatment with pepsin; the lyophilized powder is reconstituted as a 3, 6, or 12% solution (Sandoglobulin; Sandoz Pharmaceuticals [Novartis], East Hanover, NJ). Since then, several other IVIGs have been introduced by different manufacturers (Table 14-2). Some are 5 or 10% solutions; others are lyophilized powders that are reconstituted as 3-12% solutions.

Although these products vary slightly, they are generally therapeutically equivalent and usually are selected on the basis of cost and convenience. There are minor IgA and IgG subclass differences.[13] Antibody titers may also vary from lot to lot as well as among different IVIGs. Products very low in IgA content, such as Gammagard SD (or Polygam-SD), are used to minimize reactions in selective,

273

antibody-deficient patients with concurrent IgA deficiency or recipients who have IgA antibodies. Profoundly antibody-deficient patients with IgA deficiency can receive IgA-containing Ig products without risk of IgA sensitization. Some patients may not tolerate any IVIG. Premixed liquids have the advantage of convenience because the reconstitution step is not required; however, most liquid forms must be kept refrigerated.

All currently available IVIG products have adequate serum half-lives (15-25 days), a wide spectrum of antibody activity, minimal anticomplementary activity, and are said to be free of bacterial and viral contamination.

Intravenous Immune Globulin in Primary Antibody Deficiencies

IVIG was licensed in 1981 for the treatment of patients with primary and secondary antibody deficiency (Table 14-3). Its use permits much larger doses of IgG to be given so that the IgG level can be normalized (ie, reach trough levels of 500 mg/dL or greater). Several studies have documented the value of these higher doses and indicate collectively that a high dose of IVIG is associated with fewer minor and severe infections, decreased frequency and days of hospitalizations, fewer days of antibiotic therapy, improved pulmonary function, lessened sinus disease, and improved growth and well-being.[13]

Table 14-3. Immunodeficiencies in Which Intravenous Immune Globulin May Be Beneficial

Antibody deficiencies
  X-linked agammaglobulinemia
  Common variable immunodeficiency
  Immunodeficiency with hyper-IgM
  Transient hypogammaglobulinemia of infancy (sometimes)
  IgG subclass deficiency ± IgA deficiency (sometimes)
  Antibody deficiency with normal immunoglobulin levels
Combined deficiencies
  Severe combined immunodeficiencies (all types)
  Wiskott-Aldrich syndrome
  Ataxia-telangiectasia
  Short-limbed dwarfism
  X-linked lymphoproliferative syndrome
Secondary immunodeficiencies
  Malignancies with antibody deficiencies; multiple myeloma, chronic lymphocytic leukemia, other
  Protein-losing enteropathy with hypogammaglobulinemia
  Nephrotic syndrome with hypogammaglobulinemia
  Pediatric-acquired immunodeficiency syndrome
  Intensive care patients—trauma/surgery/shock
  Posttransplantation period
  Burns
  Prematurity

Ig = immunoglobulin

Used with permission from Stiehm ER.[14]

The IVIG dose necessary to achieve serum trough levels of IgG ≥500 mg/dL has been determined. Immediately (within hours) after an infusion, the IgG level increases by 200-300 mg/dL for every 100 mg/kg of IVIG infused.[13] After 3-4 weeks, because of IVIG's half-life of 15-25 days and its redistribution to the tissues, the IgG level has fallen significantly to a trough level of approximately 100 mg/dL higher than the preinfusion level for each 100 mg/kg of IVIG administered. However, the trough level increases gradually with regular high-dose therapy until a steady-state level is achieved after 4-8 months. Because of individual variation in IgG distribution and catabolism, IgG trough levels should be determined at bimonthly intervals for the first 8 months of therapy. Because most antibody-deficient patients have initial IgG levels of less than 200 mg/dL, UCLA Children's Hospital starts infusions at a dose of 400 mg/kg, repeats the dose after 3-7 days, and then gives 400 mg/kg every 28 days. This regimen usually results in a trough level of more than 500 mg/dL after 6-8 months of therapy. These therapeutic guidelines are summarized in Table 14-4.

Practical Considerations

To minimize cost, infusion time, and multiple trips to the clinic or hospital, home infusion, self-administration, and rapid infusion of 10-12% IVIG have been used with safety and efficacy.[15,16] However, this should be done only after several uneventful infusions under medical supervision have been completed and after assurance that individuals giving such therapy are trained in IVIG administration and can recognize and treat side effects. Infusions should never be done without a responsible adult available for assistance. Patients receiving home or self-infusions should have regularly scheduled physician appointments to monitor IgG trough levels and clinical status. Transaminase levels and a complete blood count should be done every 6 months while a patient is on IVIG therapy.[15]

The choice of brand of IVIG usually depends on local availability and cost. The dose, brand, and lot number should be recorded in case of late side effects. Several preparations from different manufacturers are available with different strengths, solvents, and forms (powder or liquid), and they are generally equivalent in antibody content and clini-

---

Table 14-4. Recommendations for the Use of Intravenous Immune Globulin (IVIG) in Primary Antibody Immunodeficiencies

1. Record brand, lot number, dose, infusion rate, and side reactions
2. Maintain the IgG trough levels over 500 mg/dL
3. IgG trough levels gradually increase for 4-8 months on high-dose IVIG therapy
4. For every 100 mg/kg of IVIG given, IgG peak levels increase 200-250 mg/dL and trough levels increase 100 mg/dL (after 28 days)
5. Usual maintenance dose is 400-500 mg/kg every 4 weeks
6. Check IgG trough level every 2 months until stable; then every 6 months
7. Check blood count and liver function tests twice yearly
8. IgG half-life varies in different patients so dosage must be individualized
9. Consider extra doses with infection, stress, and gastrointestinal or genitourinary loss
10. Home infusions, slow subcutaneous infusions, and rapid infusion of 10-12% IVIG can be used for convenience, economy, and shortened administration time in some patients

Used with permission from Stiehm ER.[13]

cal efficacy (Table 14-2). Some patients develop reactions to one brand but can tolerate another preparation. Increased frequency of side effects has been recorded with certain brands.[17]

Side Effects of Intravenous Immune Globulin

The side effects of IVIG administration are summarized in several reviews[18-20] and in Table 14-5. Mild side effects are common and occur in about 10% of infusions. They often can be prevented or modified by the administration of oral aspirin (15 mg/kg/dose) or acetaminophen (15 mg/kg/dose), oral diphenhydramine (Benadryl, Warner-Lambert, Morris Plains, NJ, 1 mg/kg/dose), and/or IV hydrocortisone (6 mg/kg/dose, maxi-

mum 100 mg) 1 hour before infusion.[5] For pr longed infusions in patients with a history of si effects, the premedication can be repeated after hours of infusion.[13]

Many adverse effects are associated with th rapid infusion of large quantities of IVIG, partic larly to nonimmunodeficient subjects who hav autoimmune or inflammatory disease (Table 14-5 The most striking complication is aseptic mening tis occurring within 24 hours of infusion, assoc ated with severe headache, nuchal rigidity, and sp nal fluid pleocytosis.[21-24] A history of migraines h been identified as a risk factor for the developmer of aseptic meningitis.[22] A few cases of aseptic me ingitis with a second infusion[23] have been o served, even when the brand has been switche

Table 14-5. Proven and Possible Side Effects of Intravenous Immune Globulin Administration

Common	Rare (Multiple Reports)	Very Rare (Isolated Reports)	Potential (No Reports)
Chills*	Chest pain or tightness*	Anaphylaxis*	Creutzfeldt-Jakob
Headache*	Dyspnea*	Acrodynia	disease
Backache*	Migraine headaches*	Arthritis	HIV infection
Malaise*	Aseptic meningitis	Thrombosis	
Fever*	Renal failure*	Death	
Pruritis*	Hepatitis C	Direct Coombs' test	
Rash*		Fulminant infection	
Nausea*		Cryoglobulinemia	
Tingling*		Neutropenia	
Hypo- or hypertension*		Alopecia	
Fluid overload*		Uveitis + retinal vasculitis and antineutrophil cytoplasmic antibody	
		Noninfectious hepatitis	
		Hypothermia	
		Pulmonary insufficiency*	
		Desquamation*	

*Personally observed by author.

Used with permission from Stiehm ER.[13]

The duration of meningitis is short, and long-term sequelae are minimal.[24] The etiology of aseptic meningitis is unclear but may relate to osmotic changes within the brain. Of interest is the fact that very few cases of aseptic meningitis have been reported in immunodeficient subjects.

Hepatitis C

Hepatitis C has been reported after the administration of certain lots of IVIG[25-32] and IM Rh immunoglobulin.[33,34] Hepatitis C was first reported after the administration of some experimental lots of IVIG in Sweden,[30] Italy,[28] and the United States.[27] Most cases appeared after hepatitis C antibody-positive patients were excluded from the donor pools (around 1992), suggesting that the presence of hepatitis C antibodies in older lots neutralized the virus in the occasional hepatitis C virus-positive plasma present in the donor pool. Indeed, early preparations of human IG were of some value in the prevention of non-A, non-B (presumably hepatitis C virus) hepatitis.[35] The use of new solvent/detergent treatment and/or pasteurization steps in the manufacture of IVIG and the testing of the product by RNA-polymerase chain reaction for hepatitis C antigen should reduce the risk of transmission of hepatitis C (and other viruses).[24] Excellent reviews are available.[36,37]

Human Immunodeficiency Virus and Creutzfeldt-Jakob Disease

Several lots of IVIG derived from the plasma of subjects at risk for Creutzfeldt-Jakob disease have been recalled by the manufacturer.[38] No cases of Creutzfeldt-Jakob disease have been reported after IVIG infusions.[38] No cases of HIV have been transmitted by IVIG.

Intravenous Immune Globulin in Combined Immunodeficiencies

Many, indeed most, primary T-cell immunodeficiencies have an antibody defect as a component of their immunologic deficiency (Table 14-3). The recommendation for the use of IVIG in these patients is similar to that in primary antibody deficiencies, but its use will, of course, not correct these patients' basic T-cell deficiency. Many children with combined immunodeficiency after successful T-cell reconstitution remain antibody deficient and require lifelong IVIG therapy.

Intravenous Immune Globulin in Secondary Antibody Deficiencies

Many metabolic, hematologic, or infectious illnesses are associated with transient or permanent immunodeficiency.[39] While most secondary immunodeficiencies have a T-cell defect, some of these patients have low serum immunoglobulins, poor antibody responses to antigenic challenge, or low levels of natural antibodies. This may result from the loss of immunoglobulin, the loss of immune cells, or the toxic effect of therapy or infection on the immune system. Table 14-1 includes those diseases and conditions in which secondary antibody deficiencies have been identified. Laboratory criteria in secondary immunodeficiency that support the use of IVIG include 1) significant hypogammaglobulinemia (serum IgG <200 mg/dL or a total immunoglobulin level [IgG + IgM + IgA] <400 mg/dL), 2) absent or low natural antibodies, 3) absent or poor response to antigenic challenge (eg, tetanus, pneumococcal vaccines), and 4) lack of an antibody response to the infecting organism.[40]

Hematologic/Oncologic Diseases

Antibody deficiencies can occur with multiple myeloma, chronic lymphocytic leukemia, lymphoma and advanced cancer. A double-blind multicenter study concluded that the prophylactic infusion of 400 mg/kg of IVIG every 3 weeks reduced the incidence of bacterial infections in adults with chronic lymphocytic leukemia.[41] The treatment group had fewer infections with *Streptococcus pneumoniae* and *Haemophilus influenzae*, but there was no difference in infections caused by other gram-negative bacteria or in fungal or viral infections. This beneficial effect was confirmed in a subsequent study[42] although concerns have been raised about its cost effectiveness.[43] IVIG has also been shown to reduce the incidence of infections in patients with multiple myeloma[44] and in patients with lung cancer who are receiving chemotherapy.[45]

Protein-Losing Enteropathy and Nephrotic Syndrome

Some patients develop antibody deficiency associated with massive proteinuria (nephrosis) or severe diarrhea (protein-losing enteropathy) with accelerated IgG catabolism. Many of these patients have minimal trouble with recurrent infection, given that antibody synthesis is intact and probably accelerated; however, if immunoglobulin loss exceeds the synthetic capacity, severe symptomatic hypogammaglobulinemia may result. IVIG can be used diagnostically in such cases; a large IV infusion, followed by serial measurements of serum IgG level, can document an accelerated IgG half-life (ie, <10 days). Such patients are candidates for IVIG therapy if they have recurrent infections and low IgG levels (<200 mg/dL). Large and repeated doses are necessary. Weekly subcutaneous IVIG has been used in one patient with maintenance of a therapeutic trough level of IgG not achieved by monthly IVIG infusions.[7]

Intensive Care Patients: Trauma/Surgery/Shock

Patients undergoing severe stress associated with trauma or extensive surgery have increased exposure and susceptibility to infection and a broad spectrum of immunodeficiencies, including cutaneous anergy, leukocyte dysfunction, hypogammaglobulinemia, and transiently impaired antibody synthesis.[46-48] Bowel stasis and hypotension may promote gram-negative sepsis and/or endotoxemia with the development of severe and often irreversible shock. Studies by Ziegler et al[48] and Baumgartner et al[50] suggest that when antisera to a mutant J5 *Escherichia coli* endotoxin with antilipid A activity were used in bacteremic and surgical intensive care unit (ICU) patients, the incidence

and severity of severe shock could be reduced. However, Calandra et al[51] used a human IVIG to J5 *E. coli* in 71 patients with gram-negative infections and shock but could not confirm these results. After giving a single infusion of 200 mg/kg and a similar dose of regular IVIG to a control group, they found no difference in mortality, onset of time to shock, or complications.

Just el al[52] used regular IVIG and antibiotics in 50 ICU patients suspected of infection and compared their outcome against that of 54 control patients who received antibiotics alone. Although there was no difference in survival, there was a trend to indicate that the IVIG-antibiotic group had a shortened ICU stay, a shorter period of time necessitating respirator therapy, and improved renal function, and that there was a favorable effect on infection (ie, infections were a less likely cause of death in these patients). A multicenter study of 352 postsurgical patients confirmed the observation that standard IVIG (400 mg/kg at weekly intervals) reduced the incidence of infections and shortened the stay in the ICU compared with that for placebo or hyperimmune core-lipopolysaccharide immunoglobulin-treated patients.[53]

Other studies of IVIG in trauma/surgery patients[46,54] and head trauma patients[55] have shown questionable efficacy. In sum, these studies provide no compelling evidence for the routine use of IVIG in trauma/surgical/ICU patients.

Prematurity

All premature infants have low levels of maternally derived IgG at birth, and most develop IgG levels approaching 100 mg/dL in the first months of life.[56] These IgG levels may be depressed further by pulmonary disease (with IgG transudation into the lung), stress (with increased IgG catabolism), and multiple blood drawing.[57] In addition, their sluggish antibody responses, their concurrent IgM and IgA deficiency, and their immature complement, phagocytic, and T-cell systems make them extraordinarily susceptible to infection.[58] Although the routine use of IG in premature infants has been of doubtful value, the availability of IVIG and the increasing number of surviving premature infants have reawakened interest in the routine use of IVIG in tiny premature infants.

The results of six single-institution controlled studies on the use of IVIG to prevent infection in premature infants are available.[1] Four of the six studies showed a statistically significant benefit in the prevention of sepsis, and two studies showed diminished mortality. On the basis of these encouraging results, four groups undertook larger, multi-center studies.[1] Only one of these studies[59] showed a significant benefit in decreasing bacterial infections but revealed no significant difference in survival or duration of hospitalization.

Thus, the evidence to date supports the National Institutes of Health Consensus Statement (1990) that concluded that IVIG should not be given routinely to infants of low birthweight.[60] A recent meta-analysis suggested a marginal benefit of IVIG given prophylactically to premature infants.[61]

However, IVIG may benefit selected septic newborns who do not respond to antibiotics, particularly in the presence of neutropenia and possibly with the concomitant use of granulocyte colony-stimulating factor or granulocyte-macrophage colony-stimulating factor. The future use of monoclonal antibodies or high-titered IVIGs to specific infectious agents (eg, Group B streptococci) may also be forthcoming.[62] A recent meta-analysis suggested that IVIG was of some benefit in the treatment of newborns with sepsis.[61]

After Transplantation

Conditioning regimens to eliminate or reduce the host's hematopoietic and immune systems during transplantation (marrow and solid organ) render these patients extremely susceptible to infection. The use of IVIG to prevent these infections, particularly sepsis, pneumonia, or gastrointestinal infections, has met with limited success,[63,64] with the exception of preventing complications from CMV infection.

One report did demonstrate some benefit from IVIG infusions in a controlled trial on 382 bone marrow transplant recipients.[65] The study patients received 500 mg/kg IVIG weekly for 90 days, then monthly for 1 year, with a resultant decrease in the number of infections, number of platelet transfusions, and the incidence of graft-vs-host disease. A recent review concluded that IVIG has reduced septicemia, interstitial pneumonia, fatal CMV disease, acute graft-vs-host disease, and transplantation-related mortality in adult recipients of related marrow transplants.[66] Thus, IVIG has been recommended for allogeneic marrow transplant recipients[67,68] but not for autologous transplantation.[69,70]

Burns

Bacterial sepsis, particularly *Pseudomonas* and *E. coli* sepsis, is the leading cause of death in the 300,000 patients hospitalized annually in the United States for burns.[71] These patients develop hypogammaglobulinemia because of protein loss in proportion to the severity of the burn. High-dose IVIG has prolonged survival in experimentally burned mice infected with *Pseudomonas*, and preliminary studies of IG and plasma in human burn patients have been encouraging.[72-74] IVIG with high titers against *Pseudomonas* has been prepared and is under evaluation; proof of efficacy is lacking.[75]

Intravenous Immune Globulin in Infection

Cytomegalovirus Infection

IVIG or enriched IVIG (CMV-IVIG, CytoGam) has proved of benefit in treating symptomatic CMV infection in transplantation patients and in preventing infection in CMV-negative recipients. In combination with ganciclovir, IVIG may be more efficacious than either drug alone in treating established CMV infections in marrow transplantation recipients.[76] Other studies have shown some benefit of IVIG in preventing symptomatic CMV infection in CMV-negative kidney[77] and liver transplantation recipients.[78] The optimal dose and dose scheduling regimens for CMV-IVIG are yet to be established, but they likely will be high, frequent, and expensive. Furthermore, the increasing use of ganciclovir in prevention has decreased dramatically the need for IVIG in CMV infection.

Other Herpes Viruses

IVIG has been used in chronic Epstein-Barr virus (EBV) infection and in patients with X-linked lymphoproliferative syndrome to prevent EBV infection.[79] However, controlled studies are lacking, and one report described an initially seronegative college student with this syndrome who died from overwhelming EBV infection while receiving monthly IVIG prophylaxis.[80] IVIG can also be used prophylactically in immunodeficient patients after exposure to varicella-zoster infection if varicella-zoster immune globulin is unavailable.[81]

Human Immunodeficiency Virus Infections

The rationale for the use of IVIG in HIV-infected patients includes their increased susceptibility to common bacterial infections (particularly in children) and the increased incidence of HIV-induced ITP. A large National Institutes of Health double-blind, placebo-controlled study confirmed that IVIG was effective in preventing infections in HIV-infected children with CD4 counts greater than 200 cells/mm^3.[82] Infections were less frequent, and more patients were free of infection longer in the treatment group than in the placebo group; however, there was no difference in survival between the two groups. In a continuation of this study, the placebo group was allowed to cross over to receive IVIG, with a subsequent drop in the rate of serious infections and hospitalizations.[83] IVIG is less effective in preventing infection if the HIV-infected children receive continuous trimethoprim-sulfamethoxazole prophylaxis for *Pneumocystis carinii* pneumonia.[84]

Parvovirus Infections

Parvovirus B19 can cause aplastic anemia in sickle cell anemia and in immunodeficiency patients. High-dose IVIG can cure parvovirus B19 infection with reversal of the anemia.[85]

Respiratory Syncytial Virus Infections

RSV causes considerable morbidity in very young children, premature infants, and children with pre-existing pulmonary, cardiac, or immune disease. A multicenter study that used RSV-IVIG in high-risk infants (eg, those with bronchopulmonary dysplasia, congenital heart disease, or prematurity) was conducted comparing high-dose (750 mg/kg/month) vs low-dose (150 mg/kg/month) vs no treatment in the prevention of RSV infection. The high-dose group experienced fewer lower-respiratory-tract infections, fewer hospitalizations, fewer hospital days, fewer days in the neonatal ICU, and less use of the antiviral drug ribavirin than the low-dose or placebo groups.[10] RSV-IVIG (Respi-Gam, MedImmune) was licensed by the Food and Drug Administration in January 1996.

Other Respiratory Virus Infections

IVIG contains antibodies against numerous respiratory viruses, including adenovirus, influenza, and parainfluenza viruses. Although IVIG has been used to prevent or treat these respiratory infections, proof of efficacy is lacking. Lack of standardized or high-titered products makes it difficult to evaluate the effectiveness of treatment. Furthermore, as in other viral infections, IVIG is unlikely to eradicate entrenched infections.

Bacterial Infections

Passive immunity for bacterial infections or toxins has been used for nearly a century.[86] In the preantibiotic era, antiserum was used for whooping cough and bacterial meningitis (*Haemophilus influenzae* and *Neisseria meningitides*). Antitoxin is still necessary in infections that produce toxins (eg, diphtheria and tetanus).[1] Effective vaccines and antibiotics have diminished the need for passive immunity. Nevertheless, there are certain clinical situations in which IVIG or hyperimmune IVIG may be useful; these include toxic shock syndrome, gram-negative sepsis, and *Pseudomonas* infections. However, improved products and conrolled studies are required. IVIG has been used in the pulmonary infections of cystic fibrosis with transient benefit.[87]

Intravenous Immune Globulin as an Immunomodulator

High-dose IVIG has immunosuppressive and anti-inflammatory effects that make it a valuable agent in the treatment of several autoimmune or inflammatory disorders[88] (Table 14-6). High-dose IVIG (1-2 g/kg/wk) may work by the following mechanisms:

1. It inhibits antibody synthesis (eg, ITP), (possibly by a direct effect on proliferating B cells).
2. It combines directly with autoimmune antibodies (eg, Factor VIII autoantibody) (because it contains idiotypic antibodies).
3. It blocks the uptake of antibody-coated cells in the spleen and liver (eg, ITP) (through an Fc receptor blockade of antibody-dependent cellular cytotoxicity).
4. It down regulates immune activation by decreasing inflammatory cytokine release or action (eg, Kawasaki syndrome).
5. It combines with bacterial superantigens that may be present in certain inflammatory disorders (eg, toxic shock syndrome).
6. It inhibits complement-mediated tissue injury (eg, dermatomyositis).

The best-documented uses of high-dose IVIG as an immunoregulator are in the treatment of Kawasaki syndrome and ITP. In most other disorders, the reports of efficacy are based on small, uncontrolled studies or case studies, as shown in Table 14-6. Some guidelines for the use of IVIG as an immunomodulator are given in Table 14-7.

Intravenous Immune Globulin in Kawasaki Syndrome

Kawasaki syndrome is an acute, inflammatory febrile childhood disorder of unknown cause. Generalized vasculitis is common, but coronary artery obstruction or aneurysm can cause long-term morbidity and, on occasion, death. The major goal

---

Table 14-6. Uses of Human Intravenous Immunoglobulin in Inflammatory and Autoimmune Disorders

Proven benefit*
 Kawasaki syndrome
 Immune thrombocytopenic purpura
 Guillain-Barré syndrome
 Dermatomyositis
 Chronic inflammatory demyelinating
  polyneuropathy
Probable benefit[†]
 Neonatal isoimmune or autoimmune
  thrombocytopenic purpura
 Postinfectious thrombocytopenic purpura
 Immune neutropenia (including neonatal)
 Autoimmune hemolytic anemia
 Myasthenia gravis
 Multifocal motor neuropathy
Possible benefit[‡]
 Anticardiolipin antibody syndrome
 Toxic shock syndrome
 Coagulopathy with Factor VIII inhibitor
 Bullous pemphigoid
 Churg-Strauss vasculitides
 Other types of vasculitis
 Graves' ophthalmopathy
 Multiple sclerosis
Unproven benefit[§]
 Intractable epilepsy
 Steroid-dependent asthma
 Eczema (atopic dermatitis)
 Juvenile rheumatoid arthritis
 Lupus erythematosus
 Recurrent abortion
 Hemolytic-uremic syndrome
 Viral myocarditis
 Chronic fatigue syndrome
 Rasmussen's encephalitis
 Sydenham's chorea
 Type I diabetes mellitus
 Inflammatory bowel disease
 Infantile autism

---

*Controlled studies show efficacy.

[†]Several case reports or uncontrolled studies are convincing.

[‡]Preliminary studies are encouraging but incomplete.

[§]Preliminary studies are limited or equivocal.

Modified from Stiehm ER.[13]

Table 14-7. Guidelines for Intravenous Immune Globulin (IVIG) Use as an Immunomodulator

---

1. Illnesses for possible treatment: a) noninfectious fever or inflammation, b) evidence of immune activation (eg, cytokines, activated T cells), etiology not understood, d) prior response to corticosteroids or plasmapheresis.
2. Large IVIG dose is needed (eg, 2 g/kg over 1-5 days).
3. IVIG side effects (eg, fluid overload, aseptic meningitis, etc, should be watched for [see Table 14-5]).
4. Patient may require treatment in 3-6 weeks.
5. No particular IVIG brand is more effective than another.
6. Therapeutic goals (eg, objective clinical improvement, decreased dose of steroids or other drugs, normalization of laboratory tests, etc) should be identified before therapy.
7. Proof of benefit requires dramatic clinical response or a double-blind, controlled study.
8. Treatment failure should be considered if no response is seen after 3 months or 5 treatments.

---

of therapy is to reduce the rate of coronary artery disease. IVIG was initially shown to reduce coronary artery complications and to shorten the febrile period.[89] A large US multicenter study compared aspirin alone with high-dose IVIG (400 mg/kg/day for 4 days) plus aspirin.[90] The IVIG-aspirin combination was superior to aspirin alone in preventing coronary artery abnormalities. A subsequent controlled study showed that a single 2 g/kg dose of IVIG was superior to four daily 400 mg/kg doses (with both groups receiving aspirin) in reducing the rate of coronary artery disease.[91] Thus, current optimal treatment includes a single, high-dose of IVIG (1-2 g/kg) together with aspirin.

Intravenous Immune Globulin in Immune Thrombocytopenic Purpura

High-dose IVIG (1-2 g over 1-4 days) rapidly reverses the thrombocytopenia in pediatric patients with acute ITP, probably by interfering with the reticuloendothelial uptake of antibody-coated plate-

lets.[92] It is at least as effective as corticostero[l] therapy and has a more rapid onset of action. B[e]cause acute ITP in children is a self-limiting diso[r]der, IVIG probably does not affect the basic cause [of] the disease nor decrease the likelihood of chron[ic] ITP. Although IVIG is less effective in chronic ITP, [it] may be of special value in such cases for the shor[t] term correction of thrombocytopenia during eme[r]gencies.[92] Other forms of immune thromboc[y]topenia have been managed with IVIG, includi[ng] postinfectious thrombocytopenia, the thromboc[y]topenia of acquired immune deficiency syndrom[e], and autoimmune and isoimmune thromboc[y]topenia of newborns. IVIG also has been used [in] the treatment of immune neutropenia and autoi[m]mune hemolytic anemia.[39,88,94]

Intravenous Immune Globulin in Guillain-Barré Syndrome

IVIG is effective in the treatment of Guillain-Bar[ré] syndrome, possibly by interfering with the synth[e]sis of neuronal antibodies. A large Dutch stud[y] compared plasmapheresis with IVIG in moderately to severely affected adult patients.[95] Both treatment groups improved, but those treated with IVIG responded faster and had greater improvement. Because IVIG is much easier to use and less expensive than plasmapheresis, a trial of IVIG should be used before plasmapheresis is undertaken.

Intravenous Immune Globulin in Dermatomyositis

Dermatomyositis is an autoimmune, inflammatory disease of muscles, small blood vessels, and skin. A recent small double-blind, placebo-controlled study involving 15 patients (ages 18-55 years) with treatment-resistant disease concluded that IVIG was safe and effective in treating dermatomyositis.[96]

Other Diseases

IVIG has been used in a number of neurologic disorders. It has been of particular value in myasthenia gravis[97] and chronic inflammatory demyelinating polyneuropathy.[98] IVIG has also been used in chronic fatigue syndrome, multiple sclerosis, Sydenham's chorea, and other neurologic disorders with equivocal results.[39,88,94]

High-dose IVIG has been used in systemic lupus erythematosus and juvenile rheumatoid arthritis with mixed results.[39] IVIG was used in a patient with Churg-Strauss syndrome (pulmonary vasculitis) with anecdotal benefit.[99] Patients with bullous pemphigoid, a skin disease characterized by epidermal antibodies, improved with high-dose IVIG.[39]

IVIG has been used in women with recurrent spontaneous abortions,[100] although a therapeutic effect could not be verified in a randomized, double-blind, multicenter trial in comparison with 5% human albumin, which was used as a placebo.[101] IVIG has been used in asthma and eczema without proven efficacy.

Special Preparations for Noninfectious Use

Rho (D) Immune Globulin

Intramuscular Rho (D) Immune Globulin (RhIG) is a high-titer, human anti-D immune serum globulin used in the prevention of Rh hemolytic disease of newborns. It is given to D-negative mothers at 28 weeks of gestation and after the delivery of an D-positive infant, after a miscarriage or abortion, or when feto-maternal hemorrhage is documented to occur during pregnancy. It should also be used after the transfusion of a D-negative individual with D-positive cellular blood components. Rho (D) Immune Globulin Intravenous (WinRho; Cangene) has been used successfully in the treatment of ITP in Rh-positive individuals.[11,12] Salama and Mueller-Eckhardt[102] proposed that the anti-D coats red cells, which in turn cause reticuloendothelial blockade, similar to the effect of high-dose IVIG in this disorder. The use of RhIG to prevent hemolytic disease of the newborn has been recently addressed in the American Association of Blood Banks Association Bulletin 98-2 (Appendix 14-1).

Immunosuppressive Antibodies

Three antibodies—a mouse monoclonal antibody directed against CD3 T lymphocytes (OKT3-Muromonab; Ortho Biotech, Raritan, NJ), a humanized immune monoclonal antibody against CD25 on activated lymphocytes (Zenapak-Daclimizumab; Roche, Branchburg, NJ), and a polyclonal equine antithymocyte globulin (Atgam; Upjohn, Kalamazoo, MI)—are available for immunosuppression, particularly for transplantation procedures.

Digoxin Antibody

An ovine (sheep) antibody fragment (Fab portion of IgG) that binds to digoxin and digitoxin (Digibind; Burroughs Wellcome, Research Triangle Park, NC) is valuable in the treatment of digitalis toxicity or overdose by accidental ingestion. Fragmentation of the antibody results in rapid catabolism; after IV infusion of the fragment, it combines with the drug and removes it rapidly from the serum.

Immunoglobulin Use by Unusual Routes

The administration of immune globulin orally to provide antimicrobial activity to the gastrointestinal tract mimics the action of antibody-rich colostrum and breast milk. In humans, little or no ingested immune globulin is absorbed intact into the systemic circulation. Some oral immune globulin traverses the entire gastrointestinal tract undigested, particularly in premature infants.[103] Oral immune globulin may neutralize microorganisms, inhibit their colonization, and prevent their attachment to the gastrointestinal mucosa.

Oral Immunoglobulin

Barnes et al[104] fed either human immune globulin for 7 days or a placebo to premature infants in a nursery in which rotavirus was endemic. Rotavirus-associated diarrhea developed in six of the 11 infants given placebo and in one of the 14 given oral immune globulin. The prevention of rotavirus also has been reported with oral cow colostrum and infant formula supplemented with bovine antibodies. Losonsky et al[105] used oral human immune globulin successfully to interrupt the excretion of rotavirus in immunodeficient patients chronically infected with rotavirus.

Eibl et al[106] were able to prevent necrotizing enterocolitis in all 90 infants given oral immune globulin rich in serum IgA; there were six cases, however, among 91 control infants. Bovine colostrum has been used successfully to treat cryptosporidia diarrhea in HIV-infected patients. Borowitz and Saulsbury[107] used oral immune globulin to successfully treat cryptosporidia infection in a child with acute leukemia.

Aerosolized and Intrathecal Immune Globulin

Human immunoglobulin has been used intrathecally in the treatment of viral encephalomyelitis in antibody deficiency.[108] Tetanus antitoxin has been used intrathecally with questionable benefit.[1] IVIG has been used as a respiratory aerosol in RSV infection.[109]

Future Directions

Several high-titered human immune globulins are being tested for clinical efficacy; these include a group B streptococcal IVIG (for premature infants), a bacterial polysaccharide immune globulin (for high-risk infants), a *Pseudomonas* IVIG (for burn patients), and an HIV IVIG (for HIV treatment and prevention).

The use of monoclonal antibodies, both human and murine, to treat specific infections should be forthcoming. These monoclonal antibodies may be used alone or added to polyvalent IVIG to increase the titer to a specific microorganism. The use of monoclonal antibodies to neutralize cells, bind to receptors, and detoxify certain drugs will also be forthcoming. Monoclonal idiotypic antibodies also may be used to suppress autoimmune disease or inhibit a specific harmful autoantibody. The use of monoclonal antibodies directed to specific tumor cells or organs to deliver radioisotopes or chemotherapeutic agents has been shown to be feasible. Such antibodies also could be used diagnostically for tumor cell or infection localization.

Chimeric antibodies containing the antigen-reactive site of a mouse monoclonal antibody attached to the constant regions of a human antibody can be made, and two are commercially available (Table 14-1). These humanized monoclonals are less antigenic, have a longer half-life, and have better complement-fixation ability than the intact mouse monoclonal antibody. Finally, engineered antibodies, made by DNA recombinational techniques from selected light and heavy chain genes, may permit the synthesis of high-titered therapeutic antibodies.[110]

References

1. Stiehm ER. Passive immunization. In: Feigin R, Cherry JD, eds. Textbook of pediatric in

fectious diseases. 4th ed. Philadelphia: WB Saunders Co., 1997:2769-802.

2. American Academy of Pediatrics. Active and passive immunization. In: Peter G, ed. 1997 red book: Report of the Committee on Infectious Diseases. Elk Grove Village, IL: American Academy of Pediatrics, 1997:1-68.

3. Medical Research Council Working Party. Hypogammaglobulinemia in the United Kingdom. Lancet 1969;1:163-9.

4. Conley ME, Stiehm ER. Immunodeficiency disorders: General considerations. In: Stiehm ER, ed. Immunologic disorders in infants and children. 4th ed. Philadelphia: WB Saunders Co., 1996:201-52.

5. Siber GR, Werner BG, Halsey NA, et al. Interference of immune globulin with measles and rubella immunization. J Pediatr 1993; 122:204-11.

6. Matheson DS, Clarkson TW, Gelfand EW. Mercury toxicity (acrodynia) induced by long-term injection of gamma globulin. J Pediatr 1980;97:153-5.

7. Stiehm ER, Casillas AM, Finkelstein JZ, et al. Slow subcutaneous human intravenous immune globulin (IVIG) in the treatment of antibody immunodeficiency: Use of an old method with a new product. J Allergy Clin Immunol 1998;101:848-9.

8. Gardulf A, Anderson V, Bjorkander J, et al. Subcutaneous immunoglobulin replacement in patients with primary antibody deficiencies: Safety and costs. Lancet 1995;345:365-9.

9. Bowden RA, Sayers M, Flournoy N, et al. Cytomegalovirus immune globulin and seronegative blood products to prevent primary cytomegalovirus infection after marrow transplantation. N Engl J Med 1986;314:1006-10.

10. Meissner HC, Welliver RC, Chartrand SA, et al. Prevention of respiratory syncytial virus infection in high risk infants: Consensus opinion on the role of immunoprophylaxis with respiratory syncytial virus hyperimmune globulin. Pediatr Infect Dis J 1996;15:1059-68.

11. Andrew M, Blanchette VS, Adams M, et al. A multicenter study of the treatment of childhood chronic idiopathic thrombocytopenic purpura with anti-D. J Pediatr 1992;120:522-7.

12. Scaradavou A, Woo B, Woloski BM, et al. Intravenous anti-D treatment of immune thrombocytopenic purpura: Experience in 272 patients. Blood 1997;89:2689-700.

13. Stiehm ER. Human intravenous immunoglobulin in primary and secondary antibody deficiencies. Pediatr Infect Dis J 1997;16:696-707.

14. Stiehm ER. Recent progress in the use of intravenous immunoglobulins. Curr Probl Pediatr 1992;22:337.

15. Kobayashi RH, Kobayashi AD, Lee N, et al. Home self-administration of intravenous immunoglobulin therapy in children. Pediatrics 1990;85:705-9.

16. Schiff RI, Sedlak D, Buckley RH. Rapid infusion of Sandoglobulin in patients with primary humoral immunodeficiency. J Allergy Clin Immunol 1991;88:61-7.

17. Rosenfeld EA, Schulman ST, Corydon KE, et al. Comparative safety and efficacy of two immune globulin products in Kawasaki disease. J Pediatr 1995;126:1000-3.

18. Misbah SA, Chapel HM. Adverse effects of intravenous immunoglobulin. Drug Saf 1993;9:254-62.

19. Buckley RH, Schiff RI. The use of intravenous immune globulin in immunodeficiency diseases. N Engl J Med 1991;325:110-7.

20. Duhem C, Dicato MA, Ries F. Side-effects of intravenous immune globulins. Clin Exp Immunol 1994;97(Suppl 1):79-83.

21. Kata E, Shindo S, Eto Y, et al. Administration of immune globulin associated with aseptic meningitis. JAMA 1988;259:3269-70.

22. Sekul EA, Cupler EJ, Dalakas MC. Aseptic meningitis associated with high-dose intravenous immunoglobulin therapy: Frequency and risk factors. Ann Intern Med 1994;121:259-62.

23. Scribner CL, Kapit RM, Phillips ET, et al. Aseptic meningitis and intravenous immunoglobulin therapy. Ann Intern Med 1994;121: 305-6.

24. Brannagan TH, Nagle KJ, Lange DJ, et al. Complications of intravenous immune globulin treatment in neurologic disease. Neurology 1996;47:674-7.

25. Schiff RI. Transmission of viral infections through intravenous immune globulin. N Engl J Med 1994;331:1649-50.

26. Lever AM, Webster AD, Brown D, et al. Non-A, non-B hepatitis occurring in agammaglobulinaemic patients after intravenous immunoglobulin. Lancet 1964;2:1062-4.

27. Ochs H, Fisher SH, Virant FS, et al. Non-A, non-B hepatitis and intravenous immunoglobulin. Lancet 1965;1:404-5.

28. Trepo C, Hantz O, Vitvitaki L. Non-A, non-B hepatitis after intravenous gammaglobulin. Lancet 1966;1:322.

29. Bjorklander J, Cunningham-Rundles C, Lundin P, et al. Intravenous immunoglobulin prophylaxis causing liver damage in 16 of 77 patients with hypogammaglobulinemia or IgG subclass deficiency. Am J Med 1988;84: 107-11.

30. Bjoro K, Froland SS, Yun Z, et al. Hepatitis C infection in patients with primary hypogammaglobulinemia after treatment with contaminated immune globulin. N Engl J Med 1994;331:607-11.

31. Centers for Disease Control. Outbreak of hepatitis C associated with intravenous immunoglobulin administration: United States, October 1993-June 1994. MMWR 1994;43:505-9.

32. Taliani G, Guerra E, Rosso R, et al. Hepatitis C virus infection in hypogammaglobulinemic patients receiving long-term replacement therapy with intravenous immunoglobulin. Transfusion 1995;35:103-7.

33. Meisel H, Reip A, Faltus B, et al. Transmission of hepatitis C virus to children and husbands by women infected with contaminated anti-D immunoglobulin. Lancet 1995; 345:1209-11.

34. Power JP, Lawlor E, Davidson F, et al. Molecular epidemiology of an outbreak of infection with hepatitis C virus in recipients of anti-D immunoglobulin. Lancet 1995;345:1211-3.

35. Sanchez Quijano A, Pireda JA, Lissen E, et al. Prevention of posttransfusion non-A, non-B hepatitis by nonspecific immunoglobulin in heart surgery. Lancet 1988;1:1245-9.

36. Jonas MM, Baron MJ, Bresee JS, et al. Clinical and virologic features of hepatitis C virus infection associated with intravenous immunoglobulin. Pediatrics 1996;98:211-5.

37. Slade HB. Human immunoglobulins for intravenous use and hepatitis C viral transmission. Clin Diagn Lab Immunol 1994;1:613-9.

38. Food and Drug Administration. Revised precautionary measures to reduce the possible risk of transmission of Creutzfeldt-Jakob disease (CJD) by blood and blood products (letter). December 11, 1996. Rockville, MD: Office of Communications, Training and Manufacturers Assistance, 1996.

39. Dickler HB, Gelfand EW. Current perspectives on the use of intravenous immunoglobulin. Adv Intern Med 1996;41:641-80.

40. Stiehm ER. Use of immunoglobulinemia in secondary anti-body deficiencies. In: Imbach P, ed. Immunotherapy with intravenous immunoglobulins. London: Academic Press, 1991:115-26.

41. Cooperative Group for the Study of Immunoglobulin in Chronic Lymphocytic Leukemia. Intravenous immunoglobulin for the prevention of infection in chronic lymphocytic leukemia. N Engl J Med 1988;319:902-7.

42. Gamm H, Huber CH, Chapel H, et al. Intravenous immune globulin in chronic lymphocytic leukemia. Clin Exp Immunol 1994;97 (Suppl):17-20.

43. Weeks JC, Tierney MR, Weinstein MC. Cost-effectiveness of prophylactic intravenous immune globulin in chronic lymphocytic leukemia. N Engl J Med 1991;325:81-6.

44. Chapel HM, Lee M, Hargreaves R, et al. Randomized trial of intravenous immunoglobulin as prophylaxis against infection in

plateau-phase multiple myeloma. Lancet 1994;343:1059-63.

45. Schmidt RE, Harlapp JH, Niese D, et al. Reduction of infection frequency by intravenous gammaglobulins during intensive induction therapy for small cell carcinoma of the lung. Infection 1984;12:167-70.

46. Glinz W, Grob PVJ, Nydegger UE, et al. Polyvalent immunoglobulins for prophylaxis of bacterial infections in patients following multiple trauma. Intensive Care Med 1985;11:288-94.

47. Munster AM. Infections in burns. In: Morell A, Nydegger UE, eds. Clinical use of intravenous immunoglobulins. New York: Academic Press, 1986:339-44.

48. Wilson NW, Ochs HD, Peterson B, et al. Abnormal primary antibody responses in pediatric trauma patients. J Pediatr 1989;115:424-7.

49. Ziegler EJ, McCutchan JA, Fierer J, et al. Treatment of gram-negative bacteremia and shock with human antiserum to a mutant Escherichia coli. N Engl J Med 1982;307:1225-30.

50. Baumgartner JD, Glauser MP, McCutchan JA, et al. Prevention of gram-negative shock and death in surgical patients by antibody to endotoxin core glycolipid. Lancet 1985;2:59-63.

51. Calandra T, Glauser MP, Schellekens J, et al. Treatment of gram-negative septic shock with human IgG antibody to Escherichia coli J5: A prospective, double-blind, randomized trial. J Infect Dis 1988;158:312-9.

52. Just HM, Voge W, Metzger M, et al. Treatment of intensive care unit patients with severe nosocomial infection. In: Morell A, Nydegger UE, eds. Clinical use of intravenous immunoglobulins. New York: Academic Press, 1986:346-52.

53. The Intravenous Immunoglobulin Collaborative Study Group. Prophylactic intravenous administration of standard immune globulin as compared with core-lipopolysaccharide immune globulin in patients at high risk of postsurgical infection. N Engl J Med 1992;327:234-40.

54. DeSimone C, Delogu G, Corbetta G. Intravenous immunoglobulins in association with antibiotics: A therapeutic trial in septic intensive care unit patients. Crit Care Med 1988;16:23-6.

55. Gooding AM, Bastian JF, Peterson BM, et al. Safety and efficacy of intravenous immunoglobulin prophylaxis in pediatric trauma patients: A double-blind controlled trial. J Crit Care 1993;4:212-6.

56. Ballow M, Cates KL, Rowe JC, et al. Development of the immune system in very low birth weight (less than 1500 g) premature infants: Concentrations of plasma immunoglobulins and patterns of infections. Pediatr Res 1986;20:899-904.

57. Ruderman JW, Peter JB, Gall RC, et al. Prevention of hypogammaglobulinemia of prematurity with intravenous immune globulin. J Perinatol 1988;10:150-5.

58. Wilson CB, Lewis DB, Penix LA. The physiologic immunodeficiency of immaturity. In: Stiehm ER, ed. Immunologic disorders in infants and children. 4th ed. Philadelphia: WB Saunders, 1996:253-95.

59. Baker CJ, Melish ME, Hall RT, et al. Intravenous immune globulin for the prevention of nosocomial infection in low-birth-weight neonates. N Engl J Med 1992;327:213-9.

60. National Institutes of Health Consensus Development Conference. Diseases, doses, recommendations for intravenous immunoglobulin. HLB Newslett Natl Inst Heart Lung Blood Dis 1990;6:73-8.

61. Jenson HB, Pollock BH. Meta-analyses of the effectiveness of intravenous immune globulin for prevention and treatment of neonatal sepsis. Pediatrics,1997;99:e2.

62. Hill HR. Intravenous immunoglobulin use in the neonate: Role in prophylaxis and therapy of infection. Pediatr Infect Dis J 1993;12:549-59.

63. Graham-Pole J, Camitta B, Casper J, et al. Intravenous immunoglobulin may lessen all

forms of infection in patients receiving allogeneic bone marrow transplantation for acute lymphoblastic leukemia: A Pediatric Oncology Group Study. Bone Marrow Transplant 1988;84:632-9.

64. Sullivan KM. Immunoglobulin therapy in bone marrow transplantation. Am J Med 1987; 83(Suppl 4A):34-5.

65. Sullivan KM. Intravenous immune globulin prophylaxis in recipients of a marrow transplant. J Allergy Clin Immunol 1989;84:632-9.

66. Sullivan KM, Kopecky KJ, Jocom J, et al. Immunomodulatory and antimicrobial efficacy of intravenous immunoglobulin in bone marrow transplantation. N Engl J Med 1990; 323:705-12.

67. Keller T, McGrath J, Newland A, et al. Indications for use of intravenous immunoglobulin: Recommendations of the Australian Society of Blood Transfusion Consensus Symposium. Med J Aust 1993;159:204-6.

68. Rowe JM, Cioganu N, Ascensao J, et al. Recommended guidelines for the management of autologous and allogeneic bone marrow transplantation. Ann Intern Med 1994;120:143-58.

69. Guglielmo BJ, Wong-Beringer A, Linker CA. Immune globulin therapy in allogeneic bone marrow transplant: A critical review. Bone Marrow Transplant 1994;13:499-510.

70. Wolff SN, Fay JW, Herzig RH, et al. High-dose weekly intravenous immunoglobulin to prevent infections in patients undergoing autologous bone marrow transplantation or severe myelosuppressive therapy: A study of the American Bone Marrow Transplant Group. Ann Intern Med 1993;118:937-42.

71. Munster AM. Immunologic response of trauma and burns. An overview. Am J Med 1984; 76:142-5.

72. Jones RJ, Roe EA, Gupta JL. Controlled trial of *Pseudomonas* immunoglobulin and vaccine in burn patients. Lancet 1980;2:1263-5.

73. Kafalides NA, Arana JA, Gazan A, et al. Role of infection in mortality from severe burns: Evaluation of plasma, gamma globulin, albumin, and saline solution therapy in a group of Peruvian children. N Engl J Med 1962;267:317-23.

74. Shirani KZ, Vaughan GM, McManus AT, et al. Replacement therapy with modified immunoglobulin G in burn patients: Preliminary kinetic studies. Am J Med 1984;76:175-80.

75. Pollack M. Antibody activity against *Pseudomonas aeruginosa* in immune globulins prepared for intravenous use in humans. J Infect Dis 1983;147:1090-8.

76. Winston DJ. Intravenous immunoglobulins as therapeutic agents: Use in viral infections. Ann Intern Med 1987;107:367-82.

77. Steinmuller DR, Graneto D, Swift C, et al. Use of intravenous immunoglobulin prophylaxis for primary cytomegalovirus infection post living-related-donor renal transplantation. Transplant Proc 1989;21:2069-71.

78. Bell R, Shei A, McDonald JA, et al. The role of CMV immune prophylaxis in patients at risk for primary CMV infection following orthoptic liver transplantation. Transplant Proc 1989;21:3781-2.

79. Tobi M, Strauss SE. Chronic Epstein-Barr virus disease: A workshop held by the National Institute of Allergy and Infectious Diseases. Ann Intern Med 1985;103:951-3.

80. Okano M, Pirruccello SJ, Grierson HL, et al. Immunovirological studies of fatal infectious mononucleosis in a patient with X-linked lymphoproliferative syndrome treated with intravenous immunoglobulin and inter- feron-a. Clin Immunol Immunopathol 1990;54:410-8.

81. Paryani SG, Arvin AM, Koropchak CM, et al. Comparison of varicella-zoster antibody titers in patients given intravenous immune serum globulin or varicella-zoster immune globulin. J Pediatr 1984;105:200-5.

82. The National Institute of Child Health and Human Development Intravenous Immunoglobulin Study Group. Intravenous immune globulin for the prevention of bacterial infections in children with symptomatic human

immunodeficiency virus infection. N Engl J Med 1991;325:73-80.

83. Mofenson LM, Moye J, Korelitz J, et al. Cross-over of placebo patients to intravenous immunoglobulin confirms efficacy for prophylaxis of bacterial infections and reduction of hospitalization in human immunodeficiency virus-infected children. Pediatr Infect Dis J 1994;13:477-84.

84. Spector SA, Gelber RD, McGrath N, et al. A controlled trial of intravenous immune globulin for the prevention of serious bacterial infections in children receiving zidovudine for advanced human immunodeficiency virus infection. N Engl J Med 1994;331: 1181-7.

85. Kurtzman G, Frickhofen N, Kimball J, et al. Pure red cell aplasia of 10 years duration due to persistent parvovirus B19 infection and its cure with immunoglobulin treatment. N Engl J Med 1989;321:519-23.

86. Casadevall A, Scharff MD. Return to the past: The case for antibody-based therapies in infectious diseases. Clin Infect Dis 1995;21: 150-61.

87. Winnie GB, Cowan RG, Wade NA. Intravenous immune globulin treatment of pulmonary exacerbations in cystic fibrosis. J Pediatr 1989;114:309-14.

88. Ballow M. Mechanisms of action of intravenous immune serum globulin in autoimmune and inflammatory diseases. J Allergy Clin Immunol 1997;100:151-7.

89. Furusho K, Nakano H, Shinomya K, et al. High-dose intravenous immunoglobulins for Kawasaki disease. Lancet 1984;2:1055-8.

90. Newburger JW, Takahashi M, Burns JC, et al. The treatment of Kawasaki syndrome with intravenous gammaglobulin. N Engl J Med 1986;315:341-7.

91. Newburger JW, Takahashi M, Beiser AS, et al. A single intravenous infusion of gamma-globulin as compared with 4 infusions in the treatment of acute Kawasaki syndrome. N Engl J Med 1991;324:1633-9.

92. Imbach T, D'Apuzzo V, Hirt A. High-dose intravenous gammaglobulin for idiopathic thrombocytopenic purpura in childhood. Lancet 1981;1:1228-31.

93. Bussel JB, Pham LC. Intravenous treatment with gammaglobulin in adults with immune thrombocytopenic purpura: Review of the literature. Vox Sang 1987;52:206-12.

94. Mobini N, Sarela A, Ahmed AR. Intravenous immunoglobulins in the therapy of autoimmune and systemic inflammatory disorders. Ann Allergy Asthma Immunol 1995;74:119-28.

95. VanDerMeche FG, Schmitz PI. A randomized trial comparing intravenous immunoglobulin and plasma exchange in Guillain-Barré syndrome. N Engl J Med 1992;326: 1123-9.

96. Dalakas MC, Illa I, Dambrosia JM, et al. A controlled trial of high-dose intravenous immune globulin infusions as treatment for dermatomyositis. N Engl J Med 1993;329:1993-2000.

97. Arsura E. Experience with intravenous immunoglobulin in myasthenia gravis. Clin Immunol Immunopathol 1989;53:S170-9.

98. Faed JM, Day B, Pollock M, et al. High-dose intravenous human immunoglobulin in chronic inflammatory demyelineating polyneuropathy. Neurology 1989;39:422-5.

99. Hamilos DL, Christensen J. Treatment of Churg-Strauss syndrome with high-dose intravenous immunoglobulin. J Allergy Clin Immunol 1991;88:823-4.

100. Coulam C, Peters A, MacIntyre J, et al. The use of IVIG for the treatment of recurrent spontaneous abortion. In: Imbach P, ed. Immunotherapy with intravenous immunoglobulins. London: Academic Press 1991: 394-400.

101. Heine O, Mueller-Eckhardt G. Intravenous immune globulin in recurrent abortion. Clin Exp Immunol 1994;97(Suppl 1):39-42.

102. Salama A, Mueller-Eckhardt C. Use of Rh antibodies in the treatment of autoimmune

thrombocytopenia. Transfus Med Rev 1992; 6:17-25.

103. Blum PM, Phelps DL, Ank BJ, et al. Survival of oral human immune serum globulin in the gastrointestinal tract of low birth weight infants. Pediatr Res 1981;15:1256-60.

104. Barnes GL, Doyle LW, Hewson PH, et al. A randomised trial of oral gammaglobulin in low-birth-weight infants infected with rotavirus. Lancet 1982;1:1371-3.

105. Losonsky GA, Johnson J, Winkelstein JA, et al. Oral administration of human serum immunoglobulin in immunodeficient patients with viral gastroenteritis: A pharmacokinetic and functional analysis. J Clin Invest 1985; 76:2362-7.

106. Eibl MM, Wolf HM, Furnkranz H, et al. Prevention of necrotizing enterocolitis in low-birth-weight infants by IgA-IgG feeding. N Engl J Med 1988;319:1-7.

107. Borowitz SM, Saulsbury FT. Treatment of chronic cryptosporidial infection with orally administered human serum immune globulin. J Pediatr 1991;119:593-5.

108. Erlendsson K, Swartz T, Dwyer JM. Successful reversal of echovirus encephalitis in X-linked hypogammaglobulinemia by intraventricular administration of immunoglobulin. N Engl J Med 1985;312:351-3.

109. Rimensberger PC, Schaad UB. Clinical experience with aerosolized immunoglobulin treatment of respiratory syncytial virus infection in infants. Pediatr Infect Dis J 1994; 13:328-30.

110. Burton DR, Pyti J, Koduri R, et al. Efficient neutralization of primary isolates of HIV-1 by a recombinant human monoclonal antibody. Science 1994;266:1024-7.

Appendix 14-1. Association Bulletin #98-2

PRENATAL/PERINATAL TESTING and Rh IMMUNE GLOBULIN

ADMINISTRATION

I. Initial visit

A. All women should have ABO and D testing performed as early as possible during each pregnancy. D typing should include a test for weak D,[2,3(p 619-20)] if initial typing appears to be D negative. ABO and D types must match historical records. Discrepant results must be fully investigated and resolved.

B. All pregnant women should be tested at least once during each pregnancy for unexpected alloantibodies, preferably at their first prenatal visit. The antibody screen should include an antiglobulin phase using anti-IgG antihuman globulin following incubation at 37°C. [3(p 223-3, 464)]

1. If the antibody screen is negative for anti-D,

a. For D-negative women:

1) If the first prenatal visit is earlier than 26 weeks' gestation, consider a repeat antibody screen at 26 weeks prior to administration of RhIG.

2) If the first prenatal visit is at 26 weeks or later, ADMINISTER RhIG.[*]

b. For D-positive women: Do <u>NOT</u> administer RhIG. No further investigation is required.

2. If the antibody screen is positive, antibody identification must be performed. If a clinically significant alloantibody is identified, close clinical evaluation and additional studies are indicated. This pregnancy and all subsequent ones should be managed as high risk as described in Section II B below.

---

[*]RhIG, either intravenous (IV) or intramuscular (IM), should be administered according to manufacturer's directions.

(continued)

Appendix 14-1. Association Bulletin #98-2 (continued)

      a.   For D-negative women:

          1)   If the alloantibody is <u>NOT</u> anti-D

              a)   ADMINISTER RhIG.

              b)   Manage as a high-risk pregnancy.

          2)   If the alloantibody is anti-D, manage as a high-risk pregnancy.

      b.   For D-positive women:

          1)   Do NOT administer RhIG.

          2)   Manage as a high-risk pregnancy.

    C.   Once an alloantibody has been identified, repeat identification is not necessary. A selected cell panel should be performed to exclude the presence of other alloantibodies.

    D.   Titration of clinically significant alloantibodies found early in pregnancy may be appropriate to establish a baseline for comparison to subsequent samples. Consultation with clinical experts is recommended for titration of alloantibodies other than anti-D. Retention of samples for repeat subsequent testing is prudent.

II. Follow-up visits

    A.   **Uncomplicated:** *Mothers who are not alloimmunized and who are NOT at increased risk of FMH*

        1.   No repeat ABO/D testing is necessary (unless required for some other purpose such as for transfusion).

        2.   If the first antibody screen was negative,

            a.   A repeat antibody screen should be considered <u>only for D-negative</u> women at 26-28 weeks' gestation.

                1)   If the antibody screen is (or remains) negative for anti-D at 26-28 weeks' gestation, ADMINISTER RhIG.

                2)   If the antibody screen becomes positive for anti-D or any other clinically significant alloantibody, the pregnancy should be managed as a high risk.

Appendix 14-1. Association Bulletin #98-2 (continued)

3. If the first antibody screen was (or now is) positive due to a clinically significant alloantibody, the pregnancy should be managed as a high risk.

NOTE: D-negative women who lack evidence of allo-anti-D and have received RhIG antenatally often have subsequent positive antibody screens due to passively acquired anti-D. A selected cell panel should be run to exclude clinically significant alloantibodies other than anti-D. If no other clinically significant alloantibodies are found, except passive allo-anti-D, these pregnancies do not need to be handled as high risk.

B. **High Risk**: *Women who are alloimmunized with a clinically significant alloantibody or who are at an increased risk of FMH*

1. No repeat ABO/D testing is necessary (unless required for some other purpose such as for transfusion).

2. If there is no indication of active alloimmunization to D, ADMINISTER RhIG to all D-negative women within 72 hours for any indication that may increase the risk of FMH, such as: cessation of pregnancy at >/= 13 weeks' gestation; after amniocentesis, chorionic villus sampling, PUBS or external version; or if there is a clinical suspicion of placental pathology.

   a. If the pregnancy is at or after 26 weeks' gestation, the need for additional doses of RhIG should be determined using an appropriate method to test maternal blood for the presence of excessive FMH.

NOTE: Testing for weak D is NOT recommended for detection of excessive FMH.

3. If the antibody screen is positive for a clinically significant alloantibody (in either D-negative or D-positive women), careful monitoring during this and subsequent pregnancies will be required.

   a. Repeat testing and possibly additional studies may be indicated if the alloantibody identified is clinically significant. All serologic testing should be performed after consultation between a transfusion service physician and the clinical caregiver.

(continued)

Appendix 14-1. Association Bulletin #98-2 (continued)

4. Once an alloantibody has been identified, it need not be reidentified. A selected cell panel should be run to exclude the presence of other clinically significant alloantibodies. Identification of any new alloantibodies is indicated.

5. Periodic repeat titration of clinically significant alloantibodies may be appropriate during the continuation of pregnancy. Consultation with clinical experts is recommended for titration of alloantibodies other than anti-D. Each new sample should be tested in parallel with the immediately preceding sample or with the original sample. [3(p 646)]

III. At delivery

A. Mother

1. If the delivering facility has a verified record of a negative antibody screen during the current pregnancy, repeat maternal testing is not routinely required unless a question of HDN arises.

2. If the delivering facility has a verified record of alloimmunization to D, it is not necessary to administer RhIG.

3. If the mother is known to be D-negative and not alloimmunized to D,

    a. And if the infant's cord blood is tested for D (including a test for weak D) when the cord blood is

        1) D (including weak D) negative, do NOT give maternal RhIG and do no further testing.

        2) D (including weak D) positive, perform a test for excessive FMH to determine RhIG dosage. *NOTE: Testing for weak D is NOT recommended for detection of excessive FMH.*

Appendix 14-1. Association Bulletin #98-2 (continued)

       b.   And if cord blood is not tested,

          1)   Perform a test for excessive FMH to determine RhIG dosage. NOTE: Testing for weak D is NOT recommended for detection of excessive FMH.

          2)   ADMINISTER RhIG in appropriate doses.

B. Infant

    1.   No cord blood testing is required except to establish candidacy of mother to receive RhIG or unless a question of HDN arises.

    2.   If a question of HDN arises when the mother has clinically significant alloantibodies, ABO/D and direct antiglobulin testing should be performed on infant's cord blood. In the absence of a maternal sample, eluate testing may be useful to confirm an alloantibody implicated in HDN.

REFERENCES

1. Judd WJ, Luban NLC, Ness PM, et al. Prenatal and perinatal immunohematology: Recommendations for serologic management of the fetus, newborn infant, and obstetric patient. Transfusion 1990;30:175-83.

2. Klein HG, ed. Standards for blood banks and transfusion services, 18th ed. Bethesda, MD: American Association of Blood Banks, 1996: 44.

3. Vengelen-Tyler V, ed. Technical manual, 12th ed. Bethesda, MD: American Association of Blood Banks, 1996:

(continued)

Appendix 14-1. Association Bulletin #98-2 (continued)

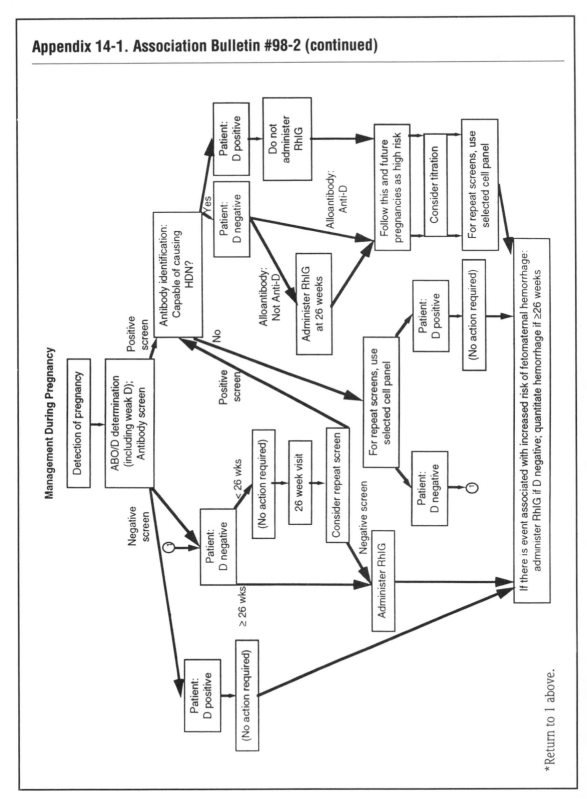

Appendix 14-1. Association Bulletin #98-2 (continued)

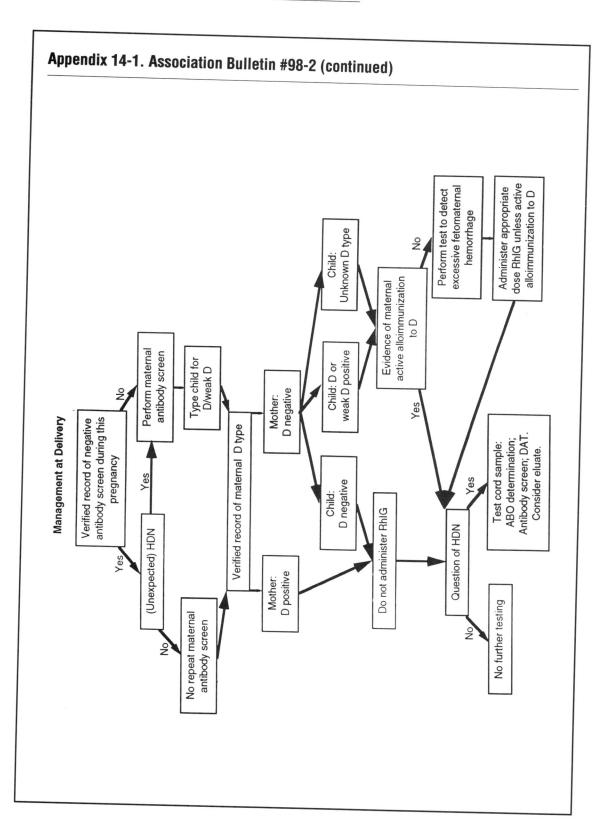

Management at Delivery

In: Mintz PD, ed.
Transfusion Therapy: Clinical Principles and Practice
Bethesda, MD: AABB Press, 1999

15

Neonatal and Intrauterine Transfusion

LINDA A. CHAMBERS, MD, AND NAOMI C. LUBAN, MD

 THE CONDITIONS NECESSITATING transfusion and the characteristics of transfusion are different in fetuses and neonates as compared with adult patients. Furthermore, infants have important physiologic features that require different criteria for transfusion. These distinctions mandate that we bring special insight and knowledge to our consideration of the risks and requirements for safe and effective transfusion therapy in this group of patients. A summary of transfusion issues for neonates is presented in Table 15-1.

Neonates as Transfusion Recipients

The portion of hospitalized neonates who are transfused is high and nearly 100% for very-low-birthweight premature infants.[2,3] The accumulated transfusion volumes over the course of a hospitali-

zation often approach the total blood volumes of the patients. Total donor exposures (the number of different donor components to which the patient is exposed) easily exceed five unless special steps are taken to obtain more than one transfusion from each donor unit for a given neonate.[4-7] Because of the small total blood volumes of infants relative to the volumes in bypass circuits, blood storage bags, and blood recovery equipment, most perioperative practices designed to limit blood loss and avoid allogeneic transfusion—including autologous donation, intraoperative blood recovery, isovolemic hemodilution, and asanguinous cardiopulmonary bypass priming—cannot be used. Blood components need to be subdivided to provide appropriate dose volumes for neonates. These special preparations may entail the transfer of blood to bags and syringes that are not suitable for product storage, or may require opening of the aseptic system in which

Linda A. Chambers, MD, Medical Director of Transfusion Services, Children's Hospital; Clinical Associate Professor of Pathologhy, The Ohio State University, Columbus, Ohio, and Naomi C. Luban, MD, Director of Transfusion Medicine, Children's Hospital, Washington, District of Columbia

Table 15-1. Summary of Transfusion Issues for Hospitalized Neonates

Observation	Implications	Recommendation
A high proportion of patients are transfused.	High total donor exposures per patient.	Limited donor programs and assigned unit practices are effective.
	Increased risk of transfusion-acquired infection.	Routine screening for transfusion-related infections and complications may be fruitful.
Routine transfusion volumes are relatively large.	Potassium, citrate, volume, cold temperature, and preservative toxicity might be increased.	Give routine transfusions over 2-3 hours. Specially select and prepare components for rapid or massive transfusions.
Recipient's blood volume small relative to standard blood components and equipment.	Subdivision of components required.	Carefully coordinate component preparation with intended transfusion.
	Plasma-incompatible platelet transfusion may be more likely to cause hemolysis.	ABO-identical or plasma-compatible platelets are preferred.[1]
	Blood loss through phlebotomy for laboratory tests is a noticeable cause of anemia.	Replacement transfusions are required, most frequently for smaller and sicker infants.
Red-cell-reactive antibodies passively are acquired from mother or by transfusion.	Anti-A and anti-B may not correspond to the neonate's ABO group.	Test for anti-A and anti-B if non-group-O red cells are to be given, or if non-group-AB plasma or platelets have been transfused and potentially incompatible red cells are to be given.
	There is risk of hemolytic anemia in antigen-positive newborns.	Crossmatch with maternal sample whenever possible. Select and prepare transfusion as if for mother and neonate simultaneously.
Recipient has a long posttransfusion life expectancy.	Increases the likelihood of surviving long enough to develop disease from transfusion-acquired infection.	Lowest infectious risk donors, components, and preparations are preferred.
Recipient has defective humoral immune response.	Recipients are unlikely to form red cell antibodies.	May assume negative antibody detection test results through neonatal period if initial test results are negative.
Recipient has defective cellular immune response.	Recipient's ability to contain donor lymphocytes may be limited.	Gamma irradiation is recommended, as discussed in text.
	Viral infections acquired as a neonate are more likely to progress to systemic illness.	CMV-reduced-risk transfusion is recommended, as discussed in text.

the component is manufactured. Consequently, careful timing of blood preparation with planned time of administration is required, and transfusions for use in the operating room may need to be prepared on an as-needed basis rather than in advance.

Routine transfusion volumes on a milliliter-per-kilogram body weight basis are high in newborns. The "standard" 15 mL/kg aliquot transfusion of red blood cells with a hematocrit of 60-85% is the equivalent of about three units for an adult. The net increase in the infant's total blood volume is about half of the transfused amount, as the infant's plasma volume shifts into the extracellular space.[8] If administered rapidly to a neonate in whom the usual compensatory mechanisms are not functional, this relative volume of red cell transfusion might result in circulatory overload or the delivery of excessive amounts of potassium, citrate, or other constituents of the preservative-anticoagulant solution. Fortunately, multiple observational studies show that the typical 10-15 mL/kg transfusion, when administered over 2-3 hours, is well tolerated and nontoxic.[5,7,9-11] Exclusive use of fresh (eg, less than 7-day-old) units or avoidance of newer preservative-anticoagulation preparations (eg, AS-1) are therefore not necessary. It is only when the neonate receives massive transfusion—for example, during cardiopulmonary bypass or exchange transfusion—that special attention needs to be paid to red cell integrity and additive toxicity when selecting red cell components.

The small blood volume of the neonate probably does change the relative risk of giving ABO plasma-incompatible platelets. A single, 40-mL platelet concentrate from a group O donor is unlikely to cause hemolysis if transfused to a group A adult because the anti-A in the component is diluted into 2-3 L of recipient plasma. However, a 3-kg neonate has a total plasma volume of only about 150 mL, so 40 mL of ABO-incompatible donor plasma in a platelet concentrate represents a substantial exposure. A special effort to use only group-identical or plasma-compatible platelets for small recipients is warranted to obviate possible hemolysis. If such products are not available, centrifugation and plasma removal prior to transfusion

are alternative approaches. Hemolysis generates bilirubin, which is particularly harmful to the neonate. If ABO-incompatible plasma is transfused in the course of giving platelet transfusions, a crossmatch should be performed before potentially incompatible red blood cells are transfused.

Newborns may have maternally acquired pathologic antibodies directed against red cells, platelets, or granulocytes, causing hemolytic disease, isoimmune thrombocytopenia, or neonatal granulocytopenia, respectively.[12-14] Compatibility testing and identification of effective transfusion components for the affected neonate must therefore deal simultaneously with the antibodies of the mother and special transfusion issues of the infant. The ABO antibodies in the newborn will likewise be maternal in origin, so they may not correspond to the newborn's red cell ABO antigen group. When non-group O red cells are going to be transfused to a neonate, it is necessary to test for the presence of anti-A/anti-B (including an antiglobulin test) rather than infer their presence or absence from the infant's ABO group. To ensure compatibility of blood for the newborn, the product should be compatible with the ABO group and Rh type, as well as unexpected red cell antibodies in the maternal serum.[15]

A large number of transfusions to neonates are given for anemia of prematurity, an anemia that develops over the first 2-3 weeks of life as the hemoglobin concentration decreases. During this time frame, erythropoiesis converts from hemoglobin F to hemoglobin A production, and the infant's red cell mass alters as the infant doubles in birthweight.[3] In the healthy term neonate, this expected decrease in hemoglobin is usually not problematic because the nadir is at about 10 g/dL and the infant with normal cardiorespiratory reserve can oxygenate effectively. The premature neonate, on the other hand, has lower iron and protein reserves and thus is at a greater risk for this anemia. If hemoglobin levels decrease to the 7- to 9-g/dL range and the infant is hospitalized with resultant iatrogenic blood loss, he or she may be additionally compromised. When this moderate anemia coincides with poor oxygenation from respiratory distress or other serious illness, transfusion is typically given to bring the hemoglobin up to the 10- to 12-g/dL range. The benefits and need for transfusion in this setting are not conclusively demonstrated, however. Even the classic signs and symptoms of anemia in this patient population (apnea, tachycardia, bradycardia, poor weight gain), when examined critically, do not closely correlate with the degree of anemia and may not improve with transfusion in all patients.[16-19] Premature neonates with anemia of prematurity do not increase their endogenous erythropoietin production as efficiently as older children and adults with the same degree of anemia.[20,21] Whether the quantitatively low concentration is a cause of anemia of prematurity or simply a feature of the condition is not yet clear. Several thought-provoking studies suggest that, at the hemoglobin nadir typically seen in this condition, most neonates compensate well, ensuring tissue oxygenation.[13,22] A diminished endogenous erythropoietin response may therefore, be normal and appropriate. Transfusion under these circumstances lessens the neonate's dependence on cardiovascular compensatory response but might not change oxygen delivery or improve any functions dependent on oxygen delivery.[22]

Whether or not inadequate erythropoietin is pathogenic to anemia of prematurity, neonates do respond to exogenous recombinant erythropoietin (rEPO) therapy with increases in hemoglobin production and higher nadir hemoglobin levels than found in untreated control subjects.[21,23,24] For programs that transfuse neonates to maintain a set hemoglobin level, rEPO, especially if started early in life, reduces transfusion frequency and volume with minimal toxicity. Combined with efforts to reduce blood loss from phlebotomy for laboratory tests, rEPO has a place in the management of premature newborns whose families wish to avoid blood transfusion.[23,25] The use of rEPO in the anemia of prematurity is discussed in detail in Chapter 20.

Adverse Effects of Transfusion

Neonates have a relatively long posttransfusion expected survival. Therefore, transfusion complications with long intervals before presentation are more likely to develop in these patients than in adult recipients. Posttransfusion chronic hepatitis C, for example, which may take 10 or more years to progress to cirrhosis and liver failure, may not affect mortality in an adult,[26-28] but it might appreciably shorten life expectancy if acquired by a neonate or young child. Hepatitis C virus, if acquired in the neonatal period, likely has the same propensity as in the adult to establish chronic infection; cause persistent, low-grade liver function abnormalities; and result in significant morbidity.[29,30] Because of their long expected survival, then, neonates as a group derive a proportionally greater benefit from reducing the risks of long-term adverse effects of transfusion.

Neonates have primarily passive, maternally transmitted, immunity to transfusion-transmissible agents such as hepatitis A, Epstein-Barr virus, and cytomegalovirus (CMV) because of a lack of intrauterine exposure and a limited capacity for innate antibody production in the fetus. As the passively acquired antibody titers drop, neonates may become susceptible to these more unusual transfusion-acquired infections while most adult recipients are actively immune.[31] Cell-mediated immunity—notably, T-lymphocyte response and cytokine production—is also not fully established in newborns.[32,33] Thus, the transfused neonate's ability to control and eliminate the viable, functioning donor lymphocytes contained in blood components may be compromised. If allowed to engraft, transfused lymphocytes can proliferate to mediate life-threatening transfusion-associated graft-vs-host disease (TA-GVHD).[34]

Gamma irradiation of cellular blood components and preparations should be done for neonatal granulocyte transfusions, for neonates with suspected or confirmed T-cell immune deficiencies, for all familial donations as discussed in Chapter 17, and, as discussed below, for intrauterine transfusions and transfusions to neonates who have received intrauterine transfusions. It is not necessary to irradiate blood for neonates on extracorporeal membrane oxygenation (ECMO), or for neonates with human immunodeficiency virus infection.

The need for irradiation for neonates under 1500g and for routine exchange transfusions remains under evaluation (see Chapter 17).

Defects in cell-mediated immunity also contribute to the increased toxicity of viral infections in the neonatal period. In hospitalized newborns of CMV-seronegative mothers, transfusion is the primary route by which CMV is acquired, whereas newborns of seropositive mothers often acquire CMV perinatally.[35] Most adult transfusion recipients are either immune from naturally acquired infection or able to handle new transfusion-transmitted infection with little or no disease.[36,37] Indeed, it is only the most immunologically damaged adult patients, such as hematopoietic stem cell transplant recipients, who develop significant disease from CMV, and it is reactivation of preexisting infection rather than new infection from transfusion that is most often the source.[38,39] The consequent disease from perinatal CMV, perhaps because it coincides with some degree of passive humoral immunity, is usually mild.[40] However, the transfusion-acquired infections, particularly in a sick or premature neonate without passive immunity, may progress to hepatitis, viral sepsis, or highly lethal CMV pneumonia. These infections are preventable through the use of CMV-reduced-risk blood components and preparations.[41,42]

CMV-seronegative neonates weighing less than 1200 g should receive CMV-reduced-risk cellular blood components and preparations. These may be either CMV-seronegative or leukocyte-reduced products. AABB Association Bulletin 97-2[43] suggests that all neonates weighing less than 1200 g should receive CMV-reduced-risk products owing to loss of passively acquired immunity over time in seropositive neonates. This is a reasonable practice, although the available evidence is that seropositive low-birthweight infants are not at increased risk of transfusion-transmitted CMV disease. Intrauterine transfusions should be CMV-reduced-risk, as should transfusions to CMV-seronegative pregnant women. (Primary CMV infection during pregnancy may pose significant risk to the fetus.) However, it is not necessary for neonates who are on ECMO or are receiving routine exchange transfusions to receive CMV-reduced-risk transfusions. Leukocyte reduction of blood products and CMV-reduced-risk transfusions are discussed in Chapter 16.

As with adult red cell transfusions, the indications for and benefits of blood administration to neonates are not founded in strong scientific observations and clinical trials but rather reflect experience and example. As a result, while there are several thoughtfully prepared sets of guidelines for neonatal transfusion, most are based on common practice and best guesses, and the authors would agree with the continuing need for critical assessment and reevaluation of the indications for transfusion in newborns.[18,44-46]

The Storage Lesion and Neonatal Transfusion

Acute complications are most often the result of metabolic changes that result from product storage and infusion of the anticoagulant/preservative solution. A storage lesion, which increases over time, occurs for both stored red blood cells and platelets. Selection of blood and blood products for both small and massive transfusions is often predicated on concerns over the storage lesion.

Potassium

The potassium (K^+) level in plasma in 35-day-old, refrigerator-stored, red blood cells may reach 78.5 mmoL/L in blood collected in standard anticoagulant solutions. The K^+ is lower, ranging from 45.6 to 50 mmoL/L at 42 days, in the newer anticoagulant/preservative solutions. In Red Blood Cells (RBCs) irradiated and stored at refrigerator temperature for 28 days, the potassium may reach even higher values. When administered as small-volume transfusions of 10-15 mL/kg, this quantity of K^+ is relatively insignificant, but fatal cardiac arrhythmias have been associated with hyperkalemia during neonatal exchange transfusion and following rapid infusion during surgery.[47-51] If a relatively large quantity of irradiated blood is going to be transfused, it should be irradiated as close to the time of transfusion as possible.

In adults receiving more than one blood volume during a 24-hour period, hypokalemia has been noted. After red blood cells have been transfused and rewarmed to body temperature, Na-K-dependent adenosine triphosphate shifts are activated and red blood cells exchange intracellular sodium for extracellular K^+, resulting in a "sink" for K^+.[52,53] Alkalosis from metabolized citrate can result in further potassium shifts into cells in exchange for hydrogen ions. Similar phenomena have not been reported in infants to date.

2,3-Diphosphoglycerate

Levels of intra-erythrocytic 2,3-diphosphoglycerate (2,3-DPG) affect the ability of red cells to release oxygen at any given pH. With progressive storage, 2,3-DPG levels decrease by more than 50%,[53] resulting in a decreased ability to off-load oxygen in the tissues. In adults, 2,3-DPG is gradually restored over several hours following routine transfusion.[54] In one study of premature infants receiving small-volume transfusions, quantitative 2,3-DPG was measured weekly. Results were similar in infants transfused with fresh citrate phosphate dextrose adenine (CPDA-1) and stored AS-1 RBCs, suggesting that, at least in this setting, infants can effectively maintain 2,3-DPG at an adult level. Of note, untransfused infants in this study had higher 2,3-DPG levels, as would be expected in infants with higher fetal hemoglobin concentrations.[11]

Cold Storage

RBCs are stored at 4-6 C. Rapid infusion of cold RBCs can result in hypothermia and cardiac arrhythmia/asystole. In infants, transfusion of cold blood has been associated with apnea, hypotension, and hypoglycemia. While small-volume transfusions are rarely associated with physiologic instability induced by cold, massive transfusion, including exchange transfusion and intraoperative transfusion, calls for blood-warming devices, which use wet and dry heat to bring the temperature of the blood up to body temperature. ECMO systems and cardiovascular bypass systems usually have in-line blood warmers. Microwave ovens and other devices that do not have strict quality checks on the heating device should never be used because heating may be inconsistent and hemolysis may result.

Dilutional Hemostatic Dysfunction

Dilutional hemostatic dysfunction results from the transfusion of many units of RBCs from which platelets and plasma have been removed. The few platelets remaining in RBCs have poor in-vivo survival and are dysfunctional. Dilutional hemostatic dysfunction is characterized by thrombocytopenia, hypofibrinogenemia, and prolongation of both the prothrombin time and partial thromboplastin time; fibrin degradation products are often present, and quantitation of coagulation factor proteins demonstrates variable reduction of all factors except Factor VIII. The neonatal liver is less able to prevent hypofibrinogenemia than the adult liver. Clinically, the patient may present with microvascular bleeding or oozing from sites of injury, venipuncture sites, and mucosal surfaces. Dilutional hemostatic dysfunction is most often manifest in the acutely bleeding patient who also has evidence of disseminated intravascular coagulation.

Adverse Effects of Anticoagulant/ Preservative Solutions

The RBC (adenine-saline added) anticoagulant/preservative solutions (AS-1, AS-3, and AS-5) permit storage of RBCs to 42 days and allow for maximum plasma extraction. They contain citrate, which binds ionized calcium to prevent coagulation of the donor's blood; dextrose and adenine to maintain intracellular adenosine triphosphate and therefore the red cell's integrity; and sodium biphosphate to prevent an excessive decrease in pH during storage, which would result in hemolysis and poor in-vivo survival. The concentration of the anticoagulant/preservative solution is highest in the freshest blood and decreases over time as the constituents diffuse into the red blood cells and are used to maintain red cell integrity. The average hematocrit of RBCs (adenine-saline added) is approximately 60%; the flow rate during infusion is more rapid because the product is less viscous than RBCs stored with other preservative solutions. The metabolic and physiologic safety of AS-1 in small-volume transfusions has been demonstrated in very-low-birthweight infants in several studies.[10,11] However, the lower hematocrit of the RBCs stored in additive solutions mandates an increase in the transfusion volume to achieve a hemoglobin increment comparable to that achieved by transfusing an RBC product with a hematocrit of 75 ± 5%. In massive transfusion, theoretical concerns of osmotic load and diuresis, hyperglycemia, hypernatremia, and hypoalbuminemia remain; no clinical trials confirming the safety of the different AS-added solutions have been performed to date in neonates in this setting. Hypoalbuminemia has been reported when RBCs (Adenine-Saline Added) were used in exchange transfusion.[55]

Decreasing Donor Exposure

While most infants weighing more than 1500 g will not require transfusion during their neonatal stay, almost all infants less than 1000 g have a transfusion requirement that results in one or several donor exposures. Attempts to decrease the number of donor exposures have resulted in several changes to standard neonatal practices. For several years, fresh (eg, less than 7-day-old) group O, Rh-negative blood was the preferred product; theoretically, this provided a product enriched in 2,3-DPG with optimal oxygen off-loading characteristics and a low supernatant potassium concentration. Donor exposure number and unit wastage were high, however. By using a sterile connecting device and multiple aliquot bags and by dedicating a unit to one or more infants and using RBCs until outdate, practitioners can reduce donor exposure without adverse clinical outcome, as reported in several studies.[4-7,10] In one large study of 40 infants, Strauss et al[10] attempted to determine if a single AS-1 red cell unit could be assigned its outdate to support the total needs of low-birthweight infants safely, as compared with CPDA-1 units stored for 7 days. Do-

nor exposure was reduced to 1.6, compared with 3.7 in the CPDA-1 arm of that study. Hyperkalemia and hypernatremia were not seen, and no adverse physiologic findings were documented. Several infants (6 of 14) required a second donor exposure because of either technical issues with the blood unit (3) or the timing of the transfusion (3).[10]

For small-volume transfusions, blood collected in either CPDA-1 or additive solutions, at a dose of 10-15 mL/kg, stored until outdate of the unit and with a hematocrit ranging from 60 to 85%, appears to be efficacious and without adverse clinical outcome. The use of washed RBC units should be limited to infants with IgA deficiency or T activation of red blood cells, or to those in renal failure for whom the anticoagulant/preservative solution and K^+ load would be detrimental. Adjustment of unwashed RBCs to a specific hematocrit or to replace coagulation factors with frozen thawed plasma should be avoided.

Massive Transfusion of the Neonate

For massive transfusion, the safety and efficacy of AS-added RBCs have not undergone the same kind of clinical trials that have been conducted for small-volume transfusions. Mathematical models would suggest that toxicities are likely.[56] CPDA-1-preserved RBCs could be used in this situation or, in those areas of the United States where RBCs are preserved exclusively in AS solutions, washing or removal of the AS solution by inverted centrifugation would be prudent. Hypocalcemia should be avoided by careful measurement of ionized calcium, particularly early in the course of an exchange transfusion and throughout the procedure in a surgical or trauma resuscitation. The rate of citrate clearance by the liver and kidneys is decreased when hypothermia or acidosis coexist. The potential for dilutional hemostatic dysfunction also mandates laboratory assessment for abnormal coagulation test results and platelet counts, and treatment with plasma and platelets when clinical symptoms ensue.

The setting of massive transfusion presents a particular serologic dilemma. Occasionally, a massive transfusion recipient may receive group O, Rh-negative, or Rh-specific red blood cells during an acute resuscitation. When the ABO group and Rh type of the individual are known, it is advantageous to switch back to group-specific and type-compatible products to conserve blood group O resources. If the patient has received plasma-containing products, however, such switching may be problematic; a full crossmatch should be performed with a fresh patient sample to identify incompatibility and avoid possible hemolysis in the recipient resulting from anti-A and anti-B isoagglutinins present in group O donor plasma. If exclusively group O cells have been used, group A, B, or AB recipients receiving out-of-group, plasma-containing components should not receive their own blood group if anti-A or anti-B are evident in the recipient's plasma as stipulated in AABB Standards for Blood Banks and Transfusion Services.

When leukocyte-reduced blood products are a part of the inventory of the transfusion service, certain patients requiring massive transfusion may benefit. This includes infants undergoing cardiothoracic surgery who are at risk for reperfusion injury[57] and those known or suspected to be severely immunocompromised who are at risk for CMV. Routine leukocyte reduction for exchange transfusion, acute surgical procedures, or medical resuscitation is not indicated.

As noted, irradiated red blood cells induce a more rapid leakage of potassium during storage than unirradiated red cells. Care should be taken to avoid the transfusion of multiple units of irradiated, refrigerator-stored RBCs in neonates and children because of the potential for hyperkalemic cardiac arrhythmia.

The theoretical risks of hypokalemic metabolic alkalosis from the metabolism of citrate during massive transfusion were noted in the section on potassium.

Intrauterine Transfusion

Extending transfusion support to the fetus in utero provides an opportunity to correct critical anemia and thrombocytopenia, which could otherwise re-

sult in fetal complications or intrauterine death. Red cell transfusion can be accomplished by instill ing red cells into the peritoneal space.[59] The red cells migrate to the circulation across the mesothe lial lining, provided there is no local disease such a ascites, hemorrhage, or massive congestion. Alte nately and more effectively, platelets as well as re cells can be introduced directly to the fetal circula tion by cannulating and infusing them into the un bilical vein. Direct access allows for sampling an testing of fetal blood, which can be important t document the degree of cytopenia and characteriz the offending antibody when the fetal disease i due to fetal-maternal incompatibility.[60] Intrauterin transfusions are typically started after about 2 weeks' gestation, when the fetus and umbilica cord can be visualized by ultrasound to permit sa manipulation and cannulation.[61] Depending on th severity of the condition being treated, a typic course might include three transfusions of red cel 1-2 weeks apart, although some centers have give as many as 11 intrauterine transfusions for sever hemolytic disease.[62-65] Platelets may need to b given every several days owing to their short lif span.

Fetal red cell transfusion corrects severe an mia, reverses the consequent congestive heart fai ure (hydrops), and has been used not only fo hemolytic disease in fetuses of mothers sensitize to red cell antigens, but also for fetal anemia secor dary to intrauterine parvovirus infection, twin-to twin transfusion, large-volume fetal hemorrhag and alpha thalassemia major.[66-70] Intrauterine plate let transfusion is used primarily to correct fet thrombocytopenia in an effort to avoid centra nervous system hemorrhage during gestation i pregnancies affected by neonatal isoimmun thrombocytopenia.[71]

Compatibility testing of blood for fetal transfi sion must take into account the ABO group of th mother, given that the fetal anti-A and anti-B will b maternal in origin, as will be other red-cell-reactiv antibodies acquired from the maternal circulatior whether or not they are pathologic in the fetus. Th most direct method to ensure compatibility is to s lect red cell group and antigen types appropriate fc transfusion to the mother, ideally by crossmatching with a maternal blood sample. Selection of blood to be used for intrauterine transfusion must take into account that the mother may have been exposed to transfused cells either as a result of the cordocentesis procedure or from posttransfusion feto-maternal hemorrhage.[72] As noted previously, the use of CMV-reduced-risk cellular components and preparations for intrauterine transfusion is recommended, as is the use of CMV-reduced-risk cellular components for CMV-seronegative pregnant women. The transfusion volumes to the fetus may be large enough to ensure that a substantial portion of the posttransfusion fetal red cell mass will be allogeneic. The half-life and ability of the transfused cells to off-load oxygen, which correlates with the 2,3-DPG level and therefore inversely with the storage age of the blood component, become important considerations. When the fetus is hydropic, unnecessary donor plasma can be removed from the component by concentrating the red cells to a high hematocrit. For nonhydropic fetuses, the high viscosity of plasma-reduced red cell transfusions may be counterproductive to posttransfusion tissue perfusion, and suspensions at more physiologic hematocrits (50-55%) are preferred.[73]

One must be particularly concerned with the immune status and risk of TA-GVHD in these patients. The fetus has less mature cellular and humoral immunity than the premature neonate and term neonate.[74] When the number of donor lymphocytes transfused is high, either because of the total volume or a high level of contamination of the component (eg, pooled platelets), the ability of the fetal system to prevent TA-GVHD may be overwhelmed. Intrauterine transfusion in and of itself also compromises the cellular immunologic response in the neonatal period, increasing the risk of TA-GVHD.[75] Gamma irradiation of cellular components both for intrauterine transfusion and for neonatal transfusion in recipients of intrauterine transfusion is, therefore, advisable.

The neonate who has had intrauterine transfusion of red cells may have peculiar compatibility testing results due to the mixed population of red cells and plasma dilution resulting from the transfu-sions. Intrauterine transfusion causes the suppression of erythropoiesis in the fetus, which can persist into the neonatal period and occasionally cause sufficient hypoproliferative anemia to require red cell transfusion several weeks after birth (so-called late anemia). The degree of suppression is greater when the last intrauterine transfusion occurs close to the time of delivery and the cord blood hemoglobin level is high.[76] Suppressed neonates have low levels of erythropoietin and reticulocytes, and erythropoiesis may not readily resume even when anemia triggers a rise in erythropoietin production.[77] As with the anemia of prematurity, the marrow will respond to exogenous erythropoietin, and rEPO treatment can be used in place of transfusion until normal production is reestablished.[78,79]

Summary

Advances in the care of critically ill newborns and fetuses have necessitated dramatic changes in the transfusion service's response to the needs of these infants. The premature infant in particular must be considered a major consumer of blood and blood products. The special selection, packaging, and administration of blood and blood products must be altered to suit the unique physiologic and pathologic aspects of the fetus's and infant's needs.

References

1. Menitove JE, ed. Standards for blood banks and transfusion services, 18th ed. Bethesda, MD: American Association of Blood Banks, 1997:37.
2. Luban NL. Review of neonatal red cell transfusion practices. Blood Rev 1994;8:148-53.
3. Strauss RG. Case analysis approach to neonatal transfusions. Lab Med 1992;23:239-43.
4. Cook S, Gunter J, Wissel M. Effective use of a strategy using assigned red cell units to limit donor exposure for neonatal patients. Transfusion 1993;33:379-83.
5. Wood A, Wilson N, Skacel P, et al. Reducing donor exposure in preterm infants requiring

multiple blood transfusions. Arch Dis Child 1995;72:F29-33.

6. Wang-Rodrigues J, Mannino FL, Liu E, Lane TA. A novel strategy to limit blood donor exposure and blood waste in multiply transfused premature infants. Transfusion 1996;36:64-70.

7. Liu EA, Mannino FL, Lane TA. Prospective, randomized trial of the safety and efficacy of a limited donor exposure transfusion program for premature neonates. J Pediatr 1994;125:92-6.

8. Bauer K, Linderkamp O, Versmold HT. Short-term effects of blood transfusion on blood volume and resting peripheral blood flow in preterm infants. Acta Paediatr 1993;82:1027-33.

9. Nose Y, Tamia H, Shimada S, Funato M. Haemodynamic effects of differing blood transfusion rates in infants less than 1500 g. J Paediatr Child Health 1996;32:177-82.

10. Strauss RG, Burmeister LF, Johnson K, et al. AS-1 red cells for neonatal transfusions: A randomized trial assessing donor exposure and safety. Transfusion 1996;36:873-8.

11. Goodstein MH, Locke RG, Wlodarczyk D, et al. Comparison of two preservative solutions for erythrocyte transfusions in newborn infants. J Pediatr 1993;123:783-8.

12. Cartron J, Tchernia G, Celton JL, et al. Alloimmune neonatal neutropenia. J Pediatr Hematol Oncol 1991;13:21-5.

13. Bussel JB, Berkowitz RL, McFarland JG, et al. Antenatal treatment of neonatal alloimmune thrombocytopenia. N Engl J Med 1988;319:1374-8.

14. Bowman JM. Treatment options for the fetus with alloimmune hemolytic disease. Transfus Med Rev 1990;4:191-207.

15. Judd WJ, Luban NLC, Silberstein LE, et al. Prenatal and perinatal immunohematology: Recommendations for serologic management of the fetus, newborn infant and obstetric patient. Transfusion 1990;30:175-83.

16. Keyes WG, Donohue PK, Spivak JL, et al. Assessing the need for transfusion of premature infants and role of hematocrit, clinical signs and erythropoietin levels. Pediatrics 1989;84:412-7.

17. Izraeli S, Ben-Sira L, Harell D, et al. Lactic acid as a predictor for erythrocyte transfusion in healthy preterm infants with anemia of prematurity. J Pediatr 1993;122:629-31.

18. Batton DG, Goodrow D, Walker RN. Reducing neonatal transfusion. J Perinatol 1992;12:152-5.

19. Ross MP, Christensen RD, Rothstein G, et al. A randomized trial to develop criteria for administering erythrocyte transfusions to anemic preterm infants 1 to 3 months of age. J Perinatol 1989;9:246-53.

20. Yamashita H, Kukita J, Ohga S, et al. Serum erythropoietin levels in term and preterm infants during the first year of life. J Pediat Hematol Oncol 1994;16:213-8.

21. Attias D. Pathophysiology and treatment of the anemia of prematurity. J Pediatr Hematol Oncol 1995;17:13-8.

22. Lachance C, Chessex P, Fouron JC, et al. Myocardial, erythropoietic and metabolic adaptation to anemia of prematurity. J Pediatr 1994;125:278-82.

23. Obladen M, Maier RF. Recombinant erythropoietin for prevention of anemia in preterm infants. J Perinat Med 1995;23:119-26.

24. Maier RF, Obladen M, Scigalla P, et al. The effect of epoetin beta (recombinant human erythropoietin) on the need for transfusion in very low birth weight infants. N Engl J Med 1994;330:1173-8.

25. Fernandes CH, Hagan R, Frieberg A, et al. Erythropoietin in very preterm infants. J Paediatr Child Health 1994;30:356-9.

26. Seef LB, Baskell-Bales Z, Wright EC, et al. Long-term mortality after transfusion associated non-A, non-B hepatitis. N Engl Med 1992;327:1906-11.

27. Ljungman P, Johansson N, Aschan J, et al. Long-term effects of hepatitis C virus infection in allogeneic bone marrow transplant recipients. Blood 1995;86:1614-8.

28. Alter HJ, Purcell RH, Shih JW, et al. Detection of antibody to hepatitis C virus in prospec

tively followed transfusion recipients with acute and chronic non-A non-B hepatitis. N Engl J Med 1989;321:1494-500.

29. Bortolotti F, Vajro P, Barbera C, et al. Hepatitis C in childhood: Epidemiological and clinical aspects. Bone Marrow Transplant 1993;12 (Suppl 1):21-3.

30. Maniwa H, Mitake Y, Hamada M, et al. Clinical and serological courses of a newborn with post-transfusion hepatitis C. J Viral Hepat 1995; 2:303-5.

31. Noble RC, Kane MA, Reeves SA, Roeckel I. Posttransfusion hepatitis A in a neonatal intensive care unit. JAMA 1984;252:2711-5.

32. Quie PG. Antimicrobial defenses in the neonate. Semin Perinatol 1990;14 (4 Suppl 1):2-9.

33. Wilson CB, Lewis DB. Basis and implications of selectively diminished cytokine production in neonatal susceptibility to infection. Rev Infect Dis 1990;12 (Suppl 4):S410-20.

34. Sanders MR, Graeber JE. Posttransfusion graft-versus-host disease in infancy. J Pediatr 1991;117:159-63.

35. de Cates CR, Gray J, Roberton NR, Walker J. Acquisition of cytomegalovirus infection by premature neonates. J Infect Dis 1994;28: 25-30.

36. Tegtmeier GE. Posttransfusion cytomegalovirus infections. Arch Pathol Lab Med 1989; 113:236-45.

37. Kelsey SM, Newland AC. Cytomegalovirus seroconversion in patients receiving intensive induction therapy prior to allogeneic bone marrow transplantation. Bone Marrow Transplant 1989;4:543-6.

38. Winston DJ, Huang ES, Miller MJ, et al. Molecular epidemiology of cytomegalovirus infections associated with bone marrow transplantation. Ann Intern Med 1985;102:16-20.

39. Bowden RA, Sayers M, Flournoy N, et al. Cytomegalovirus immune globulin and seronegative blood products to prevent primary cytomegalovirus infection after marrow transplantation. N Engl J Med 1986;314:1006-10.

40. Snydman DR, Werner BG, Meissner HC, et al. Use of cytomegalovirus immunoglobulin in multiply transfused premature neonates. Pediatr Infect Dis J 1995;14:34-40.

41. Ballard RA, Drew WL, Hufnagle KG, Riedel PA. Acquired cytomegalovirus infection in preterm infants. Am J Dis Child 1979;133: 482-5.

42. Yeager AS, Grumet FC, Hafleigh EB, et al. Prevention of transfusion-acquired cytomegalovirus infections in newborn infants. J Pediatr 1981;98:281-7.

43. Leukocyte reduction for the prevention of transfusion-transmitted cytomegalovirus (TT-CMV). Association Bulletin 97-2. Bethesda, MD: American Association of Blood Banks, 1997.

44. Warwick R, Modi N. Guidelines for the administration of blood products. Arch Dis Child 1995;72:379-81.

45. Davies SC, Kinsey SE. Clinical aspects of paediatric blood transfusion: Cellular components. Vox Sang 1994;67(Suppl 5):50-3.

46. Voak D, Cann R, Finney RD, et al. Guidelines for administration of blood products: Transfusion of infants and neonates. British Committee for Standards in Haematology, Blood Transfusion Task Force. Transfus Med 1994; 4:63-9.

47. Scanlon JW, Krakaur R. Hyperkalemia following exchange transfusion. J Pediatr 1980;96: 108-10.

48. Brown KA, Bissonnette B, MacDonald M, Poon AO. Hyperkalemia during massive blood transfusion in pediatric craniofacial surgery. Can J Anaesth 1990;37:401-8.

49. Brown KA, Bissonnette B, McIntyre B. Hyperkalemia during rapid blood transfusion and hypovolaemic cardiac arrest in children. Can J Anaesth 1990;37:747-54.

50. Hall TL, Barnes A, Miller JR, et al. Neonatal mortality following transfusion of red cells with high plasma potassium levels. Transfusion 1993;33:606-9.

51. Blanchette VS, Grey E, Hardic MJ, et al. Hyperkalemia following exchange transfusion:

Risk eliminated by washing red cell concentrates. J Pediatr 1993;123:285-8.

52. Wood L, Beutler E. Temperature dependence of sodium-potassium activated erythrocyte adenosine triphosphatase. J Lab Clin Med 1967;70:287-94.

53. Beutler E, Meul A, Wood L. Depletion and regeneration of 2,3-diphosphoglyceric acid in stored red blood cells. Transfusion 1969;9: 109-14.

54. Heaton A, Keegan T, Holm S. In vivo regeneration of red cell 2,3-diphosphoglycerate following transfusion of DPG depleted AS-1, AS-3 and CPDA-1 red cells. Br J Haematol 1989;71:131-6.

55. Tuchschmid T, Mieth D, Burger R, Duc G. Potential hazard of hypoalbuminemia in newborn babies after exchange transfusion with ADSOL red blood cell concentrates. Pediatrics 1990;85:234-5.

56. Luban NLC, Strauss RG, Hume HA. Commentary on the safety of red blood cells preserved in extended storage media for neonatal transfusions. Transfusion 1991;31:229-35.

57. Allen BS, Rahman S, Ilbawi MN, et al. Detrimental effects of cardiopulmonary bypass in cyanotic infants: Preventing the reoxygenation injury. Ann Thorac Surg 1997;64:1387-8.

58. Moise KJ Jr. Intrauterine transfusion with red cells and platelets. West J Med 1993;159: 318-24.

59. Schumacher B, Moise KJ Jr. Fetal transfusion for red blood cell alloimmunization in pregnancy. Obstet Gynecol 1996;88:137-50.

60. Ryan G, Morrow RJ. Fetal blood transfusion. Clin Perinatol 1994;21:573-89.

61. Sampson AJ, Permezel M, Doyle LW, et al. Ultrasound-guided fetal intravascular transfusions for severe erythroblastosis, 1984–1993. Aust N Z J Obstet Gynaecol 1994;34:125-30.

62. Plockinger B, Strumpflen I, Deutinger J, Bernaschek G. Diagnosis and treatment of fetal anemia due to isoimmunization. Arch Gynecol Obstet 1994;255:195-200.

63. Goodrum LA, Saade GR, Belfort MA, et al. The effect of intrauterine transfusion on fetal bilirubin in red cell alloimmunization. Obstet Gynecol 1997;89:57-60.

64. Kanhai HH, Porcelign L, van Zoeren D, et al. Antenatal care in pregnancies at risk of alloimmune thrombocytopenia: Report of 19 cases in 16 families. Eur J Obstet Gynecol Reprod Biol 1996;68:67-73.

65. Merchant RH, Lulla CP, Gupte SC, Krishnani RH. Fetal outcome following intrauterine intravascular transfusion in rhesus alloimmunization. Indian Pediatr 1995;32:971-7.

66. Carr S, Rubin L, Dixon D, et al. Intrauterine therapy for homozygous alpha-thalassemia. Obstet Gynecol 1995;85:876-9.

67. Mielke G, Enders G. Late onset of hydrops fetalis following intrauterine parvovirus B19 infection, Fetal Diagn Ther 1997;12:40-2.

68. Lipitz S, Achiron R, Horoshovski D, et al. Fetomaternal haemorrhage discovered after trauma and treated by fetal intravascular transfusion. Eur J Obstet Gynecol Reprod Biol 1997;71:21-2.

69. Fairley CK, Smoleniec JS, Caul OE, Miller E. Observational study of effort of intrauterine transfusion on outcome of fetal hydrops after parvovirus B19 infection. Lancet 1995;346: 1335-7.

70. Montgomery LD, Belfort MA, Adam K. Massive fetomaternal hemorrhage treated with serial combined intravascular and intraperitoneal fetal transfusions. Am J Obstet Gynecol 1995;173:234-5.

71. Bussel J, Berkowitz R, McFarland AD, et al. In-utero platelet transfusion for alloimmune thrombocytopenia. Lancet 1988;2:1307-8.

72. Vietor HE, Kanhai HH, Brand A. Induction of additional red cell alloantibodies after intrauterine transfusions. Transfusion 1994;34: 970-4.

73. Welch R, Rampling MW, Anwar A, et al. Changes in hemorheology with fetal intravascular transfusion. Am J Obstet Gynecol 1994; 170:726-32.

74. Yankowitz J, Weiner CP. Blood transfusion for haemolytic disease as a cause of leukocytosis in the fetus. Prenat Diagn 1996;16:719-22.

75. Parkman R, Mosier D, Umansky I, et al. Graft-versus-host disease after intrauterine and exchange transfusions for hemolytic disease of the newborn. N Engl J Med 1974;290: 359-63.

76. Saade GR, Moise KJ Jr, Belfort MA, et al. Fetal and neonatal hematologic parameters in red cell alloimmunization: Predicting the need for late neonatal transfusions. Fetal Diagn Ther 1993;8:161-4.

77. Dallacasa P, Ancora G, Miniero R, et al. Erythropoietin course in newborns with Rh hemolytic disease transfusion and not transfused in utero. Pediatr Res 1996;40:357-60.

78. Ovali F, Samanci N, Dagoglu T. Management of late anemia in rhesus hemolytic disease: Use of recombinant human erythropoietin (a pilot study). Pediatr Res 1996;39:831-4.

79. Scaradavou A, Inglis S, Peterson P, et al. Suppression of erythropoiesis by intrauterine transfusions in hemolytic disease of the newborn: Use of erythropoietin to treat the late anemia. J Pediatr 1993;123:297-84.

In: Mintz PD, ed.
Transfusion Therapy: Clinical Principles and Practice
Bethesda, MD: AABB Press, 1999

16

Leukocyte-Reduced and Cytomegalovirus-Reduced-Risk Blood Components

JOHN P. MILLER, MD, PhD, AND JAMES P. AuBUCHON, MD

GROWING EVIDENCE INDICATES that leukocytes and their metabolic products (cytokines) are associated with many of the adverse outcomes of transfusion, although these cells may have beneficial effects in selected clinical situations (Table 16-1). Febrile reactions to the transfusion of blood components may occur as a result of the presence of donor leukocytes or cytokines released during blood storage. Alloimmunization to HLA antigens present on leukocytes can lead to refractoriness to platelet transfusion, but it also also may induce an immune tolerance that facilitates organ transplantation. Engraftment of donor T lymphocytes following hematopoietic progenitor cell transplanta-

tion causes graft-vs-host disease (GVHD), yet these same cells are responsible for the beneficial graft-vs-leukemia effect and are used in the treatment of relapsed leukemia that occurs following marrow transplantation. Removal of leukocyte-associated viruses (eg, cytomegalovirus) may prevent their transmission by transfusion, and leukocyte reduction also may prevent virus reactivation in patients infected already. While controversial, leukocyte transfusion has immunomodulatory effects that may affect the incidence of postoperative infection and tumor recurrence. Filtration of white blood cells (WBCs) shortly after blood collection may help reduce bacterial growth in contaminated components. Neutrophils are involved in the patho-

John P. Miller, MD, PhD, Medical Director, American Red Cross, Northern Ohio Region, Cleveland, Ohio; and James P. AuBuchon, MD, Professor of Pathology and Medicine, Department of Pathology, Dartmouth-Hitchcock Medical Center, Lebanon, New Hampshire

Table 16-1. Potential Adverse Effects of Leukocytes

Immunologically mediated effects

   Alloimmunization to HLA

      Febrile nonhemolytic transfusion reactions

      Platelet refractoriness

      Transplant rejection

   Graft-vs-host disease

   Immunosuppression

   Viral disease reactivation

Infectious disease transmission

   Viruses (eg, cytomegalovirus, human T-cell lymphotropic virus types I and II, Epstein-Barr virus)

   Bacteria

Reperfusion injury

physiology of the reperfusion injury seen following periods of cardiac ischemia; hence, their removal during coronary artery bypass surgery may minimize the amount of myocardial damage. This review focuses on the evidence for the clinical effectiveness of leukocyte reduction of blood components and concludes with recommendations for its use.

Leukocyte Removal: Mechanisms, Timing, and Potential Adverse Effects

The effectiveness and ease of use of leukocyte-reduction filters have led to the use of filtration as the most common method to remove leukocytes from blood components, superseding other methods such as differential centrifugation, sedimentation, washing, and freezing/thawing.[1] Leukocyte-reduction filters remove WBCs primarily on the basis of their larger size compared with red blood cells (RBCs) and platelets and also by WBC adherence to the fibers of the filter; other forces contribute as

well, including adhesion through cell-cell interactions.[2] Current filters remove between 3 and 5 $\log_{10}$ (99.9-99.999%) of WBCs from RBC and platelet components, reducing a unit's WBC content to less than 5×10^6 per unit, the threshold for many of the adverse effects of transfused leukocytes.[1,3-6] The metabolic activity and function of RBCs and platelets appear not to be affected by filtration, and storage without the presence of leukocytes has been shown to improve biochemical parameters and posttransfusion recovery.[7-9] On the other hand, filtration may result in the loss of up to 15-25% of RBCs and platelets, thereby reducing the dose administered and potentially incurring the costs of additional transfusion.[9-11]

Leukocyte filtration may be performed in three settings: 1) in the blood center during the collection of apheresis platelets,[12] or shortly after collection and preparation of blood components (prestorage); 2) in the laboratory (poststorage); or 3) at the time of transfusion (bedside, poststorage). Prestorage filtration appears to have several advantages over bedside filtration, including better quality control of the physical variables that affect filter performance, a lower incidence of febrile reactions and alloimmunization, and (possibly) diminished immunomodulation that may result from the transfusion of leukocytes or their membrane fragments.[13-16]

Two rare types of reactions have tentatively been attributed to the effects of leukocyte reduction filtration. Several hypotensive reactions have been reported in patients taking angiotensin-converting enzyme (ACE) inhibitors following the administration of leukocyte-reduced blood components prepared with the use of negatively, not positively, charged filters.[17-21] These reactions are similar to those that have been observed during therapeutic apheresis with albumin replacement and during hemodialysis when patients have been taking ACE inhibitors. The etiology is thought to be activation of the kallikrein system with the generation of bradykinin triggered by the exposure of plasma to negatively charged surfaces.[22] As the ACE is responsible for the metabolism of bradykinin, patients taking an inhibitor of this enzyme may be particularly sensitive to bradykinin generation during filtration.

The other reaction type is a novel one not associated with transfusion previously. Since November 1997, the Centers for Disease Control and Prevention have received more than 50 reports of a transfusion-related "red eye" syndrome consisting of severe conjunctival injection, ocular pain, periorbital edema, arthralgias, and headache.[23] These reactions have occurred only after the transfusion of leukocyte-filtered components prepared with a particular filter, but the underlying mechanism remains to be determined. Given the anecdotal nature of the reports of both types of reaction, further investigation is necessary to define their exact mechanisms and to document that filtration is responsible for the adverse effects.

Febrile, Nonhemolytic Transfusion Reactions

Fever, a common consequence of the transfusion of allogeneic leukocytes, occurs in approximately 1% of RBC[24] and up to 30% of platelet[24-26] transfusions. A febrile, nonhemolytic transfusion reaction (FNHTR) is defined as a rise in patient temperature of 1 C, with or without chills and rigors, once other causes of fever (eg, infection or hemolysis) have been ruled out.[27] Besides the patient discomfort associated with these symptoms, the laboratory and clinical evaluations of these reactions increase the cost and delay the benefits of transfusion.[28] Fortunately, many, but not all, FNHTRs may be prevented through the use of leukocyte-reduced blood components. The management of FNHTRs is discussed in Chapter 18.

Several mechanisms have been proposed to explain the role of donor leukocytes in the pathogenesis of fever in the transfusion recipient.[2] In all three of the proposed models, the final common pathway for the production of fever is the release of inflammatory cytokines (eg, interleukin [IL]-1, IL-6, and tumor necrosis factor [TNF]) from leukocytes. These mediators stimulate the prostaglandin synthesis in the hypothalamus that results in fever.[29] In the first model of an FNHTR, recipient antibodies

are directed against HLA or non-HLA antigens on donor leukocytes. Fever results when antibody binds to the transfused leukocytes, causing the release of pyrogens such as IL-1 from *donor* leukocytes. While plausible, however, this mechanism fails to explain all situations in which FNHTRs occur. Antibodies directed against HLA, granulocyte-specific, and platelet-specific antigens have been detected in the sera of patients experiencing FNHTRs,[30-33] but more severe reactions have been associated with granulocyte[33] antibodies. This first model fails to explain the occurrence of FNHTRs to leukocyte-reduced platelet units because the target antigen is borne only on a cell incapable of producing a pyrogen (eg, a platelet).[28, 34-36] In the second model, formation of antigen-antibody complexes causes complement activation, with C5a stimulating the release of inflammatory cytokines from *recipient* monocytes.[37-39] Recent evidence now supports a third model for the occurrence of FNHTRs following transfusion: the accumulation of inflammatory cytokines in blood components through active synthesis during storage.[26,40-42]

Several clinical observations suggest that cytokines (eg, IL-1, IL-6, and TNF) generated during blood storage may be a major cause of FNHTRs.[26,40] First, FNHTRs are more common after the transfusion of platelets (which are stored at 20-24 C) than after the transfusion of RBCs, even though the latter contain more leukocytes.[25,26,34] Second, the incidence of FNHTRs increases with the age of the component.[26,40-43] Third, FNHTRs occur in patients who lack a history of pregnancy or prior transfusion and who, therefore, should not have a previously generated antibody to trigger the reaction.[25,40] Fourth, leukocyte reduction, even with high-efficiency filters, does not prevent all reactions. Fifth, Heddle and colleagues[40] observed a higher frequency of FNHTRs following transfusion of the plasma rather than of the cellular component of whole blood-derived platelet concentrates (PCs). In fact, only about 10% of FNHTRs are associated with the presence of HLA antibodies in the recipient.[40,44] Taken together, these observations are consistent with the accumulation of soluble, donor-derived, inflammatory cytokines during blood component storage that are not removed by leukocyte-reduction filters.

Since Muylle and colleagues[45] first reported that concentrations of IL-1, IL-6, and TNF increased with component storage time, numerous investigators have confirmed the higher levels of cytokines in blood components following storage.[40,41,46-49] The exponential increase in cytokine concentration suggests active synthesis rather than passive leakage from leukocytes.[50] Increased levels of cytokines are correlated with length of storage, initial leukocyte count, and storage temperature. These variables and IL-6 concentrations are clinically correlated with an increased incidence of FNHTRs.[40-42] Levels of IL-6 can increase between 10- and 1000-fold by day 5 of storage in PCs,[40,41,48,49,51-53] and a similar, 10-fold increase in FNHTRs is seen following transfusion of buffy coat PCs at day 5 compared with day 1.[42] PCs prepared by the platelet-rich plasma method are associated with higher cytokine levels and FNHTRs than are buffy coat-derived PCs that contain fewer WBCs.[41,54] Less cytokine accumulation is seen with RBCs than with PCs stored at room temperature, and the generation of IL-1, IL-6, and TNF may be prevented by PC storage at 4 C.[48] As expected, prestorage leukocyte reduction is effective in preventing cytokine accumulation in blood components during storage, whereas poststorage filtration is not.[46,47,49,51,55]

The clinical efficacy of leukocyte-reduced RBCs in the prevention of FNHTRs is well documented. Removal of 75-90% of the leukocytes from a unit of RBCs to below 5×10^8 prevents most FNHTRs in multitransfused patients with a history of recurrent FNHTRs.[37,44,56-58] In such patients, the incidence of these reactions diminished from 10.3% to 1.3% following microaggregate filtration, an older leukocyte-reduction technique with about 90% removal efficiency.[58] In transfusion-dependent thalassemia patients who experience a high incidence of FNHTRs, leukocyte-reduction filtration decreased the incidence of these reactions from 13% to 0.5%.[56,57] In patients with hematologic malignancy, the exclusive use of poststorage, leukocyte-reduced RBCs resulted in an FNHTR rate of 2.15%.[44] Prestorage filtration appears to be more ef-

fective than poststorage filtration in preventing FNHTRs but does not eliminate these reactions entirely. Federowicz and colleagues[55] found that the incidence of FNHTRs following the transfusion of prestorage, leukocyte-reduced RBCs was 1.1% compared with 2.15% when leukocytes were removed after storage.

The role of leukocyte-reduced platelets in the prevention of FNHTRs remains controversial. Initial reports found a decreased incidence of FNHTRs, but the small number of patients and transfusions that were evaluated limits their conclusions.[59-64] Mangano and colleagues[34] found a lower incidence of FNHTRs with poststorage leukocyte-reduced platelet units; the rate of febrile reactions in this group of patients dropped from 27% to 17% for those receiving PCs and from 14% to 7% for those receiving plateletpheresis units. In contrast, Goodnough et al[65] found that bedside filtration caused no difference in the reaction rates to platelet transfusion. Similarly, a prospective, clinical study of patients with hematologic malignancies showed no difference in the incidence of FNHTRs with the use of leukocyte-reduced components.[36] The role of prestorage leukocyte reduction in decreasing the rates of FNHTRs is suggested by a lower incidence of such reactions in patients receiving buffy coat PCs than in those receiving platelet-rich, plasma-derived PCs.[41] Also, FNHTRs occur more often with the transfusion of older, buffy coat PCs (0.45% when transfused on day 1 of storage vs 8.62% on day 5).[42] The clinical effectiveness of prestorage leukocyte reduction in diminishing FNHTRs to platelet transfusion also may exceed that of poststorage leukocyte reduction; in a study of hematology/oncology patients with a history of at least two prior febrile reactions, those who subsequently received poststorage leukocyte-reduced plateletpheresis units had a 3.5-fold higher reaction rate (4.50%) than those who received leukocyte-reduced plateletpheresis units prior to storage (1.28%).[66]

Leukocyte reduction can be achieved today by the filtration of RBC or platelet components and also by special apheresis collection techniques for plateletpheresis components. Certain collection instruments incorporate methodology that reliably yields a therapeutic dose of platelets accompanied by fewer than 1×10^6 leukocytes. In fact, most of these instruments turn out components with one or two orders of magnitude fewer leukocytes than those required for the component to be considered leukocyte reduced. Some researchers have noted slight differences in the distribution of leukocyte types in filtered plateletpheresis components vs those components produced through special collection techniques. While the clinical implications of these differences remain to be ascertained, the very low levels of residual leukocytes of any type make it unlikely that these two approaches to leukocyte reduction will have clinically discernible differences in their effects.

Prevention of Alloimmunization and Platelet Refractoriness

Alloimmunization to Class I HLA antigens on platelets is a major cause of refractoriness to platelet transfusion, which occurs in 30-70% of multitransfused patients.[67-69] A poor 1-hour posttransfusion corrected count increment suggests that alloimmunization is present.[70,71] A poor corrected count increment may also be due to other clinical factors, including fever, infection, disseminated intravascular coagulation, veno-oclusive disease, amphotericin therapy, or ABO incompatibility.[72] Refractoriness to platelet transfusion because of the presence of HLA alloantibodies may be managed in many patients with the use of HLA-matched or crossmatched platelets.[73] In patients with broadly reactive antibodies, the efficacy of these techniques may be limited, and life-threatening thrombocytopenia may persist in spite of multiple platelet transfusions. (The frequency with which refractoriness causes hemorrhagic morbidity or mortality remains to be determined.[2]) Therefore, the prevention of alloimmunization in patients who are likely to be multitransfused is preferable to the management of refractoriness once it develops.

Methods to prevent alloimmunization include the use of leukocyte-reduced or ultraviolet (UV)-irradiated components. Platelets express only Class I antigens and are a poor stimulus of primary alloimmunization.[74] Exposure to HLA Class II antigens present on leukocytes by transfusion or pregnancy appears to be necessary for antibodies to HLA Class I antigens to develop on the same cell.[75] Further, the development of HLA antibodies requires Class I and II antigens to be present on the same cell, as third-party leukocytes fail to produce alloimmunization.[75] UV irradiation of platelet components reduces the recipient's humoral immune response by interfering with antigen presentation to helper T lymphocytes.[76] Although not licensed in the United States, UV irradiation is effective in preventing alloimmunization[77-80] with no deleterious effect on platelet function or in-vivo survival.[81]

Numerous studies have evaluated the clinical efficacy of leukocyte reduction in the prevention of alloimmunization and platelet refractoriness (Table 16-2).[82-100] Most of these investigations found a lower incidence of alloimmunization and refractoriness in patients transfused with leukocyte-reduced components. The development of alloantibodies appears to have a dose-response relationship, as studies with more efficient leukocyte removal are associated with less alloimmunization. The threshold number of leukocytes per component to reduce alloantibody formation appears to be approximately $1-5 \times 10^6$. In fact, two of the studies that failed to show an effect of leukocyte reduction involved transfused components with WBC concentrations above this level.[84,85]

Recent evidence suggests that leukocyte reduction prevents primary alloimmunization but is less efficacious in avoiding an anamnestic response and refractoriness in previously sensitized patients.[77,90,97,100] The development of alloantibodies and refractoriness is 2- to 10-fold higher and occurs sooner in women with a history of pregnancy than in immunologically unexposed patients. The Trial to Reduce Alloimmunization to Platelets study[77] found that the use of leukocyte-reduced components did not lower the incidence of refractoriness in patients with a history of pregnancy compared with control patients; however, their use halved the rate of alloantibody formation in previously pregnant women. In contrast, in a study of female

Table 16-2. Prevention of Alloimmunization by Leukocyte Reduction

Reference	Number of Patients	HLA Alloimmunity (%)		Platelet Refractoriness (%)	
		Control No. (%)	Leukocyte-reduced No. (%)	Control No. (%)	Leukocyte-reduced No. (%)
Eernisse, 1981[82]	96*	10/16 (63)	19/68 (28)	26/28 (93)	16/68 (24)
Schiffer, 1987[85]	56	13/31 (42)	5/25[†] (20)	6/31 (19)	4/25[†] (16)
Fisher, 1985[83]	24	5/12 (42)	0/12 (0)	NA	NA
Murphy, 1986[84]	50	13/31 (42)	3/19 (16)	7/31 (23)	1/19[†] (5)
Sniecinski, 1988[91]	40	10/20 (50)	3/20 (15)	10/20 (50)	3/20 (15)
Andreu, 1988[86]	69	11/35 (31)	4/34 (12)	14/30 (47)	6/28 (21)
Brand, 1988[87]	335	NA	69/335 (21)	NA	31/335 (9)
Saarinen, 1990[88]	47*	NA	NA	11/21 (52)	0/26 (0)
Oksanen, 1991[90]	31	3/15 (20)	2/16 (13)	1/15 (7)	0/16 (0)
van Marwijk Kooy,1991[89]	53	11/26 (42)	2/27 (7)	12/26 (46)	3/27 (11)
Saarinen, 1993[92]	60*‡	3/10 (30)	0/50[§] (0)	1/10 (10)	0/50[§] (0)
Bedford Russell, 1993[93]	42	7/23 (30)	0/19 (0)	ND	ND
Williamson, 1994[36]	123	21/56 (38)	15/67[†] (22)	8/27 (30)	6/23[†] (26)
	53	15/24 (62)	9/29 (31)		
Oksanen, 1994[94]	135	16/42 (38)	5/30[†] (17)	14/68 (21)	2/67 (3)
Hogge, 1995[95]	117	10/50 (20)	10/67[†] (15)	19/50 (38)	19/67[†] (28)
Abou-Elella, 1995[96]	170	ND	17/170 (10)	ND	ND
Sintnicolaas, 1995[97]	62	9/21 (43)	11/25[†‖] (44)	14/34 (41)	8/28 (29)
Novotny, 1995[98]	194	ND	3/112[¶]** (2.7) 16/52[‖] (31)	ND	42/194 (22)
Killick, 1997[99]	16	ND	2/16** (12)	ND	0/16 (0)
Legler, 1997[100]	145		17/145 (12)		40/145 (28)
TRAP, 1997[77]	530	45%	17-18%	13%	3-4%

All p<0.05 unless otherwise noted; NA = not available; ND = not determined
*Not randomized
†p >0.05
‡Reference group received mostly leukocyte-reduced components
§p not determined
‖Secondary alloimmunization
¶Primary alloimmunization
**Prestorage leukocyte reduction

patients with hematologic malignancies and a history of prior pregnancy, Sintnicolaas and colleagues[97] found no difference in lymphocytotoxic antibody formation or refractoriness through the use of leukocyte-reduced blood components. These results are supported by observations that prestorage leukocyte reduction virtually eliminates primary sensitization but not a secondary response.[98] The transfusion of platelets (which express Class I, but not Class II, HLA antigens) may stimulate an anamnestic response leading to lymphocytotoxic antibody formation. Further study is necessary to determine if patients who have been pregnant or transfused previously will benefit from leukocyte-reduced blood components to prevent refractoriness to platelet transfusion.

Leukocyte reduction with current technology does not prevent all primary alloimmunization from occurring as a result of platelet transfusions. Alloimmunization may result from the transfusion of WBC fragments that accumulate during platelet,[101] but not RBC,[102] storage and may pass through poststorage leukocyte-reduction filters. In an animal model, prestorage leukocyte reduction is associated with less alloimmunization and refractoriness than poststorage leukocyte reduction.[103] In addition, the removal of plasma and leukocytes is more effective than leukocyte reduction alone.[104] It remains to be seen if prestorage filtration will be more effective in preventing alloimmunization in the clinical setting. In addition, residual WBCs in the leukocyte-reduced PCs may contribute to primary alloimmunization.

Leukocyte reduction prevents primary alloimmunization, but is it cost-effective? Added expenses associated with the procedure include the cost of the filter (prestorage or poststorage) and the extra labor required of clinical or laboratory staff. Also, one cannot predict accurately which patients are most susceptible to forming alloantibodies, so leukocyte-reduced components must be provided to all patients at risk of becoming refractory. On the other hand, the management of refractoriness is expensive, and the mean cost of hemotherapeutic support for marrow transplantation patients who become refractory may be as much as $15,000.[105]

Cost savings through the use of leukocyte-reduced components has been reported in patients with leukemia and lymphoma.[91,106,107] The savings were realized through decreased platelet use, decreased use of HLA or crossmatched platelets, and shortened hospital stays. Additional savings may result from a more rapid hematopoietic recovery and lower infection rate following transplantation in acute myelogenous leukemia (AML)-patients receiving leukocyte-reduced blood components.[90] These studies are encouraging and may indicate that leukocyte reduction is cost-effective in the patient populations studied. With additional information to delineate the benefits and the clinical cost savings related to avoiding alloimmunization and refractoriness, clinicians may be better able to identify those patients most likely to benefit from this approach.

Use of Cytomegalovirus-Reduced-Risk Blood Products

Cytomegalovirus (CMV) is a leukocyte-associated virus that may be transmitted by blood components. Infection in immunocompromised patients may be associated with considerable morbidity and mortality (pneumonitis, gastroenteritis, retinitis) and is best avoided. Persons at demonstrable risk for the adverse sequelae of infection are listed in Table 16-3.[108] Transfusion-associated CMV (TA-CMV) may be minimized through the use of seronegative blood components. For example, such components have reduced the infection rate in CMV-seronegative marrow transplantation patients to 1-4% compared with an incidence of 23-37% associated with the transfusion of CMV-unscreened blood components.[109-112]

The possibility of leukocyte reduction as an alternative to the use of CMV- seronegative products is intriguing. First, the seroprevalence of CMV in the US donor population is high (50-80%), which would limit the number of seronegative units available for transfusion.[108] Second, the cost of CMV screening would be eliminated in patients already receiving leukocyte-reduced blood components for other indications, such as the prevention of

Table 16-3. Indications for Cytomegalovirus (CMV)-Reduced-Risk Blood Components[108]

Category*	Clinical Circumstance	CMV-Seronegative Blood (Unmodified)	Leukocyte-Reduced (LR) Blood (CMV-Unscreened)
I	CMV+ patient	Not indicated	Not indicated
	CMV– patient	Not indicated	Not indicated
II	CMV+ patient	Not indicated	Use of LR blood to prevent virus re-activation awaits further research
	CMV– patient	Either CMV– blood or LR blood is indicated	Either CMV– blood or LR blood is indicated
III	CMV+ recipient	Not indicated	Not indicated
	CMV– recipient of CMV+ organ donor	Not indicated	Not indicated
	CMV– recipient of CMV– organ donor	Either CMV– blood or LR blood is indicated	Either CMV– blood or LR blood is indicated
IV	CMV+ recipient	Not indicated	Use of LR blood to prevent virus reactivation awaits further research
	CMV– recipient of CMV+ donor	Either CMV– blood or LR blood is indicated	Either CMV– blood or LR blood is indicated
	CMV– recipient of CMV– donor	Either CMV– blood or LR blood is indicated	Either CMV– blood or LR blood is indicated
V	CMV+ recipient	Either CMV– blood or LR blood is indicated	Either CMV– blood or LR blood is indicated
	CMV– recipient	Either CMV– blood or LR blood is indicated	LR blood may be slightly preferred to CMV– blood (passive CMV immunoglobulin)

*Category I patients:
General hospital patients and general surgery patients (including cardiac surgery)
Patients receiving chemotherapy that is not intended to produce severe neutropenia (adjuvant therapy for breast cancer, treatment of chronic lymphocytic leukemia, etc).
Patients receiving corticosteroids (patients with immune thrombocytopenic purpura, collagen vascular diseases, etc)
Full-term infants
Category II patients:
Patients receiving chemotherapy that is intended to produce severe neutropenia (leukemia, lymphoma, etc)
Pregnant patients
HIV-infected individuals
Category III patients:
Solid organ allograft patients who do not require massive transfusion support
Category IV patients:
Patients receiving allogeneic and autologous hematopoietic progenitor cell transplants
Category V patients:
Low-birth-weight (<1200 g) premature infants

FNHTRs or alloimmunization. Third, leukocyte reduction might prevent the transmission of CMV by seronegative units that are either falsely negative or were donated during the seronegative window period.

Numerous studies have examined the efficacy of leukocyte reduction in the prevention of TA-CMV (Table 16-4). Although many of these studies were limited in design, they provide strong support for the prevention of TA-CMV by leukocyte-reduction filtration. The prospective, multicenter study of 502 marrow transplantation patients by Bowden and colleagues[112] supports the efficacy of leukocyte reduction in preventing TA-CMV. However, the conclusion that leukocyte-filtered blood components are as effective as CMV-seronegative blood components remains controversial.[108,124] In the primary analysis of the results, the rates of CMV infection and disease occurring in the period of 21-100 days after transplant were equivalent. Infec-

Table 16-4. Prevention of Cytomegalovirus (CMV) Transmission by Leukocyte Reduction (LR)

Reference	No. of Patients	Diagnosis	Posttransfusion CMV (%)		
			Control	LR	Seronegative
Verdonck, 1987[113]	29	Bone marrow transplant	NA	0/29 (0)	NA
Murphy, 1988[114]	20	Acute leukemia	2/9 (22)	0/11 (0)	NA
Gilbert, 1989[115]	72	Neonates	9/42 (21)	0/30 (0)	NA
De Graan-Hentzen, 1989[116]	145	Leukemia, lymphoma	10/86 (12)	0/59 (0)	NA
Bowden, 1989[117]	17	Bone marrow transplant	NA	0/17 (0)	NA
De Witte, 1990[118]	28	Bone marrow transplant	NA	0/28 (0)	NA
Bowden, 1991[119]	65	Bone marrow transplant	7/30 (23)	0/35 (0)	NA
Eisenfeld, 1992[120]	48	Neonates	NA	0/48 (0)	NA
van Prooijen, 1994[121]	48	Bone marrow transplant	ND	0/48	ND
Xu, 1995[122]	27	Neonates	9/12	2/15*	ND
Bowden, 1995[112]	502	Bone marrow transplant	ND	3/250	2/252[†]
				3/250	0/252[‡]
				6/250	4/252[§]
				6/250	0/252[‖]
Preiksaitis, 1997[123]	76	Children with malignancy	0/32	ND	0/30

NA = not available; ND = not determined

*Equivalent to background seroconversion in infants (>90% of mothers are seropositive)

[†]Infection at day 21-100 after marrow transplant, p=1.0.

[‡]Disease at day 21-100 after marrow transplant, p=0.25.

[§]Infection at day 0-100 after marrow transplant, p=0.5.

[‖]Disease at day 0-100 after marrow transplant, p=0.03.

tions observed before day 21 were considered either to be acquired prior to entry into the study or to reflect false-negative CMV screening test results upon study entry. In contrast, a secondary analysis of the data from the date of transplant (days 0-100) showed equivalent rates of CMV *infection* but a higher incidence of CMV *disease* in the filtered group, although the numbers were small (n=6 filtered, n=0 seronegative, p=0.03). In spite of the debate over the data analysis, the results of this study clearly demonstrate that the use of leukocyte-reduced blood components can decrease TA-CMV to levels seen with seronegative blood components. Prestorage leukocyte reduction may reduce TA-CMV further, but this remains to be demonstrated.

Although the American Association of Blood Banks (AABB) guideline (Table 16-3) supports the equivalent efficacy of leukocyte-reduced and CMV-seronegative blood components in preventing TA-CMV,[108] the US Food and Drug Administration (FDA) Blood Products Advisory Committee failed to support a statement of equivalent *safety* for these two approaches.[125] In a recent meeting with the AABB, FDA representatives indicated that before the agency could recommend the use of leukocyte-reduced products, filter manufacturers must submit data proving equal efficacy. In the meantime, "the state of the art right now is CMV screened products," according to Jay Epstein, MD.[126] Apart from these licensing issues, many institutions are using leukocyte reduction instead of or in conjunction with CMV seronegativity to reduce the risk of CMV transmission by blood components, a practice with which the authors and editor agree.

Table 16-3 enumerates the patients who are most likely to benefit from CMV-reduced-risk blood components. It is recognized that, in contrast to the guidelines, some clinicians provide CMV-reduced-risk components only to neonates weighing less than 1200 g who were born to CMV-seronegative mothers rather than to all such low-birth-weight neonates and also only to CMV-seronegative hematopoietic progenitor cell transplant recipients who receive CMV-seronegative

transplants rather than to all CMV-seronegative recipients. Such practices are acceptable. As a practical point because all hematopoietic progenitor cell transplant recipients are likely to be receiving leukocyte-reduced blood components, they are all likely to be transfused with CMV-reduced-risk components.

Second-Strain Infection

Restriction endonuclease analysis has been used to demonstrate that the transplantation of seropositive solid organs into seropositive recipients may result in recipient infection with a second strain of CMV.[127-130] Although second-strain infections occur, they are associated with less symptomatic disease than seen with primary infection.[130-132] By analogy with solid organ transplantation, one might expect the transmission of second-strain infection by the transfusion of CMV-unscreened blood components, but this has not been reported. Adler[133,134] found equivalent rates of CMV infection in seropositive cardiac surgery patients who received either CMV-unscreened (7/48) or seronegative (5/46) blood. Similarly, Winston and colleagues[135] found no second-strain infections in a small study of marrow transplant patients, but, rather, symptomatic disease that represented the reactivation of latent infection. Given the lack of evidence of transmission by transfusion and the lower morbidity associated with second-strain infections in solid organ transplantation, the use of CMV-reduced-risk blood components to prevent recipient infection with a different strain of CMV is not recommended.[108]

Virus Reactivation

The reactivation of latent CMV infection occurs in immunocompromised patients and may also be associated with blood transfusion. In rodent models, the culture of allogeneic cells or the transfusion of allogeneic blood stimulated the reactivation of CMV infection.[136-138] The effect of a transfusion may depend on immune status, as one study demonstrated reactivation only in animals that had received total body irradiation.[136] In cardiac surgery patients, Adler[134] found increased CMV titers following the transfusion of CMV-seronegative and CMV-unscreened units. CMV reactivation correlated with the number of units transfused and was not seen in nontransfused patients. Two small studies of CMV-seropositive heart transplant patients have demonstrated that the use of leukocyte-reduced blood components is associated with less CMV disease (0/17, 0%) than the use of non-leukocyte-reduced components (14/36, 43%).[139,140] While these studies are encouraging, the multicenter Viral Activation Transfusion Study (VATS) under way should help clarify the role of leukocyte-reduced blood components in minimizing CMV reactivation in immunocompromised individuals.[141] (The reactivation of human immuno- deficiency virus [HIV] infection is discussed in the next section.)

Immunomodulation by Allogeneic Transfusion

The immunosuppressive effect of allogeneic transfusion on renal allograft survival was observed by Opelz 25 years ago, and this beneficial effect is still seen with current immunosuppressive regimens.[142,143] In addition, allogeneic transfusion has been shown to have a favorable effect on the recurrence rates of spontaneous abortion[144] and inflammatory bowel disease,[145,146] and it may enhance engraftment and survival in marrow transplant patients.[90] On the other hand, the deleterious effects of transfusion-induced immunosuppression may include the reactivation of viral infections and increases in postoperative bacterial infection and tumor recurrence. The immunomodulation seen with allogeneic transfusion likely relates to a decrease in cell-mediated immunity along with an increase in humoral immunity. The observed effects of allogeneic transfusion include a shift from a Th1 to a Th2 immune response, as well as decreases in natural killer cell activity, the CD4/CD8 ratio, and lymphocyte blastogenesis.[147]

The role of leukocytes in mediating the immunomodulatory effects of allogeneic transfusion remains controversial despite numerous animal, observational, and randomized clinical trials. Blajchman and colleagues[104,148,149] have demonstrated that mice and rabbits receiving allogeneic blood before or after inoculation with fibrosarcoma cells have increased pulmonary metastases compared with animals receiving syngeneic blood. This tumor growth-promoting effect could be transferred to naive animals by the infusion of splenic T cells derived from animals that had received allogeneic transfusion previously. The effect on tumor growth was eliminated in animals receiving prestorage but not poststorage leukocyte-reduced blood. This observation suggests that cytokines may mediate the immunosuppressive effect, an observation that is supported also by the fact that enhanced tumor growth was seen with stored syngeneic blood, not with fresh syngeneic blood. Further, the intraperitoneal injection of spleen cells enclosed in diffusion chambers also was associated with increased tumor growth. Thus, animal models support the hypothesis that the transfusion of leukocytes present in allogeneic blood enhances tumor growth through soluble inflammatory mediators.

The results of human observational and randomized studies that have examined the effect of allogeneic transfusion on malignancy and postoperative infection rates are less clear. While approximately two-thirds of the nearly 100 observational studies have demonstrated that allogeneic transfusion is associated with increased cancer recurrence, a large number of studies have failed to observe this effect.[147] The conclusions of these studies are limited by their design: they used statistical techniques to control for the effects of confounding variables on recurrence rates.[150] Several meta-analyses of the literature have been performed in an attempt to reach a conclusion from these studies by increasing the number of patients included in the analysis and by addressing the issue of confounding variables.[150,151] Chung[151] found a cumulative odds ratio for cancer recurrence of 1.8 (95% confidence interval [CI] = 1.30-2.51). Vamvakas[150] found a smaller effect; the relative risk for colorectal cancer recurrence was 1.60 (95% CI =

1.27-2.02), although the effect was eliminated when only prospective studies, which showed a relative risk of 1.18, were included in the analysis (95% CI = 0.93-1.51).

Two randomized clinical trials have examined the effect of allogeneic transfusion on cancer recurrence by comparing patients who received either allogeneic or autologous units.[152,153] Busch[152] found no difference in cancer recurrence in a study of 475 patients randomized to receive either an allogeneic or autologous transfusion. However, transfused patients, regardless of whether they received allogeneic or autologous blood, had a worse prognosis than patients who did not require transfusion. On the other hand, Heiss[153] found a lower rate of cancer recurrence in patients receiving autologous rather than allogeneic blood. If it is assumed that autologous transfusions have no immunosuppressive effect, which might not be the case, studies comparing the risks of autologous and allogeneic blood might fail to recognize the effect of allogeneic transfusion.[154] In a multicenter clinical study of 871 patients, Houbiers and colleagues[155] compared the transfusion of leukocyte-reduced and buffy coat-depleted RBCs on colorectal cancer recurrence and did not find a significant difference between the two groups. Nevertheless, a clinical trial examining the effect of leukocyte reduction on cancer recurrence has not been performed in the United States, where some components have higher leukocyte concentrations because PCs are prepared by the platelet-rich plasma method. Thus, the immunosuppressive effect of allogeneic transfusion on cancer recurrence and the efficacy of leukocyte-reduced components to minimize this risk remain a matter of debate.

The majority of more than 30 observational studies have demonstrated that perioperative transfusion is associated with increased postoperative infections.[150] Six randomized clinical trials have studied the effect of allogeneic, autologous, and leukocyte-reduced blood transfusions on postoperative infections.[152,155-159] While Heiss[156] found a significantly decreased postoperative infection rate in patients transfused with autologous compared with buffy-coat-depleted blood (12% vs 27%), in

another study Busch[152] found similar rates of infection (27% vs 25%). Three of four prospective studies that examined the effect of leukocyte-reduced blood compared with allogeneic blood found the former to have a beneficial effect on postoperative infection.[157-159] While the fourth study, by Houbiers,[155] failed to demonstrate the benefits of leukocyte reduction, this may relate to its multicenter design. Vamvakas[160] performed a meta-analysis of four of the six clinical trials and found a relative risk for allogeneic transfusion of 1.03 (95% CI = 0.81-1.30). However, the authors caution that this analysis would fail to detect an increase in infections of 32% or less. For perspective, the clinically accepted practice of using allogeneic leukocytes to prevent recurrent spontaneous abortions is effective in only 10% of patients.[161] As is the case with cancer recurrence, the effect of leukocyte reduction of blood components prepared by the platelet-rich plasma method should be examined before conclusions can be made about transfusion practice in the United States. Thus, the answer to the question about the potential beneficial effect of leukocyte reduction on postoperative infection rates remains elusive.

Although the debate over the magnitude and clinical significance of perioperative allogeneic transfusion continues, it is acknowledged that even a small effect will have a profound impact on morbidity, mortality, and the costs associated with transfusion in surgical patients. Jensen[162] found substantial savings in total hospital charges for colorectal cancer patients receiving either leukocyte-reduced whole blood ($7867) or no transfusion ($7037) compared with those receiving transfusion with allogeneic blood ($12,347). Similarly, among 140 hip surgery patients, Blumberg[147] found a dose-dependent increase in length of stay and total hospital charges for patients receiving allogeneic transfusion (15.2 days, $26,490) compared with patients receiving autologous or no transfusion (9.4 days, $19,295). In a theoretical analysis, Blumberg[147] estimated that 2150 deaths per year in the United States would be attributable to the immunosuppressive effect of transfusion if only 10% of the reported increases in tumor recurrence and postoperative infection were causal. However, these studies have significant methodologic limitations in their handling of financial data and their estimates of infection rates attributable to transfusion. Hence, in the absence of definitive data, financial and clinical factors must be considered in the decision to use leukocyte-reduced blood components in an attempt to decrease the immunosuppressive effect of allogeneic transfusion in the surgical setting.

Finally, allogeneic transfusion may have an adverse effect on disease progression in HIV-positive patients through immunosuppression or virus reactivation. The transfusion of patients infected with HIV may lead to a more rapid progression to acquired immune deficiency syndrome (AIDS) and result in a higher death rate.[163-166] Although these epidemiologic findings may indicate that the need for transfusion is related to more severe disease, several findings suggest it may be due to immunomodulation or virus reactivation. The expression of HIV by infected T cells appears to require immunologic stimulation of these cells.[167-169] Busch and colleagues[170] found that allogeneic leukocytes stimulated a dose-dependent rise in HIV expression in infected cells in culture. Recently, Mudido et al[171] reported an increase in HIV p24 antigen and HIV RNA following transfusion in nine patients. In a small prospective study, however, Groopman[172] demonstrated that leukocyte reduction did not eliminate HIV reactivation by transfusion. It is hoped that the results of the VATS,[141] in progress, will provide some answers regarding virus reactivation and the efficacy of leukocyte reduction to alleviate this adverse effect of transfusion.

Bacterial Contamination of Blood Components

The transfusion of blood components contaminated with bacteria may cause septic transfusion reactions. These reactions may be characterized by a combination of fever, rigors, hypotension, tachycardia, hemoglobinuria, and disseminated intravascular coagulation. As the risks of virus transmission by transfusion continue to decrease, attention has focused on bacterial contamination as a significant cause of transfusion-associated morbidity and mortality. The incidence of septic transfusion reactions may be as high as 1 in 700 pooled, random-donor PCs, 1 in 4000 single-donor PCs, and 1 in 31,000 RBC transfusions.[173,174] During the period of 1986 to 1991, bacterial contamination was implicated in 16% (29/182) of all transfusion-related fatalities reported to the FDA.[175]

Bacterial contamination of blood components occurs mainly at the time of venipuncture (a result of inadequate skin preparation or asymptomatic bacteremia). Contaminating organisms from the skin appear to be in the first 5-10 mL of blood collected, so diversion of this volume may reduce inoculation of the blood entering the collection bag.[176] The most common organism contaminating platelets is *Staphylococcus epidermidis*.[177] *Yersinia enterocolitica*, which can grow at refrigerated temperatures, is the most common pathogen associated with septic reactions to RBC transfusion.[177] The management of septic reactions to blood component transfusion is discussed in Chapter 18.

Several in-vitro studies have demonstrated that leukocyte-reduction filters are capable of removing bacteria from inoculated RBCs or whole blood.[177-183] Units spiked with *Y. enterocolitica* and leukocyte-reduced by filtration several hours after collection had lower bacterial contamination than unfiltered components. On the other hand, leukocyte-reduction filtration is less efficacious in removing bacteria from platelets. Wenz and colleagues[184] demonstrated a delay in bacterial growth in leukocyte-reduced platelets, but no difference in contamination was seen after day 1 of postfiltration storage. Similarly, molecular analysis of bacterial RNA showed equivalent growth rates in platelets containing *S. epidermidis*.[185]

Leukocyte-reduction filters may remove bacteria by two mechanisms. First, filtration may remove bacteria directly, given that *Staphylococcus xylosus* can be extracted from components that have been leukocyte reduced previously.[186] Filters have removed bacteria from saline but not from 5% albumin, which apparently alters the interaction of organisms with the filter surface.[187] The direct removal of bacteria from Fresh Frozen Plasma but not from heat-inactivated plasma suggests that bacterial adherence to the filter surface may be complement dependent.[188] Second, leukocyte filters also may remove phagocytized bacteria present within WBCs.[65,189] These bacteria might have been released back into the blood if the leukocytes underwent cell death and fragmentation before the bacteria were killed. The optimal time for filtration is probably between 2 and 12 hours after collection, a period that would permit phagocytosis and removal of leukocytes prior to the later release of viable organisms, a mechanism that has been cited to explain bacterial growth in a unit previously found to be sterile.[190,191] Thus, the removal of small amounts of bacteria may be an added benefit of prestorage leukocyte reduction. However, sterility cannot be guaranteed, and filtration cannot be expected to serve as a remedy for bacterial contamination.

Graft-vs-Host Disease and the Graft-vs-Leukemia Effect

In hematopoietic progenitor cell transplant patients, the engraftment of donor T lymphocytes may cause GVHD. Similarly, the transfusion of cellular blood components containing viable donor lymphocytes may cause transfusion-associated graft-vs-host disease (TA-GVHD). This is a more severe form of the disease because TA-GVHD is characterized by pancytopenia caused by the engrafted cells attacking the recipient's marrow. The majority of cases are fatal.[192] Fortunately, TA-GVHD is quite rare in immuno-competent transfusion recipients as usually donor lymphocytes are cleared rapidly by recipient cytotoxic (CD 8) T cells.[193] The majority of donor cells (99.9%) are removed by day 2 following transfusion; however, a small number of lymphocytes may persist in the circulation for a month or more.[194,195]

Immunocompromised individuals at risk for TA-GVHD include marrow transplant recipients, patients with hematologic malignancies or solid tumors, patients with T-cell immunodeficiencies, and fetuses receiving intrauterine transfusions.[196] In ad-

dition, numerous cases of TA-GVHD have been reported in neonates. In a recent review of the Japanese literature, the majority of neonatal TA-GVHD cases (24/27) were associated with the transfusion of fresh blood.[197] These observations indicate that the transfused lymphocytes must be viable to achieve engraftment and cause tissue damage.

TA-GVHD also may occur in immunocompetent transfusion recipients who are heterozygous for an HLA haplotype for which the donor is homozygous.[198] The risk of TA-GVHD is higher in directed donations from relatives and may be increased as much as 21-fold in donations from parents to children.[199] The effect of donations from close relatives is noted again in the Japanese data where, in one series, 22 of 27 TA-GVHD cases occurred following the transfusion of blood from relatives.[197] The necessary combination of HLA types can occur in situations where the donor and recipient are unrelated, of course. Although this chance occurrence is more likely in a society in which there is less genetic diversity, the chance of it occurring in a transfusion pair in the United States is surprisingly high: approximately 1/22,000.[199]

The prevention of TA-GVHD is accomplished by gamma irradiation of cellular blood components, which inactivates T lymphocytes. Irradiation must occur in a quality-controlled setting to ensure a midplane dose of at least 25 Gy.[200] In fact, TA-GVHD has been reported in a child with acute myelogenous leukemia who received blood components that had been irradiated at 15 Gy.[201] The threshold number of leukocytes capable of causing TA-GVHD appears to be 10^4/kg.[202,203] Currently available leukocyte-reduction filters are capable of approaching this level of leukocyte reduction, which suggests that they may decrease TA-GVHD. Dzik and Jones were able to demonstrate a dose-dependent exponential decrease in the mixed lymphocyte reaction model of GVHD using leukocyte-reduced blood.[203] However, a case of TA-GVHD has been reported in a patient receiving exclusively components prepared by leukocyte-reduction filtration (with the use of a less-effective filter than is currently available).[204] Therefore, leukocyte reduction must not be relied upon as a substitute for gamma irradiation of blood components to prevent TA-GVHD.

Failure to eradicate all malignant cells can lead to leukemia relapse following marrow transplantation. The relapse rate is lower in patients who develop GVHD and higher in patients who receive T cell-depleted marrow.[205] Further, complete remission of relapsed leukemia following marrow transplantation has been achieved by the transfusion of donor-specific buffy coats.[205,206] These findings suggest that donor T cells may have an antitumor effect, which is referred to as the graft-vs-leukemia effect. This subject is discussed in detail in Chapter 13.

As a result of these observations, it has been postulated that the removal of T cells by leukocyte reduction of blood components may have a deleterious effect on malignancy recurrence. However, several reports have demonstrated no difference in disease-free survival among leukemia patients receiving either leukocyte-reduced or standard blood components.[207-210] On the other hand, Oksanen and colleagues[90] observed a *favorable* effect of leukocyte reduction on disease-free survival, hematopoietic recovery, and posttransplantation infection. Thus, leukocyte-reduced components may be used for their beneficial effects in marrow transplant patients without adversely affecting malignancy recurrence.

Reperfusion Injury

The restoration of blood flow to ischemic tissues increases the structural and functional damage caused by anoxia alone. Tissue damage is the result of neutrophil binding to endothelial cells and migration into underlying structures with subsequent release of oxygen-free radicals and proteases. Pharmacologic blockade of the endothelial or neutrophil receptors has been shown to attenuate the ultrastructural damage seen in reperfused organs. Thus, it has been postulated that the removal of leukocytes from reperfused blood may reduce the harmful effects of neutrophils on ischemic tissue.[211,212]

Several studies have examined the effect of leukocyte reduction on myocardial reperfusion injury. In animal models, the use of leukocyte-reduced blood components resulted in better left ventricular function, fewer arrhythmias, and smaller infarct size.[213-218] In heart transplant patients, Pearl and colleagues[219] observed less ultrastructural damage in patients receiving leukocyte-reduced blood. The removal of leukocytes is also effective in decreasing biochemical markers of myocardial damage, including creatine kinase MB, thromboxane B_2, and malondialdehyde.[220,221] Leukocyte removal may also improve pulmonary function, as fewer neutrophils are sequestered or activated in the lungs of dogs when filtered blood is used.[222] Although Gu et al[223] observed improved pulmonary gas exchange in postoperative cardiac patients receiving leukocyte-reduced reperfusate, two other reports failed to demonstrate a positive effect on pulmonary function.[224,225] Thus, while these initial results are encouraging, it remains to be determined if leukocyte reduction improves clinical outcome in cardiac bypass patients.

Summary/Clinical Recommendations

It is clear that, in almost all clinical situations, passenger leukocytes (lymphocytes in particular) do not convey any benefits to transfusion recipients. Questions about the role of leukocyte reduction center around the harm that leukocytes may cause. Febrile reactions are certainly far less common when sensitized patients receive leukocyte-reduced components. Leukocytes facilitate primary alloimmunization and lead to refractoriness in patients who have not been pregnant previously or sensitized otherwise. Removing leukocytes from blood components for these patients may have clinical and even financial benefits, but leukocyte reduction for previously sensitized patients may provide only an illusion of benefit. Leukocyte reduction appears to be as effective as the use of CMV-seronegative components in avoiding CMV transmission. Given that many of the patients requiring CMV-reduced-risk components also may benefit from avoiding alloimmunization, two benefits may be achieved for a single expenditure in a simple process. The possibility of avoiding immunomodulation through leukocyte reduction of allogeneic components is intriguing. If it can be demonstrated conclusively that malignancies recur earlier or that more postoperative infections occur after the transfusion of leukocyte-replete allogeneic components, these benefits of leukocyte reduction probably will drive clinical practice toward total conversion to leukocyte-reduced components, and the additional filtration costs will be overwhelmed by the savings experienced from avoiding complications.

The lack of data to analyze the outcomes of applying leukocyte reduction in the above clinical situations hinders firm conclusions regarding the most appropriate applications of this technology. As the consequences of exposure to allogeneic leukocytes are usually not perceived as life-threatening, most clinicians are willing to wait for definitive proof of benefit before implementing a wider use of leukocyte reduction. Those convinced of the immunosuppressive consequence of allogeneic exposure may have sufficient rationale to provide all or nearly all transfusions as leukocyte reduced.

While the clinical indications for leukocyte reduction remain debatable at present, the timing of the removal of passenger leukocytes has been shown clearly to be prior to storage. Not only does prestorage leukocyte reduction allow for better quality assurance, but also removal before the fragmentation of leukocyte membranes and the production of pyrogenic and immunomodulatory cytokines can be achieved. Therefore, while the "if" question remains for leukocyte reduction, the "when" has been established already.

References

1. Bruil A, Beugeling T, Feijen J, van Aken WG. The mechanisms of leukocyte removal by filtration. Transfus Med Rev 1995;9(2):45-66.
2. Dzik WH. Leukoreduced blood components: Laboratory and clinical aspects. In: Rossi EC, Simon TL, Moss GS, Gould SA, eds. Principles of transfusion medicine. Baltimore, MD: Williams & Wilkins, 1996;353-73.
3. Pietersz RNI, Steneker I, Reesink HW, et al. Comparison of five different filters for the removal of leukocytes from red cell concentrates. Vox Sang 1992;62:76-81.
4. Heaton WA, Holme S, Smith K, et al. Effects of 3-5 $\log_{10}$ prestorage leukocyte depletion on red cell storage and metabolism. Br J Haematol 1994;87:363-8.
5. AuBuchon JP, Elfath MD, Popovsky MA, et al. Prestorage 5 $\log_{10}$ leukoreduction filtration of red blood cells (abstract). Transfusion 1995;35(Suppl):56S.
6. Müller-Steinhardt M, Janetzko K, Kandler R, et al. Impact of various red cell concentrate preparation methods on the efficiency of prestorage white cell filtration and on red cells during storage for 42 days. Transfusion 1997;37:1137-42.
7. Sweeney JD, Holme S, Heaton WAL, Nelson E. White cell-reduced platelet concentrates prepared by in-line filtration of platelet-rich plasma. Transfusion 1995;35:131-6.
8. Sweeney JD, Holme S, Stromberg RR, Heaton WAL. In vitro and in vivo effects of prestorage filtration of apheresis platelets. Transfusion 1995;35:125-30.
9. Boomgaard MN, Gouwerok CWN, Palfenier CH, et al. Pooled platelet concentrates prepared by the platelet-rich-plasma method and filtered with three different filters and stored for 8 days. Vox Sang 1995;68:82-9.
10. Kao KJ, Mickel M, Braine HG, et al. White cell reduction in platelet concentrates and packed red cells by filtration: A multicenter clinical trial. Transfusion 1995;35:13-9.
11. Weisbach V, Putzo A, Zingsem J, et al. Leukocyte depletion and storage of single-donor platelet concentrates. Vox Sang 1997;72:20-5.
12. Zingsem J, Zimmermann R, Weisbach V, et al. Comparison of COBE white cell-reduction and standard plateletpheresis protocols in the same donors. Transfusion 1997;37:45-9.

13. Popovsky M. Quality of blood components filtered before storage and at the bedside: Implications for transfusion practice. Transfusion 1996;36:470-4.

14. Sirchia G, Rebulla P, Sabbioneda L. Optimal conditions for white cell reduction in red cells by filtration at the patient's bedside. Transfusion 1996;36:322-7.

15. Sprogue-Jakobsen U, Saetre AM, Georgsen J. Preparation of white cell-reduced red cells by filtration: Comparison of a bedside filter and two blood bank filter systems. Transfusion 1995;35:421-6.

16. Ledent E, Berlin G. Factors influencing white cell removal from red cell concentrates by filtration. Transfusion 1996;36:714-8.

17. Fried MR, Eastlund T, Christie B, et al. Hypotensive reactions to white cell-reduced plasma in a patient undergoing angiotensin-converting enzyme inhibitor therapy. Transfusion 1996;36:900-3.

18. Hume HA, Popovsky MA, Benson K, et al. Hypotensive reactions: A previously uncharacterized complication of platelet transfusion? Transfusion 1996;36:904-9.

19. Moore SB. Hypotensive reactions: Are they a new phenomenon? Are they related solely to transfusion of platelets? Does filtration of components play a role? Transfusion 1996; 36:852-3.

20. Takahasi TA, Abe H, Hosoda M, et al. Bradykinin generation during filtration of platelet concentrates with a white cell reduction filter (letter). Transfusion 1995; 35:967.

21. Shiba M, Tadokoro K, Sawanobori M, et al. Activation of the contact system by filtration of platelet concentrates with a negatively charged white cell-removal filter and measurement of venous blood bradykinin level in patients who received filtered platelets. Transfusion 1997;37:457-62.

22. Owen HG, Brecher ME. Atypical reactions associated with use of angiotensin-converting enzyme inhibitors and apheresis. Transfusion 1994;34:891-4.

23. Adverse ocular reactions following transfusions. MMWR Morb Mortal Wkly Rep 1998;47:49-50.

24. Menitove JE, McElligott MC, Aster RH. Febrile transfusion reaction: What component should be given next? Vox Sang 1982;42:318-21.

25. Chambers LA, Donovan LM, Pacini DG, Kruskall MS. Febrile reactions after platelet transfusion: The effect of single versus multiple donors. Transfusion 1990;30:219-21.

26. Heddle NM, Klama LN, Griffith L, et al. A prospective study to identify the risk factors associated with acute reactions to platelet and red cell transfusions. Transfusion 1993; 33:794-7.

27. Vengelen-Tyler V, ed. Technical manual. 12th ed. Bethesda, MD: American Association of Blood Banks, 1996:548.

28. Miller JP, Mintz PD. The use of leukocyte-reduced blood components. Transfusion 1995;35:69-90.

29. Dinarello CA, Wolff SM. Molecular basis of fever in humans. Am J Med 1982;72:799-819.

30. Perkins HA, Payne R, Ferguson J, Wood M. Nonhemolytic febrile transfusion reactions. Quantitative effects of blood components with emphasis on isoantigenic incompatibility of leukocytes. Vox Sang 1966;11:578-600.

31. Decary F, Ferner P, Giavedoni L, et al. An investigation of non-hemolytic transfusion reactions. Vox Sang 1984;46:277-85.

32. de Rie MA, van der Plas-van Dalen CM, Engelfriet CP, von dem Borne AEGK. The serology of febrile transfusion reactions. Vox Sang 1985;49:126-34.

33. Brubaker DB. Clinical significance of white cell antibodies in febrile nonhemolytic transfusion reactions. Transfusion 1990;30:733-7.

34. Mangano MM, Chambers LA, Kruskall MS. Limited efficacy of leukopoor platelets for prevention of febrile transfusion reactions. Am J Clin Pathol 1991;95:733-8.

35. Gong J, Högman CF, Hambraeus A, et al. Transfusion-transmitted *Yersinia enterocolitica* infection: Protection through buffy coat removal and failure of the bacteria to grow in platelet-rich or platelet-poor plasma. Vox Sang 1993;65:42-6.

36. Williamson LM, Wimperis JZ, Williamson P, et al. Bedside filtration of blood products in the prevention of HLA alloimmunization—a prospective randomized study. Blood 1994; 83:3028-35.

37. Mintz PD. Febrile reactions to platelet transfusions. Am J Clin Pathol 1991;95:609-12.

38. Dzik WH. Is the febrile response to transfusion due to donor or recipient cytokine? (letter) Transfusion 1992;32:594.

39. Okusawa S, Dianrella CA, Endres S, et al. C5a induction of human interleukin-1: Synergistic effect with endotoxin or interferon-a. J Immunol 1987;139:2635-40.

40. Heddle NM, Klama L, Singer J, et al. The role of the plasma from platelet concentrates in transfusion reactions. N Engl J Med 1994; 331:625-8.

41. Muylle L, Wouters E, Peetermans ME. Febrile reactions to platelet transfusion: The effect of increased interleukin 6 levels in concentrates prepared by platelet-rich plasma method. Transfusion 1996;36:886-90.

42. Riccardi D, Raspollini E, Rebulla P, et al. Relationship of the time of storage and transfusion reactions to platelet concentrates from buffy coats. Transfusion 1997;37:528-30.

43. Muylle L, Wouters E, DeBock R, et al. Reactions to platelet transfusion: The effect of the storage time of the concentrate. Transfus Med 1992;2:289-93.

44. Dzieczkowski JS, Barrett BB, Nester D, et al. Characterization of reactions after exclusive transfusion of white cell-reduced cellular blood components. Transfusion 1995;35: 20-5.

45. Muylle L, Joos M, Wouters E, et al. Increased tumor necrosis factor a (TNFα), interleukin 1, and interleukin 6 (IL-6) levels in the plasma of stored platelet concentrates: Relationship between TNFα and IL-6 levels and febrile transfusion reactions. Transfusion 1993;33:195-9.

46. Aye MT. Production of cytokines in platelet concentrates. In: Freedman JJ, Blajchman MA, McCombie N, eds. Canadian Red Cross Society Symposium on Leukodepletion: Report of proceedings. Transfus Med Rev 1994;8:8.

47. Stack G, Baril L, Napychank P, Snyder EL. Cytokine generation in stored, white cell-reduced, and bacterially contaminated units of red cells. Transfusion 1995;35:199-203.

48. Currie LM, Harper JR, Allan H, Connor J. Inhibition of cytokine accumulation and bacterial growth during storage of platelet concentrates at 4 C with retention of in vitro functional activity. Transfusion 1997;37:18-24.

49. Shanwell A, Kristiansson M, Remberger M, Ringdén O. Generation of cytokines in red cell concentrates during storage is prevented by prestorage white cell reduction. Transfusion 1997;37:678-84.

50. Ferrara JLM. The febrile platelet transfusion reaction: A cytokine shower. Transfusion 1995;35:89-90.

51. Muylle L, Peetermans ME. Effect of prestorage leukocyte removal on the cytokine levels in stored platelet concentrates. Vox Sang 1994;66:14-7.

52. Wadhwa M, Thorpe R, Bird C, et al. Cytokine levels in platelet concentrates: Quantitation by bioassays and immunoassays. Br J Haematol 1996;95:755-6.

53. Fujihara M, Takahashi TA, Ogiso C, et al. Generation of interleukin 8 in stored apheresis platelet concentrates and the preventative effect of prestorage ultraviolet B radiation. Transfusion 1997;37:468-75.

54. Flegel WA, Wiesneth M, Stampe D, Koerner K. Low cytokine in buffy coat-derived platelet concentrates without filtration. Transfusion 1995;35:917-20.

55. Federowicz I, Barrett BB, Andersen JW, et al. Characterization of reactions after transfu-

sion of cellular blood components that are white cell reduced before storage. Transfusion 1996;36:21-8.

56. Sirchia G, Rebulla P, Parravicini A, et al. Leukocyte depletion of red cell units at the bedside by transfusion through a new filter. Transfusion 1987;27:402-5.

57. Sirchia G, Wenz B, Rebulla P, et al. Removal of white cells from red cells by transfusion through a new filter. Transfusion 1990;30: 30-3.

58. Wenz B. Microaggregate blood filtration and the febrile transfusion reaction, a comparative study. Transfusion 1983;23:95-8.

59. Dan ME, Stewart S. Prevention of recurrent febrile transfusion reactions using leukocyte poor platelet concentrates prepared by the "leukotrap" centrifugation method (abstract). Transfusion 1986;26:569.

60. Kalmin ND, Orell JE, Villarreal IG. An effective method for the preparation of leukocyte-poor platelets. Transfusion 1987;27:281-3.

61. Schiffer CA. Prevention of alloimmunization against platelets (editorial). Blood 1991;77: 1-4.

62. Slichter SJ, O'Donnell MR, Weiden PL, et al. Canine platelet alloimmunization: The role of donor selection. Br J Haematol 1986;63: 713-27.

63. Stec N, Kickler TS, Ness PM, et al. Effectiveness of leukocyte (WBC) depleted platelets in preventing febrile reactions in multi-transfused oncology patients (abstract). Transfusion 1986;26:569.

64. Sternbach M, Champagne J, Rybka W, et al. Leukotrap, a device for white cell poor platelets. Quality control studies in vitro and in vivo. Transfus Sci 1989;10:57-62.

65. Goodnough LT, Riddell J, Lazarus H, et al. Prevalence of platelet transfusion reactions before and after implementation of leukocyte-depleted platelet concentrates by filtration. Vox Sang 1993;65:103-7.

66. Muir JC, Herschel L, Pickard C, AuBuchon JP. Prestorage leukocyte reduction decreases the risk of febrile reactions in sensitized platelet recipients (abstract). Transfusion 1995;35(Suppl):45S.

67. Dutcher JP, Schiffer CA, Aisner J, et al. Long-term follow-up of patients with leukemia receiving platelet transfusions: Identification of a large group of patients who do not become alloimmunized. Blood 1981;58:1007.

68. Lee EJ, Schiffer CA. Serial measurement of lymphocytotoxic antibody and response to non-matched platelet transfusions in alloimmunization patients. Blood 1987;70: 1727-9.

69. Schiffer CA, Lichtenfeld JL, Wiernik PH, et al. Antibody response in patients with acute non-lymphocytic leukemia. Cancer 1976; 37:2177-82.

70. Daly PA, Schiffer CA, Aisner J, et al. Platelet transfusion therapy. One hour post-transfusion increments are valuable in predicting the need for HLA-matched preparations. JAMA 1980;243:435-8.

71. O'Connell B, Lee EJ, Schiffer CA. The value of 10-minute posttransfusion platelet counts. Transfusion 1988;28:66-7.

72. Bishop JF, McGrath K, Wolf MM, et al. Clinical factors influencing the efficacy of pooled platelet transfusions. Blood 1988;71:383-7.

73. Sintnicolaas K, Sizoo W, Haije WG, et al. Delayed alloimmunisation by random single donor platelet transfusions. A randomised study to compare single donor and multiple donor platelet transfusions in cancer patients with severe thrombocytopenia. Lancet 1981;1:750-4.

74. Lane TA, Anderson KC, Goodnough LT, et al. Leukocyte reduction in blood component therapy. Ann Intern Med 1992;117:151-62.

75. Welsh KI, Burgos H, Batchelor JR. The immune response to allogeneic rat platelets: Ag-B antigens in matrix form lacking 1a. Eur J Immunol 1977;7:267-72.

76. Confer DL. The prevention of HLA alloimmunization. In: Kurtz JR, Brubaker DB, eds. Clinical decisions in platelet therapy. Bethesda, MD: American Association of Blood Banks, 1992:105-19.

77. The Trial to Reduce Alloimmunization to Platelets Study Group. Leukocyte reduction and ultraviolet B irradiation of platelets to prevent alloimmunization and refractoriness to platelet transfusions. N Engl J Med 1997; 337:1861-9.

78. Buchholz DH, Miripol J, Aster RH, et al. Ultraviolet irradiation of platelets to prevent recipient alloimmunization (abstract). Transfusion 1988;28:26S.

79. Menitove JE, Kagen LR, Aster RH, et al. Alloimmunization is decreased in patients receiving UV-B irradiated platelet concentrates and leukocyte-depleted red cells. Blood 1990; 76:1607.

80. Pamphilon DH, Blundell EL. Ultraviolet B irradiation of platelet transfusions: A strategy to reduce recipient alloimmunization. Semin Hematol 1992;29:118-21.

81. Kahn RA, Duffy BF, Rodey GG. Ultraviolet irradiation of platelet concentrate abrogates lymphocyte activation without affecting platelet function in vitro. Transfusion 1985; 25:547-50.

82. Eernisse JG, Brand A. Prevention of platelet refractoriness due to HLA antibodies by administration of leukocyte-poor blood components. Exp Hematol 1981;9:77-83.

83. Fisher M, Chapman JR, Ting A, et al. Alloimmunisation to HLA antigens following transfusion with leucocyte-poor and purified platelet suspensions. Vox Sang 1985;49: 331-5.

84. Murphy MF, Metcalfe P, Thomas H, et al. Use of leucocyte-poor blood components and HLA-matched-platelet donors to prevent HLA alloimmunization. Br J Haematol 1986;62(3):529-34.

85. Schiffer CA, Patten E, Reilly J, et al. Effective leukocyte removal from platelet preparations by centrifugation in a new pooling bag. Transfusion 1987;27:162-4.

86. Andreu G, Dewailly J, Leberre C, et al. Prevention of HLA immunization with leukocyte-poor packed red cells and platelet concentrates obtained by filtration. Blood 1988; 72:964-9.

87. Brand A, Claas FHJ, Voogt PJ, et al. Alloimmunization after leukocyte-depleted multiple random donor platelet transfusions. Vox Sang 1988;54:160-6.

88. Saarinen UM, Kekomäki R, Siimes MA, et al. Effective prophylaxis against platelet refractoriness in multitransfused patients by use of leukocyte-free blood components. Blood 1990;75:512-7.

89. van Marwijk Kooy M, van Prooijen HC, Moes M, et al. Use of leukocyte-depleted platelet concentrates for the prevention of refractoriness and primary HLA alloimmunization: A prospective, randomized trial. Blood 1991;77:201-5.

90. Oksanen K, Kekomäki R, Ruutu T, et al. Prevention of alloimmunization in patients with acute leukemia by use of white cell-reduced blood components—a randomized trial. Transfusion 1991;31:588-94.

91. Sniecinski I, O'Donnell MR, Nowicki B, et al. Prevention of refractoriness and HLA-alloimmunization using filtered blood products. Blood 1988;71:1402-7.

92. Saarinen UM, Koskimies S, Myllylä G. Systematic use of leukocyte-free blood components to prevent alloimmunization and platelet refractoriness in multitransfused children with cancer. Vox Sang 1993;65:286-92.

93. Bedford Russell AR, Rivers RPA, Davey N. The development of anti-HLA antibodies in multiply transfused preterm infants. Arch Dis Child 1993;68:49-51.

94. Oksanen K. Leukocyte-depleted blood components prevent platelet refractoriness in patients with acute myeloid leukemia. Eur J Haematol 1994;53:100-7.

95. Hogge DE, McConnell M, Jacobson C, et al. Platelet refractoriness and alloimmunization in pediatric oncology and bone marrow transplant patients. Transfusion 1995;35: 645-52.

96. Abou-Elella AA, Camarillo TA, Allen MB, et al. Low incidence of red cell and HLA anti-

body formation by bone marrow transplant patients. Transfusion 1995; 35:931-5.

97. Sintnicolaas K, van Marwijk Kooij M, van Prooijen HC, et al. Leukocyte depletion of random single-donor platelet transfusions does not prevent secondary human leukocyte antigen—alloimmunization and refractoriness: A randomized study. Blood 1995;85: 824-8.

98. Novotny VMJ, van Doorn R, Witvliet MD, et al. Occurrence of allogeneic HLA and non-HLA antibodies after transfusions of prestorage filtered platelets and red blood cells: A prospective study. Blood 1995;85:1736-41.

99. Killick SB, Win N, Marsh JC, et al. Pilot study of HLA alloimmunization after transfusion with prestorage leucodepleted blood products in aplastic anaemia. Br J Haematol 1997;97:677-84.

100. Legler TJ, Fischer I, Dittmann J, et al. Frequency and causes of refractoriness in multiply transfused patient. Ann Hematol 1997; 74:185-9.

101. Ramos RR, Curtis BR, Duffy BF, Chaplin H. Low retention of white cell fragments by polyester fiber white cell-reduction platelet fibers. Transfusion 1994;34:31-4.

102. Dzik S, Szuflad P, Eaves S. HLA antigens on leukocyte fragments and plasma proteins: Prestorage leukoreduction by filtration. Vox Sang 1994;66:104-11.

103. Blajchman MA, Bardossy L, Carmen RA, et al. An animal model of allogeneic donor platelet refractoriness: The effect of the time of leukodepletion. Blood 1992;79:1371-5.

104. Bordin JO, Bardossy L, Blajchman MA. Growth enhancement of established tumors by allogeneic blood transfusion in experimental animals and its amelioration by leukodepletion: The importance of the timing of the leukodepletion. Blood 1994;84:344-8.

105. Lill M, Snider C, Calhoun L, et al. Analysis of utilization and cost of platelet transfusions in refractory hematology/oncology patients. Transfusion 1997;37(Suppl):26S.

106. Blumberg N, Heal JM, Kirkley SA, et al. Leukodepleted-ABO-identical blood components in the treatment of hematologic malignancies: A cost analysis. Am J Hematol 1995; 48:108-15.

107. Balducci L, Benson K, Lyman GH, et al: Cost-effectiveness of white cell-reduction filters in treatment of adult acute myelogenous leukemia. Transfusion 1993;33:665-70.

108. Leukocyte reduction for the prevention of transfusion-transmitted cytomegalovirus (TT-CMV). Association Bulletin 97-2. Bethesda, MD: American Association of Blood Banks, 1997.

109. Bowden RA, Sayers M, Flournoy N, et al. Cytomegalovirus immune globulin and seronegative blood products to prevent primary cytomegalovirus infection after marrow transplantation. N Engl J Med 1986;314: 1006-10.

110. Miller WJ, McCullough J, Balfour HH Jr, et al. Prevention of cytomegalovirus—infection following bone marrow transplantation: A randomized trial of blood product screening. Bone Marrow Transplant 1991;7:227-34.

111. Bowden RA, Sayers M, Gleaves CA, et al. Cytomegalovirus-seronegative blood components for the prevention of primary cytomegalovirus infection after marrow transplantation: Considerations for blood banks. Transfusion 1987;27:478-81.

112. Bowden RA, Slichter SJ, Sayers M, et al. A comparison of filtered leukocyte-reduced and cytomegalovirus (CMV) seronegative blood products for the prevention of transfusion-associated CMV infection after marrow transplant. Blood 1995;86:3598-603.

113. Verdonck LF, de Graan-Hentzen YC, Dekker AW, et al. Cytomegalovirus seronegative platelets and leukocyte-poor red blood cells from random donors can prevent primary cytomegalovirus infection after bone marrow transplantation. Bone Marrow Transplant 1987;2:73-8.

114. Murphy MF, Grint PC, Hardiman AE, et al. Use of leukocyte-poor blood components to prevent primary cytomegalovirus (CMV) infection in patients with acute leukemia. Br J Haematol 1988;70:253-5.

115. Gilbert GL, Hayes K, Hudson IL, et al. Prevention of transfusion-acquired cytomegalovirus infection in infants by blood filtration to remove leucocytes. Lancet 1989;1:1228-31.

116. DeGraan-Hentzen YCE, Gratama JW, Mudde GC, et al. Prevention of primary cytomegalovirus infection in patients with hematologic malignancies by intensive white cell depletion of blood products. Transfusion 1989;29:757-60.

117. Bowden RA, Sayers MH, Cays M, et al. The role of blood product filtration in the prevention of transfusion associated cytomegalovirus (CMV) infection after marrow transplant (abstract). Transfusion 1989;29(Suppl):57S.

118. De Witte T, Schattenberg A, van Dijk BA, et al. Prevention of primary cytomegalovirus infection after allogeneic bone marrow transplantation by using leukocyte-poor random blood products from cytomegalovirus-unscreened blood-bank donors. Transplantation 1990;50:964-8.

119. Bowden RA, Slichter SJ, Sayers MH, et al. Use of leukocyte-depleted platelets and cytomegalovirus-seronegative red blood cells for prevention of primary cytomegalovirus infection after marrow transplant. Blood 1991;78:246-50.

120. Eisenfeld L, Silver H, McLaughlin J, et al. Prevention of transfusion-associated cytomegalovirus infection in neonatal patients by the removal of white cells from blood. Transfusion 1992;32:205-9.

121. van Prooijen HC, Visser JJ, van Oostendorp WR, et al. Prevention of primary transfusion-associated cytomegalovirus infection in bone marrow transplant recipients by the removal of white cells from blood components with high-affinity filters. Br J Haematol 1994;87:114-7.

122. Xu D, Yonetani M, Uetani Y, Nakamura H. Acquired cytomegalovirus infection and blood transfusion in preterm infants. Acta Paediatr Jpn 1995;37:444-9.

123. Preiksaitis JK, Desai S, Vaudry W, et al. Transfusion- and community-acquired cytomegalovirus infection in children with malignant disease: A prospective study. Transfusion 1997;37:941-6.

124. Landaw EM, Kanter M, Petz LD. Safety of filtered leukocyte-reduced blood products for prevention of transfusion-associated cytomegalovirus infection. Blood 1996;87:4910-9.

125. Safety and equivalence claims for leukocyte-reduced products. Faxnet No. 330, April 16, 1997. Bethesda, MD: American Association of Blood Banks, 1997.

126. Leukocyte reduction and CMV prevention. Faxnet No. 357, December 10, 1997. Bethesda, MD: American Association of Blood Banks, 1977.

127. Chou S. Acquisition of donor strains of cytomegalovirus by renal-transplant recipients. N Engl J Med 1986;314:1418-23.

128. Chou S. Cytomegalovirus infection and reinfection transmitted by heart transplantation. J Infect Dis 1987;155:1054-5.

129. Chou S. Reactivation and recombination of multiple cytomegalovirus strains from individual organ donors. J Infect Dis 1989;160:11-5.

130. Grundy JE, Super M, Sweny P, et al. Symptomatic cytomegalovirus infection in seropositive kidney recipients: Reinfection with donor virus rather than reactivation of recipient virus. Lancet 1988;2:132-5.

131. Chou S. Neutralizing antibody responses to reinfecting strains of cytomegalovirus in transplant patients. J Infect Dis 1989;160:16-21.

132. Falagas ME, Werner BG, Griffith J, et al. Primary cytomegalovirus infection in liver transplant recipients: Comparison of infections transmitted via donor organs and via

transfusions. Clin Infect Dis 1996;23(2): 292-7.

133. Adler SP, Lawrence LT, Baggett J, et al. Prevention of transfusion-associated cytomegalovirus infection in very low-birth-weight infants using frozen blood and donors seronegative for cytomegalovirus. Transfusion 1984;24:333-5.

134. Adler SP, McVoy MM. Cytomegalovirus infections in seropositive patients after transfusion: The effect of red cell storage and volume. Transfusion 1989;29:667-71.

135. Winston DJ, Huang ES, Miller MJ, et al. Molecular epidemiology of cytomegalovirus infections associated with bone marrow transplantation. Ann Intern Med 1985;102: 16-20.

136. Bruggerman CA. Reactivation of latent CMV in the rat. Transplant Proc 1991;23(Suppl 3):22-4.

137. Cheung K-S, Lang DJ. Transmission and activation of cytomegalovirus with blood transfusion: A mouse model. J Infect Dis 1977; 135:841-5.

138. Olding LB, Jensen FC, Oldstone MBA. Pathogenesis of cytomegalovirus infection. J Exp Med 1975;141:561-72.

139. Bracey A, Radovancevic R, Radovancevic B, et al. Effect of leukocyte-depleted blood on CMV disease after heart transplant. XXIIIrd Congress of the ISBT Abstracts 1994:13.

140. Thompson KS, Plapp FV, Long ND, et al. CMV infection in heart transplant recipients. Transfusion 1992;32(Suppl):65S.

141. Busch MP, Collier A, Gernsheimer T, et al. The Viral Activation Transfusion Study (VATS): Rationale, Objectives, and Design Overview. Transfusion 1996;36:854-9.

142. Opelz G, Sengar DPS, Mickey MR, et al. Effect of blood transfusions on subsequent kidney transplants. Transplant Proc 1973; V5(1):253-9.

143. Opelz G, Vanrenterghem Y, Kirste G, et al. Prospective evaluation of pretransplant blood transfusions in cadaver kidney recipients. Transplantation 1997;63:964-7.

144. Clark DA, Gunby J, Daya S. The use of allogeneic leukocytes or IV IgG for the treatment of patients with recurrent spontaneous abortions. Transfus Med Rev 1997;11:85-94.

145. Peters WR, Fry RD, Fleshman JW, et al. Multiple blood transfusions reduce the recurrence rate of Crohn's disease. Dis Colon Rectum 1989;32:749-53.

146. Williams JG, Hughes LE. Effect of perioperative blood transfusion on recurrence of Crohn's disease (letter). Lancet 1989;2: 1524.

147. Blumberg N. Allogeneic transfusion and infection: Economic and clinical implications. Semin Hematol 1997:34(3 Suppl 2):34-40.

148. Blajchman MA, Bardossy L, Carmen R, et al. Allogeneic blood transfusion-induced enhancement of tumor growth: Two animal models showing amelioration by leukodepletion and passive transfer using spleen cells. Blood 1993;81:1880-2.

149. Dzik S, Blajchman MA, Blumberg N, et al. Current research on the immunomodulatory effect of allogeneic blood transfusion. Vox Sang 1996;70:1987-94.

150. Vamvakas EC. Transfusion-associated cancer recurrence and postoperative infection: Meta-analysis of randomized, controlled clinical trials. Transfusion 1996;36:175-86.

151. Chung M, Steinmetz OK, Gordon PH. Perioperative blood transfusion and outcome after resection for colorectal carcinoma. Br J Surg 1993;80:427-32.

152. Busch ORC, Hop WCJ, van Papendrecht MAWH, et al. Blood transfusions and prognosis in colorectal cancer. N Engl J Med 1993;328:1372-6.

153. Heiss MM, Mempel W, Delanoff C, et al. Blood transfusion-modulated tumor recurrence: First results of a randomized study of autologous versus allogeneic blood transfusion in colorectal cancer surgery. J Clin Oncol 1994;12:1859-67.

154. Heiss MM, Fraunberger P, Delanoff C, et al. Modulation of immune response by blood transfusion: Evidence for a differential effect

of allogeneic and autologous blood in colorectal cancer surgery. Shock 1997;8:402-8.

155. Houbiers JGA, Brand A, van de Watering LMG, et al. Randomised controlled trial comparing transfusion of leucocyte-depleted or buffy-coat-depleted blood in surgery for colorectal cancer. Lancet 1994;344:573-8.

156. Heiss MM, Mempel W, Jauch KW, et al. Beneficial effect of autologous blood transfusion on infectious complications after colorectal cancer surgery. Lancet 1993;342:1328-33.

157. Jensen LS, Andersen AJ, Christiansen PM, et al. Postoperative infection and natural killer cell function following blood transfusion in patients undergoing elective colorectal surgery. Br J Surg 1992;79:513-6.

158. Jensen LS, Kissmeyer-Nielson P, Wolff B, Qvist N. Randomised comparison of leucocyte-depleted versus buffy-coat-poor blood transfusion and complications after colorectal surgery. Lancet 1996;348:841-5.

159. van de Watering LM. Beneficial effects of leukocyte depletion of transfused blood on postoperative complications in patients undergoing cardiac surgery: A randomized clinical trial. Circulation 1998;97:562-8.

160. Vamvakas EC, Carven JH, Hibberd PL. Blood transfusion and infection after colorectal cancer surgery. Transfusion 1996;36:1000-8.

161. Blajchman MA. Allogeneic blood transfusions, immunomodulation, and postoperative bacterial infection: Do we have the answers yet? Transfusion 1997;37:121-5.

162. Jensen LS, Grunnet N, Hanberg-Sorensen F, Jorgensen J. Cost-effectiveness of blood transfusion and white cell reduction in elective colorectal surgery. Transfusion 1995;35:719-22.

163. Sloand E, Kumar P, Klein HG, et al. Transfusion of blood components to persons infected with human immunodeficiency virus type 1: Relationship to opportunistic infection. Transfusion 1994;34:48-53.

164. Vamvakas E, Kaplan HS. Early transfusion and length of survival in acquired immune deficiency syndrome: Experience with a population receiving medical care at a public hospital. Transfusion 1993;33:111-8.

165. Ward JW, Bush TJ, Herbert BS, et al. The natural history of transfusion-associated infection with human immunodeficiency virus. N Engl J Med 1989;321:947-52.

166. Whyte BM, Swanson CE, Cooper DA. Survival of patients with the acquired immunodeficiency syndrome in Australia. Med J Aust 1989;150:358-62.

167. Folks TM, Justement J, Kinter A, et al. Cytokine-induced expression of HIV-1 in a chronically infected promonocyte cell line. Science 1987;238:800-2.

168. Margolick JB, Volkman DJ, Folks TM, et al. Amplification of HTLV-III/LAV infection by antigen-induced activation of T cells and direct suppression by virus of lymphocyte blastogenic responses. J Immunol 1987;138:1719-23.

169. Zagury D, Bernard J, Leonard R, et al. Long-term cultures of HTLV-III-infected T cells: A model of cytopathology of T-cell depletion in AIDS. Science 1986;231:850-3.

170. Busch MP, Lee T-H, Heitman J. Allogeneic leukocytes but not therapeutic blood elements induce reactivation and dissemination of latent human immunodeficiency virus type 1 infection: Implications for transfusion support of infected patients. Blood 1992;80:2128-35.

171. Mudido PM, Georges D, Dorazio D, et al. Human immunodeficiency virus type 1 activation after blood transfusion. Transfusion 1996;36:860-5.

172. Groopman JE. Impact of transfusion on viral load in human immunodeficiency virus infection. Semin Hematol 1997;34(Suppl 2):27-33.

173. Barrett BB, Andersen JW, Anderson KC. Strategies for the avoidance of bacterial contamination of blood components. Transfusion 1993;33:228-33.

174. Morrow JF, Braine HG, Kickler TS, et al. Septic reactions to platelet transfusions. A persistent problem. JAMA 1991;266:555-8.

175. Hoppe PA. Interim measures for detection of bacterially contaminated red cell components. Transfusion 1992;32:199-201.

176. Klein HG, Dodd RY, Ness PM, et al. Current status of microbial contamination of blood components: Summary of a conference. Transfusion 1997;37:95-101.

177. Wagner SJ, Friedman LI, Dodd RY. Transfusion-associated bacterial sepsis. Clin Microbiol Rev 1994;7:290-302.

178. Buchholz DH, AuBuchon JP, Snyder EL, et al. Removal of *Yersinia enterocolitica* from AS-1 red cells. Transfusion 1992;32:667-72.

179. Gong J, Högman CF, Hambraeus A, et al. Transfusion-associated *Serratia marcescens* infection: Studies of the mechanism of action. Transfusion 1993;33:802-8.

180. Högman CF. *Yersinia enterocolitica* and blood transfusion (letter). Transfusion 1993;33:534.

181. Kim DM, Brecher ME, Bland LA, et al. Prestorage removal of *Yersinia enterocolitica* from red cells with white cell-reduction filters. Transfusion 1992;32:658-62.

182. Pietersz RNI, Reesink HW, Pauw W, et al. Prevention of *Yersinia enterocolitica* growth in red-blood-cell concentrates. Lancet 1992; 340:755-6.

183. Wenz B, Burns ER, Freundlich LF. Prevention of growth of *Yersinia enterocolitica* in blood by polyester fiber filtration. Transfusion 1992;32:663-6.

184. Wenz B, Ciavarella D, Freundlich L. Effect of prestorage white cell reduction on bacterial growth in platelet concentrates. Transfusion 1993;33:520-3.

185. Brecher ME, Boothe G, Kerr A. The use of a chemiluminescence-linked universal bacterial ribosomal RNA gene probe and blood gas analysis for the rapid detection of bacterial contamination in white cell-reduced and nonreduced platelets. Transfusion 1993; 33:450-7.

186. Goldman M. The removal of microbiological agents by leukodepletion. In: Freedman JJ, Blajchman MA, McCombie N. Canadian Red Cross Society Symposium on Leukodepletion: Report on proceedings. Transfus Med Rev 1994;8:6.

187. AuBuchon JP, Pickard C. White cell reduction and bacterial proliferation. Transfusion 1993;33:533.

188. Rawal BD, Vyas G. Complement-mediated bactericidal action and the removal of *Yersinia enterocolitica* by white cell filters (letter). Transfusion 1993;33:536.

189. Högman CF, Gong J, Hambraeus A, et al. The role of white cells in the transmission of *Yersinia enterocolitica* in blood components. Transfusion 1992;32:654-7.

190. Glaser A, Erpenbeck T, Böck M, et al. Effectiveness of white cell reduction by filtration with respect to blood storage time. Transfusion 1993;33:536-7.

191. Högman CF, Gong J, Eriksson L, et al. White cells protect donor blood against bacterial contamination. Transfusion 1991;31:620-6.

192. Anderson KC, Weinstein HJ. Transfusion-associated graft-versus-host disease. N Engl J Med 1990;323:315-21.

193. Fast LD. Recipient DC8+ cells are responsible for the rapid elimination of allogeneic donor lymphoid cells. J Immunol 1996;157: 4805-10.

194. Lee TH, Donegan E, Slichter S, Busch MP. Transient increase in circulating donor leukocytes after allogeneic transfusions in immunocompetent recipients compatible with donor cell proliferation. Blood 1995;85: 1207-14.

195. Goodarzi MO, Busch MP, Donegan EA, et al. Unusual kinetics of white cell clearance in transfused mice. Transfusion 1995;35: 145-9.

196. Linden JV, Pisciotto PT. Transfusion-associated graft-versus-host disease and blood irradiation. Transfus Med Rev 1992; 6:116-23.

197. Ohto H, Anderson KC. Posttransfusion graft-versus-host disease in Japanese newborns. Transfusion 1996;36:117-23.

198. Benson K, Marks AR, Marshall MJ, et al. Fatal graft-versus-host disease associated with transfusions of HLA-matched, HLA-homozygous platelets from unrelated donors. Transfusion 1994;34:432-7.

199. Wagner FF, Flegel WA. Transfusion-associated graft-versus-host disease: Risk due to homozygous HLA haplotypes. Transfusion 1995;35:284-91.

200. Moroff G, Leitman SF, Luban NLC. Principles of blood irradiation, dose validation, and quality control. Transfusion 1997;37:1084-92.

201. Lowenthal RM, Challis DR, Griffiths AE, et al. Transfusion-associated graft-versus-host disease: Report of an occurrence following the administration of irradiated blood. Transfusion 1993;33:524-9.

202. Rubinstein A, Radl J, Cottier H, et al. Unusual combined immunodeficiency syndrome exhibiting kappa-IgD paraproteinemia, residual gut immunity and graft-versus-host reaction after plasma infusion. Acta Paediatr Scand 1973;62:365-72.

203. Dzik WH, Jones KS. The effects of gamma irradiation versus white cell reduction on the mixed lymphocyte reaction. Transfusion 1993;33:493-6.

204. Akahoshi M, Takanashi M, Masuda M, et al. A case of transfusion-associated graft-versus-host disease not prevented by white cell-reduction filters. Transfusion 1992;32:169-72.

205. Collins RH Jr, Pineiro LA, Nemunaitis JJ, et al. Transfusion of donor buffy coat cells in the treatment of persistent or recurring malignancy after allogeneic bone marrow transplantation. Transfusion 1995;35:891-8.

206. Tzeng CH, Lin JS, Lee JCI, et al. Transfusion of donor peripheral blood buffy coat cells as effective treatment for relapsed acute leukemia after transplantation of allogeneic bone marrow or peripheral blood stem cells from the same donor. Transfusion 1996;36:685-90.

207. Lopez J, Fernandez-Villalta MJ, Gomez-Reino F, et al. Absence of graft-versus-leukemia effect of standard hemotherapy in patients with acute myeloblastic leukemia. Transfusion 1990;30:191-2.

208. Norol F, Parquet N, Kuentz M, et al. Absence of graft-versus-leukaemia (GVL) effect by leucocytes transfused: A prospective randomized trial in acute myeloid leukaemia (AML) patients. Br J Haematol 1991;78:591-2.

209. Rebulla P, Pappalettera M, Barbui T, et al. Duration of first remission in leukaemic recipients of leucocyte-poor blood components. Br J Haematol 1990;75:441-2.

210. Copplestone JA, Williamson P, Norfolk DR. Wider benefits of leukodepletion of blood products. Blood 1995;86:409-10.

211. Thiagarajan RR, Winn RK, Harlan JM. The role of leukocyte and endothelial adhesion molecules in ischemia—reperfusion injury. Thromb Haemost 1997;78:310-14.

212. Appleyard RF, Cohn LH. Myocardial stunning and reperfusion injury in cardiac surgery. J Card Surg 1993;8(2 Suppl):316-24.

213. Byrne JG, Appleyard RF, Lee CC, et al. Controlled reperfusion of the regionally ischemic myocardium with leukocyte-depleted blood reduces stunning, the no-reflow phenomenon, and infarct size. J Thorac Cardiovasc Surg 1992;103:66-72.

214. Wilson IC, Gardner TJ, DiNatale JM, et al. Temporary leukocyte depletion reduces ventricular dysfunction during prolonged postischemic reperfusion. J Thorac Cardiovasc Surg 1993;106:805-10.

215. Kutsumi Y, Misawa T, Tada H, et al. Effect of a leukocyte-platelet removal filter on ischemic induced reperfusion injury. ASAIO Trans 1990;36:M723-6.

216. Breda MA, Drinkwater DC, Laks H, et al. Prevention of reperfusion injury in the neonatal heart with leukocyte-depleted blood. J Thorac Cardiovasc Surg 1989;97:654-5.

217. Litt MR, Jeremy RW, Weisman HF, et al. Neutrophil depletion limited to reperfusion reduces myocardial infarct size after 90 minutes of ischemia. Evidence for neutrophil-mediated reperfusion injury. Circulation 1989;80:1816-27.

218. Kofsky ER, Julia PL, Buckberg GD, et al. Studies of controlled reperfusion after ischemia. XXII Reperfusate composition: Effects of leukocyte depletion of blood and blood cardioplegic reperfusates after acute coronary occlusion. J Thorac Cardiovasc Surg 1991;101:350-9.

219. Pearl JM, Drinkwater DC Jr, Laks H, et al. Leukocyte-depleted reperfusion of transplanted human hearts: A randomized, double-blind clinical trial. J Heart Lung Transplant 1992;11:1082-92.

220. Pearl JM, Drinkwater DC Jr, Laks H, et al. Leukocyte-depleted reperfusion of transplanted human hearts prevents ultrastructural evidence of reperfusion injury. J Surg Res 1992;52:298-308.

221. Sawa Y, Taniguchi K, Kadoba K, et al. Leukocyte depletion attenuates reperfusion injury in patients with left ventricular hypertrophy. Circulation 1996;93:1640-6.

222. Bando K, Pillai R, Cameron DE, et al. Leukocyte depletion ameliorates free radical-mediated lung injury after cardiopulmonary bypass. J Thorac Cardiovasc Surg 1990;99:873-7.

223. Gu YJ, deVries AJ, Boonstra PW, van Oeveren W. Leukocyte depletion results in improved lung function and reduced inflammatory response after cardiac surgery. J Thorac Cardiovasc Surg 1996;112:494-500.

224. Lust RM, Bode AP, Yang L, et al. In-line leukocyte filtration during bypass. Clinical results from a randomized prospective trial. ASAIO 1996;42:M819-22.

225. Mihaljevic T, Tönz M, von Segesser LK, et al. The influence of leukocyte filtration during cardiopulmonary bypass on postoperative lung function. A clinical study. J Thorac Cardiovasc Surg 1995;109:1138-45

In: Mintz PD, ed.
Transfusion Therapy: Clinical Principles and Practice
Bethesda, MD: AABB Press, 1999

17

Transfusion-Associated Graft-vs-Host Disease

JED B. GORLIN, MD, AND PAUL D. MINTZ, MD

IRRADIATION OF CELLULAR BLOOD components prevents transfusion-associated graft-vs-host-disease (TA-GVHD) in recipients at risk. Although a relatively rare complication, TA-GVHD is usually fatal within 3 weeks of occurrence. Therefore, preventive efforts are paramount. Since a sufficient dose of gamma irradiation administered to component effectively prevents this complication, why not irradiate all cellular components—ie, those components that can mediate this complication? Before this question is answered, it must be understood that irradiation is not without drawbacks, both economically and with respect to effects on the irradiated component. This chapter assists the reader in establishing the preventive policies and procedures for TA-GVHD that are most appropriate for his or her own institution.

History

The American Association of Blood Banks (AABB) and many blood centers are celebrating 50th anniversaries as the practice of large-scale collection and transfusion of blood and blood components moves into its second half-century. Yet TA-GVHD as a profound complication of blood transfusion has only recently been fully recognized. In part, this stems from its relatively infrequent occurrence. Furthermore, acquired conditions that place one at greatest risk for TA-GVHD, such as the profound immunosuppression associated with hematopoie-

Jed B. Gorlin, MD, Medical Director, Memorial Blood Centers of Minnesota, and Assistant Professor of Pediatrics, Laboratory Medicine, and Pathology, University of Minnesota School of Medicine, Minneapolis, Minnesota and Paul D. Mintz, MD, Associate Chair and Professor of Pathology, Professor of Internal Medicine, and Director, Clinical Laboratories and Blood Bank, University of Virginia Health Sciences Center, Charlottesville, Virginia

tic stem cell transplantation, have been more common following advances in the therapy of malignancies since the 1970s.

In 1955, Shimoda first reported a patient with "postoperative erythroderma."[1] This clinical syndrome, which was later recognized frequently, is now known to be a form of TA-GVHD. The initial report of recognized TA-GVHD cited the occurrence of erythroderma, hepatomegaly, and fatal aplastic anemia in two infants treated with multiple transfusions of "fresh" blood.[2] Simonsen defined the required elements for a graft-vs-host reaction to include 1) immunologically competent donor cells, 2) an antigenic difference between graft and host detectable by the donor cells, and 3) an inability of the host to reject the graft effectively.[3] Hathaway et al described both chronic wasting disorders and more acute presentations.[4,5] Subsequently, TA-GVHD was recognized in patients with acquired immunosuppression from intensive chemotherapy or marrow transplantation.[6-11] Later, the disease was observed in immunocompetent transfusion recipients,[12] who were demonstrated to be at risk of TA-GVHD if the donor was homozygous for HLA antigens for which the recipient was heterozygous.[13]

Clinical Manifestations

Pathophysiology, Signs, and Symptoms

The development of TA-GVHD depends on the recognition of immunologic disparity by donor T cells. Many of the clinical manifestations are believed to result from cytokine dysregulation including overproduction of interleukin (IL)-1, IL-2, γ-interferon, and tumor necrosis factor.[14,15]

TA-GVHD typically begins 2-50 days after transfusion.[16] Its characteristic signs and symptoms include rash, diarrhea, fever, and elevated bilirubin and hepatic enzymes. An intense pancytopenia resulting from hematopoietic failure is also often present, and this phenomenon distinguishes TA-GVHD from the GVHD that may occur following

hematopoietic stem cell transplantation. In this latter process, the hematopoietic tissue is derived from the donor and is spared from attack by donor-derived lymphocytes.

The frequent occurrence in Japan of a rash in patients following cardiopulmonary bypass surgery earned it the title of cardiac bypass erythroderma.[1] This phenomenon is now known to have been caused by GVHD from the transfusion of fresh blood collected from the patients' relatives. The pathophysiology of this process is discussed below. The rash of TA-GVHD usually begins as a central maculopapular eruption, subsequently spreads to the extremities, and may progress to bullae formation.

TA-GVHD has a reported mortality in excess of 90%. Patients have usually died of overwhelming infection resulting from hematopoietic failure.[16] Yet even initial reports have included some nonfatal cases, such as that reported by Cohen et al in 1979.[17]

Pathology

Organs at greatest risk of attack during GVHD are those rich in HLA antigens, including the spleen, liver, gastrointestinal tract, marrow and lymph nodes, and skin. Pathologic examination, most conveniently performed by simple skin biopsy, reveals aggressive lymphocytic infiltration.

Genetic Documentation of TA-GVHD

Definitive diagnosis entails documentation that lymphocytes from a given donor are present in the recipient in association with the clinical condition. Various techniques have been used to produce such documentation, including HLA typing, cytogenetic testing, and genomic amplification. Most conveniently, peripheral blood cells are studied; however, tissue diagnoses may also be performed.[16,18-21] Polymerase chain reaction of Y chromosome regions has been used to document circulating cells responsible for TA-GVHD from male donors in female recipients.[22]

Incidence

Until some recent large Japanese series were published, the total number of TA-GVHD cases reported in the world's literature was fewer than 200. The actual incidence of TA-GVHD is not known; any estimation must be based on retrospective reports of cases. Although the disease is usually fatal, there is reason to believe that it has been relatively underreported.[23] Furthermore, because of the comorbidities in many patients and the diagnostic difficulty, it is undoubtedly underrecognized.

Treatment

Treatment with a wide variety of immunosuppressive regimens, including steroids, cytoxan, and antithymocyte globulin, has been tried without obvious benefit. Often the diagnosis of TA-GVHD is not made until severe multiorgan damage has already occurred. While milder cases are increasingly being recognized, and recovery from TA-GVHD has been reported, it is not clear that a specific therapeutic regimen has been particularly responsible for recovery from these less aggressive versions of TA-GVHD.[22]

Irradiation

How It Works

Irradiation with high energy results in ionization that produces chemical crosslinks within the DNA of the irradiated cell. If the dose is high enough to damage the DNA but not less sensitive parts of the cell, normal cellular functions may remain unaffected but cellular reproduction is prevented. Since part of the mechanism of TA-GVHD requires cellular proliferation of the donor lymphocytes, prevention of proliferation effectively precludes a significant graft-vs-host response.[24]

Although irradiation may result in the malignant transformation of nucleated cells, and existing data are not sufficient to prove that this risk does not exist in irradiated blood components, available data do indicate that this risk is very small.[25-27] In addition, gamma irradiation may theoretically activate latent viruses. No reports exist of this occurrence from irradiated blood components, and the amount of radiation used likely exceeds the amount that could cause this to occur.[28(p9)]

Types of Units

Freestanding

Freestanding irradiators contain a source of radioactive material that undergoes a constant rate of decay. As the source decays, it continually releases a stream of radioactive particles and rays. The sources typically used in freestanding irradiators are cesium (Cs-137) or cobalt (Co-60). Cs-137 is the most commonly used source because of its longer half-life (30 vs 5.2 years) and its higher energy. A longer half-life means that dose adjustments are required less often, and a higher energy requires shorter irradiation time to achieve a fixed dose. To protect those in the vicinity of the irradiators, the source is massively shielded by lead, resulting in both extremely expensive ($50-150,000/unit) and heavy (2-3 ton) devices. In addition, costs of maintaining freestanding units are substantial for licensing, quality control, and safety monitoring.

Linear Accelerator

For centers that are without access to a freestanding irradiator but are associated with an institution that provides therapeutic irradiation, the components may be subjected to irradiation by a linear accelerator. This method results in an equivalent component. However, if the component is required during hours when the therapeutic unit is not normally open, the logistics of calling in a team to provide an irradiated component preclude this as a practical option for centers that often require irradiated components.

Dosage

The optimal dose for TA-GVHD prophylaxis has yet to be determined. Doses as low as 5 Gy significantly attenuate (2/3 decrease) ^{3}H thymidine uptake in mixed lymphocyte culture assays.[29] However, recipients of components that were irradiated in devices where the intended dose to the midplane was as high as 15 and 20 Gy have acquired TA-GVHD.[30,31] Consequently, the US Food and Drug Administration (FDA) has suggested a midplane dose of 25 Gy with the minimum dose of 15 Gy to any point within the container.[28(p11)] The AABB Standards require the intended dose of irradiation to be at least 25 Gy delivered to the midplane of the canister if a freestanding irradiator is used or to the central midplane of the field if a radiotherapy instrument is used. The minimum dose at any point in the canister or field must be 15 Gy.[32(p14)] There have been no reports of TA-GVHD resulting from the transfusion of components treated at this dosage. Pelszynski et al used a sensitive in-vitro assay for T-cell proliferation and concluded that a gamma-irradiation dose of 25 Gy may be required to inactivate completely the T cells in units of Red Blood Cells (RBCs).[33] Rosen et al used mixed lymphocyte cultures and mitogen stimulation assays and concluded that a dose of 2898 cGy eliminated all detectable T-lymphocyte proliferation, whereas the next lower dose tested (2415 cGy) resulted in a small residual response to concanavalin A.[34] Currently, most centers irradiate to an intended dose of 25 Gy to the midplane.

The FDA has stated that the maximum irradiation dose should be 50 Gy.[35] Thus, a dose of 25 Gy would permit a blood component to be irradiated twice and released for transfusion, whereas if a higher dose were used, a component irradiated twice could not be transfused.

Adverse Effects and Storage

The 24-hour posttransfusion recovery of irradiated red cells, after storage, is decreased compared with that of nonirradiated cells. Published data have indicated that red cells irradiated within 24 hours of collection maintain acceptable viability for up to 28 days.[36,37] The FDA has stated that the dating period for RBCs should be not more than 28 days from the date of irradiation but also not more than the dating period of the nonirradiated product.[28(pp12-13)]

Significant changes in cell function have not been shown in platelets subject to irradiation at 20 Gy or 30 Gy on the day of collection and kept for 5 days.[38,39] No change in storage time is necessary for platelet concentrates.[28(p13)]

Although high irradiation doses may impair cell function, one study suggests the lack of any adverse consequences to red cells, platelets, or granulocytes up to 50 Gy.[29] A 1997 report observed lipid peroxidation and hemoglobin oxidation at clinically used doses, but the clinical significance of these findings is unclear.[40]

Irradiated units of RBCs contain approximately twice as much extracellular potassium as unirradiated units of similar age as well as greater levels of cell-free hemoglobin.[41-44] Although the clinical significance of these changes for recipients has been debated, some hospitals have elected not to store irradiated cells for more than 48 hours prior to transfusion to a neonate or infant, and they try to use irradiated units for exchange transfusions to neonates immediately after irradiation.

Jin et al demonstrated that gamma irradiation of RBCs from donors with sickle cell trait did not result in any differences in plasma potassium or red cell adenosine triphosphate (ATP) compared with units from donors with hemoglobin AA.[45] Samuel et al showed that irradiated units could be rejuvenated comparably to nonirradiated units. Red cell ATP and 2,3-diphosphoglycerate (2,3-DPG) levels were restored equally in the irradiated and unirradiated units.[46] Miraglia et al showed that autologous 24-hour posttransfusion recoveries of frozen irradiated red cells were acceptable.[47]

The increasingly global distribution of blood components raises the practical question of whether there are any adverse effects from the irradiation dose used by conventional airport security scanners. The average dose is 5 logs lower than the 25 Gy to which blood is exposed for prevention of TA-GVHD. Indeed, it is questionable whether the low airport scanner dose would have any measurable effect on hematopoietic progenitor cells; however, as a matter of caution, the standards of the National Marrow Donor Program (I9.140), the Foundation for the Accreditation of Hematopoietic Cellular Therapy (D7.174), and the AABB (G4.350) specifically require that cells collected for hematopoietic reconstitution not be irradiated by devices designed to detect metal objects.

Quality Control and Quality Assurance

The 1993 FDA memorandum regarding blood product irradiation states that the dose of irradiation delivered should be 25 Gy targeted to the central portion of the container and that 15 Gy should be the minimum dose at any other point. It further states that validation studies should be performed to establish that the irradiator performs within the above limits and that maintenance procedures should be established to ensure that satisfactory performance continues. The validation studies should be performed annually and after mechanical repairs, and the use of indicator devices to signal exposure of the product to irradiation is recommended.[28(p11)]

AABB *Standards* states that a method to ensure the exposure of each blood component to irradiation should be used.[32(p14)] Irradiation indicators should be considered qualitative. Since there is a considerable range in dosing throughout an irradiation canister (possibly up to 25% attenuation of the beam as it passes through an aqueous medium), it is most practical to use indicators that require only the minimum acceptable dose (ie, 15 Gy), to avoid being faced with the quandary of an incompletely changed indicator on a unit from the bottom of the canister.

AABB *Standards* requires that when any component has been irradiated, it should be so labeled.[32(p22)] As noted, the expiration date of irradiated RBCs needs to be changed not to exceed 28 days if more than this time remains until the original day of outdate. Training of those individuals performing irradiation must include safety proce-dures and be appropriately documented. The irradiator must be monitored for leakage.

As noted, irradiating with 25 Gy ensures the availability of the product for transfusion if a second dose is given for any reason.

General Indications for Irradiation

TA-GVHD is fundamentally an immunologic battle between the invading transfused T cells and the host's immune defense. Indeed, Lee et al have demonstrated the existence of an in-vivo mixed lymphocyte reaction that occurs following transfusion of leukocytes into a normal host.[48] Specifically, the number of donor leukocytes rapidly decreases as the cells are removed from the circulation over several days, followed on days 3-5 by a 1-log expansion of donor cells. In the normal setting, host immune mechanisms are able to clear the remaining cells; in some cases, it is possible to demonstrate long-term stable chimeras.[49] In military parlance, the likely winner of the skirmish between donor and host immune cells is determined by multiple factors, including the relative number of troops on each side (ie, the dose of transfused leukocytes vs host numbers), the level of training and equipment of each combatant (the immune competence of the donor and host), and the fatigue of each army (fresh vs stored donor cells; previous host exposure to immunosuppressive irradiation and/or chemotherapy, disease). Hence, increased risk of TA-GVHD is associated with relatively large transfusions of lymphocytes (eg, exchange transfusions in premature infants or granulocyte transfusions) or an immunosuppressed host (congenital or acquired).

An exception to TA-GVHD requiring a compromised host is when the donor cells appear sufficiently immunologically (HLA) identical to the cells of the recipient but the recipient's cells appear foreign to the donor. This may result when a donor is homozygous for a given HLA haplotype for which the recipient is heterozygous,[13] and it occurs most commonly 1) with a relatively high-frequency HLA haplotype in a given population (eg, Japan), and 2) following related donor transfusions. This situation is discussed below.

Which Components May Cause TA-GVHD?

Cytotoxic T cells mediate TA-GVHD. Hence, any component that contains sufficient, viable cytotoxic T cells can, in theory, mediate TA-GVHD. In practice, only cellular components contain sufficient viable cells to be of concern. While there have been reported cases of TA-GVHD following fresh plasma infusion,[50-52] no cases have been reported following administration of Fresh Frozen Plasma (FFP). Other components known to have caused TA-GVHD include Whole Blood (fresh and stored), RBCs, granulocytes, and platelet concentrates.[53] Frozen components, including frozen washed red cells, FFP, and cryoprecipitate, have not been associated with TA-GVHD.

Indications for Irradiating Cellular Blood Components

Table 17-1 details indications for receiving irradiated cellular components. These are divided into categories of absolute indications, probable indications, controversial indications, and indications where irradiated products are not required. What follows is a discussion of selected indications from each of the categories.

Absolute Indications

Congenital Cellular Immunodeficiency

Many of the earliest reports of TA-GVHD described infants and children with congenital disorders of cellular immunity who developed complications following blood transfusion.[2,54-56] Early reports included TA-GVHD in severe combined immunodeficiency patients,[54-56] thymic hypoplasia,[57] and Wiskott-Aldrich syndrome.[50] All three of these diagnoses are problematic in that the underlying diagnosis is often not made in a timely fashion, so that treatment for some severe infectious complication may require transfusion support before irradiation of blood components is implemented. In addition, thymic hypoplasia may occur in conjunction with congenital cardiac anomalies, (ie, DiGeorge syn-

drome), placing the infant at high likelihood of requiring cardiac surgery before an opportunistic infection may have occurred. Hence, many pediatric cardiac surgery programs require that all infants with congenital cardiac aortic arch defects or intracardiac anomalies (eg, tetralogy of Fallot, truncus arteriosus, pulmonary and aortic valve defects) receive irradiated blood until the chromosomal defect associated with DiGeorge syndrome is excluded. Congenital immunodeficiencies as parts of rare syndromes may be difficult to recognize. For example, a case of TA-GVHD was reported in a patient with multiple intestinal atresias, now known to be associated with a congenital immunodeficiency.[58]

Hematopoietic Stem Cell Transplant Recipients

Both allogeneic and autologous recipients of hematopoietic stem cell transplants have developed TA-GVHD.[10,11] The profound immunosuppression, especially following total body irradiation, appears to put the recipient at particular risk. It is universal practice to provide irradiated cellular components during treatment. More controversial is whether these recipients should continue to require irradiated products on subsequent admissions. In practice, most centers leave the requirement for special components (eg, leukocyte-reduced, irradiated) as part of the patient requirements indefinitely since immunocompetence may not be fully restored following recovery.

Hodgkin's Disease

There are many reports of TA-GVHD in patients with Hodgkin's disease.[18,59-67] This may follow from an underlying defect in immune regulation. Hence, irradiation of cellular components for patients with Hodgkin's disease is accepted practice.[68]

Granulocyte Transfusions

Granulocyte transfusions involve large numbers of very fresh leukocytes (including lymphocytes) being infused into typically immunologically compromised hosts; consequently, multiple reports

Table 17-1. Indications for Irradiation of Cellular Blood Components for Prevention of Transfusion-Associated Graft-vs-Host Disease

ABSOLUTE INDICATIONS

Patients with congenital cellular immune deficiency[2,50,54-58]

Allogeneic hematopoietic stem cell recipients[10]

Autologous hematopoietic stem cell recipients[11]

Patients with Hodgkin's disease[18,59-67]

Granulocyte transfusions[59,69-72]

Intrauterine transfusions[73-76]

Transfusions to neonates who have received intrauterine transfusions[74]

Transfusions from biologic relatives[13,23,77-80]

PROBABLE INDICATIONS

Transfusions to premature infants < 1500 g[82-86]

Patients with hematologic malignancies (other than Hodgkin's disease) treated with cytotoxic agents[6-9,69-72,88-91]

Patients receiving high-dose chemotherapy, radiation therapy, and/or aggressive immunosuppressive therapy[59,92-96]

HLA-matched and/or crossmatch-compatible platelet concentrate transfusions[100,102,103]

CONTROVERSIAL INDICATIONS

Solid organ transplant recipients[105,106]

Large-volume transfusions and exchange transfusions to term neonates who did not receive intrauterine transfusions

Aplastic anemia patients not receiving aggressive immunosuppressive therapy[98]

Term neonates on extracorporeal membrane oxygenation[107]

IRRADIATION NOT INDICATED

Patients infected with the human immunodeficiency virus

Patients with hemophilia

Small-volume transfusions to term neonates who did not receive intrauterine transfusions

Elderly patients

Patients receiving immunosuppressive medications (see text)

Immunocompetent surgical patients

Pregnant patients

Patients with membrane, metabolic, or hemoglobin red blood cell disorders (eg, thalassemia, sickle cell disease)

associate this component with TA-GVHD.[59,69-72] Thus, granulocyte concentrates must be irradiated prior to transfusion.

Intrauterine Transfusions and Transfusions to Neonates Who Have Received Intrauterine Transfusions

All intrauterine transfusions must be irradiated. In 1969, Naiman et al reported a case of fatal TA-GVHD in an 8-week-old infant who had received three intrauterine transfusions,[73] one of which was implicated by cytogenetic studies. In 1974, Parkman et al reported fatal TA-GVHD in two infants after intrauterine transfusion and exchange transfusion.[74] In both of these patients, the lymphocytes causing the GVHD were demonstrated to have come from an exchange transfusion donor. The authors commented that in the preceding 27 years, no infants treated with exchange transfusion alone had had fatal TA-GVHD. They speculated that the introduction of lymphocytes by intrauterine transfusion had rendered the infants susceptible to TA-GVHD from the exchange transfusion. They suggested that irradiating blood used for exchange transfusion would be appropriate in this circumstance. Subsequent to the reports of Naiman and Parkman, others noted TA-GVHD caused by intrauterine transfusions that were not irradiated.[75,76] In practice, irradiation of all cellular components transfused to neonates and infants who have received intrauterine transfusions is recommended.

Since prenatal care that may have involved an intrauterine transfusion may have occurred at a different institution, many transfusion services simply find it practical to provide irradiated blood for all exchange transfusions. In the absence of a prior intrauterine transfusion, however, there is no compelling reason to irradiate an exchange transfusion for a term neonate who has no other indication for receiving irradiated components.

Transfusions from Biologic Relatives

TA-GVHD has been reported in immunocompetent recipients. Most of the patients have received blood from a donor homozygous for an HLA haplotype for which the recipient was heterozygous (either HLA-A and -B or HLA-A, -B, and -DR). This situation, first reported in detail by Thaler et al, allows the donor cells to react against the foreign recipient while the host's immune system views the donor lymphocytes' "Trojan Horse" as self and does not reject them.[13] Previously, the syndrome "postoperative erythroderma" was recognized in Japan among patients who had received fresh blood typically from relatives.[1] In a study reported 33 years later, but prior to Thaler's report, a similar situation with respect to HLA types had been noted.[77] In a subsequent review of TA-GVHD among immunocompetent Japanese recipients, the majority of cases (62%) occurred with the use of fresh blood (< 72 hours from donation) but in only a minority of cases (29%) were the donor and recipient related.[23] Among donors and recipients who were studied, in 93% of cases, the donor was HLA homozygous for a haplotype shared with the recipient. Petz et al comprehensively reviewed the English-language literature regarding TA-GVHD in immunocompetent recipients.[78] They noted the use of fresh blood (<96 hours from donation) in 87% of cases, a family relationship between donor and recipient in 44%, and an HLA homozygous donor for a haplotype shared by the recipient in 87% of cases.

Kanter has calculated that the probability of this situation existing among relatives is greatest for transfusions between parents and children, next most likely for transfusions between grandparents and grandchildren or between aunts/uncles and nieces/nephews, and third most likely among siblings.[79] Wagner and Flegel calculated that the risks for this occurrence between parents and children is increased at least 21-fold for US whites, 18-fold for Germans, and 11-fold for Japanese compared with the risks from nonrelated transfusions.[80]

In practice, cellular blood components from all biological relatives are irradiated. Many hospitals will irradiate blood from all directed donors because eliciting whether a directed donor is related by blood to a particular recipient is fraught with uncertainty.

Probable Indications

Transfusions to Premature Infants Weighing Less Than 1500 g

Whether transfusions to premature infants require irradiation has been the subject of conflicting opinions. Many centers have established policies to ensure that extremely premature infants receive irradiated blood. Specifically, in a neonatal transfusion practices survey, a majority of the responding institutions reported that they provide irradiation for at least some neonates.[81] While as a practical matter some institutions choose to irradiate all cellular components dispensed to their own neonatal intensive care unit, the report concluded that it was questionable whether gamma irradiation of blood components is needed for neonates other than those in the recognized high-risk groups of congenital cellular immunodeficiency diseases, recipients of intrauterine transfusions with or without subsequent exchange transfusion, and recipients of blood components from blood relatives.[81] It is difficult to interpret the published literature of TA-GVHD in premature infants. Most case reports have had additional confounding risk factors, including underlying immunodeficiencies, related donors, and/or prior intrauterine transfusions. Only a few reports document TA-GVHD in a premature infant without other risk factors from an HLA-disparate donor.

Nevertheless, premature infants represent one of the most frequently reported groups at risk for TA-GVHD.[82] In addition, premature infants weighing less than 1500 g have relatively poorly developed cell-mediated immunity.[83] In fact, the empirical observation is that premature infants with TA-GVHD without confounding risk factors were usually under 1500 g at birth.[82,84,85] While it must be emphasized that these case reports represent exceptions to the great number of uneventfully transfused premature infants, in aggregate they represent a substantial portion of the total case reports of TA-GVHD.[86] Therefore, the authors strongly recommend irradiation of cellular components for extremely premature infants (< 1500 g) as a prudent precaution. However, the routine irradiation of cellular blood products for all neonates is not recommended.[87]

Patients With Hematologic Malignancies (Other Than Hodgkin's Disease) Treated With Cytotoxic Agents

Irradiation of cellular components for patients with non-Hodgkin's lymphoma and leukemias is often categorized as a probable indication; that is, multiple cases have been reported, but it is not yet universal practice to provide irradiated components for these patients.[6-9,69-72,88-91] In short, the risk for TA-GVHD is less in patients with hematologic malignancies other than Hodgkin's disease.

Patients Receiving High-Dose Chemotherapy, Radiation Therapy, and/or Aggressive Immunosuppressive Therapy

Transfusion following aggressive chemotherapy for other malignancies especially neuroblastoma, has been associated with TA-GVHD.[92-94] Patients with rhabdomyosarcoma,[95] glioblastoma,[59] and renal adenocarcinoma[96] have also reportedly developed TA-GVHD. The glioblastoma case followed a granulocyte transfusion, which, as discussed above, is now considered an absolute indication for irradiation. Thus, irradiated cellular blood components are recommended for patients with malignancies who are receiving therapy that may cause severe immune deficiency. The authors agree with those who suggest that routine irradiation of blood products is not indicated for patients with solid tumors in the absence of intensive immunosuppressive therapy.[97(p261)]

Because TA-GVHD has been reported in patients with aplastic anemia,[98-99] it is appropriate to irradiate cellular products for such patients who are receiving intensive immunosuppressive regimens. However, for patients not receiving such treatment, the authors do not believe that irradiation of these components is necessary.

In short, any highly immunosuppressive regimen appears to increase the risk of TA-GVHD.

Platelet Donors Chosen for HLA Matching or Crossmatch Compatibility

The authors recommend irradiating all platelet concentrates selected on the basis of crossmatch compatibility and/or HLA matching. Donors homozygous for HLA haplotypes may be overrepresented among those selected as HLA matches for recipients, because such homozygous donors will express fewer HLA antigens and will be more likely not to express antigens found in the recipient. Grishaber et al noted that in their experience with patients who received platelets matched for Class I HLA antigens, in 5% of transfusions the recipient received lymphocytes from a donor exhibiting no foreign antigens but the patient had antigens not present on donor lymphocytes.[100] Twenty-three percent of patients received at least one such transfusion. Takahashi et al calculated that the risk of receiving a one-way HLA-matched blood transfusion from an unrelated donor in the United States among caucasians is 1 in 797 and in Japan, 1 in 312.[101]

TA-GVHD has been reported in recipients of HLA-matched nonirradiated platelets from unrelated donors, but such cases are relatively rare.[102,103] This may be because the process is not recognized, because minor histocompatibility incompatibilities may be more likely to exist among unrelated recipients and could lead to donor lymphocyte clearance, or because idiotypic antibody to the T-cell receptor is present in multitransfused patients.[103,104]

Controversial Indications

Solid Organ Transplantation

Immunosuppressive regimens following solid organ transplantation are historically not as aggressive as those associated with hematopoietic stem cell transplantation. Nonetheless, especially with advances in immunosuppression for liver transplantation, the regimens have grown more potent. TA-GVHD following liver transplantation, possibly associated with underlying host cytopenias, has been reported in cases documented to have mutually discordant HLA types.[105-106] Nonetheless, it is

not routine practice to irradiate blood for solid organ allograft recipients.

Aplastic Anemia Patients Not on Aggressive Immunosuppressive Therapy

TA-GVHD has occurred following treatment for aplastic anemia.[98,99] As noted, the authors do not believe that patients with this disease require irradiated cellular blood components unless they are receiving aggressive immunosuppressive therapy.

Term Neonates Undergoing Extracorporeal Membrane Oxygenation

While thousands of neonates have been treated using extracorporeal membrane oxygenation and have required massive transfusion support, TA-GVHD is exceedingly rare in these patients. Nonetheless, there is at least one published case of TA-GVHD in a full-term infant treated for neonatal respiratory distress following meconium aspiration.[107] On day 17, the child developed a florid rash and fever. Skin biopsy was consistent with GVHD. Despite treatment with steroids and cyclosporine, multiorgan failure ensued and the child died. No underlying immune defect could be demonstrated including documentation of normal number of T cells and mitogen stimulation studies. The specific donor mediating the TA-GVHD was not identified; hence, the possibility of a one-way HLA match by chance could not be ruled out in this case.

Nonindications

Human Immunodeficiency Virus Infection

That no case of TA-GVHD has occurred following acquisition of human immunodeficiency virus (HIV) infection despite the numerous unirradiated transfusions to which this patient group has undoubtedly been exposed, illustrates that the risk factors for TA-GVHD are more complex than simple immunodeficiency. Since the primary immunodeficiency of acquired immune deficiency syndrome is in the CD4+ T cells, it might be posited that the cytotoxic T cells responsible for host defense against

TA-GVHD remain unscathed. An animal model confirms the importance of CD8+, as opposed to CD4+, cells being critical for host defense against TA-GVHD. Indeed, it took far more donor cells to cause GVHD when CD4+ cells were depleted in the host than when host CD8+ cells were depleted.[108] Alternatively, HIV infection of donor CD4+ cells could prevent them from mounting GVHD.

Small-Volume Transfusions to Term Neonates Who Did Not Receive Intrauterine Transfusion

With the exception of the child treated with extracorporeal membrane oxidation described above, there are no reports of full-term neonates without other risk factors developing TA-GVHD.[107] Term neonotes do not routinely require irradiated cellular components. As noted, some programs will irradiate all exchange transfusions to term neonates rather than attempt to rule out who has received an intrauterine transfusion.

Elderly Patients

Elderly recipients do not appear to be at increased risk of TA-GVHD solely on the basis of age. Since a considerable proportion of blood transfused is received by individuals aged 60 or older, it must be presumed that an adequate opportunity exists to detect a significantly increased risk. Hence, blood should not be irradiated solely because the recipient is elderly.

Patients Receiving Immunosuppressive Medications

Patients with autoimmune diseases who have received immunosuppressive medications have not been reported to have developed TA-GVHD. Therefore, irradiation of cellular blood products for these patients is not indicated.

Alternatives to Irradiation

Leukocyte Reduction

In theory, since the risk of TA-GVHD is a function of the dose of infused immunocompetent T cells, the effective removal of these cells should prevent this complication. In practice, the use of leukocyte reduction for prophylaxis against TA-GVHD is precluded by the variable efficiency observed in leukocyte reduction with current technology and the variable number of leukocytes required to mediate this complication.[109(pp562-3)] Indeed, documented cases of TA-GVHD have occurred despite transfusion of solely leukocyte reduced units to the recipients.[110-112]

Ultraviolet Pathogen Inactivation Methods

Alternatively, while not yet licensed for this application, photochemical inactivation of bacterial and viral pathogens in blood components using psoralens and ultraviolet (UV)-A light irradiation may also serve as prophylaxis against TA-GVHD. Several reports document the efficacy of this process to inactivate T cells that mediate TA-GVHD using both in-vitro and in-vivo models.[113,114] Most recently, prevention of TA-GVHD by photochemical inactivation of donor T cells has been demonstrated in a model using immunocompromised mice.[115] Hence, when this proess gains acceptance as a method to reduce transfusion-related infectious risks, it may have the side benefit of obviating the need to irradiate products for individuals at risk of TA-GVHD.

Alternatively, simply irradiating leukocyte-containing components with the less intense UV-B light may prevent TA-GVHD. A mouse model documented prevention of GVHD using UV-B irradiated donor leukocytes.[116] Again, since licensed devices to irradiate components using UV-B light are not available, and since the presence of red cells in the irradiated product complicates the efficacy of this treatment, further advances in this technology are required before it can be routinely applied to prevent TA-GVHD.

Conclusion

TA-GVHD is a devastating complication of cellular blood component transfusion. Although TA-GVHD typically occurs in immunocompromised patients, the development of this process in immunocompetent patients who received blood from relatives was an unexpected consequence of the demand for directed donations. The relatively low-cost, low-risk procedure of 25 Gy of gamma irradiation has afforded a reliable prevention.

References

1. Shimoda T. The case report of post-operative erythroderma. Geka 1955;17:487.

2. Hathaway WE, Githens JH, Blackburn WR, et al. Aplastic anemia, histiocytosis and erythroderma in immunologically deficient children. N Engl J Med 1965;273:953-8.

3. Simonsen M. Graft versus host reactions: Their natural history and applicability as tools of research. Prog Allergy 1962;6:349-467.

4. Hathaway WE, Brangle RW, Nelson TL, Roeckel IE. Aplastic anemia and alymphocytosis in an infant with hypogammaglobulinemia: Graft-versus-host reaction? J Pediatr 1966;68:713-22.

5. Hathaway WE, Fulginiti VA, Pierce CW, et al. Graft-vs-host reaction following a single blood transfusion. JAMA 1967;201:1015-20.

6. Szaley F, Buki B, Kalouics I, Keleman E. Post transfusion GVHR in an adult with acute leukemia and aplastic anemia. Orv Hetil 1972; 113:1275-80.

7. Rosen RC, Heustis DW, Corrigan JJ Jr. Acute leukemia and granulocyte transfusion: Fatal graft versus host reaction following transfusion of cells obtained from normal donors. J Pediatr 1978;93:268-70.

8. Lowenthal RM, Menon C, Challis DR. Graft-versus-host-disease in consecutive patients with acute myeloid leukemia treated with blood cells from normal donors. Aust N Z J Med 1981;11:179-83.

9. Nikoskelainen J, Soderstrom K-O, Rajamaki A, et al. Graft versus host reaction in 3 adult leukemia patients after transfusion of blood cell products. Scand J Haematol 1983;31: 403-9.

10. Fagiolo E, D'Addosio AM. Post-transfusion graft-vs-host disease (GVHD): Immunopathology and prevention. Haematologica 1985; 70:62-74.

11. Postmus PE, Mulder NH, Elema JD. Graft versus host disease after transfusions of non-irradiated blood cells in patients having received autologous bone marrow: A report of 4 cases following ablative chemotherapy for solid tumors. Eur J Cancer Clin Oncol 1988; 24:889-94.

12. Sakakibara T, Juji T. Post-transfusion graft-versus-host disease after open heart surgery. Lancet 1986;2:1099.

13. Thaler M, Shamiss A, Orgad S, et al. The role of blood from HLA-homozygous donors in fatal transfusion-associated graft-versus-host disease after open-heart surgery. N Engl J Med 1989;321:25-8.

14. Vogelsang GB, Hess AD. Graft-versus-host disease: New directions for a persistent problem. Blood 1994;84:2061-7.

15. Antin JH, Ferrara JLM. Cytokine dysregulation and acute graft-versus-host disease. Blood 1992;80:2964-8.

16. Suzuki K, Akiyama H, Takamoto S, et al. Transfusion-associated graft-versus-host disease in a presumably immunocompetent patient after transfusion of stored packed red cells. Transfusion 1992;32:358-60.

17. Cohen D, Weinstein H, Mihm M, Yankee R. Nonfatal graft-versus-host disease occurring after transfusion with leukocytes and platelets obtained from normal donors. Blood 1979;53:1063-7.

18. Kunstmann E, Bocker T, Roewer L, et al. Diagnosis of transfusion-associated graft-versus-host disease by genetic fingerprinting and polymerase chain reaction. Transfusion 1992;32:766-70.

19. Hayakawa S, Chishima F, Sakata H, et al. A rapid molecular diagnosis of posttransfusion graft-versus-host disease by polymerase chain reaction. Transfusion 1993;33:413-7.

20. Wang L, Juji T, Tokunaga K, et al. Polymorphic microsatellite markers for the diagnosis

of graft-versus-host disease. N Engl J Med 1994;330:398-401.

21. Zulian GB, Roux E, Tiercy JM, et al. Transfusion-associated graft-versus-host disease in a patient treated with cladribine (2-chlorodeoxyadenosine): Demonstration of exogenous DNA in various tissue extracts by PCR analysis. Br J Haematol 1995;89:83-9.

22. Mori S, Matsushita H, Ozaki K, et al. Spontaneous resolution of transfusion-associated graft-versus-host disease. Transfusion 1995; 35:431-5.

23. Ohto H, Anderson KC. Survey of transfusion-associated graft-versus-host disease in immunocompetent recipients. Transfus Med Rev 1996;10:31-43.

24. Butch S. Principles of irradiation. In: Butch S, Tiehan A, eds. Blood irradiation: A user's guide. Bethesda, MD: AABB Press, 1996: 41-64.

25. Little JB. Mechanisms of malignant transformation of human diploid cells. Carcinogenesis 1985;10:337-53.

26. Brach MA, Hass R, Sherman ML, et al. Ionizing radiation induces expression and binding activity of the nuclear factor kappa-B. J Clin Invest 1991;88:691-5.

27. Linden JV, Pisciotto PT. Transfusion-associated graft-versus-host disease and blood irradiation. Transfus Med Rev 1992;6:116-23.

28. Food and Drug Administration. Memorandum: Recommendations regarding license amendments and procedures for gamma irradiation of blood products (July 22, 1993). Rockville, MD: Office of Communication, Training, and Manufacturing Assistance, 1993.

29. Button LN, DeWolf WC, Newburger PE, et al. The effects of irradiation on blood components. Transfusion 1981;21:419-26.

30. Lowenthal RM, Challis DR, Griffiths AE, et al. Transfusion-associated graft-versus-host disease: Report of an occurrence following the administration of irradiated blood. Transfusion 1993;33:524-9.

31. Sproul AM, Chalmers EA, Mills KI, et al. Third party mediated graft rejection despite irradiation of blood products. Br J Haematol 1992;80:251-62.

32. Menitove JE, ed. Standards for blood banks and transfusion services, 18th edition. Bethesda, MD: American Association of Blood Banks, 1997.

33. Pelszynski MM, Moroff G, Luban NLC, et al. Effect of a γ irradiation of red blood cell units on T-cell inactivation as assessed by limiting dilution analysis: Implications for preventing transfusion-associated graft-versus-host disease. Blood 1994;83:1683-9.

34. Rosen NR, Weidner JG, Boldt HD, Rosen DS. Prevention of transfusion-associated graft-versus-host disease: Selection of an adequate dose of gamma radiation. Transfusion 1993; 33:125-7.

35. FDA panel defers recommendations to reduce donor deferral period for men who have had sex with other men but agrees that HIV risk deferral criteria need changing: Blood product irradiation. ABC Newsletter 1997;47:14.

36. Friedman KD, McDonough WC, Cimino DF. The effect of prestorage gamma irradiation on post-transfusion red blood cell recovery (abstract). Transfusion 1991;31:50S.

37. Davey RJ, McCoy NC, Yu M, et al. The effect of prestorage irradiation on post-transfusion red cell survival. Transfusion 1992;32:525-8.

38. Rock G, Adams GA, Labow RS. The effects of irradiation on platelet function. Transfusion 1988;28:451-5.

39. Duguid JK, Carr R, Jenkins JA, et al. Clinical evaluation of the effects of storage time and irradiation on transfused platelets. Vox Sang 1991;60:151-4.

40. Anand AJ, Dzik WH, Imam A, Sadrzadeh SMH. Radiation-induced red cell damage: Role of reactive oxygen species. Transfusion 1997;37:160-5.

41. Ramirez AM, Woodfield DG, Scott R, et al. High potassium levels in stored irradiated blood. Transfusion 1987;27:444-5.

42. Rivet C, Baxter A, Rock G. Potassium levels in irradiated blood (letter). Transfusion 1989;29:185.

43. Anderson G, Mintz PD. Vitamin E and the potassium leak lesion (letter). Transfusion 1991; 31:476.

44. Mintz PD, Anderson G. Effect of gamma irradiation on the *in vivo* recovery of stored red blood cells. Ann Clin Lab Sci 1993;23:216-20.

45. Jin YS, Anderson G, Mintz PD. Effects of gamma irradiation on red cells from donors with sickle cell trait. Transfusion 1997;37:804-8.

46. Samuel LH, Anderson G, Mintz PD. Rejuvenation of irradiated AS-1 red cells. Transfusion 1997;37:25-8.

47. Miraglia CC, Anderson G, Mintz PD. Effect of freezing on the in vivo recovery of irradiated red cells. Transfusion 1994;34:775-8.

48. Lee T-H, Donegan E, Slichter S, Busch MP. Transient increase in circulating donor leukocytes after allogeneic transfusions in immunocompetent recipients compatible with donor cell proliferation. Blood 1995;85:1207-14.

49. Lee T-H, Ohto H, Paglieroni T, et al. Survival kinetics of specific donor leukocyte subsets in transfused immunocompetent patients (abstract). Transfusion 1996;36:45S.

50. Douglas SD, Fudenberg HH. Graft-versus-host reaction in Wiskott-Aldrich syndrome: Antemortem diagnosis of human GvH in an immunologic deficiency disease. Vox Sang 1969;16:172-8.

51. Rubinstein A, Radl J, Cottier H, et al. Unusual combined immunodeficiency syndrome exhibiting kappa-IgD paraproteinemia, residual gut-immunity and graft-versus-host reaction after plasma infusion. Acta Paediatr Scand 1973;62:365-72.

52. Park BH, Good RA, Gate J, Burke B. Fatal graft-vs.-host reaction following transfusion of allogeneic blood and plasma in infants with combined immunodeficiency disease. Transplant Proc 1974;6:385-7.

53. Roberts GT, Sacher RA. Transfusion-associated graft-versus-host disease. In: Rossi EC, Simon EL, Moss GS, Gould SA, eds. Principles of transfusion medicine. Baltimore, MD: Williams and Wilkins, 1996:785-801.

54. Hong R, Kay EM, Cooper MD, et al. Immunological reconstitution in lymphopenic immunological deficiency syndrome. Lancet 1968;1:503-6.

55. Jacobs JC, De Capoa A, McGilvray E, et al. Complement deficiency and chromosomal breaks in case of Swiss-type agammaglobulinaemia. Lancet 1968;1:499-503.

56. Gatti RA, Platt N, Pomerance H, et al. Hereditary lymphopenic agammaglobulinemia associated with distinctive form of short-linked dwarfism and ectodermal dysplasia. J Pediatr 1969;75:675-84.

57. McCarty JR, Raimer SS, Jarratt M. Toxic epidermal necrolysis from graft-versus-host disease. Occurrence in a patient with thymic hypoplasia. Am J Dis Child 1978;132:282-4.

58. Walker MW, Lovell MA, Kelly TE, et al. Multiple areas of intestinal atresia associated with immunodeficiency and posttransfusion graft-versus-host disease. J Pediatr 1993;123:93-5.

59. Schmidmeir W, Feil W, Gebhart W, et al. Fatal graft-versus-host reaction following granulocyte transfusions. Blut 1982;45:115-9.

60. Dinsmore RE, Straus DJ, Pollack MS, et al. Fatal graft-versus-host disease following blood transfusion in Hodgkin's disease documented by HLA typing. Blood 1980;55:831-4.

61. Burns LJ, Wesbury MW, Burns CP, et al. Acute graft versus host disease resulting from normal donor blood transfusion. Acta Haematol 1984;71:270-6.

62. Von Fliedner V, Higby DJ, Kim U. Graft-versus-host reaction following blood product transfusion. Am J Med 1982;72:951-61.

63. Kessinger A, Armitage JO, Klassen LW, et al. Graft vs host disease following transfusion of

normal blood products to patients with malignancies. J Surg Oncol 1987;36:206-9.

64. Spitzer TR, Cahill R, Cotler-Fox M, et al. Transfusion induced graft-versus-host disease in patients with malignant lymphoma: A case report and review of the literature. Cancer 1990;66:2346-9.

65. Groff P, Torhorst J, Speck B, et al. Die graft-versus-host-krankheit, eine wenig bekannte komplikation der bluttransfusion. Schweiz Med Wochenschr 1976;106:634-9.

66. Stutzman L, Nisce L, Friedman M. Increased toxicity of total nodal irradiation (TNI) following combination chemotherapy (abstract). Proc Am Soc Clin Oncol 1979; 20:391.

67. Mathe G, Schwartzenberg L, deVries MJ, et al. Les divers aspects du syndrome secondaire compliquant les transfusions allogeniques du moelle osseuse ou de leukocytes chez des sujets atteints d'hemopathies malignes. Eur J Cancer 1965;1:75-113.

68. Anderson KC, Weinstein HJ. Transfusion-associated graft-versus-host disease. N Engl J Med 1990;323:315-21.

69. DeDobbeleer GP, Ledoux-Corbusier MH, Achten GA. Graft versus host reaction. An ultrastructural study. Arch Dermatol 1975; 3:1597-602.

70. Ford JM, Lucey JJ, Cullen MH, et al. Fatal graft-versus-host disease following transfusion of granulocytes from normal donors. Lancet 1976;2:1167-9.

71. Weiden PL, Zuckerman N, Hansen JA, et al. Fatal graft-versus-host disease in a patient with lymphoblastic leukemia following normal granulocyte transfusions. Blood 1981; 57:328-32.

72. Tolbert B, Kaufman CE Jr, Burgdorf WHC, Brubaker D. Graft versus host disease from leukocyte transfusions. J Am Acad Dermatol 1983;9:416-9.

73. Naiman JL, Punnett HH, Lischner HW, et al. Possible graft-versus-host reaction after intrauterine transfusion for Rh erythroblastosis fetalis. N Engl J Med 1969;281:697-701.

74. Parkman R, Mosier D, Umansky I, et al. Graft-versus-host disease after intrauterine and exchange transfusions for hemolytic disease of the newborn. N Engl J Med 1974; 290:359-63.

75. Bohm N, Kleine W, Enzel U. Graft-versus-host disease in two newborns after repeated blood transfusions because of rhesus incompatibility. Beitr Pathol 1977;160:381-400.

76. Hentschel R, Broecker EB, Kolde G, et al. Intact survival with transfusion-associated graft-versus-host disease proved by human leukocyte antigen typing of lymphocytes in skin biopsy specimens. J Pediatr 1995;126: 61-4.

77. Ito K, Yoshida H, Yanagibashi K, et al. Change of HLA phenotype in postoperative erythroderma. Lancet 1988;1:413-4.

78. Petz LD, Calhoun L, Yam P, et al. Transfusion-associated graft-versus-host disease in immunocompetent patients: Report of a fatal case associated with transfusion of blood from a second-degree relative, and a survey of predisposing factors. Transfusion 1993; 33:742-50.

79. Kanter MH. Transfusion-associated graft-versus-host disease: Do transfusions from second-degree relatives pose a greater risk than those from first-degree relatives? Transfusion 1992;32:323-7.

80. Wagner FF, Flegel WA. Transfusion-associated graft-versus-host disease: Risk due to homozygous HLA haplotypes. Transfusion 1995;35:284-91.

81. Strauss RG, Levy GJ, Sotelo-Avila C, et al. National survey of neonatal transfusion practices, II: Blood component therapy. Pediatrics 1993;91:530-6.

82. Ohto H, Anderson KC. Posttransfusion graft-versus-host disease in Japanese newborns. Transfusion 1996;36:117-23.

83. Pahwa S, Sia C, Harper R, Pahwa R. T-lymphocyte subpopulations in high-risk infants: Influence of age and blood transfusions. Pediatrics 1985;76:914-7.

84. Sanders MR, Graeber JE. Posttransfusion graft-versus-host disease in infancy. J Pediatr 1990;117:159-63.

85. Flidel O, Barak Y, Lifschitz-Mercer B, et al. Graft versus host disease in extremely low birth weight neonates. Pediatrics 1992;89:689-90.

86. Anderson KC, Goodnough LT, Sayers M, et al. Variation in blood component irradiation practice: Implications for prevention of transfusion-associated graft-versus-host disease. Blood 1991;77:2096-102.

87. Strauss RG. Practical issues in neonatal transfusion practice. Am J Clin Pathol 1997;107:S57-63.

88. Schmitz N, Kayser W, Gassmann W, et al. Ten cases of graft-versus-host disease following transfusion of irradiated blood products. Blut 1982;44:83-8.

89. Siimes MA, Koskimies S. Chronic graft versus host disease after blood transfusions by incompatible HLA antigens in bone marrow (letter). Lancet 1982;1:42-3.

90. Pflieger H. Graft-versus-host disease following blood transfusions. Blut 1983;46:61-6.

91. Gossi U, Bucher U, Brun del Re G, et al. Acute graft versus host disease following a single transfusion of erythrocytes. Schweiz Wochenschr 1985;115:34-40.

92. Woods WG, Lubin BH. Fatal graft-versus-host disease following a blood transfusion in a child with neuroblastoma. Pediatrics 1981;67:217-21.

93. Remlinger K, Buckner CD, Clift RA, et al. Fatal graft versus host disease and probable graft versus host reaction due to an unradiated granulocyte transfusion after allogeneic bone marrow transplant. Transplant Proc 1983;15:1725-8.

94. Kennedy JS, Rickets RR. Fatal graft-versus-host disease in a child with neuroblastoma following a blood transfusion. J Pediatr Surg 1986;21:1108-9.

95. Labotka RJ, Radvany R. Graft vs host disease in rhabdomyosarcoma following transfusion with nonirradiated blood products. Med Pediatr Oncol 1985;13:101-4.

96. Capon SM, DePond WD, Tyan DB, et al. Transfusion-associated graft-versus-host disease in an immunocompetent patient. Ann Intern Med 1991;114:1025-6.

97. McCullough J, ed. Transfusion medicine. New York, NY: McGraw-Hill, 1998.

98. Lowenthal RM, Grossman L, Goldman JM, et al. Granulocyte transfusions in treatment of infection in patients with acute leukemia and aplastic anemia. Lancet 1975; 1:353-8.

99. Weschler A, Magnin PH, Casas JG, et al. Post transfusion graft versus host reaction in aplastic anemia. Med Cutan Ibero Lat Am 1984;12:203-7.

100. Grishaber JE, Birney SM, Strauss RG. Potential for transfusion-associated graft-versus-host disease due to apheresis platelets matched for HLA Class I antigens. Transfusion 1993;33:910-4.

101. Takahashi K, Juji T, Miyazaki H. Post-transfusion graft-versus-host disease occurring in non-immunosuppressed patients in Japan. Transfus Sci 1991;12:281-9.

102. Benson K, Marks AR, Marshall MJ, Goldstein JD. Fatal graft-versus-host disease associated with transfusions of HLA-matched, HLA-homozygous platelets from unrelated donors. Transfusion 1994;34:432-7.

103. Takanashi M, Nishimura M, Tadokoro K, Juji T. Graft-versus-host disease associated with transfusions of HLA-matched, HLA-homozygous platelets. Transfusion 1995;35:276-7.

104. Nishimura M, Sakai K, Akaza T, et al. Anti-idiotypic antibody to T-cell receptor in multiply transfused patients may play a role in resistance to graft-versus-host disease. Transfusion 1992;32:719-28.

105. Wisecarver JL, Cattral MS, Langnas AN, et al. Transfusion-induced graft-versus-host disease after liver transplantation. Transplantation 1994;58:269-71.

106. Klein HG. Transfusion in transplant patients: The good, the bad, and the ugly. J Heart Lung Transplant 1993;12:S7-12.

107. Hatley RM, Reynolds M, Paller AS, Chou P. Graft-versus-host disease following ECMO. J Pediatr Surg 1991;26:317-9.

108. Fast LD, Valeri CR, Crowley JP. Immune responses to major histocompatibility complex homozygous lymphoid cells in murine F_1 hybrid recipients: Implications for transfusion-associated graft-versus-host disease. Blood 1995;86:3090-6.

109. Brubaker DB. Transfusion-associated graft-versus-host disease. In: Anderson KC, Ness PM, eds. Scientific basis of transfusion medicine—implications for clinical practice. Philadelphia, PA: WB Saunders Co, 1994: 544-79.

110. Akahoshi M, Takanashi M, Masuda M, et al. A case of transfusion-associated graft-versus-host disease not prevented by white cell-reduction filters. Transfusion 1992;32:169-72.

111. Heim MU, Munker R, Sauer H, et al. Graft-versus-host krankheit (GVH) mit letalem ausgang nach der gabe von gefilterten erythrozytenkonzentraten (EK), abstracted. Infusiontherapie 1991;(Suppl)18:8.

112. Hayashi H, Nishiuchi T, Tamura H, Takeda K. Transfusion-associated graft-versus-host disease caused by leukocyte-filtered stored blood. Anesthesiology 1993;79:1419-21.

113. Grass J, Hei D, Wiesehahn GP, et al. Inactivation of T-cells with psoralens and UVA in human platelet concentrates (abstract). Blood 1995;86:542a.

114. Grass J, Wafa T, Reames A, et al. Prevention of transfusion-associated graft versus host disease (TA-GVHD) by photochemical treatment (PCT) (abstract). Blood 1996;88:627a.

115. Grass J, Delmonte J, Wages D, et al. Prevention of transfusion-associated graft vs. host disease (TA-GVHD) in immunocompromised mice by photochemical treatment (PCT) of donor T cells (abstract). Blood 1997;90:207a.

116. del Rosario MLU, Zucali JR, Kao KJ. Prevention of GVHD by induction of immune tolerance with UVB-irradiated leukocytes in H-2 disparate bone marrow donor (abstract). Blood 1997;90:207a.

In: Mintz PD, ed.
Transfusion Therapy: Clinical Principles and Practice
Bethesda, MD: AABB Press, 1999

18

Management of Transfusion Reactions

ROBERTSON D. DAVENPORT, MD

TRANSFUSION REACTIONS ARE A diverse group of adverse reactions to transfusion that usually present during or shortly after transfusion. The diversity of transfusion reactions means that no single algorithm can encompass all types of reactions, but there are some common general principles. Foremost, prompt clinical evaluation of the patient is the most important aspect in the management of these reactions. The work-up and treatment of a transfusion reaction must be predicated on the clinical picture, especially in atypical cases. If a transfusion reaction occurs while a transfusion is in progress, the transfusion should be stopped immediately and the IV line should be kept open with saline. The issue of whether the unit being transfused should be removed and sent to the blood bank is a matter of clinical judgment and hospital policy. It is important to recognize, however, that the unit a patient is reacting to is not necessarily the one that is being infused. It is always good practice to reconfirm the identity of the patient and the unit or units of blood at the bedside, even in cases of mild reactions. All suspected transfusion reactions should be reported to the blood bank or transfusion service.

Febrile Nonhemolytic Reactions

Presentation and Recognition

A febrile transfusion reaction is defined as a rise in temperature of 1 C or greater. Fever may be accompanied by a sensation of chills, cold, or rigors.[1] Some reactions will present initially as rigors, and fever may not be evident for up to 30 minutes. Secondary symptoms include headache, nausea, and vomiting, but these alone do not constitute a febrile reaction without a temperature rise. Symptoms usually occur during the transfusion but may be delayed for up to 1 hour after the procedure has been

Robertson D. Davenport, MD, Associate Professor of Pathology, University of Michigan Medical School, Ann Arbor, Michigan

completed. Some patients, such as neonates or people with hypothalamic lesions, may have atypical presentations. Febrile nonhemolytic reactions are not life-threatening, but prompt clinical evaluation is important to exclude other causes of fever. Rigors in particular warrant treatment; not only are they very uncomfortable, but also they result in an increased metabolic rate that may not be well tolerated by patients with cardiovascular or pulmonary disease. A patient who is hypothermic at the start of a transfusion and then manifests an expected temperature rise to normal, without symptoms, is not having a febrile reaction.

The differential diagnosis of febrile nonhemolytic reactions includes hemolytic reactions, bacterial contamination, transfusion-related acute lung injury (TRALI), and disease- or treatment-related fevers. In some patients, it may be impossible to distinguish between a febrile transfusion reaction and disease-related fever. In general, when fever accompanies transfusion, a transfusion reaction should be ruled out. Unusually high fever or changes in vital signs, such as hypotension, should be considered evidence of a possible transfusion reaction.

Treatment

As noted above, in the event of a reaction, a transfusion in progress should be discontinued. There is controversy as to whether the unit involved should be returned to the blood bank (see below). It is important to rule out a hemolytic transfusion reaction or bacterial contamination of the unit. Antipyretics, such as acetaminophen (325-500 mg) can be administered. However, antipyretics are not necessarily required, as the fever of nonhemolytic transfusion reactions is self-limited and usually resolves within 2-3 hours. Aspirin-containing medications should be avoided because of the effect on platelet function. Diphenhydramine (50-100 mg) is commonly administered in this setting but probably has no effect on the course of febrile reactions.

Rigors will not respond promptly to antipyretic medications. Meperidine can be useful for the treatment of rigors; 25-50 mg administered intravenously will cause cessation of rigors within seconds. Care should be taken, however, in using this drug. Meperidine is a narcotic and respiratory depressant. Patients with a depressed intrinsic respiratory drive, such as those with cyanotic congenital heart disease who are chronically hypercapnic and acidotic, may become apneic. A narcotic receptor antagonist, such as naloxone (0.4-2.0 mg), should be available immediately. Most patients will become sleepy when given meperidine. If necessary, as in the setting of outpatient transfusion, naloxone can be administered to reverse sedation after completion of the transfusion.

There is controversy as to whether the transfusion can be restarted after a reaction has been diagnosed and the patient has been treated. The principal argument in favor of restarting the transfusion is the reduction in the number of donor exposures, especially if pooled platelet concentrates are involved.[2] Arguments against restarting the transfusion include the possibility that the patient may have a continued febrile reaction to the unit, and, if a hemolytic reaction or bacterial contamination has not been definitely excluded, a severe reaction may ensue.[3] The decision to restart the transfusion should be driven by the clinical condition of the patient, the results of transfusion reaction testing (see below), and the particular policy of the hospital.

Prevention

Premedication with antipyretics is often used to prevent febrile reactions. However, the efficacy of premedication has not been established. Acetaminophen in commonly used doses has few adverse effects; however, it is not generally recommended for patients who have not had previous febrile reactions. If a patient has had two or more febrile reactions, however, premedication may be indicated. It is unlikely that acetaminophen will mask a serious reaction such as immune hemolysis or bacterial contamination. The routine use of other premedications should be discouraged. Meperidine in particular should not be used without a clear indication. Other common premedications, such as diphenhydramine or steroids, play no role in preventing febrile reactions.

Febrile transfusion reactions have been associated with acquired antibodies to leukocyte antigens in the transfused unit, particularly in multitransfused or previously pregnant patients.[4] There may be a critical maximum number of residual leukocytes needed in a transfused component—5×10^6 leukocytes per unit—to prevent a febrile reaction. A level of residual leukocytes less than this is achievable with currently available filters. Although poststorage leukocyte reduction by filtration is often used to prevent febrile reactions, few data indicate its efficacy. Some studies have not been able to demonstrate a consistent reduction in febrile reactions with poststorage leukocyte reduction.[5,6] Furthermore, because these filters add significantly to the cost of transfusion and many patients do not have repeated febrile reactions, the routine use of leukocyte reduction filters needs to be examined critically.

Febrile reactions also have been attributed to the accumulation of pyrogenic cytokines in units during storage.[7] These biologic mediators are produced primarily by leukocytes. Filtration at the time of transfusion will not remove pyrogenic cytokines from blood units, although it may remove other cytokines and activated complement components.[8] The use of prestorage leukocyte reduction has been shown to reduce the generation of cytokines in stored platelets and red cells, and may be more effective than poststorage leukocyte reduction in preventing febrile reactions.[9] Preparation methods that result in low numbers of leukocytes in blood components, such as the buffy coat technique of platelet concentrate manufacture, may have less cytokine accumulation and cause fewer febrile reactions.[10] Finally, accumulated cytokines can be removed by either plasma reduction or the washing of cellular blood components.[11] However, plasma removal will not prevent all febrile reactions.

Allergic (Urticarial) Reactions

Presentation and Recognition

Mild allergic reactions to transfusion are commonplace. They may occur with any type of blood component and are associated with the amount of plasma transfused. Presenting symptoms include pruritis, urticaria, erythema, and cutaneous flushing. When the upper airway is involved because of laryngeal edema, there may be hoarseness, stridor, and a feeling of a "lump" in the throat. Lower airway involvement due to bronchoconstriction may present with wheezing, chest tightness, substernal pain, dyspnea, anxiety, or cyanosis. Gastrointestinal involvement may include nausea, vomiting, abdominal pain, and diarrhea.

Reactions to other allergens are frequent in the hospital setting. The differential diagnosis of an allergic transfusion reaction includes drug reactions, allergy to tape or latex, underlying allergic conditions such as asthma, coincident clinical conditions such as pulmonary embolism, and sensitivity to ethylene oxide. When there is dyspnea, TRALI and volume overload must be considered.

Treatment

Should an allergic reaction occur, the transfusion should be discontinued and IV access maintained. If there is upper airway involvement, prompt intubation may be necessary. Oxygen should be administered if there is dyspnea or evidence of desaturation. Mild allergic reactions usually will respond to IV antihistaminics such as diphenhydramine (50-100 mg). More severe reactions may require epinephrine (see below). In mild cutaneous reactions, the transfusion usually can be restarted after treatment without a recurrence or worsening of the symptoms. In more serious reactions, particularly if there is airway involvement, restarting the transfusion is not advisable.

Prevention

With the exception of IgA deficiency (see below), the specific antigen to which the patient is reacting cannot usually be identified. Therefore, it is usually impossible to select antigen-negative blood components. Rarely, the symptoms may be due to the passive transfer of IgE antibodies or a drug from the donor. Some patients with cryoglobulinemia or cold hemagglutinin disease will react to cold blood, in which the case use of a blood warmer may eliminate the symptoms. Other postulated mechanisms of allergic transfusion reactions include antibodies to leukocyte antigens and infusion of vasoactive substances, such as C3a and C5a, histamine, or mast cell activators such as leukotrienes.[12] Premedication with an antihistaminic, such as diphenhydramine, 25-50 mg, administered orally or IV, may prevent mild allergic reactions. Steroids such as methylprednisolone (125 mg) may help patients who manifest repeated allergic reactions, although the efficacy of steroids has not been proved. Care should be taken when administering steroids to patients who require multiple transfusions because adrenal suppression can occur.

Patients who have had repeated or significant allergic reactions may benefit from the concentration of cellular blood components through the removal of most of the plasma or by the washing of red cells and platelets. However, the routine use of washed components for patients with typical allergic reactions is unwarranted. Leukocyte reduction of cellular blood components by filtration appears to have little effect on the incidence of allergic reactions.[13] In addition to removing leukocytes, some filters have the capacity to bind anaphylatoxins and some cytokines.[14] Essentially, the clinical efficacy of leukocyte-reduction filters in preventing responses to transfused biologically active molecules has not been clearly established.

Severe Allergic (Anaphylactic) Reactions

Presentation and Recognition

In addition to the signs of typical milder allergic reactions, anaphylactic or anaphylactoid reactions manifest cardiovascular instability, including hypotension, tachycardia, loss of consciousness, cardiac arrhythmia, shock, and cardiac arrest. Respiratory involvement with dyspnea or stridor may be more pronounced than is seen usually in typical allergic reactions. The differential diagnosis

of anaphylactic transfusion reactions is similar to that of other allergic transfusion reactions, but TRALI, circulatory overload, hemolytic reactions, and bacterial contamination are stronger considerations here.

Treatment

If an anaphylactic reaction occurs, the transfusion should be discontinued and IV access maintained. Supportive care, including intubation, oxygen, IV fluids, and placement of the patient in the Trendelenburg position, should be instituted promptly. Epinephrine should be available immediately. For hypotension unresponsive to supportive measures or for significant bronchospasm, subcutaneous epinephrine 0.3-0.5 mg (0.3-0.5 mL of a 1:1000 solution) can be given. This dose can be repeated every 20-30 minutes for up to three doses. Alternatively, 0.5 mg of epinephrine may be given IV (5 mL of a 1:10,000 solution) and repeated every 5-10 minutes for refractory hypotension.

An antihistamine such as diphenhydramine, 50-100 mg, can be given IV, particularly when there are cutaneous manifestations such as urticaria. Aminophylline (6 mg/kg loading dose) may be useful when there is bronchospasm. Steroids are probably not effective in the acute situation, but if symptoms persist, a drug such as hydrocortisone (500 mg) may be given.

Prevention

Patients with IgA deficiency who develop anti-IgA can have anaphylactic reactions.[15] Those who have significant allergic reactions should be evaluated for their quantitative IgA levels. Recent transfusion may elevate serum IgA levels falsely. However, if IgA deficiency has been established, anti-IgA testing should be done, usually by a reference laboratory. IgA-deficient plasma can be obtained from rare donor registries, if necessary. Red cells and platelets can be washed to remove sufficient amounts of IgA to prevent reactions. A citrate washing procedure has been shown to remove IgA effectively.[16] However, washing with unbuffered saline has also been shown to prevent anaphylactic reactions from anti-IgA.[17] In cases of massive transfusion, the washing of red cells and platelets probably is not necessary after two blood volumes have been transfused.[17]

The IgA content of commercial immunoglobulin preparations varies considerably with the method of manufacture.[18] Patients with anti-IgA who require intravenous immune globulin (IVIG) may not react to preparations with low amounts of IgA.

Premedication with antihistamines or steroids may be as effective for severe allergic reactions as it is for milder ones (see above). Epinephrine also can be used prophylactically for patients at high risk for anaphylaxis who must be transfused. However, there is no certainty that premedication will prevent a serious allergic reaction. Patients with a history of anaphylactic reactions should be transfused only in a setting where emergency medical treatment is accessible immediately.

Acute Hemolytic Reactions

Presentation and Recognition

Acute hemolytic transfusion reactions (AHTRs), by definition, present within 24 hours of transfusion. Intravascular hemolysis is much more common in acute hemolytic reactions than is extravascular hemolysis. The presenting signs include fever and chills, nausea, vomiting, pain, dyspnea, tachycardia, hypotension, bleeding, and hemoglobinuria.[19] Renal failure is a later complication. Pain during an AHTR has been reported as localizing to the flanks, back, abdomen, chest, head, and infusion site. A subjective feeling of distress is reported sometimes. Unexpected bleeding may be due to disseminated intravascular coagulation (DIC).

Under special circumstances, the clinical presentation of an AHTR may be quite different from that in the typical patient. Patients who are unconscious or under anesthesia will, have no complaints, of course. Paralysis, either pharmacological or pathological, will prevent rigors. The support of blood pressure with inotropic agents can mask vasomotor instability. Anuric patients will not have hematuria. The initial manifestation of an AHTR may be uncontrollable bleeding due to DIC, particularly in the intraoperative setting. Decreased platelet count, low fibrinogen, and the presence of fibrin degradation products and D-dimers indicate DIC. Unfortunately, if an AHTR is not recognized early in this situation, more incompatible blood may be transfused in an attempt to keep up with blood loss.

Laboratory findings in AHTRs include hemoglobinemia, hemoglobinuria, elevated lactate dehydrogenase, hyperbilirubinemia, and low haptoglobin. The blood urea nitrogen and creatinine will be elevated if renal failure has occurred. The direct antiglobulin test (DAT) may show positive results with a mixed-field pattern if transfused incompatible red cells are present in the circulation. Red cell antibody identification studies may or may not show positive results, depending on the specificity of the antibody involved and the amount of antibody in the serum. ABO incompatibility is the most common cause of AHTRs.

Mortality from an AHTR generally depends on the amount of incompatible red cells transfused. A review of 41 hemolytic transfusion reactions causing acute renal failure indicated that no deaths occurred among patients who received fewer than 500 mL of incompatible blood, while there was a 25% mortality rate in the group that received 500-1000 mL and a 44% mortality rate among those who received more than 1000 mL of incompatible blood.[20] Transfusion of even small amounts of incompatible blood may not be safe. At least 12 deaths have been reported to the Food and Drug Administration involving the transfusion of less than one unit of blood; in fact, as little as 30 mL has been fatal.[21]

Differential Diagnosis

There are many clinical conditions in the differential diagnosis of an AHTR, including autoimmune hemolytic anemia (AIHA), cold hemagglutinin disease, congenital hemolytic anemia, nonimmune hemolysis (due to incompatible IV fluids, improper storage, malfunctioning blood warmer or infusion pump, small needles, high hematocrit), hemoglobinopathies, polyagglutination, paroxysmal nocturnal hemoglobinuria, artificial heart valve dysfunction, bleeding, microangiopathic hemolytic anemia, drug-induced hemolysis, and infections (clostridium, malaria).[19]

Any cause of hemolysis or shortened red cell survival should be considered. Improper storage or administration of Red Blood Cells may result in nonimmune hemolysis that can present similarly to an AHTR. Published descriptions of causes of non-immune hemolysis include overheating of blood in a blood warmer or microwave oven, freezing of red cells, inadequate removal of glycerol from frozen red cells, attempts to force blood through a filter or small-bore needle, transfusion of outdated blood, and use of a hypotonic solution concomitant with blood transfusion.[19] The administration of some drugs can cause hemolysis. Intravenous dimethyl-sulfoxide has been reported to mimic an AHTR.[22]

Patients with congenital hemolytic anemia, such as glucose-6-phosphate dehydrogenase deficiency, may manifest hemolysis after a blood transfusion. Conversely, blood donated by individuals with glucose-6-phosphate dehydrogenase deficiency can cause hemoglobinemia and hyperbilirubinemia in transfusion recipients.[23,24]

Treatment

In the event of an acute hemolytic reaction, the transfusion should be discontinued and IV access maintained. The identity of the patient and the unit or units of RBCs should be reconfirmed, and other units of RBCs that have been dispensed for the patient should be located and quarantined. The reaction should be reported to the blood bank promptly. If a misidentification is discovered, there may be another patient (eg, with a similar name) who may also be at risk of receiving incompatible blood.

The treatment of an AHTR must be guided by the clinical response of the patient. Patients who have minimal symptoms may be managed best by careful observation. However, in severe reactions,

early vigorous intervention may be lifesaving. It bears repeating that the severity of AHTRs is related directly to the volume of incompatible blood transfused. Thus, early recognition, discontinuation of the transfusion, and prevention of the transfusion of additional incompatible units are the essential first steps of treatment. Initial attention must be paid to cardiovascular support. If hypotension is present, fluid resuscitation and pressor support may be indicated. Care should be taken to avoid fluid overload, however, especially in patients with impaired cardiac or renal function. Pulmonary artery catheterization may be useful in selected patients to guide resuscitation.

Because the load of incompatible red cells in the circulation dictates the severity and course of AHTRs, an exchange transfusion with antigen-negative blood may be considered. Again, the decision to perform an exchange transfusion must be guided by the clinical response of the patient. It is not appropriate to expose a patient to the added risk of infectious disease if the hemolytic process is well tolerated. With ABO incompatibility, however, an exchange transfusion may reduce the chance of morbidity or death greatly.

Because renal failure is a significant problem in some patients, attention should be given to prevention. Early treatment of hypotension and DIC are the most important interventions to limit the extent of possible renal impairment. Maintenance of urine output with IV fluids and diuretics, mannitol or furosemide, early in the course of the reaction has been used successfully. Hydration with normal saline and 5% dextrose (1:1 ratio) at a rate of 3000 mL/m^2 per day and administration of sodium bicarbonate to maintain the urine pH above 7.0 have been recommended.[25] Infusion of an initial dose of 20% mannitol 100 mL/m^2 given over 30-60 minutes followed by 30 mL/m^2 per hour for the next 12 hours has also been recommended.[26] However, if oliguria in the face of normovolemia is present, fluid loading may be contraindicated. The use of vasopressor agents with direct vasodilatory effects on the renal vascular bed, such as low-dose dopamine (1-5 µ/kg/minute), may be considered also.

The prevention and treatment of DIC are controversial. Some authors have advocated heparin as a treatment option.[27] Heparin may have a direct anticomplement effect, which limits intravascular hemolysis and the sequelae of complement activation.[28] An obvious drawback of heparin therapy, however, especially in the intraoperative or postoperative patient, is the potential for hemorrhage. The use of Fresh Frozen Plasma or platelet concentrates in DIC is even more controversial. Transfusion of these components probably should be limited to those patients with active bleeding.

Further transfusion of red cells should be avoided until the cause of the reaction has been established. Foremost, however, no patient should be allowed to bleed to death for lack of serologically compatible blood. Red cells lacking known clinically significant antigens to which the patient currently has an antibody should be obtained, if possible. The results of serologic tests performed up to this point must be considered, and clinical judgment exercised. While the focus of attention in most AHTRs is on red cells, care should be taken to avoid the transfusion of plasma or platelets that may aggravate hemolysis, especially when ABO incompatibility is a possible cause. Undue haste in both serologic evaluation and decision-making must be avoided because human errors are committed most often under pressure.

Prevention

Proper identification of the transfusion recipient and the pretransfusion blood specimens is the single, most important aspect of the prevention of AHTRs, as this is the single, most common cause of AHTRs. Every transfusion service must establish and enforce the procedures to be followed in its institution. At a minimum, these procedures should include permanent and unique identification of each patient using a wristband, confirmation of the proper labeling of blood specimens by comparison with the wristband, and confirmation of the patient's identification prior to starting the transfusion. Deviation from institutional policies on patient and specimen identification should be taken very seriously.

Properly performed pretransfusion testing is essential in preventing hemolytic transfusion reactions. This complex topic is beyond the scope of this chapter. Interested readers should consult the *Technical Manual* published by the American Association of Blood Banks.[29(pp331-48)]

As an adjunct to the above measures, barrier systems have been devised that are intended to physically prevent the transfusion of blood without correct identification of the patient.[30] While such systems are promising for the prevention of erroneous transfusion, there is insufficient evidence of their effectiveness to warrant recommending them. In addition, reliance on a device to prevent the incorrect administration of blood may undermine the much more important steps involved in proper patient identification.

Delayed Hemolytic Reactions

Presentation and Recognition

By definition, delayed hemolytic transfusion reactions (DHTRs) occur at least 24 hours after transfusion of the offending unit. The time from transfusion to diagnosis of a DHTR is quite variable. Most patients present within the first 2 weeks after receiving the transfusion. However, clinical DHTR may be recognized more than 6 weeks later. Typically, hemolysis is extravascular, but intravascular hemolysis may occur also. Fortunately, these reactions tend to be much less severe than AHTRs; accordingly, they may be overlooked. Some patients will present with only unexpected anemia. Other clinical signs include fever or chills, jaundice, pain, or dyspnea.[19] Rarely renal failure may ensue. In patients with sickle cell disease, DHTRs may precipitate a sickle crisis.[31,32]

Laboratory findings in DHTRs include anemia, elevated lactate dehydrogenase, hyperbilirubinemia, low haptoglobin, leukocytosis, the presence of a new red cell antibody, and a positive reaction on a DAT. The degree of hyperbilirubinemia will depend on the rate and amount of hemolysis as well as on liver function. Typically, unconjugated bilirubin levels are elevated during active hemolysis. Depressed haptoglobin levels do not necessarily indicate intravascular hemolysis as they may be seen with extravascular hemolysis as well.

The differential diagnosis of a DHTR is similar to that of an AHTR, but with emphasis on occult infection, AIHA, cold hemagglutinin disease, congenital hemolytic anemia, polyagglutination, paroxysmal nocturnal hemoglobinuria, artificial heart valve dysfunction, bleeding, microangiopathic hemolytic anemia, and drug-induced hemolysis. Fever and leukocytosis in DHTRs may be interpreted as evidence of infection.

The diagnosis of a DHTR may be difficult to make in some patients. The finding of a red cell antibody after transfusion of antigen-positive blood does not always indicate that hemolysis has occurred.[33] Patients with underlying liver disease present a particular problem, especially this population is transfused heavily and has a high incidence of alloantibody formation. Hemoglobinemia may be difficult to recognize in icteric serum. Many patients with liver disease have a positive DAT result without active hemolysis. Hyperbilirubinemia and elevation of serum lactate dehydrogenase levels are common in both acute and chronic liver disease.

Patients with active bleeding present another diagnostic difficulty. In these patients, there is loss of transfused red cells in proportion to autologous red cells. With massive hemorrhage, it is possible that no transfused antigen-positive red cells survived, but, usually, DHTRs are not clinically important as compared with the degree of bleeding. With lesser degrees of hemorrhage, varying numbers of surviving antigen-positive red cells will be able to trigger a DHTR. One useful clue to the occurrence of a DHTR is if it can be demonstrated that transfused red cells lacking the implicated antigen persist while transfused cells bearing the antigen are absent.

The resorption of a hematoma can have manifestations very similar to a DHTR, including unconjugated hyperbilirubinemia, elevated lactate dehydrogenase, and depressed haptoglobin levels. In addition, fibrin degradation products from the hematoma that are present in the serum may be confused with DIC. In these patients, as in bleeding patients, evidence of persistent circulating antigen-positive red cells is evidence against the diagnosis of a DHTR.

Diagnosis of a DHTR in the presence of AIHA is also problematic. It is now well recognized that autoantibodies can mask alloantibodies in a patient's serum. The clinical and laboratory presentations of AIHA may be identical to that of a DHTR.[34] Concern has been raised that transfusion may aggravate hemolysis in AIHA; however, a recent study has suggested that this is not usually the case, even in the face of serologic incompatibility.[35]

Treatment

Many patients tolerate DHTRs well and may need only to be followed carefully. Generally, fluid loading and diuresis are not indicated unless there is active intravascular hemolysis. Complications, such as renal failure or sickle crisis, should be treated as such. If there is a large burden of antigen-positive red cells, an exchange transfusion should be considered. In general, transfusion should be avoided until the causative antibody can be identified and antigen-negative units obtained. However, as with AHTRs, a patient should not be allowed to have significant morbidity from anemia for the lack of serologically compatible blood. The selection of red cells for transfusion needs to be based on the results of serologic testing and good communication between the medical director of the blood bank and the patient's physician.

Because extravascular hemolysis is similar to AIHA, in which high-dose intravenous IVIG infusion may be useful, IVIG may be considered in the treatment of DHTRs also. A single dose of IVIG, 400 mg/kg, infused within 24 hours of transfusion, has been used successfully to prevent transfusion reactions in alloimmunized patients for whom compatible blood could not be obtained.[36] Five patients so treated had sustained increases in hematocrit. No transfusion reaction developed in any of the cases.

Prevention

Serologic identification of red cell antibodies is key to the prevention of all hemolytic transfusion reactions. Although beyond the scope of this chapter, this subject is presented well in the AABB *Technical Manual.*[29(pp349-78)]

It almost goes without saying that the selection of donor units lacking antigens that correspond to alloantibodies is essential for the prevention of DHTRs. However, there is controversy as to whether phenotype matching of donors and recipients is an appropriate strategy to prevent alloimmunization and DHTRs in the nonimmunized patient. Arguments in favor of this practice have been put forth regarding sickle cell disease when there is a mismatch between the donor pool and recipient phenotypes. Examination of alloimmunization rates among children in one urban area indicated that children of ethnic origins had a 42.9% incidence of alloimmunization compared with 17.6% in nonethnic patients.[37] This was not merely the result of a variation in transfusion rates because the latter group received more transfusions than the former. In another study that compared sickle cell patients to patients with other forms of chronic anemia, 30% of the patients with sickle cell anemia were alloimmunized in contrast to 5% of the patients with other forms of anemia.[38] Of the 32 alloimmunized patients with sickle cell anemia, 17 had multiple antibodies and 14 had DHTRs. Such studies suggest that phenotype matching may be beneficial for selected patients but do not provide sufficient evidence for recommending it as a routine practice.

Bacterial Contamination of Blood Components

Presentation and Recognition

The clinical presentation of a transfusion reaction caused by bacterially contaminated blood components is usually dramatic. The onset of symptoms in most cases is during the transfusion or shortly after it; delayed presentation of more than 1 day has rarely been reported with contaminated platelet transfusions.[39] Fever, chills, hypotension, nausea, and vomiting are the most commonly reported symptoms. Dyspnea and diarrhea may occur also. High fever or hypotension during or shortly after transfusion are particular clues that a contaminated unit may have been transfused. The clinical complications due to bacterial contamination are significant, often resulting in shock, renal failure, DIC, and death. The mortality rate is high and depends on the type of component involved, the identity and amount of the causative organism, and the clinical condition of the patient. The implicated unit is usually RBCs or platelet concentrates, although contamination of Fresh Frozen Plasma and Cryoprecipitated AHF during thawing has been reported.[40] The organism involved depends on the type and storage of the blood component. *Yersinia enterocolitica* and *Pseudomonas* species are found most frequently in contaminated red cells because of their ability to grow at low temperatures in a high-iron environment.[39] Both gram-positive cocci such as *Staphylococcus* and *Streptococcus*, and gram-negative rods such as *Salmonella*, *Escherichia*, and *Serratia* have been reported in platelet concentrates.[39]

The differential diagnosis includes hemolytic reactions, nonhemolytic febrile reactions, TRALI, and sepsis unrelated to blood transfusion. The diagnosis is established through culture of the implicated unit and the patient's blood, bacteriologic stains of the unit, endotoxin testing, or DNA-based microbiological methods. Usual staining methods include Gram's stain, methylene blue stain, and acridine orange stains. Interpretation of these stains may be difficult because of the presence of fibrin and cellular debris. Sealed segments from the unit are not sufficient for culture or staining, as they may be sterile when the contents of the bag are contaminated. A positive blood culture from the patient without confirmation of the same organism in the transfused component is not sufficient for diagnosis.

Treatment

Usually, treatment must be initiated before the causative organism has been identified. If a reaction occurs, the transfusion should be discontinued, the unit with its associated tubing should be removed, and any other blood bags that have been recently transfused should be recovered. The blood bank should be consulted about procedures for culture or microbiological staining, and a blood culture should be obtained from the patient from a different site than where the blood was infused. Supportive care of circulation and respiration should be initiated as required. Antibiotic therapy initially should include broad-spectrum coverage such as a β-lactam and an aminoglycoside until microbiological stains or cultures indicate the causative organism. If red cells are involved, the antibiotics should include anti-*Pseudomonas* coverage.

Prevention

Unfortunately, there is no way at the present time to detect bacterial contamination consistently before blood components are issued for transfusion. Proposed methods include visual inspection of the blood bag,[41] endotoxin testing,[42] culture or staining,[43] and a "dipstick" test.[44] Measures that have been proposed possibly to reduce the incidence of bacterial contamination include extension of donor screening,[45] limitation of storage time,[46] and prestorage leukocyte reduction.[47] There is no consensus on which of these techniques, if any, should be used.

Transfusion-Related Acute Lung Injury

Presentation and Recognition

TRALI usually presents within hours of transfusion. Its symptoms include dyspnea, hypoxemia, tachycardia, fever, hypotension, and cyanosis. Fever and hypotension, when present, are usually moderate and respond quickly to antipyretics and fluids. Characteristically, there is a lack of abnormal breath sounds. A chest x-ray usually shows pulmonary edema. By definition, there are no signs of cardiac failure. The reported mortality is approximately 20%, depending on the severity of the lung injury and the underlying clinical status of the patient. There is a wide range of severity in this transfusion reaction; milder forms may not be readily recognized.

The differential diagnosis includes circulatory overload, bacterial contamination, allergic reactions, acute respiratory distress syndrome (ARDS), pulmonary embolism, and pulmonary hemorrhage. The diagnosis is established by findings of noncardiogenic pulmonary edema. Pulmonary artery wedge pressure is not elevated. Characteristically, TRALI resolves within 48-96 hours from outset.[48] Failure of the patient to improve substantially after this time should call the diagnosis into question. Although chest x-ray findings may persist beyond 7 days, unlike ARDS, there appear to be no permanent pulmonary sequelae.

Treatment

The treatment of TRALI is supportive. If a transfusion is in progress, it should be discontinued and blood bags from recently transfused units should be recovered. The blood bank should be consulted regarding the evaluation of TRALI. Usually, oxygen is indicated. Severely affected patients may require mechanical ventilation. Corticosteroids appear to be of little, if any, value. Diuresis is not indicated in the absence of signs of fluid overload.

Prevention

TRALI has been attributed to the presence of antibodies in the plasma of the transfused unit that are directed against HLA or granulocyte antigens present on recipient leukocytes. It also has been attributed to the presence of lipid inflammatory mediators in the unit that prime recipient neutrophils to cause capillary injury and leakage.[49] There are, at present, no practical methods to screen units for either antileukocyte antibodies or lipid mediators. The first mechanism requires a particular combination of donor and recipient that is very unlikely to recur unless the unit was from a directed donor. Identification of antibodies in the transfused unit and corresponding antigen positivity in the recipient are not particularly useful for management of the acute event. Some authors have suggested that donations from individuals implicated in TRALI previously should be manufactured into components devoid of plasma, such as washed red cells.[48] However, there is no consensus on this subject.

The accumulation of lipid mediators can be reduced by prestorage leukocyte reduction or by shortening the storage time of cellular components, particularly platelet concentrates.[50] Patients who are septic may be at risk of TRALI if units containing high levels of these mediators are transfused.[51] Therefore, either prestorage filtered or fresher units may be desirable for these patients. Again, however, there is no consensus on this.

Posttransfusion Purpura

Presentation and Recognition

Posttransfusion purpura (PTP) is analogous to a DHTR. In this case, the patient makes an alloantibody in response to platelet antigens in the transfused blood. Similar to the phenomenon of red cell autoantibodies in DHTRs, an antibody is produced in the PTP patient that, for a period of time, causes the destruction of autologous, antigen-negative platelets. Patients present with thrombocytopenia typically 5-10 days after transfusion, although patients presenting more than 3 weeks from transfusion have been reported.[52] The mechanism of autologous platelet destruction is not clear but appears to be immune mediated. Three proposed mechanisms involve immune complexes that bind to autologous platelets through Fc receptors,[53] transient production of an autoantibody,[54] and adsorption of soluble platelet antigens from donor plasma.[55] The implicated transfusion may be of any blood component. The signs and symptoms are frequently profound thrombocytopenia, purpura, or

bleeding. Febrile reactions have been reported, retrospectively, with the implicated transfusion. The thrombocytopenia is self-limited in PTP, with recovery occurring within 7-48 days.[52]

The differential diagnosis of PTP includes idiopathic thrombocytopenic purpura, sepsis, DIC, marrow failure, drug-related thrombocytopenia, and heparin-associated antibodies. The identification of a platelet alloantibody and lack of the corresponding antigen on the patient's platelets establish the diagnosis. Virtually all human platelet antigens have been associated with PTP, although HPA-1 (Pl^{A1}) has been reported most commonly.[52] Antibodies with HLA specificity have been implicated rarely in PTP. PTP must be differentiated from the far more common alloimmunization to platelet antigens. This may be problematic when the patient has an underlying cause of thrombocytopenia. The definitive test is survival studies of autologous platelets, but these studies are difficult to perform. Spontaneous resolution or response to treatment may be the only way to establish the diagnosis in such cases.

Treatment

The efficacy of treatment is difficult to judge because PTP will remit spontaneously with time, and few cases have been studied closely. Plasmapheresis may be used to reduce the amount of circulating platelet antibody. Response to apheresis is variable, but it has been reported to take an average of about 12 days.[52] The choice of replacement fluid is controversial. Fresh Frozen Plasma replacement has been suggested to effect a more rapid recovery but has the added risks of infectious disease transmission.[56] More recently, high-dose IVIG infusion has been shown to be effective at doses of 400-500 mg/kg per day for up to 10 days.[52] Some patients have responded to a single infusion of IVIG. The use of corticosteriods (ie, prednisone 2 mg/kg/day) has been reported to normalize the platelet count within 1 week.[57] Splenectomy should be reserved for refractory patients or patients at a high risk of life-threatening hemorrhage, such as intracranial bleeding.

Platelet transfusion is of very little value in PTP. Because autologous platelets do not survive in circulation, there is no expectation that transfused platelets, regardless of antigen matching, will do any better. Whether platelet transfusion prolongs the course of PTP is controversial. Thus, platelet transfusion should be reserved for patients with active bleeding.

Prevention

PTP is unpredictable, so its first occurrence is not preventable. However, PTP rarely will recur with subsequent transfusion. This has led to the recommendation that for future transfusions, patients with PTP receive only components from donors lacking the implicated antigen.[58] There is, however, no clear consensus on this point. In addition, antigen-typed donors may be difficult, if not impossible, to recruit. If this policy is to be followed, typing of family members may be useful. Routine use of washed or frozen deglycerolized blood components for PTP patients is not indicated because these products have been reported to cause PTP.[59]

Hypotensive Reactions

Presentation and Recognition

Transfusion-associated hypotension is a transfusion reaction that has been described relatively recently.[60] It is defined as hypotension occurring during transfusion in the absence of signs or symptoms of other transfusion reactions, such as fever, chills, dyspnea, urticaria, or flushing. The degree of hypotension required for the diagnosis is controversial but could be defined reasonably as a drop of at least 10 mm Hg in systolic or diastolic arterial blood pressure from the pretransfusion baseline. However, if the immediate pretransfusion blood pressure is elevated from the patient's typical blood pressure and the arterial pressure does not fall below the patient's usual blood pressure, it should not be considered a hypotensive reaction. Hypotension begins during the transfusion and resolves quickly

when the transfusion is discontinued. If hypotension persists beyond 30 minutes after discontinuation of the transfusion, another diagnosis should be strongly considered. Hypotensive reactions have been associated with red cell and platelet transfusions. Some reactions have been associated with the use of leukocyte-reduction filters.[61,62]

The diagnosis is clinical, based on the degree and timing of the hypotension and the absence of other causes. The differential diagnosis includes hemolytic reactions, bacterial contamination, TRALI, allergic reactions, cardiac arrhythmia, myocardial infarction, occult bleeding, vasovagal reaction, drug reactions, and any other known causes of hypotension.

Treatment

If hypotension occurs, the transfusion should be discontinued and IV access maintained. The patient should be positioned with head down and feet elevated (Trendelenburg position), and isotonic fluids (ie, normal saline) should be administered. Pressor support is indicated only if the hypotension is severe and refractory to IV fluids.

Prevention

The cause of transfusion-associated hypotension has not been established definitively. However, the condition is most likely due to the release of bradykinin through activation of the contact pathway of coagulation. Some reactions have been associated with angiotensin-converting enzyme (ACE) inhibitor drugs or the use of leukocyte-reduction filters.[61] Angiotensin-converting enzyme is the major enzyme that breaks down bradykinin in circulation. Some filters, particularly those with a net-negative surface charge, appear to cause activation of kallikrein and cleavage of high-molecular-weight kininogen that results in the release of bradykinin.[63-65] However, there is variability because not all such filtered units show activation. The cause of this variability has not been determined to date.

Hypotensive reactions are difficult to predict. Clearly, many patients taking ACE inhibitors or receiving filtered blood components do not have hypotensive reactions. A patient who has demonstrated one reaction may be at risk of subsequent reactions. Further transfusion should be given slowly with close monitoring. If a leukocyte-reduction filter is associated with the reactions, consideration should be given to either not using a filter or using a different filter. There is at present no practical way to test for bradykinin in blood components.

Nonimmune Hemolysis

Presentation and Recognition

Lysis of red cells can occur as a result of storage, handling, or transfusion conditions. Patients who receive lysed red cells may tolerate them remarkably well. However, transient hemodynamic, pulmonary, and renal impairment may occur,[65] and death due to transfusion of lysed red cells has been reported.[21] The transfusion of autologous blood from a patient with sickle hemoglobin can result in hemolysis and death.[66] The clinical signs are usually hemoglobinemia and hemoglobinuria. Hyperkalemia may occur, particularly in patients with renal failure. Fever also may occur. Finding lysis of red cells in the transfused unit and excluding other causes, such as hemolytic transfusion reactions, establish the diagnosis. All RBC units will show a slight degree of hemolysis with prolonged storage, but this will not result in clinical signs after transfusion. The principal reported complications of nonimmune hemolysis are renal failure and cardiac arrhythmia due to hyperkalemia. Hemolytic transfusion reactions rarely can occur when no red cell antibody is identifiable.[67] Differentiation of this condition from nonimmune hemolysis may be impossible without careful investigation of the transfusion circumstances.

The differential diagnosis includes hemolytic transfusion reactions, autoimmune hemolysis, bacterial contamination, sepsis, paroxysmal nocturnal hemoglobinuria, cold hemagglutinin disease, drug-induced hemolysis, oxidative stress (due to glucose-6-phosphate dehydrogenase deficiency, abnormal hemoglobin), and causes of hematuria. The diagnosis is usually one of exclusion. Careful examination of the transfusion set and conditions is very important. Useful laboratory studies on the patient include repeat antibody screen and DAT, serial hematocrit, and conjugated and unconjugated bilirubin. Studying the contents of the implicated blood bag is unlikely to yield useful information on the cause of hemolysis. Hematocrit and plasma hemoglobin levels will document the extent of hemolysis. Culture of the blood bag in the absence of signs of bacterial contamination is not indicated. Comparison with attached segments and segments saved in the blood bank may provide clues to when the hemolysis took place.

Treatment

Should nonimmune hemolysis occur, the transfusion should be discontinued and IV access maintained. The blood bag, together with attached tubing and IV fluids, should be saved for further investigation. A hemolytic transfusion reaction needs to be ruled out (see above). The serum potassium level should be checked and an electrocardiogram obtained to assess hyperkalemia. Care is supportive. Urine output should be maintained with hydration (see treatment of hemolytic reactions) unless there is a contraindication such as renal failure.

Prevention

Nonimmune hemolysis is prevented by proper handling, storage, and transfusion practices. A complete discussion of these topics may be found elsewhere.[29(pp447-60)] In particular, IV fluids other than 0.9% sodium chloride injection (normal saline) or other FDA-approved solutions should not be administered with or mixed with red cells. Infusion pumps, blood warmers, and blood storage refrigerators should be maintained properly. Tubing through which transfusions are administered should not be exposed to patient-warming devices. Transfusion through small-bore needles under pressure should be avoided. Frozen RBC units should be checked properly for adequate deglycerolization.

Transfusion-Related Circulatory Overload

Presentation and Recognition

Circulatory overload is an all-too-common and preventable transfusion reaction. It presents as congestive heart failure during or shortly after transfusion with dyspnea, orthopnea, cyanosis, tachycardia, elevated blood pressure, pulmonary edema, jugular venous distention, pedal edema, and headache. The differential diagnosis includes TRALI, allergic reactions, and causes of congestive failure not related to transfusion, such as valvular heart disease. Clearly, patients with preexisting heart disease are at risk of circulatory overload with transfusion.

Treatment

If circulatory overload occurs, the transfusion should be discontinued and IV access maintained, but administration of further fluids should be limited. Oxygen should be given, and the patient placed in an upright position. The hypervolemia or pulmonary edema should be treated like other causes of congestive heart failure. An ancient but very effective treatment of congestive heart failure is phlebotomy. This can be combined with manual plasma removal and retransfusion of collected red cells to reduce plasma volume without reducing the red cell mass.

Prevention

Volume overload should be anticipated in at-risk patients and prevented readily. Blood should be transfused slowly. Although a transfusion should be completed within 4 hours usually, the duration may be extended if indicated medically. However, if more than 6 hours are required, alternative strategies should be considered. Small volumes can be transfused with adequate time between transfusions to allow for diuresis. To avoid additional donor exposures, a unit can be split sterilely and a portion retained in the blood bank for later transfusion. Units can also be concentrated by plasma removal. A diuretic can be administered before or during the transfusion.

Transfusion-Related Hypothermia

Presentation and Recognition

Patients receiving a large-volume transfusion of components stored at 4-6 C are at risk for developing hypothermia.[68] This may be exacerbated by poor tissue perfusion, shock, or heat loss from open body surfaces, such as the peritoneum, during surgery. During massive transfusions in the operating room, such complicating factors often occur. Signs of hypothermia include decreased core body temperature, metabolic acidosis, coagulopathy, platelet dysfunction, and cardiac arrhythmia. When the core temperature drops below 32 C, there is substantial risk of cardiac dysfunction and death.[69] Hypothermia may be induced also, as it is in open-heart surgery or some cardiovascular surgical procedures that use hypothermic circulatory arrest. Regardless of the cause of hypothermia, however, the consequences are the same.

Patients with cold-reacting autoantibodies or cold hemagglutinin disease present special problems. Red cell autoantibodies that do not cause complement fixation, as in typical cold-reacting antibodies, are not usually of concern in cardiovascular surgery. If agglutination does occur with hypothermia, it is completely reversible and does not cause hemolysis or tissue ischemia on rewarming.[70] However, patients with hemolytic or strongly agglutinating cold-reacting antibodies may need to have thermal amplitude studies performed.

Treatment

Regardless of the cause of heat loss, the treatment of hypothermia is the same: increase of the core body temperature with warming devices. The treatment of coagulation abnormalities occurring with hypothermia is controversial. Platelet transfusion may be useful, particularly if there are signs of microvascular bleeding. Plasma transfusion may correct prolonged prothrombin time or partial thromboplastin time. During controlled hypothermic bypass with circulatory arrest, substantial hemorrhage may occur during rewarming and reestablishment of circulation. The empiric use of plasma and platelet transfusion appears to be effective in controlling bleeding.[71] However, unless the core temperature is raised, any amount of transfusion is unlikely to correct the coagulopathy.

Prevention

Transfusion-induced hypothermia may be prevented with the use of appropriate blood-warming devices. Many such devices are available. It probably makes little difference what device is used as long as it has sufficient capacity to warm blood adequately at the highest transfusion rate needed, and it is maintained properly. However, only a device designed specifically for warming blood should be used because hemolysis may occur readily with improper warming. When possible, transfusions should be given slowly enough so that hypothermia is not an issue. Most important, however, is that tissue perfusion must be maintained. Patients are generally at far greater risk of serious morbidity from shock than from transfusion-induced hypothermia. If a blood-warming device is not available and the patient requires rapid transfusion, the rate should not be restricted solely out of concerns for transfusion-induced hypothermia.

Transfusion-Related Hyperkalemia

Presentation and Recognition

As red cells are stored, potassium leaks from the intracellular space. The concentration of potassium in the plasma of a unit of red cells near outdate can be quite high—as much as 78.5 mEq/L in CPDA-1 units at 35 days.[29(p138)] Although this level can appear alarming, it is seldom of clinical consequence because the plasma volume of the unit is less than 100 mL and is diluted in the patient's total plasma volume immediately upon transfusion. In addition, the transfused red cells have a net potassium deficit and begin to restore the intracellular potassium concentration as soon as normal metabolic activity returns. Nonetheless, some patients, particularly children and people with renal failure, may develop clinically significant hyperkalemia.[72,73] However, hyperkalemia occurs much more commonly for other reasons, including nonimmune hemolysis of transfused red cells (see above). The principal sign and cause of morbidity is cardiac arrhythmia. The differential diagnosis includes metabolic acidosis, renal failure, potassium administration, mineralocorticoid deficiency, and rhabomyolysis.

Treatment

The treatment of hyperkalemia is the same regardless of the cause. A glucose infusion, 200-500 mL of 10% glucose IV given over 30 minutes, can be used to drive potassium into cells. Additional glucose, 500-1000 mL of 10% glucose, may be infused over several hours. Insulin, 10 units given subcutaneously, may be administered as well, although it may not be required in patients with normal insulin responses. Generally, these measures will reduce the serum potassium by 1 mEq/L for several hours. Alkalosis will also reduce the serum potassium concentration as hydrogen ions leave the intracellular space in exchange for potassium ions. Bicarbonate, 44-132 mEq, may be added to 1L of glucose, especially if the patient is acidotic. Oral, potassium-binding resins such as sodium polystyrene sulfonate (15-30 g), or hemodialysis, have long-term effects of removing excess potassium.

Prevention

In the rare circumstances when the potassium load in transfused blood is clinically significant, hyperkalemia may be avoided by giving the transfusion over several hours or reducing the plasma potassium in the transfused cells. RBC units stored for less than 7 days have acceptable potassium levels.[74] Plasma removal will decrease the total potassium amount transfused. The washing of red cells will remove potassium further, but this is seldom necessary.

Transfusion-Related Acid-Base Abnormalities

Presentation and Recognition

RBC units become progressively acidic with increasing storage time.[74] This has led to concern that a massive transfusion may exacerbate acidosis, particularly where trauma is involved. However, there appears to be little correlation between acidosis and the amount of blood transfused.[75] Acidosis is more likely the result of poor tissue perfusion, which may be worsened by hypothermia.[76] After transfusion, a metabolic alkalosis is more common. This is partly due to the metabolism of citrate, which consumes hydrogen ions. Postoperative alkalosis can be particularly severe if bicarbonate is administered during transfusion.[75]

Treatment

In general, no specific treatment is required for acid-base changes that are associated with transfusion. If there is an underlying acid-base abnormality, it may be exacerbated transiently by transfusion. Therapy should be directed toward the underlying cause. In particular, bicarbonate should not be given as routine prophylaxis with massive transfusion.

Prevention

Temporary and mild acid-base changes are the expected result of transfusion and usually do not require intervention. When possible, transfusion over several hours will allow ample time for homeostatic correction of acid-base changes. When rapid and massive transfusion is required, attention should be directed toward resuscitation. As Collins eloquently stated, "Many of the serious toxicities attributed to the massive transfusion of stored blood are often due to giving too little blood or giving it too late."[76]

References

1. Heddle NM, Kelton JG. Febrile nonhemolytic transfusion reactions. In: Popovsky MA, ed. Transfusion reactions. Bethesda, MD: AABB Press, 1996:45-80.
2. Oberman HA. Controversies in transfusion medicine: Should a febrile transfusion response occasion the return of the blood component to the blood bank? Con. Transfusion 1994;34:353-5.
3. Widmann FK. Controversies in transfusion medicine: Should a febrile transfusion response occasion the return of the blood component to the blood bank? Pro. Transfusion 1994;34:356-8.
4. Perkins HA, Payne R, Ferguson J, Wood M. Nonhemolytic febrile transfusion reactions. Quantitative effects of blood components with emphasis on isoantigenic incompatibility of leukocyte. Vox Sang 1996;11:578-600.
5. Mangano MM, Chambers LA, Kruskall MA. Limited efficacy of leukopoor platelets for prevention of febrile transfusion reactions. Am J Clin Pathol 1991;95:733-8.
6. Tan KK, Lee WS, Liaw LC, Oh A. A prospective study on the use of leucocyte filters in reducing blood transfusion reactions in multitransfused thalassemic children. Singapore Med J 1993;34:109-11.
7. Muylle L, Joos M, Wouters E, et al. Increased tumor necrosis factor α (TNF α), interleukin 1, and interleukin 6 (IL-6) levels in the plasma of stored platelet concentrates: Relationship between TNF α and IL-6 levels and febrile transfusion reactions. Transfusion 1993;33:195-9.
8. Snyder EL, Mechanic S, Baril E, Davenport RD. Removal of soluble biologic response modifiers (complement and chemokines) by a bedside leukoreduction filter. Transfusion 1996;36:707-13.

9. Federowicz I, Barrett B, Andersen J, et al. Characterization of reactions after transfusion of prestorage leukoreduced cellular blood components (abstract). Blood 1995;86 (Suppl):608a.

10. Muylle L, Wouters E, Peetermans ME. Febrile reactions to platelet transfusion: The effect of increased interleukin 6 levels in concentrates prepared by the platelet-rich plasma method. Transfusion 1996;36:886-90.

11. Heddle NM, Klama L, Singer J, et al. The role of the plasma from platelet concentrates in transfusion reactions. N Engl J Med 1994; 331:670-1.

12. Vamvakas ED, Pineda AA. Allergic and anaphylactic reactions. In: Popovsky MA, ed. Transfusion reactions. Bethesda, MD: AABB Press, 1996:81-124.

13. Dzieczkowski JS, Barrett BB, Nester D, et al. Characterization of reactions after exclusive transfusion of white-cell-reduced cellular blood components. Transfusion 1995;35: 20-5.

14. Geiger TL, Perrotta PL, Davenport R, et al. Removal of anaphylatoxins C3a and C5a, and chemokines IL-8 and RANTES by polyester leukoreduction and plasma filters. Transfusion, 1997;37:1156-62.

15. Vyas GN, Holmadahl L, Perkins HA, Fudenberg HH. Serologic specificity of human anti-IgA and its significance in transfusion. Blood 1969;34:573-81.

16. Sloand EM, Fox SM, Banks SM, Klein HG. Preparation of IgA-deficient platelets. Transfusion 1990;30:322-6.

17. Davenport RD, Burnie KL, Barr RM. Transfusion management of patients with IgA deficiency and anti-IgA during liver transplantation. Vox Sang 1992;63:247-50.

18. Sacher RA. Intravenous gammaglobulin products: Development, pharmacology and precautions. In: Garner RJ, Sacher RA, eds. Intravenous gammaglobulin therapy. Arlington, VA: American Association of Blood Banks, 1988:8-12.

19. Davenport RD. Hemolytic transfusion reactions. In: Popovsky MA, ed. Transfusion reactions. Bethesda, MD: AABB Press, 1996: 1-44.

20. Bluemle LW Jr. Hemolytic transfusion reactions causing acute renal failure: Serologic and clinical considerations. Postgrad Med 1965;38:484-9.

21. Sazama K. Reports of 355 transfusion-associated deaths: 1976 through 1985. Transfusion 1990;30:583-90.

22. Samoszuk M, Reid ME, Toy PT. Intravenous dimethylsulfoxide therapy causes severe hemolysis mimicking a hemolytic transfusion reaction (letter). Transfusion 1983;23:405.

23. Shalev O, Manny N, Sharon R. Posttransfusional hemolysis in recipients of glucose-6-phosphate dehydrogenase-deficient erythrocytes. Vox Sang 1993;64:94-8.

24. Mimouni F, Shohat S, Reisner SH. G6PD-deficient donor blood as a cause of hemolysis in two preterm infants. Isr J Med Sci 1986;22: 120-2.

25. Nussbaumer W, Schwaighofer H, Gratwohl A, et al. Transfusion of donor-type red cells as a single preparative treatment for bone marrow transplants with major ABO incompatibility. Transfusion 1995;35:592-5.

26. Slavc I, Urban CH, Schwinger W, et al. ABO-incompatible bone marrow transplantation: Prevention of hemolysis by alkaline hydration with mannitol diuresis in conjunction with red cell reduced buffy coat bone marrow. Wien Klin Wochenschr 1992;104:93-6.

27. Rock RC, Bove JR, Nemerson Y. Heparin treatment of intravascular coagulation accompanying hemolytic transfusion reactions. Transfusion 1969;9:57-61.

28. Gray JM, Oberman HA, Beck ML. Delay in the onset of immune hemolysis in vivo apparently due to heparinization. Transfusion 1973;13:422-4.

29. Vengelen-Tyler V, ed. Technical manual. 12th ed. Bethesda, MD: American Association of Blood Banks, 1996.

30. Mercurilali F, Inghilleri F, Colotti MT, et al. One-year use of the Bloodloc system in an orthopedic institute. Transfus Clin Biol 1994; 1:227-30.

31. Mintz PD, Williams ME. Cerebrovascular accident during a delayed hemolytic transfusion reaction in a patient with sickle cell anemia. Ann Clin Lab Sci 1986;16:214-8.

32. Solanki D, McCurdy PR. Delayed hemolytic transfusion reactions. An often-missed entity. JAMA 1978; 239:729-31.

33. Ness PM, Shirey RS, Thoman SK, Buck SA. The differentiation of delayed serologic and delayed hemolytic transfusion reactions: Incidence, long-term serologic findings, and clinical significance. Transfusion 1990;30:688-93.

34. Pirofsky B. Clinical aspects of AIHA. Semin Hematol 1976;13:251-65.

35. Salama A, Berghofer H, Mueller-Eckhardt C. Red blood cell transfusion in warm-type autoimmune haemolytic anaemia. Lancet 1992; 340:1515-7.

36. Kohan AI, Niborski RC, Rey JA, et al. High-dose intravenous immunoglobulin in non-ABO transfusion incompatibility. Vox Sang 1994;67:195-8.

37. Luban NL. Variability in rates of alloimmunization in different groups of children with sickle cell disease: Effect of ethnic background. Am J Pediatr Hematol Oncol 1989; 11:314-9.

38. Vichinsky EP, Earles A, Johnson RA, et al. Alloimmunization in sickle cell anemia and transfusion of racially unmatched blood. N Engl J Med 1990;322:1617-21.

39. Goldman M, Blajchman MA. Blood product-associated bacterial sepsis. Transfus Med Rev 1991;5:73-83.

40. Rhame FS, McCullough JJ, Cameron S, et al. *Pseudomonas cepacia* infections caused by thawing cyroprecipitate in a contaminated water bath (abstract). Transfusion 1979;19: 653-4.

41. Kim DM, Brecher ME, Bland LA, et al. Visual identification of bacterially contaminated red cells. Transfusion 1992;32:221-5.

42. Arduino MJ, Bland LA, Tipple MA, et al. Growth and endotoxin production in *Yersinia enterocolitica* and *Enterobacter agglomerans* in packed erythrocytes. J Clin Microbiol 1989;27:1483-5.

43. Reik H, Rubin SJ. Evaluation of the buffy-coat smear for rapid detection of bacteria. JAMA 1981;245:357-9.

44. Burstain J, Workman K, Brecher M. Inexpensive and rapid detection of bacterially contaminated platelets using urine dipsticks (abstract). Transfusion 1995;35:64S.

45. Grossman BJ, Kollins P, Lau PM, et al. Screening blood donors for gastrointestinal illness: A strategy to eliminate carriers of *Yersinia enterocolitica*. Transfusion 1991;31:500-1.

46. Food and Drug Administration. Blood Products Advisory Committee. Prevention of transmission of *Yersinia* infection (transcript). Washington, DC: Freedom in Information Office, May 9, 1991.

47. Kim DM, Brecher ME, Bland LA, et al. Prestorage removal of *Yersinia enterocolitica* from red cells with white cell-reduction filters. Transfusion 1992;32:58-62.

48. Popovsky MA, Chaplin HC Jr, Moore SB. Transfusion-related acute lung injury: A neglected, serious complication of hemotherapy. Transfusion 1992;32:589-92.

49. Popovsky MA. Transfusion-related acute lung injury (TRALI). In: Popovsky MA, ed. Transfusion reactions. Bethesda, MD: AABB Press, 1996:167-84.

50. Silliman CC, Thurman GW, Ambruso DR. Stored blood components contain agents that prime the neutrophil NADPH oxidase through platelet-activating-factor receptor. Vox Sang 1992;63:133-6.

51. Silliman CC, Paterson AJ, Dick WO, et al. The association of biologically active lipids with the development of transfusion-related acute lung injury: A retrospective study. Transfusion 1997;37:719-26.

52. McFarland JG. Posttransfusion purpura. In: Popovsky MA, ed. Transfusion reactions. Bethesda, MD: AABB Press, 1996:205-30.

53. Shulman NR, Aster RH, Leitner A, Hiller MC. Immunoreactions involving platelets, V: Post-transfusion purpura due to a complement fixing antibody against a genetically controlled platelet antigen. A proposed mechanism for thrombocytopenia and its relevance to autoimmunity. J Clin Invest 1961;40:1597-620.

54. Stricker RB, Lewis BH, Corash L, Shuman MA. Post-transfusion purpura associated with an autoantibody directed against a previously undefined platelet antigen. Blood 1987;69: 1458-63.

55. Taaning E, Skow F. Elution of anti-Zw^a (Pl^{A1}) from autologous platelets after normalization of platelet count in post-transfusion purpura. Vox Sang 1991;60:40-4.

56. Kroll H, Kiefel V, Mueller-Eckhardt C. Postransfusionelle Purpura: Klinische und immunologische Untersuchungen bei 38 Patientinnen. Infusionsther Transfusionsmed 1993; 20: 198-204.

57. Weisberg LJ, Linker CA. Prednisone therapy of post-transfusion purpura. Ann Intern Med 1984;100:76-7.

58. Budd JL, Wieyers SE, O'Hara JM. Relapsing post-transfusion purpura: A preventable disease. Am J Med 1985;78:361-2.

59. Christie D, Pulkrabek S, Putnam J, et al. Post-transfusion purpura due to an alloantibody reactive with glycoprotein Ia/IIa (anti HPA-5b). Blood 1991;77:2785-9.

60. Hume HA, Popovsky MA, Benson K, et al. Hypotensive reactions: A previously uncharacterized complication of platelet transfusion? Transfusion 1996;36:904-9.

61. Fried MR, Eastlund T, Christie B, et al. Hypotensive reactions to white cell-reduced plasma in a patient undergoing angiotensin-converting enzyme inhibitor therapy. Transfusion 1996;36:900-3.

62. Abe H, Ikebuchi K, Shimbo M, Sidiguchi S. Hypotensive reactions with a white cell-reduction filter: Activation of kallikrein-kinin cascade in a patient (abstract). Transfusion 1997;37(Suppl):39S.

63. Davenport RD, Penezina OP. Cleavage of high molecular weight kininogen induced by filtration of platelet concentrates (abstract). Transfusion 1997;37(Suppl):104S.

64. Shiba M, Tadokoro K, Sawanobori M, et al. Activation of the contact system by filtration of platelet concentrates with a negatively charged white cell-removal filter and measurement of venous blood bradykinin level in patients who received filtered platelets. Transfusion 1997;37:457-62.

65. Mair B, Leparc GF. Hypotensive reactions associated with platelet transfusions and angiotensin-converting enzyme inhibitors. Vox Sang 1998;74:17-30.

66. DeChristopher PJ, Orlina AR. Sudden death associated with autologous transfusion in a surgical patient with hemoglobin SC disease. ISBT & AABB 1990 Joint Congress: Book of Abstracts. Bethesda, MD: American Association of Blood Banks, 1990:119.

67. Davey RJ, Gustafson M, Holland PV. Accelerated immune red cell destruction in the absence of serologically detectable alloantibodies. Transfusion 1980;20:348-53.

68. Luna GK, Maier RV, Pavlin EG, et al. Incidence and effect of hypothermia in seriously injured patients. J Trauma 1987;27:1014-8.

69. Jurkovich GJ, Greiser WB, Luterman A, Curreri PW. Hypothermia in trauma victims: An ominous predictor of survival. J Trauma 1987; 27:1019-24.

70. Holman WL, Smith SH, Edwards R, Huang ST. Agglutination of blood cardioplegia by cold-reacting autoantibodies. Ann Thorac Surg 1991;51:833-6.

71. Kouchoukos NT, Daily BB, Rokkas CK, et al. Hypothermic bypass and circulatory arrest for operations on the descending thoracic and thoracoabdominal aorta. Ann Thorac Surg 1995; 60:76-7.

72. Linko K, Tigerstedt I. Hyperpotassemia during massive blood transfusions. Acta Anaesthesiol Scand 1984;28:220-1.

73. Hall TL, Barnes A, Miller JR, et al. Neonatal mortality following transfusion of red cells with high potassium levels. Transfusion 1993; 33:616-9.

74. Latham JT, Bove JR, Weirich FL. Clinical and hematologic changes in stored CPDA-1 blood. Transfusion 1982;22:128-60.

75. Miller RD, Tong MJ, Robbins TO. Effects of massive transfusion of blood on acid-base balance. JAMA 1971;216:1762-5.

76. Collins JA. Problems associated with the massive transfusion of stored blood. Surgery 1974; 174:274-95.

In: Mintz PD, ed.
Transfusion Therapy: Clinical Principles and Practice
Bethesda, MD: AABB Press, 1999

19

Alternatives to Allogeneic Transfusion in Patients With Surgical Anemia

LAWRENCE T. GOODNOUGH, MD

 THE LAST DECADE HAS SEEN EX-plosive growth in the use of alterna-tives to the transfusion of allogeneic blood, arising primarily from concern over the risk of transfusion-transmitted diseases.[1] Numerous professional organizations and federal agencies have endorsed autologous blood transfu-sion, and recombinant human erythropoietin (EPO) therapy has been approved around the world for use in the perioperative setting. How-ever, advances in blood safety and the increased costs that are associated with blood conservation have caused autologous blood procurement and the role of EPO therapy to be reevaluated in the sur-gical setting. This review summarizes these devel-opments and provides perspective on emerging blood conservation strategies.

Preoperative Autologous Blood Donation

Table 19-1 summarizes the advantages and disad-vantages of preoperative autologous blood dona-tion (PAD). In selected patient subgroups, preoperative collection of autologous blood can re-duce exposure to allogeneic blood significantly. Pa-tients are considered candidates for PAD when they are scheduled for procedures for which a blood transfusion is considered likely. For proce-dures that are unlikely to require transfusion (ie, when a maximal surgical blood order schedule does not suggest that blood be set up for cross-match[2]), preoperative blood collection has not been recommended. More than 10 years' experi-ence with PAD has resulted in emerging issues that

Lawrence T. Goodnough, MD, Professor of Medicine and Pathology, Washington University School of Medicine; and Director, Transfusion Services, Barnes-Jewish Hospital, St. Louis, Missouri

Table 19-1. Autologous Blood Donation

Advantages	Disadvantages
1. Prevents transfusion-transmitted disease	1. Does not affect risk of bacterial contamination
2. Prevents red cell alloimmunization	2. Does not affect risk of ABO-incompatibility error
3. Supplements the blood supply	3. Costs more than allogeneic blood
4. Provides compatible blood for patients with alloantibodies	4. Wastes blood not transfused
5. Prevents some adverse transfusion reactions	5. Increases prevalence of adverse reactions to autologous donation
	6. Subjects patient to preoperative anemia and increased likelihood of perioperative transfusion

include reevaluation of its safety, its efficacy, and its cost-effectiveness.[3]

Selection of Patients

Several recently published guidelines provide recommendations for selecting patients suitable for autologous blood donation.[4-7] Table 19-2 details the guidelines published in 1993 by the British Committee for Standards in Hematology.[7] The American Association of Blood Banks recommends that patients with evidence of systemic infection or unstable angina be excluded, but units from patients with positive viral markers may be collected with the approval of the patient's physician and the transfusion facility.[8] The first unit collected from a given patient during a 30-day period must undergo the same testing as allogeneic units for infectious disease markers; however, subsequent units need not be tested.[9] Because iron-restricted erythropoiesis is a limiting factor in the successful collection of multiple units of blood over a short interval,[10] ideally, supplemental iron is prescribed before the first blood collection, in time to allow maximal iron in-

take. Oral iron may be insufficient to maintain iron saturation in the setting of enhanced erythropoiesis.[11]

Autologous blood collection can be performed for patients who would not normally be considered for allogeneic donation. With suitable volume modification and parental cooperation, pediatric patients can participate in preoperative collection programs.[12] Patients with significant cardiac disease are generally considered poor risks for autologous collection. Despite reports of safety in small numbers of patients scheduled for coronary artery bypass grafting who underwent autologous blood donation,[13] the risks associated with autologous blood donation[14] in these patients are probably greater than current estimated risks of allogeneic transfusion.[15]

Collecting blood from pregnant women is rarely indicated.[16] In routine pregnancy and delivery or uncomplicated cesarean section, blood is needed so infrequently that autologous collection is considered inappropriate. However, potential candidates for autologous blood collection include women with alloantibodies to multiple or high-incidence antigens, or with placental previa or other condi-

Table 19-2. Patients Who Should Be Deferred From Autologous Blood Donation[7]

1. Evidence of infection and risk of bacteremia
2. Scheduled for surgery to correct aortic stenosis
3. Unstable angina
4. Active seizure disorder
5. Myocardial infarction or cerebrovascular accident within 6 months of donation
6. Patients with significant cardiac or pulmonary disease who have not yet been cleared for surgery by their treating physician
7. High-grade left main coronary artery disease
8. Cyanotic heart disease
9. Uncontrolled hypertension

tions placing them at high risk for ante- or intrapartum hemorrhage.[17]

Efficacy

Preoperative autologous collections are most beneficial for patients undergoing procedures incurring substantial blood loss, such as orthopedic joint replacement, vascular surgery, cardiac or thoracic surgery, and radical prostatectomy.[3] Autologous blood should not be collected for procedures that seldom require transfusion, such as transurethral resection of the prostate, cholecystectomy, herniorrhaphy, vaginal hysterectomy, and uncomplicated obstetric delivery.[18] A hospital's maximal surgical blood order schedule for blood crossmatch can provide estimates of transfusion needs for specific procedures; the generally accepted cutoff where transfusion is "unlikely" is when 10% or fewer patients are transfused.[18]

It is important to establish guidelines for the appropriate number of units to be collected. A sufficient number of units should be drawn whenever possible so that the patient can avoid exposure to allogeneic blood. Collection for liquid blood storage should be scheduled as far in advance of surgery as possible to allow compensatory erythropoiesis[19-23] to prevent anemia (Table 19-3).[24] The efficacy of PAD depends on the degree to which the patient's erythropoiesis increases the production of red blood cells. Studies have shown that the endogenous EPO response is suboptimal at the level of mild anemia produced under "standard" conditions—that is, 1 blood unit donated weekly. A computer model has predicted that if the erythropoietic response to autologous blood phlebotomy is not able to maintain the patient's level of hematocrit during the donation interval, the drawing of autologous blood may be harmful[25]; this outcome was confirmed in a 1996 study of patients undergoing hysterectomy,[26] in which the authors demonstrated that PAD resulted in perioperative anemia and an increased likelihood of blood transfusion.

The relationship between autologous blood ordering and collection and subsequent allogeneic blood transfusion in orthopedic surgical patients has been examined.[27] When autologous blood-ordering guidelines that are the same as those established for ordering crossmatched allogeneic blood are used, 68% of patients donate the number of units requested successfully, and only 10% of these patients subsequently receive allogeneic blood. In contrast, of those who are unable to store the number of autologous blood units requested, 27% subsequently receive allogeneic blood. Donation success depends primarily on whether donors are anemic (HCT ≤ 39%) at first donation. Thus, the likelihood of allogeneic blood exposure is related to blood-ordering practices in nonanemic autologous blood donors, whereas success in blood collection (ie, effective erythropoietic replacement of blood lost or donated) determines the likelihood of allogeneic blood exposure in patients who are anemic. Table 19-4 summarizes selected studies that have reported rates of allogeneic blood exposure in autologous blood donors undergoing elec-

Table 19-3. Compensatory Red Blood Cell Production during Autologous Blood Donation

Reference	Units		Interval (weeks)	Red Blood Cell (mL) Production Mean (range)
	Requested	Donated		
Toy[19]	2	2	2	100
Kasper, Gerlich, Buzello[20]	3	2.7	3	351 (9-719)
Gesemann, Gentner, Scheirmann[21]	4	4	4	390 (64-716) Female 495 (0-766) Male
Goodnough, Prize, Rudnick, Soegiarso[22]	6	4.1	3	549 (499-599) Female 602 (564-640) Male
Mercuriali, Zanella, Barosi, et al[23]	6	2.6	3	328 (250-406) Oral iron
	6	3.3	3	432 (353-511) Intravenous iron

Reprinted with permission from Goodnough and Mercuriali.[24]

tive surgery.[28-35] In contrast to autologous blood donation under standard conditions, studies of "aggressive" autologous blood phlebotomy (twice weekly for 3 weeks, beginning 25-35 days before surgery) have demonstrated that endogenous EPO levels do increase. Studies of exogenous (pharmacologic) EPO therapy to stimulate EPO recovery further during autologous phlebotomy or surgical blood loss were reviewed in 1997.[36]

Cost-Effectiveness

While the most important indicator for autologous blood procurement is effectiveness in reducing allogeneic transfusions, the "wastage" rate of autologous units is an index of its efficiency and costs. Even for procedures such as joint replacement or radical prostatectomy, a well-designed program may result in discard rates of up to 50% of collected units.[17] When autologous blood is collected for procedures that seldom require transfusion, such as vaginal hysterectomies and normal vaginal deliveries, 50-90% of units collected for these procedures are wasted.[17,18,26] While autologous blood collections have become popular, the additional costs associated with the collection of autologous units compared with those for allogeneic blood, the inherent wastage rate of these units, advances in the safety of allogeneic blood, and the pressure to reduce health-care costs now make the preoperative donation of autologous blood poorly cost-effective.[29,37-39] Some suggestions to make autologous blood programs less costly include abbreviating the donor interview for collection, using only whole blood and discontinuing component production, limiting the use of frozen autologous blood, applying the same transfusion guidelines for autologous and allogeneic blood, and testing only the first autologous blood unit donated for infectious disease markers.

A mathematical model published in 1996 illustrates in Fig 19-1 the relationship between anticipated surgical blood losses, the level of hematocrit that the physician may want to maintain perioperatively, and the need for autologous blood donation for individual patients.[3] This model would be used

Table 19-4. Efficacy of Autologous Blood Procurement in Elective Surgery

Reference	Allogeneic Blood Exposure	
	Preoperative Autologous Donation, % (3 units)	Acute Hemodilution, % (up to 4 units)
Goodnough, Shaffron, Marcus[28]	17	—
Goodnough, Grishaber, Birkmeyer, et al[29]	16	33
Toy, Menozzi, Strauss, et al[30]	14	—
Monk, Goodnough, Brecher[31]	—	21
Monk, Goodnough, Brecher, et al[32]	15	23
Ness, Bourke, Walsh[33]	3	0
Monk, Goodnough, Birkmeyer, et al[34]	10	10
Colberg, Monk, Goodnough, Andriole[35]	—	29

to: 1) measure the patient's initial hematocrit; 2) set the minimum tolerable hematocrit (transfusion trigger), taking into account individual patient characteristics such as age and medical status; 3) apply these values to the graph shown in Fig 19-1 to derive the estimated blood loss (EBL) necessary to reach this transfusion trigger; and 4) compare this EBL to the standard EBL for the particular surgical procedure. If the EBL for the procedure exceeds the EBL required for transfusion, it is likely that a transfusion will be needed and that PAD would be beneficial to this patient. If the EBL for the procedure is less than the EBL for transfusion, it is likely that transfusion will not be required and that PAD is unnecessary.

Acute Normovolemic Hemodilution

Acute normovolemic hemodilution (ANH) is a technique that involves removing whole blood from a patient while restoring the circulating blood volume with a cellular fluid shortly before an anticipated significant surgical blood loss. Blood is collected in standard blood bags containing anticoagulant on a tilt-rocker with automatic cutoff

via volume sensors. The blood is stored at room temperature and reinfused in the operating room after major blood loss has ceased, or sooner if indicated. For the cellular fluid, simultaneous infusions of crystalloid (3 mL crystalloids for each 1 mL blood withdrawn) and colloid (dextrans, starches, gelatin, albumin, 1 mL for each 1 mL of blood withdrawn) have been recommended. Subsequent intraoperative fluid management is based on the usual surgical requirements. Blood units are reinfused in the reverse order of collection: the first unit collected, and therefore the last unit transfused, has the highest hematocrit and concentration of coagulation factors and platelets.

Efficacy

The chief benefit of hemodilution has been recognized to be the reduction of red cell losses when whole blood is shed perioperatively at lower hematocrit levels after ANH is complete.[40] Mathematical modeling has suggested that severe hemodilution to preoperative hematocrit levels of less than 20%, accompanied by substantial blood losses, would be required before the red cell volume "saved" by he-

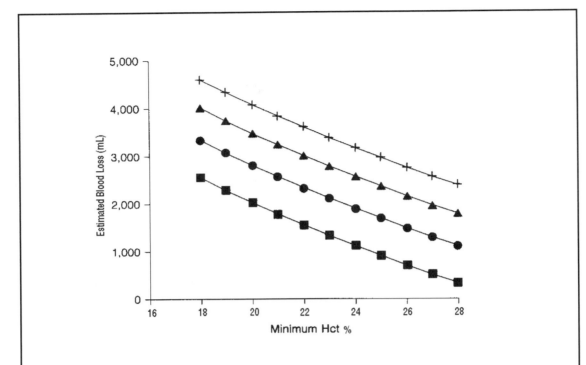

Figure 19-1. Relationship of estimated blood loss and minimum (nadir) hematocrit during hospitalization at various initial hematocrit levels (30, 35, 40, and 45%) in a surgical patient with a whole blood volume of 5000 mL. ■ = initial hematocrit 30%; ● = initial hematocrit 35%; ▲ = initial hematocrit 40%; + = initial hematocrit 45%. Reprinted with permission from Cohen and Brecher.[25]

modilution became clinically important.[41] A case study analysis of patients who had undergone "minimal" ANH (representing 15% of patients' blood volume) estimates that only 100 mL red cells (the equivalent of 1/2 unit of blood) is saved under these conditions.[42] With moderate hemodilution (target hematocrit levels of 28%), the savings become more substantial. The removal of 3 blood units in a patient who subsequently undergoes a blood loss of 2600 mL results in an estimated 732 mL red cells lost, compared with 947 mL of RBCs that would have been lost if hemodilution had not been performed. Thus, the surgical red cell losses saved in this instance by hemodilution are 215 mL, or the equivalent of 1 allogeneic blood unit.[43]

The withdrawal of whole blood and its replacement with crystalloid or colloid solution decrease the arterial oxygen content, but compensatory hemodynamic mechanisms and the existence of surplus oxygen-delivery capacity make ANH safe. A sudden drop in red cell mass increases cardiac output and lowers blood viscosity, thereby decreasing peripheral resistance. If cardiac output can compensate effectively, oxygen delivery to the tissues at a hematocrit of 25-30% is as good as, but no better than, delivery at a hematocrit of 35-45%.[44] The safety and efficacy of more extensive hemodilution are controversial,[45] and may provide little additional blood conservation.

Because blood collected by ANH is stored at room temperature and usually is returned to the patient within 8 hours of collection, there is little deterioration of platelets or coagulation factors. The hemostatic value of the blood collected by ANH is of questionable benefit for orthopedic or urologic surgery because plasma and platelets are rarely indicated in this setting. Its value in protecting plasma and platelets from the acquired coagulopathy of extracorporeal circulation in cardiac surgery (known as "blood pooling") is better established.[46]

Clinical Studies Comparing Acute Normovolemic Hemodilution and Preoperative Autologous Donation

Two prospective, randomized trials[32,33] and a case-controlled, retrospective comparison[34] of ANH and PAD in patients undergoing radical prostatectomy demonstrated that subsequent allogeneic blood exposure was not different (10-20%) for patients undergoing either method of autologous blood procurement. However, patients who donated blood prior to radical prostatectomy presented with significantly lower hematocrit levels on the day of surgery.[31] A study of PAD prior to elective hysterectomy also found that the net clinical effect of PAD was to cause preoperative anemia and, as a result, to expose patients to a more liberal transfusion policy.[26]

It has been recommended that patients scheduled for radical prostatectomy donate 3 units of autologous blood preoperatively; data have shown that this reduces the prevalence of allogeneic exposure from 66-70% to 14-16%.[29,30] A prospective study of moderate ANH reported in 1997 that for patients who underwent ANH without PAD, 21% of them received allogeneic blood[31] (Table 19-4); this is comparable to the allogeneic blood exposure rates for 3 units of PAD and for the 17-20% allogeneic blood exposure rates in previously published series of elective surgery patients for which PAD has been regarded as the standard of care.[28-30]

The benefit of ANH can be illustrated in a mathematical model (Fig 19-2) published in 1998. An adult with an estimated 5-L blood volume, an initial hematocrit of 40%, and surgical blood losses of up to 3000 mL would end up with a level of hematocrit that would remain at or about 25% postoperatively without an autologous blood intervention.[47] Generally, this level of hematocrit is considered safe for patients without known risk factors.[48] Patients undergoing radical prostatec-

tomy procedures at the Washington University School of Medicine undergo surgical blood losses estimated by the anesthesiologist to be 1632 ± 751 mL. However, recent calculations show that, typically, actual blood losses for surgical procedures are underestimated by a factor of two.[49] Moreover, these procedures are accompanied by a 2% risk of perioperative myocardial infarction.[50] Note that in this model, the performance of ANH with initial hematocrit levels of 40-45% would allow up to 2500-3500 mL of surgical blood loss, yet the nadir level of hematocrit could be maintained at or above 28%. The benefit of ANH in this model is to protect patients who have substantial blood losses that cannot be predicted and to maintain perioperative hematocrit levels that minimize risks related to ischemia. Blood conservation strategies need to address both of these issues.[51,52]

In addition to an efficacy equivalent to PAD, ANH represents "point-of-care" autologous blood procurement and, therefore, is less costly than PAD. First, autologous blood units procured by ANH are retransfused by on-site personnel before the patient leaves the operating room and require no inventory or testing costs. ANH therefore eliminates the possibility of an administrative error that could lead to an ABO-incompatible blood transfusion and death, whereas PAD does not eliminate this risk; the estimated risk of death from a hemolytic transfusion reaction[53] now approximates the risk of mortality from HIV or hepatitis infection from blood transfusion.[15] Since ANH and reinfusion are accomplished in the operating room by on-site personnel, procurement and administration costs are minimized. In addition, blood obtained during ANH does not require transportation, the commitment of the patient's time, and the loss of work associated with PAD. Finally, the wastage[17] of autologous blood units, which is inevitable because the number of units requested for donation is based on the cumulative percentage (eg, up to 90%) of anticipated blood needs, whereas the number of units reinfused subsequently reflects the mean (approximately 50%) transfusion needs,[3] is eliminated with ANH. A pro and con debate on the merits of ANH was published in 1998.[54,55]

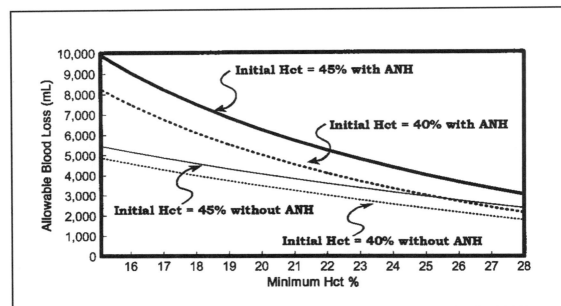

Figure 19-2. The maximum allowable blood loss in a patient with a blood volume of 5000 mL and an initial hematocrit level of 45% (the solid lines) or 40% (the dotted lines), with and without acute normovolemic hemodilution. Hct = hematocrit; ANH = acute normolovemic hemodilution. Reprinted with permission from Goodnough, Monk, and Brecher.[47]

Intraoperative Blood Recovery

The term intraoperative blood recovery describes the technique of recovering and reinfusing blood lost by a patient during surgery. The oxygen-transport properties of recovered red blood cells are equal to or better than those of stored allogeneic red cells, and the survival of recovered red cells appears to be at least comparable to that of transfused allogeneic red cells.[50] Intraoperative blood recovery is contraindicated when certain procoagulant materials (eg, topical collagen) are applied to the surgical field, as systemic activation of coagulation may result. Relative contraindications include malignant neoplasm, infection, and contaminants in the operative field. Microaggregate filters (40 μ) are used most often to filter the blood before reinfusion, as recovered blood may contain tissue debris, small blood clots, or bone fragments. Cell-washing devices can provide the equivalent of 12 units of banked blood per hour to a massively

bleeding patient. Because washing does not remove bacteria from recovered blood, however, intraoperative recovery should not be used if the operative field has gross bacterial contamination. Aspiration of other body fluids, such as amniotic or ascitic fluid, should be avoided. The incidence of adverse events resulting from the reinfusion of recovered blood is not known. Hemolysis of recovered blood can occur during suctioning from the surface instead of from deep pools of shed blood, particularly when blood is aspirated at vacuum settings greater than 100 mm Hg. The clinical importance of free hemoglobin in the concentrations usually seen has not been established, although excess free hemoglobin may indicate inadequate washing.[56] Positive bacterial cultures from recovered blood are not unusual, but clinical infection is rare, even with massive contamination.[57] Dilutional coagulopathy may occur if large volumes of recovered blood are administered. Most programs use machines that collect shed blood, wash it, and concentrate the RBCs. This process typically results in 225-mL units of saline-suspended red blood cells with a hematocrit of 50-60%. The infusate contains minimal coagulation factors and platelets.

As with PAD and acute normovolemic hemodilution, intraoperative autologous blood recovery should undergo scrutiny regarding both safety and cost-effectiveness. A controlled study in cardiothoracic surgery has demonstrated a lack of efficacy for intraoperative recovery when transfusion requirements and clinical outcome were followed.[57] A second study has found that only a minority of patients undergoing major orthopedic and cardiac surgery achieved cost equivalence with intraoperative recovery using semiautomated instruments compared with banked blood.[58] While the recovery of a minimum of 1 blood unit equivalent is possible for less expensive methods (ie, those with unwashed blood), it is generally agreed that at least 2 blood unit equivalents need to be recovered using the cell-saver (with washed blood) to achieve cost-effectiveness.[58-60]

Postoperative Blood Recovery

Postoperative blood recovery denotes the collection of blood from surgical drains followed by reinfusion, with or without processing. In some programs, postoperative shed blood is collected into sterile canisters and reinfused without being processed through a microaggregate filter. The blood collected is dilute, partially hemolyzed, and defibrinated, and it may contain high concentrations of cytokines. The concentration of fibrin degradation products can be very high, especially in shed mediastinal blood. If blood transfusion has not begun within 6 hours of initiating the collection, the blood must be discarded.

The evolution of cardiac surgery has been accompanied by broad experience in the postoperative conservation of blood. Postoperative autologous blood recovery and reinfusion are practiced widely, but not uniformly. Prospective and controlled trials have shown conflicting results over the efficacy of postoperative blood recovery in cardiac surgery patients; at least three such studies

have demonstrated a lack of efficacy[61-63] while at least two have shown a benefit.[64,65] The disparity of the results in these studies may be explained, in part, by differences in transfusion practices because the reports cited above incorporated criteria for blood transfusion into their protocols. Additionally, these studies were not blind, so modification of physicians' transfusion practices may have been an uncredited intervention in them.

In the postoperative orthopedic surgical setting, a number of reports have described similarly the successful recovery and reinfusion of washed[66] and unwashed[67,68] wound drainage from patients undergoing arthroplasty. The volume of reinfused drainage blood has been reported to be as much as 3000 mL and to average more than 1100 mL in patients undergoing cementless knee replacement.[68]

The safety of reinfused unwashed orthopedic wound drainage has been controversial. Theoretical concerns have been expressed regarding the infusion of potentially harmful materials in recovered blood, including free hemoglobin, red cell stroma, marrow fat, toxic irritants, tissue or methacrylate debris, fibrin degradation products, and activated coagulation factors and complement. Although two small series have reported complications,[69,70] several larger studies have reported no serious adverse effects when drainage was passed through a standard 40-µ blood filter.[67,68,71]

The potential for decreasing exposure to allogeneic blood among orthopedic patients undergoing postoperative blood recovery, whether washed or unwashed, is greatest for patients undergoing cementless bilateral total knee replacement, revision hip or knee replacement, and long-segment spinal fusion. As in the case of intraoperative recovery, blood loss must be sufficient to warrant the additional cost of processing technology.[72] The prospective identification of patients who can benefit from intra- and postoperative autologous blood recovery is possible if anticipated surgical blood losses and the perioperative "transfusion trigger" are taken into account (Fig 19-1).

Recombinant Human Erythropoietin Therapy

Recombinant human EPO therapy has been approved for use in patients undergoing PAD in Japan, the European Union, and Canada since 1993, 1994, and 1996, respectively. Approval was granted for perisurgical adjuvant therapy without PAD in Canada in 1996 and for nonvascular, noncardiac procedures in the United States in 1996.[39] EPO (and, also, iron, B_{12}, or folic acid) has been recommended as therapy that should be used instead of blood transfusion if appropriate and if the clinical condition of the patient permits sufficient time for the prescribed agent to promote erythropoiesis.[73(p10)] Emerging issues for EPO therapy in the surgical setting that are addressed below include "low-dose" EPO therapy, EPO therapy coupled with ANH, and EPO therapy in patients undergoing cardiac surgery. EPO therapy in the nonsurgical setting is discussed in Chapter 20.

Early Clinical Trials

Patients donating autologous blood under standard conditions (ie, 1 blood unit weekly)[74,75] have an inadequate response of endogenous EPO to blood loss anemia, suggesting that EPO therapy might be able to facilitate autologous blood donation by enhancing compensatory erythropoiesis; this was confirmed subsequently in a clinical trial of aggressive autologous blood donation (up to 6 units over a 3-week preoperative interval), with or without EPO therapy, in patients undergoing orthopedic surgery.[76] Subsequent clinical trials[22,77-79] in orthopedic patients demonstrated that for autologous blood donors who were not anemic (hematocrit 39%) at first donation, no clinical benefit (defined as reduced allogeneic blood exposure) was seen with EPO therapy. Thus, for nonanemic patients, autologous blood donation remains an option if they can tolerate aggressive blood phlebotomy and thereby achieve stimulation of erythropoiesis via their endogenous EPO response.[3]

For anemic (hematocrit ≤ 39%) autologous blood donors, a European clinical trial demon-

strated that EPO therapy (300 or 600 U/kg taken intravenously in six doses) reduced exposure to allogeneic blood during orthopedic surgery when compared with placebo-therapy.[23] However, this result was achieved only with the concurrent administration of both intravenous and oral supplemental iron. A subsequent US trial with supplemental oral iron and EPO therapy (600 U/kg taken intravenously in six doses) did not reduce allogeneic blood transfusions when compared with placebo-therapy,[80] in large part because a substantial percentage of the patients were either severely anemic (hematocrit <33%) or iron-deficient.

Several studies have evaluated perisurgical EPO therapy in nonanemic orthopedic surgical patients without autologous blood procurement. Both a Canadian[81] and a US study[82] were able to show that EPO-treated (300 U/kg injected subcutaneously for 14 days, beginning 9 days preoperatively) patients had one half the rate of exposure (approximately 25%) to allogeneic blood as had the placebo-treated patients (approximately 50%), even though the mean initial hemoglobin levels exceeded 130 g/L for patients in both studies. On the basis of these clinical trials, EPO therapy was approved for perisurgical use in anemic surgical patients in Canada and the United States in 1996.

Safety and the Role of EPO Therapy in Cardiac Surgery

The safety of EPO therapy in patients undergoing noncardiac surgery has been demonstrated by the equal distribution of adverse concomitant events between patients treated with EPO or placebo in more than 1000 patients participating in clinical trials. Thrombotic events in patients with renal failure described in early trials have not been seen in clinical trials of EPO in these surgical settings.[76]

An unresolved question is the safety of EPO therapy in cardiac surgery patients and its role in this setting. In a European trial,[83] the authors found no differences in mortality, thrombotic events, or serious adverse events among their 76 patients, whether treated with EPO or given placebo, nor any differences in hemostatic parameters during the 14-day preoperative interval in which increased levels of hematocrit (from $42 \pm 3\%$ to $48 \pm 3\%$) were demonstrated.[84] In fact, the investigators were able to demonstrate that, when compared with placebo-treated patients, EPO-treated patients had an improved extractable oxygen perioperatively, which also was associated with a lower incidence of lactic acidosis.[85] A US study also concluded that no differences in adverse events between EPO- and placebo-treated patients were observed and that EPO therapy was well tolerated (Table 19-5).[86] However, the descriptions of adverse events and mortalities in this report indicate that an uneven distribution of these events between the two treatment groups could not be ruled out to any degree of certainty. For example, even if the true mortality rate was 0% in the placebo group and 6% in the combined EPO groups, the probability is only 23% (power of 0.229) that the resulting data would produce a statistically significant p value of less than 0.05.[87]

What is the current role of EPO therapy in cardiac surgery, particularly in the United States, where cardiac and vascular surgeries are excluded as indications for its use? This approach remains a valuable tool for patients with special requirements, such as Jehovah's Witness patients for whom blood transfusion is not an option.[88] Future trials of EPO therapy in cardiac surgery in other countries will be helpful in providing additional information on its safety in this setting. Until additional safety data are forthcoming, however, the off-label use of EPO in patients undergoing cardiac or vascular surgery in the United States cannot be recommended. Emerging data on the use of EPO in noncardiac procedures, such as elderly men undergoing radical prostatectomy procedures,[32,89] may provide additional evidence that perioperative elevations of hematocrit, even in patients at risk for ischemic heart disease, are safe and well-tolerated. Red blood cell expansion is seen with an increase in reticulocyte count by day 3 of treatment in nonanemic patients treated with EPO who are iron replete.[4] As illustrated in Fig 19-3, the equivalent of 1 blood unit is produced by day 7 (visit three) and the equivalent of 5 blood units are produced over 26 days (visit eight).[22] If 3-5 blood units are necessary to minimize allogeneic blood exposure in patients undergoing complex procedures such as orthopedic joint replacement surgery,[90,91] the preoperative interval necessary for EPO-stimulated erythropoiesis can be estimated to be 3-4 weeks.

Table 19-5. Serious Adverse Events (SAE) in Two Clinical Trials of Cardiac Surgical Patients, With or Without Erythropoietin (EPO) Therapy

| | European* | | USA[†] | |
	Placebo (n=38)	EPO (n=38)	Placebo (n=56)	EPO (n=126)
Thrombosis/SAE	5	2	17	35
Mortality	4	4	0	7

*Sowade, Warnke, and Scigalla.[83]
[†]D'Ambra, Gray, Hillman, et al.[86]

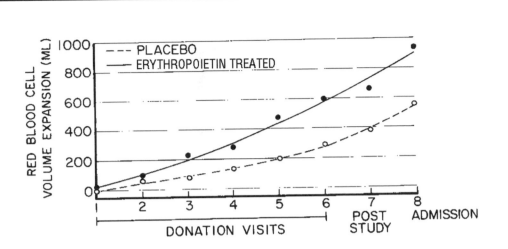

Figure 19-3. Red cell volume expansion during autologous blood donation in 23 placebo-treated (o) and 21 erythropoietin-treated (●) patients. Data points represent the calculated volume (mL) of red blood cell expansion at donation visits 1 through 6, the poststudy visit, and hospital admission. Red blood cell production is indicated by a polynomial regression curve for each treatment group (n=44 at each point). The rate of red blood cell expansion can be derived for any preoperative interval. The mean cumulative interval since donation visit 1 was 3.5 days to visit 2, 7.2 days to visit 3, 10.6 days to visit 4, 14.2 days to visit 5, 17.6 days to visit 6, 20.9 days to visit 7 (poststudy visit), and 26.3 days to visit 8 (hospital admission). Reprinted with permission from Goodnough, Price, Rudnick, and Soegiarso.[22]

Costs of EPO Therapy

The costs associated with EPO therapy and the potential impact of reimbursement policies are important issues in the setting of surgical anemias, as has been the case in medical anemias.[92,93] Costs associated with EPO therapy may be lowered by strategies that improve the dose-response relationship. The pharmacoeconomics of subcutaneous administration is superior to that of intravenous administration.[94] A 1996 study[95] demonstrated that four weekly injections of subcutaneous EPO (600 U/kg) were less costly but just as effective as a daily dose of EPO (300 U/kg for 14 doses The costs of EPO therapy ($0.01/U)[31] for a 70-kg patient in selected clinical trials are summarized in Table 19-6. However, these regimens[32,80-2] remain expensive and, when unaccompanied by autologous blood procurement, are still associated with an allogeneic exposure rate of 16-25%.

Emerging Strategies: Low-Dose EPO Coupled With Hemodilution

An alternative method of perioperative autologous blood procurement is ANH. The rationale for the use of hemodilution is that perisurgical red blood cell loss is reduced if whole blood is shed at a lower (25-30%) rather than a higher (39-45%) level of intraoperative HCT.[40] Because this blood is reinfused in the operating room, the costs of blood procurement are much lower than those of procuring preoperatively donated autologous blood. Two studies in patients undergoing radical prostatectomy concluded that moderate ANH is less costly but just as effective as autologous blood donation, resulting in an approximate allogeneic exposure rate of 20%.[31,41]

One way to enhance the efficacy of hemodilution is to couple this technique with EPO therapy. In one study, a three-arm trial of moderate hemodi-

Table 19-6. Costs* of Perisurgical Erythropoietin Therapy

Reference	Dose	Cost
Canadian Orthopedic Study Group[81] Faris, Ritter, Abels[82]	300 U/kg × 14 days	$2940
Sowade, Warnke, Scigalla, et al[83]	500 U/kg × 5 over 14 days	$1750
Monk, Goodnough, Brecher, et al[32]	600 U/kg D-21, D-14, and 300 U/kg day of surgery	$1050
Goldberg, McCutchen, Jove, et al[95]	600 U/kg × 4 weekly	$1680

*For a 70-kg patient, at $0.01/unit.

lution with EPO therapy (1500 U/kg in three divided doses over 3 weeks) was compared with hemodilution alone and also with the PAD of 3 units in patients undergoing radical prostatectomy.[32] Four percent of patients treated with EPO and ANH required allogeneic blood, compared with 16% of patients in the other two groups. In the EPO-treated patients, mean hematocrit levels were greater than 30% throughout the surgical hospitalization. This benefit may be clinically important because radical prostatectomy is a procedure that is associated with a 2% risk of perioperative myocardial infarction.[50] Using this approach, the cost of three weekly doses for a 70-kg man was $1050 (Table 19-6). When the transfusion costs associated with ANH ($100) are added, the total costs may be estimated at $1150, or approximately twice the cost associated with donation of 3 units of autologous blood.[96] A clinical trial of reduced doses of weekly subcutaneous EPO (450 U/kg × 2 and 300 U/kg × 2 beginning 14 days before surgery), coupled with hemodilution, has been completed in patients undergoing radical prostatectomy[35]; the use of low-dose EPO (300 U/kg) in this trial, along with hemodilution, was cost-equivalent to the donation of 3 autologous blood units or the transfusion of 2 allogeneic blood units.[96]

The most cost-effective use of EPO may be to increase the level of hematocrit in patients who are anemic and are anticipated to have substantial surgical blood losses. A target preoperative hematocrit of 45% should minimize the need for allogeneic blood transfusions, especially when accompanied by prudent transfusion practice.[97,98] Patients undergoing more complex surgeries with substantial blood needs may require a combination of EPO therapy and autologous blood procurement, such as ANH. Low-dose EPO therapy coupled with ANH may be shown ultimately to be cost-equivalent to the collection of 3 autologous blood units before elective surgery.

Other Alternatives to Allogeneic Transfusion

Iron Therapy

In the setting of blood loss, normal individuals have been shown to have difficulty providing sufficient iron to support rates of erythropoiesis that are greater than three times basal.[90,91] An analysis of endogenous erythropoietin response from phlebotomy (see the placebo group in Fig 19-4) or from recombinant human EPO therapy (see the other groups in Fig 19-4) on red cell production has dem-

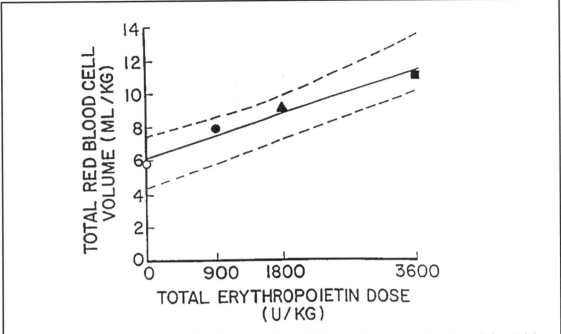

Figure 19-4. The dose-response relationship between the total (cumulative) amount of erythropoietin administered (units per kilogram body weight for six treatments over 3 weeks) and the red blood cell volume increase (milliliters per kilogram body weight) during the preoperative interval for patients treated intravenously with placebo (O), 150 U/kg (●), 300 U/kg (▲), and 600 U/kg(■). The dotted lines indicate the 95% confidence interval. Reprinted with permission from the American College of Surgeons (Journal of the American College of Surgeons), 1994;179:171-6.[91]

onstrated a good correlation.[91] EPO-stimulated erythropoiesis is independent of age and gender,[99] and the variability in response among patients is most likely due to iron-restricted erythropoiesis.[11] A 1998 study estimates that the maximum marrow response seen in EPO-treated iron-replete patients is approximately four times that of basal marrow red blood cell production.[11] Previous investigators have shown that conditions associated with enhanced plasma iron and transferrin saturation, such as in patients with hemochromatosis[100] or in patients supplemented with intravenous iron administration,[23] are necessary to produce an even greater marrow response. In hemochromatosis, marrow response has been estimated to increase by 6- to 8-fold over baseline red blood cell production with aggressive phlebotomy.[100] According to

Finch,[101] relative iron deficiency occurs in individuals when the iron stores are normal, but the increased erythron iron requirements exceed the supply of iron.

A previous study demonstrated with ferrokinetic studies that iron supplementation with at least 100 mg elemental iron per day taken with food can cover the increased iron needs in autologous blood donors.[102] For all patients, initial storage iron status is not a clinically important limitation for red blood cell production in the presence of oral iron supplementation.[11] However, as illustrated in Fig 19-5, in iron-replete patients receiving EPO therapy, there is a significant relationship between storage iron and marrow response. This finding illustrates the relevance of storage iron for maintaining sufficient plasma transferrin saturation for optimal erythropoiesis in the surgical setting.

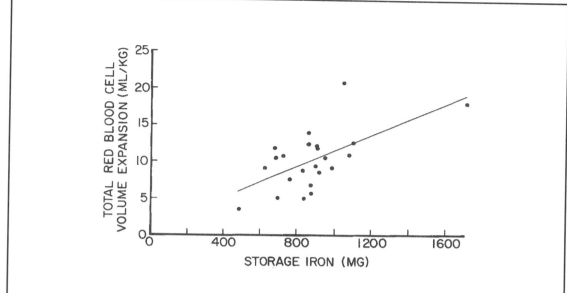

Figure 19-5. The relationship between initial storage iron (mg) and red blood cell volume expansion (mL/kg) in iron-replete EPO-treated patients. Storage iron is derived for each patient on the basis of the initial serum ferritin level. Linear regression analysis demonstrated a significant correlation ($r=0.6$, $p=0.02$). Reprinted with permission from Goodnough and Marcus.[11]

A 1996 trial of intravenous iron dextran therapy coupled with EPO therapy demonstrated rapid erythropoietic responses in patients undergoing surgical repair of hip fracture.[103] However, intravenous iron dextran therapy can be associated with significant toxicities that may preclude its routine use in the surgical setting. Yet, intravenous iron preparations could be used in this setting to enhance erythropoiesis if higher plasma transferrin saturations were maintained than with oral ferrous sulfate supplementation. A European trial demonstrated that intravenous iron saccharate and EPO therapy promoted increased erythropoiesis when compared with EPO therapy with oral iron supplementation alone.[23] The significant rate of allogeneic blood exposure for both iron-depleted (21%) and iron-replete (18%) patients, despite aggressive autologous blood procurement,[11] underscores the potential value of intravenous iron supplementation in the surgical setting.

Vitamin K

Vitamin K is required for the final synthetic step in the production of calcium-binding coagulation Factors II (prothrombin), VII, IX, and X. Serious bleeding can result from vitamin K deficiency, whether due to dietary deficiencies, to the effects of antibiotics on intestinal bacteria that produce usable vitamin K, or to treatment with vitamin K antagonists such as warfarin. Treatment with intravenous vitamin K_1 (Aquamephyton, 10-15 mg) results in rapid correction; usually, an improvement in prothrombin time can be seen within 12 hours and full correction within 24-48 hours. Although Fresh Frozen Plasma supplies active factors and can correct vitamin K deficiency, it should be reserved for situations in which life-threatening bleeding is a risk. The circular of information for blood products[73,p18] states that Fresh Frozen Plasma is contraindicated "when coagulation can be corrected more effectively with specific therapy, such as vitamin K."

References

1. Wallace EL, Churchill WH, Surgenor DM, et al. Collection and transfusion of blood and blood components in the United States, 1992. Transfusion 1998;38:625-36.
2. Mintz PD, Nordine RB, Henry JB, Weble R. Expected hemotherapy in elective surgery. N Y State J Med 1976;76:532-7.
3. Goodnough LT, Monk TG, Brecher ME. A review of autologous blood procurement in the surgical setting: Lessons learned in the last 10 years. Vox Sang 1996;71:133-41.
4. National Heart, Lung, and Blood Institute Expert Panel. Transfusion alert: Use of autologous blood transfusion. Transfusion 1995:35:703-11.
5. National Heart, Lung, and Blood Institute Autologous Transfusion Symposium Working Group. Autologous transfusion: Current trends and research issues. Transfusion 1995;35:525-31.
6. Consensus Conference on Autologous Transfusion. Final consensus statement. Transfusion 1996;36:667-9.
7. British Committee for Standards in Hematology, Blood Transfusion Task Force. Guidelines for autologous transfusion. Transfus Med 1993;307-16.
8. Menitove JT, ed. Standards for blood banks and transfusion services. 18th ed. Bethesda, MD: American Association of Blood Banks. 1997:48.
9. Food and Drug Administration. Memorandum: Autologous blood collection and processing procedures (February 12, 1990). Rockville, MD: Office of Communication, Training and Manufacturers Assistance, 1990.
10. Goodnough LT, Price TH, Rudnick S. Iron restricted erythropoiesis as a limitation to autologous blood donation in the erythropoietin-stimulated bone marrow. J Lab Clin Med 1991;118:289-96.
11. Goodnough LT, Marcus RE. Erythropoiesis in patients stimulated with erythropoietin: The relevance of storage iron. Vox Sang 1998 (in press).
12. Silvergleid AJ. Safety and effectiveness of predeposit autologous transfusions in pre-teen and adolescent children. JAMA 1987; 257:3403-4.
13. Mann M, Sacks HJ, Goldfinger D. Safety of autologous blood donation prior to elective surgery for a variety of potentially high risk patients. Transfusion 1983;23:229-32.
14. Popovsky MA, Whitaker B, Arnold NL. Severe outcomes of allogeneic and autologous blood donation: Frequency and characterization. Transfusion 1995;35:734-7.
15. Schreiber GB, Busch MP, Kleinman SH, Korelitz JJ. The risk of transfusion-transmitted viral infections. N Engl J Med 1996;334:1685-90.
16. Sayers MH. Controversies in transfusion medicine. Autologous blood donation in pregnancy: Con. Transfusion 1990;30:172-4.
17. Renner SW, Howanitz PJ, Bachner P. Preoperative autologous blood donation in 612 hospitals. Arch Pathol Lab Med 1992;116:613-9.
18. Goodnough LT, Saha P, Hirschler N, Yomtovian R. Autologous blood donation in non-orthopaedic surgery as a blood conservation strategy. Vox Sang 1992;63:96-101.
19. Toy PTCY. When should the first of two autologous donations be made? (abstract) Transfusion 1994;34:14S.
20. Kasper SM, Gerlich W, Buzello W. Preoperative red cell production in patients undergoing weekly autologous blood donation. Transfusion 1997;37:1058-62.
21. Gesemann M, Gentner PR, Scheirmann P. Association of hematopoiesis during autologous blood donation with initial hemoglobin concentration and length of donation period. Infusionther Transfusionmed 1997;24:316.
22. Goodnough LT, Price TH, Rudnick S, Soegiarso RW. Preoperative red blood cell production in patients undergoing aggressive autologous blood phlebotomy with and with-

out erythropoietin therapy. Transfusion 1992;32:441-5.

23. Mercuriali F, Zanella A, Barosi G, et al. Use of erythropoietin to increase the volume of autologous blood donated by orthopedic patients. Transfusion 1993;33:55-60.

24. Goodnough LT, Mercuriali F. Compensatory erythiopoiesis during routine autologous blood donation (letter). Transfusion 1998; 38:613-4.

25. Cohen JA, Brecher ME. Preoperative autologous blood donation: Benefit or detriment? A mathematical analysis. Transfusion 1995; 35:640-4.

26. Kanter MH, Van Maanen D, Anders KH, et al. Preoperative autologous blood donation before elective hysterectomy. JAMA 1996; 276:798-801.

27. Goodnough LT, Vizmeg K, Verbrugge D. The impact of autologous blood procurement practices on allogeneic blood exposure in elective orthopaedic surgery patients. Am J Clin Pathol 1994;101:354-7.

28. Goodnough LT, Shaffron D, Marcus RE. The impact of preoperative autologous blood donation on orthopaedic surgical practice. Vox Sang 1990;598:65-9.

29. Goodnough LT, Grishaber JE, Birkmeyer JD, et al. Efficacy and cost-effectiveness of autologous blood predeposit in patients undergoing radical prostatectomy procedures. Urology 1994;44:226-31.

30. Toy PTCY, Menozzi D, Strauss RG, et al. Efficacy of preoperative donation of blood for autologous use in radical prostatectomy. Transfusion 1993;33:721-4.

31. Monk TG, Goodnough LT, Brecher ME. Acute normovolemic hemodilution can replace preoperative autologous donation as a method of autologous blood procurement in radical prostatectomy. Anesth Analg 1997; 85:953-8.

32. Monk TG, Goodnough LT, Brecher ME, et al. A prospective, randomized trial of three blood conservation strategies for radical prostatectomy. Anesthesiology (in press).

33. Ness PM, Bourke DL, Walsh PC. A randomized trial of perioperative hemodilution versus transfusion of preoperatively deposited autologous blood in elective surgery. Transfusion 1991;31:226-30.

34. Monk TG, Goodnough LT, Birkmeyer JD, et al. Acute normovolemic hemodilution is a cost-effective alternative to preoperative autologous blood donation by patients undergoing radical retropubic prostatectomy. Transfusion 1995;35:559-65.

35. Monk TG, Goodnough LT, Colberg JW, Andreole GL. A cost-effective regimen for preoperative erythropoietin therapy (abstract). Anesthesiology 1998 (in press).

36. Goodnough LT, Monk TG, Andriole GL. Eyrthropoietin therapy. N Engl J Med 1997; 336:933-8.

37. Etchason J, Petz L, Keeler E, et al. The cost-effectiveness of preoperative autologous blood donations. N Engl J Med 1995;332: 719-24.

38. Birkmeyer JD, AuBuchon JP, Littenberg B, et al. Cost-effectiveness of preoperative autologous blood donation in coronary artery bypass grafting. Ann Thorac Surg 1994;57: 161-9.

39. Birkmeyer JD, Goodnough LT, AuBuchon JP, et al. The cost-effectiveness of preoperative autologous blood donation for total hip and knee replacement. Transfusion 1993;33:544-51.

40. Messmer K, Kreimeier M, Intagliett A. Present state of intentional hemodilution. Eur Surg Res 1986;18:254-63.

41. Brecher ME, Rosenfeld M. Mathematical and computer modeling of acute normovolemic hemodilution. Transfusion 1994;34: 176-9.

42. Goodnough LT, Grishaber JE, Monk TG, Catalona WJ. Acute preoperative hemodilution in patients undergoing radical prostatectomy: A case study analysis of efficacy. Anesth Analg 1994;78:932-7.

43. Goodnough LT, Bravo J, Hsueh Y, et al. Red blood cell volume in autologous and homolo-

gous units: Implications for risk/benefit assessment for autologous blood "crossover" and directed blood transfusion. Transfusion 1989;29:821-2.

44. Zetterstrom H, Wiklund L. A new nomogram facilitating adequate haemodilution. Acta Anaesthesiol Scand 1986;30:300-4.

45. Weiskopf RB. Mathematical analysis of isovolemic hemodilution indicates that it can decrease the need for allogeneic blood transfusion. Transfusion 1995;35:37-41.

46. Petry AF, Jost T, Sievers H. Reduction of homologous blood requirements by blood pooling at the onset of cardiopulmonary bypass. J Thorac Cardiovasc Surg 1994;1097:1210-4.

47. Goodnough LT, Monk TG, Brecher ME. Acute normovolemic hemodilution in surgery. Hematology, 1997;2:413-20.

48. American Society of Anesthesiology. Practice guidelines for blood component therapy. Anesthesiology 1996;84:732-47.

49. Brecher ME, Monk TG, Goodnough LT. A standardized method for the calculation of blood loss. Transfusion 1997;37:1070-4.

50. Andriole GL, Smith DS, Rao G, et al. Early complications of contemporary anatomic radical retropubic prostatectomy. J Urol 1994;152:1858-60.

51. Faust RJ. Perioperative indications for red cell transfusion. Has the pendulum swung too far? Mayo Clin Proc 1993;68:512-4.

52. Goodnough LT, Monk TG. Evolving concepts in autologous blood procurement. Case reports of perisurgical anemia complicated by myocardial infarction. Am J Med 1996;101:12A-33S.

53. Sazama K. Reports of 355 transfusion-associated deaths: 1975 through 1985. Transfusion 1990;30:583-90.

54. Goodnough LT, Monk TG, Brecher ME. Acute normovolemic hemodilution should replace preoperative autologous blood donation before elective surgery. Transfusion 1998;38:473-7.

55. Rottman G, Ness PM. Is acute normovolemic hemodilution a legitimate alternative to allogeneic blood transfusions? Transfusion 1998;38:477-81.

56. Williamson KR, Taswell HF. Intraoperative blood recovery: A review. Transfusion 1991; 31:662-75.

57. Bell K, Stott K, Sinclair CJ, et al. A controlled trial of intra-operative autologous transfusion in cardiothoracic surgery measuring effect on transfusion requirements and clinical outcome. Transfus Med 1992;2:295-300.

58. Solomon MD, Rutledge ML, Kane LE, Yawn DH. Cost comparison of intraoperative autologous versus homologous transfusion. Transfusion 1988;28:379-82.

59. Bovill DF, Moulton CW, Jackson WS, et al. The efficacy of intraoperative autologous transfusion in major orthopedic surgery: A regression analysis. Orthopedics 1986;9: 1403-7.

60. Goodnough LT, Monk TG, Sicard G, et al. Intraoperative recovery in patients undergoing elective abdominal aortic aneurism repair. An analysis of costs and benefits. J Vasc Surg 1996;24:213-8.

61. Ward HB, Smith RA, Candis KP, et al. A prospective, randomized trial of autotransfusion after routine cardiac surgery. Ann Thorac Surg 1993;56:137-41.

62. Thurer RL, Lytle BW, Cosgrove DM, Loop FD. Autotransfusion following cardiac operations: A randomized, prospective study. Ann Thorac Surg 1979; 27:500-6.

63. Roberts SP, Early GL, Brown B, et al. Autotransfusion of unwashed mediastinal shed blood fails to decrease banked blood requirements in patients undergoing aorta coronary bypass surgery. Am J Surg 1991;162:477-80.

64. Schaff HV, Hauer JM, Bell WR, et al. Autotransfusion of shed mediastinal blood after cardiac surgery. A prospective study. J Cardiovasc Thorac Surg 1978;75:632-41.

65. Eng J, Kay PH, Murday AJ, et al. Postoperative autologous transfusion in cardiac surgery. A prospective, randomized study. Eur J Cardiovasc Thorac Surg 1990;4:595-600.

66. Semkiw LB, Schurman OJ, Goodman SB, Woolson ST. Postoperative blood recovery using the cell saver after total joint arthroplasty. J Bone J Surg (Am) 1989;71A:823-7.

67. Faris PM, Ritter MA, Keating EM, Valeri CR. Unwashed filtered shed blood collected after knee and hip arthroplasties. J Bone Joint Surg Am 1991;73A:1169-77.

68. Martin JW, Whiteside LA, Milliano MT, Reedy ME: Postoperative blood retrieval and transfusion in cementless total knee arthroplasty. J Arthroplasty 1992;7:205-10.

69. Clements DH, Sculco TP, Burke SW, et al. Salvage and reinfusion of postoperative sanguineous wound drainage. J Bone Joint Surg Am 1992;74A:646-51.

70. Woda R, Tetzlaff JE. Upper airway oedema following autologous blood transfusion from a wound drainage system. Can J Anesthesiol 1992;39:290-2.

71. Blevins FT, Shaw B, Valeri RC, et al. Reinfusion of shed blood after orthopaedic procedures in children and adolescents. J Bone Joint Surg Am 1993;75A:363-71.

72. Goodnough LT, Verbrugge D, Marcus RE. The relationship between hematocrit, blood lost, and blood transfused in total knee replacement: Implications for postoperative blood recovery and reinfusion. Am J Knee Surg 1995;8:83-7.

73. American Red Cross, America's Blood Centers, American Association of Blood Banks. Circular of information for the use of blood and blood components. April 1997.

74. Goodnough LT, Brittenham G. Limitations of the erythropoietic response to serial phlebotomy: Implications for autologous blood donor programs. J Lab Clin Med 1990;115:28-35.

75. Kickler TS, Spivak JL. Effect of repeated whole blood donations on serum immunoreactive erythropoietin levels in autologous donors. JAMA 1988;260:65-7.

76. Goodnough LT, Rudick S, Price TH, et al. Increased collection of autologous blood preoperatively with recombinant human erythropoietin therapy. N Engl J Med 1989;321:1163-7.

77. Goodnough LT, Price TH, and the EPO Study Group. A phase III trial of recombinant human erythropoietin therapy in non-anemic orthopedic patients subjected to aggressive autologous blood phlebotomy: Dose, response, toxicity, and efficacy. Transfusion 1994;34:66-71.

78. Beris P, Mermillod B, Levy G, et al. Recombinant human erythropoietin as adjuvant treatment for autologous blood donation. Vox Sang 1993;65:212-8.

79. Biesma DH, Marx JJ, Kraaijenhagen RJ, et al. Lower homologous blood requirement in autologous blood donors after treatment with recombinant human erythropoietin. Lancet 1994;344:367-70.

80. Price TH, Goodnough LT, Vogler W, et al. The effect of recombinant erythropoietin administration on the efficacy of autologous blood donation in patients with low hematocrits. Transfusion 1996;36:29-36.

81. Canadian Orthopaedic Perioperative Erythropoietin Study Group. Effectiveness of perioperative recombinant human erythropoietin in elective hip replacement. Lancet 1993;341:1227-32.

82. Faris PM, Ritter MA, Abels RI. The effects of recombinant human erythropoietin on perioperative transfusion requirements in patients undergoing major orthopaedic surgery. J Bone Joint Surg Am 1996;78-A:62-72.

83. Sowade O, Warnke H, Scigalla P, et al. Avoidance of allogeneic blood transfusions by treatment with epoetin beta (recombinant human erythropoietin) in patients undergoing open heart surgery. Blood 1997;89:411-8.

84. Sowade O, Ziemer S, Sowade B, et al. The effect of preoperative recombinant human erythropoietin therapy on platelets and hemostatis in patients undergoing cardiac surgery. J Lab Clin Med 1997;129:376-83.

85. Sowade O, Gross J, Sowade B, et al. Evaluation of oxygen availability with oxygen status

algorithm in patients undergoing open heart surgery treated with epoetin beta. J Lab Clin Med 1997;129:97-105.

86. D'Ambra MN, Gray RJ, Hillman R, et al. The effect of recombinant human erythropoietin on transfusion risk in coronary bypass patients. Ann Thorac Surg 1997;64:1686-93.

87. Goodnough LT, Despostis GJ, Parvin CA. Erythropoietin therapy in patients undergoing cardiac surgery. Ann Thorac Surg, 1997; 64:1579-80.

88. Gaudiani VA, Mason HDW. Preoperative erythropoietin in Jehovah's Witnesses who require cardiac procedures. Ann Thorac Surg 1991;51:823-4.

89. Hogue CW, Goodnough LT, Ding Y, Monk TG. Myocardial ischemic episodes in elderly patients having autologous blood procurement. Anesthesiology 1996;85:A50.

90. Coleman PH, Stevens AR, Dodge HT, Finch CA. Rate of blood regeneration after blood loss. Arch Intern Med 1953;92:341-8.

91. Goodnough LT, Verbrugge D, Marcus RE, Goldberg V. The effect of patient size and dose of recombinant human erythropoietin therapy on red blood cell expansion. J Am Coll Surg 1994;179:171-6.

92. Sisk JE, Gianfrancesco FD, Costner JM. Recombinant erythropoietin and medicare payment. JAMA 1991;266:247-52.

93. Doolittle RF. Biotechnology—The enormous cost of success. N Engl J Med 1991;324:1360-2.

94. Mc Mahon FG, Vargas R, Ryan M, et al. Pharmacokinetics and effects of recombinant human erythropoietin after intravenous and subcutaneous injections in healthy volunteers. Blood 1990;76:1718-22.

95. Goldberg MA, McCutchen JW, Jove M, et al. A safety and efficacy comparison study of two dosing regimens of erythropoietin alpha in patients undergoing major orthopedic surgery. Am J Orthop 1996;25:544-52.

96. Goodnough LT, Bodner MS, Martin JW. Blood transfusion and blood conservation: Cost and utilization issues. Am J Med Qual 1994;9:172-83.

97. Welch GH, Meehan KR, Goodnough LT. Prudent strategies for elective red blood cell transfusion. Ann Intern Med 1992;116:393-402.

98. Goodnough LT. Blood transfusion and blood conservation practices. Flip sides of the same coin? Ann Thorac Surg 1993;56:137-44.

99. Goodnough LT, Price TH, Parvin CA. The endogenous erythropoietin response and the erythropoietic response to blood loss anemia: The effects of age and gender. J Lab Clin Med 1995;126:57-64.

100. Crosby WH. Treatment of hemochromatosis by energetic phlebotomy. One patient's response to getting 55 liters of blood in 11 months. Br J Haematol 1958;4:82-8.

101. Finch CA. Erythropoiesis, erythropoietin, and iron. Blood 1982;60:1241-6.

102. Skikne BS, Cook JD. Effect of enhanced erythropoiesis on iron absorption. J Lab Clin Med 1992;120:746-51.

103. Goodnough LT, Merkel K. The use of parenteral iron and recombinant human erythropoietin therapy to stimulate erythropoiesis in patients undergoing repair of hip fracture. Int J Hematol 1996;1:163-6.

In: Mintz PD, ed.
Transfusion Therapy: Clinical Principles and Practice
Bethesda, MD: AABB Press, 1999

20

The Role of Hematopoietic Growth Factors in Transfusion Medicine

CAROLYN F. WHITSETT, MD

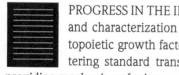
PROGRESS IN THE IDENTIFICATION and characterization of human hematopoietic growth factors is radically altering standard transfusion practices, providing mechanisms for improving the quality of existing blood components,[1,2] and making possible the development of novel and customized blood products.[3] For some patients with anemia, physicians now have the option of stimulating endogenous erythrocyte production with erythropoietin (EPO) instead of giving allogeneic transfusions. EPO can also be used to facilitate preoperative autologous donation for patients having surgery or to reduce postoperative anemia (reviewed in Chapter 19). The neutropenic patient can be treated with granulocyte colony-stimulating factor (G-CSF) or granulocyte-macrophage colony-stimulating factor (GM-CSF). When administered

to healthy blood donors, G-CSF can increase the number of granulocytes obtained with apheresis technology. Both alone and in combination with other cytokines, G-CSF can also mobilize hematopoietic progenitor cells into the peripheral blood, permitting the collection of these cells with apheresis technology. Peripheral blood progenitor cells (PBPCs) have become the preferred hematopoietic stem cell product for autologous transplantation and are under investigation for allogeneic use.[4] Finally, recombinant human interleukin-11 (IL-11, rhIL-11, Neumega, Genetics Institute, Inc, Cambridge, MA), one of several growth factors under development to stimulate megakaryocytopoiesis, has been licensed by the US Food and Drug Administration (FDA) for the prevention of severe thrombocytopenia following myelosuppressive chemotherapy in patients with nonmyeloid malignancies.

Carolyn F. Whitsett, MD, Director, Transfusion Service, Crawford Long Hospital of Emory University, Atlanta, Georgia

This chapter is devoted to hematopoietic growth factors and cytokines, with an emphasis on their role in transfusion medicine applications. More than 35 factors that influence the proliferation and differentiation of hematopoietic cells have been described. Only four recombinant growth factors—EPO, G-CSF, GM-CSF, and IL-11—have been approved for routine clinical use, but many other factors are being evaluated in preclinical studies and early clinical trials. Table 20-1 lists selected growth factors and cytokines that have documented or potential transfusion medicine applications. In addition to recombinant forms of the natural molecule, there are also fusion cytokines developed to mimic a combination of growth factors.[6]

This chapter discusses EPO, G-CSF and GM-CSF, IL-11, and thrombopoietin. The scientific literature on hematopoietic growth factors is vast, and, for some topics, it was necessary to use review articles rather than original sources when citing references.

Erythropoietin

Erythropoietin, the primary growth factor regulating the production of red blood cells, was first purified from human urine in 1977.[7] EPO is a glycoprotein with a molecular weight of 34,000 daltons. The gene for human EPO was cloned in 1985 and was assigned to chromosome 7 (7q11-q22) shortly thereafter. The results of the first clinical trials using recombinant human erythropoietin (rHuEPO) in end-stage renal disease were published in 1986,[8] and the Phase III study leading to FDA approval of rHuEPO for the treatment of the anemia of chronic renal disease was published in 1989.[9] Currently, rHuEPO is approved to treat anemia associated with cancer and cancer chemotherapy, to treat anemia developing in human immunodeficiency virus (HIV)-infected individuals treated with zidovudine, and to decrease allogeneic blood transfusions in anemic patients having nonvascular, noncardiac surgery. In Canada and Europe, rHuEPO is also approved to facilitate autologous blood donation.[10] In addition, rHuEPO

is being evaluated in the treatment of anemia of prematurity, anemia of chronic disease, myelodysplasia, and hemoglobinopathies.

Biology

The biology of EPO and the structure and function of the erythropoietin receptor are the subject of early reviews.[7,11] Progress in understanding intracellular events following the binding of EPO to its receptor are summarized in a 1997 review.[12] The protein moiety of circulating EPO consists of a 165-amino acid polypeptide chain. Three N-linked and one O-linked acidic oligosaccharide chains are attached to the native molecule. Removal of the terminal N-acetyl neuraminic acid leads to rapid clearance of EPO from the circulation, indicating that the carbohydrate component of EPO plays an important role in metabolism. In healthy individuals, the serum level of EPO is 5-25 mU/mL. In adults, EPO is produced primarily in the kidney, although in the fetus the primary production site is the liver. Hybridization studies using sense and antisense RNA probes suggest that interstitial cells in the peritubular capillary bed are the sites of EPO production. The switch from hepatic to renal production begins at about 120-140 days of gestation and is completed approximately 40 days after birth. Hypoxia is the primary stimulus causing increased production. There is often an inverse relationship between red cell mass and EPO levels, so EPO levels are very high in patients with aplastic anemia and following chemotherapy. However, in some diseases, cytokines that inhibit EPO production are elevated, and the normal EPO response to reduced red cell mass is not observed. For this reason, the EPO response may be expressed as a ratio that compares the observe EPO level with the predicted EPO value (observed/predicted log ratio) on the basis of a simple anemia such as iron deficiency anemia. Ratios of up to 0.9 are considered low.[13]

EPO exerts its effect on erythroid progenitor cells by binding to a specific membrane receptor. This receptor is a transmembrane protein belonging to the cytokine receptor superfamily. The gene coding for the EPO receptor is located on chromo-

Table 20-1. Selected Lineage-Dominant Hematopoietic Growth Factors and Cytokines

Factor	Form Available	Description	Availability	Primary Hematopoietic Effect	Transfusion Medicine Applications
Erythropoietin (EPO)	Epoetin-alpha	165 amino acids, glycosylated produced in Chinese hamster ovary cells	Worldwide	Stimulates the division and differentiation of committed erythroid progenitor cells; induces the release of reticulocytes from the bone marrow	1. Treatment of anemia when there is a relative or absolute deficiency of erythropoietin, including renal disease, cancer, HIV infection, and chronic disease
				May have some effect on megakaryocyte progenitors	2. Support perioperative autologous blood donation and reduce blood transfusions in individuals with hemoglobin ≥10 gm/dL<13 g/dL
	Epoetin-beta	Different type and degree of glycosylation than epoetin-alpha	Europe, Japan		3. Reduction in postoperative anemia
	Novel erythropoiesis- stimulating protein[5]	Hyperglycosylated analogue of recombinant erythropoietin	Clinical development		4. Reduce severity of anemia in patients declining transfusion
Granulocyte colony- stimulating factor (G-CSF)	Filgrastim	Nonglycosylated G-CSF 175 amino acids, produced in *Escherichia coli*	Worldwide	Stimulates the proliferation and differentiation of neutrophil precursors; activates mature cells	*1. Accelerate neutrophil recovery following chemotherapy or marrow transplantation
	Lenograstim	Glycosylated G-CSF 175 amino acids produced in Chinese hamster ovary cells	Europe, Japan	Mobilizes progenitor cells into peripheral blood	2. Reduce the incidence of febrile neutropenia following chemotherapy
					3. Increase the yield of granulocytes from normal apheresis donors
					4. Mobilize peripheral blood progenitor cells (PBPCs) in patients; mobilize PBPCs in related and unrelated donors

(continued)

Table 20-1. Selected Lineage-Dominant Hematopoietic Growth Factors and Cytokines (continued)

Factor	Form Available	Description	Availability	Primary Hematopoietic Effect	Transfusion Medicine Applications
Granulocyte-macrophage colony-stimulating factor (GM-CSF)	Sargramostim	Glycosylated GM-CSF of 127 amino acids produced in *Saccharomyces cerevisiae* differs from natural GM-CSF by substitution of leucine at position 23 Glycosylation pattern may also be different; three primary species with molecular mass of 19,500, 16,800, and 15,500	Worldwide	Stimulates the proliferation and differentiation of myeloid progenitor cells including neutrophils, eosinophils, monocytes Mobilizes progenitor cells into peripheral blood	1. Shorten time to neutrophil recovery following induction chemotherapy in older patients with acute myelogenous leukemia 2. For mobilization and following transplantation of PBPCs (patients) 3. For acceleration of myeloid recovery following autologous marrow transplantation 4. Treatment of graft failure or engraftment delay following autologous or allogeneic marrow transplantation
	Molgramostim	Nonglycosylated GM-CSF produced in *E. coli*	Europe, Japan		
Interleukin-11 (IL-11)	Oprelvekin	177 amino acid polypeptide differing from natural IL-11 only in lacking the aminoterminal proline residue; produced in *E. coli*	United States	Stimulates megakaryocytopoiesis including production, differentiation, and maturation of megakaryocytes Part of effect appears to be mediated through thrombopoietin (in-vitro studies)	Reduce chemotherapy-associated thrombocytopenia and decrease the need for platelet transfusions following myelosuppressive chemotherapy in patients with non-myeloid malignancies at high risk of severe thrombocytopenia
Thrombopoietin (TPO)	Thrombopoietin	Full-length 332 amino acid polypeptide	Clinical development	Stimulates megakaryopoiesis and thrombopoiesis	1. Accelerate platelet recovery following myelosuppressive chemotherapy
	Megakaryocyte growth and differentiation factor (MGDF)	Truncated thrombopoietin molecule produced in *E. coli*	Clinical development[†]		2. Increase the yield of platelets from apheresis procedures in normal donors

*Since this manuscript was submitted for publication, the FDA has approved filgrastim to reduce the time to neutrophil recovery and the duration of fever following chemotherapy in patients with acute myelogenous leukemia.
[†]Since this manuscript was submitted for publication, platelet donation clinical trials have been discontinued following the development of thrombocytopenia and neutralizing antibodies.

some 19p. Very few receptors are found on early burst-forming units–erythroid (BFU-Es), but the number increases with differentiation and appears to be maximal in the stage between colony-forming units–erythroid (CFU-Es) and proerythroblasts. EPO receptors are present in very low numbers at the orthochromatic normoblast stage and are lacking in reticulocytes and mature erythrocytes.

This traditional view of the distribution of EPO receptors is being challenged by new studies with flow cytometry, which use biotin-labeled EPO and streptavidin-RED670 conjugate.[14] These studies demonstrate EPO receptors on CD34+CD38- marrow cells. This fraction is enriched for nonlineage committed hematopoietic cells. When marrow cells committed to erythroid differentiation, as indicated by staining for glycophorin A, were evaluated, CD34+GpA+ marrow cells and CD34+CD38- cells had comparable numbers of EPO receptors (mean number/cell = 1297±431 and 1590±560, respectively). This observation was published in 1997, and additional confirmatory studies are needed. However, these results are consistent with early reports of EPO having an effect on a broad spectrum of hematopoietic progenitor cells.[6] EPO and its receptor have also been detected in neural tissue. Astrocytes produce EPO, and the receptor has been demonstrated on rat hippocampal and cortical neurons and in the central nervous system of midterm human fetuses.[15,16]

EPO is a survival and differentiation factor as well as a mitogenic factor for erythroid cells, having varying effects at different stages of maturation. It is not required for the generation of BFU-Es or for their differentiation into CFU-Es, but it is essential for the survival, proliferation, and differentiation of CFU-Es.[7] Promotion of progenitor survival is in part through inhibition of apoptosis. The intracellular signaling events leading to mitogenesis or differentiation are not fully characterized at this time. However, some biochemical events that follow the binding of EPO to its receptor are well documented, such as phosphorylation of EPO receptor and other cytoplasmic proteins[11,12] and receptor homodimerization.[17] EPO binding activates the JAK (Janus kinases)-STAT (signal transducers and acti-

vators of transcription) pathway and the RAS/RAF1/MAP kinase pathways.[18,19] The cytoplasmic domain of EPO receptor has positive and negative regulatory elements, and a truncated receptor has been associated with primary familial and congenital polycythemia.[20]

Pharmacokinetics

Two forms of rHuEPO are commercially available: epoetin-alpha and epoetin-beta. Epoetin-alpha contains 39% carbohydrate and epoetin-beta contains 24% carbohydrate. Only epoetin-alpha has been approved for use in the United States. Both produce the same biologic effect, but there are different World Health Organization standards for each. A hyperglycosylated form of rHuEPO, novel erythropoiesis-stimulating protein, has been developed by Amgen, Inc (Thousand Oaks, CA) and is in clinical development.[5] Novel erythropoiesis-stimulating protein is reported to have a longer serum half-life and greater in-vivo biologic activity than rHuEPO.

Epoetin-alpha may be administered subcutaneously or intravenously. Following intravenous administration, the elimination half-time is 4-6 hours in normal adults[21] and 4-13 hours in patients with chronic renal failure (Epogen, Professional Prescribing Information, Amgen, Inc). A monoexponential decrease in serum EPO levels is observed for 18-24 hours following administration. Studies comparing the pharmacokinetics in infants (<1.25 kg) and adults indicate that infants have a greater plasma clearance and distribution volume and significantly shorter elimination and mean residence times.[22] When EPO is administered subcutaneously to adults, the peak concentration is reached in 5-24 hours and serum concentrations gradually decline. In very-low-birthweight infants, the peak concentration is reached at 8.9 hours and the elimination half-time is 7-7.9 hours.[23] These data indicate that infants and children will require larger doses of EPO to achieve the same clinical outcome. In general, to achieve a target hematocrit, the dose of EPO administered subcutaneously is less than the dose required when EPO is administered intravenously.[24] Following treatment with EPO, an increase in reticulocyte count is usually seen in 7-10 days with an increase in hemoglobin occurring in 2-6 weeks, depending on iron stores. Specific dosage recommendations and a discussion of common adverse events are included in the section on clinical indications.

Allergic reactions, for which most populations are at equal risk, have been rare and usually very mild. The most recent prescribing information indicates that antibodies to rHuEPO have not been described. However, two recent (1996 and 1997) case reports outline the development of rHuEPO antibodies in dialysis patients previously having a good clinical response to rHuEPO.[25,26] One of these cases is from the United States, and the product administered would have been epoetin-alpha; in the US case report, the patient developed pure red cell aplasia. After discontinuation of rHuEPO, erythroid precursors and progenitors reappeared in the marrow as the antibody decreased in titer. Despite these two reports, the development of antibodies to rHuEPO is an extremely rare event.

Clinical Indications

The surgical and perioperative uses of EPO are presented in Chapter 19. Medical indications for EPO are presented in this section. In addition to chronic renal failure, EPO is FDA-approved for the treatment of anemia associated with cancer and cancer chemotherapy and of anemia in HIV-infected patients treated with zidovudine. In addition to these approved uses, there are studies that support the use of EPO in anemia of prematurity, anemia caused by chronic inflammatory diseases, and anemia associated with multiple myeloma and lymphoma. The clinical outcomes associated with the use of EPO in myelodysplasia and hemoglobinopathies are highly variable, and these are discussed briefly at the end of this section. A 1997 review summarizes the current use of EPO outside the setting of uremia.[13]

Chronic Renal Failure

Anemia in patients with chronic renal failure may be multifactorial. Although a deficiency of EPO

may be the most common etiology, blood loss from laboratory testing, gastrointestinal bleeding, and the dialysis extracorporeal circuit; hemolysis; aluminum toxicity; iron deficiency; vitamin deficiencies (especially folate); and hyperparathyroidism may also be contributing factors.[27] EPO has been available for treatment in this patient group since 1986, and a concise summary of the impact of rHuEPO on the anemia of chronic renal failure in the United States, Canada, and Western Europe has been published.[28] In the United States, 88% of hemodialysis patients and 52% of peritoneal dialysis patients receive rHuEPO (1992 data). The highest figure reported for hemodialysis patients receiving rHuEPO was from Norway, where 93% of patients were being treated. For peritoneal dialysis patients, the highest figure reported was from Austria, where 60% of patients were being treated, and the lowest figures reported were from France, where 45% of hemodialysis patients and 25% of peritoneal dialysis patients were being treated with rHuEPO. In most countries, economic factors, especially reimbursement policies, appear to play an important role in treatment decisions.

The Phase III clinical trial of rHuEPO in patients with end-stage renal disease, which ultimately led to FDA approval, established a target hematocrit of 35%.[8] Patients received either 300 or 150 U/kg intravenously three times a week. The dose was then reduced to 75 U/kg and adjusted to maintain a hematocrit of 35%. Ninety-seven percent of patients reached the target hematocrit within 12 weeks, and blood transfusions were eliminated in 2 months. Increased hematocrit was associated with improved quality of life. Similar benefits were described for predialysis and peritoneal dialysis patients.[27]

In 1989, the FDA established a target hematocrit value of 30-33% for patients treated with rHuEPO, and this figure was recently increased to 33-36%. In 1997, the National Kidney Foundation convened a panel of experts to develop clinical practice guidelines for the evaluation and treatment of anemia in the patient with chronic renal failure.[27] The guidelines developed by the expert panel are comprehensive, providing detailed recommendations for evaluation and treatment (summarized in Table 20-2), and readers are referred to the original document for clinical guidance. The published report cited statistics from the US Renal Data System 1996 Annual Report, which indicated that the mean hematocrit of EPO-treated patients in the United States was 30.2%, with 42% of patients having hematocrits below 30%. Health Care Financing Administration guidelines permit reimbursement for rHuEPO only when the rolling 3-month average hematocrit is no greater than 36.5%. After reviewing a large number of abstracts and peer-reviewed scientific reports, the panel concluded that most data suggest that patients with chronic renal failure function better with hematocrits closer to the normal range. One notable exception to this conclusion was a study sponsored by Amgen, Inc among dialysis patients with documented heart disease who were treated with epoetin-alpha. Patients with hematocrits in the normal range had more nonfatal myocardial infarctions and deaths than the group with hematocrits of 30±3%.

When EPO was administered to dialysis patients, minor side effects such as skin reaction at the injection site, arthralgia, or a mild influenza-like syndrome were observed in 11% or fewer of the patients. The most common serious side effects reported in clinical trials of rHuEPO were hypertension, access failure, and seizures.[9,27,28] The frequency of de-novo development of hypertension or an increase in blood pressure following treatment with rHuEPO is approximately 23%.[27] This side effect is seen primarily in patients with chronic renal failure and may be associated with hypertensive encephalopathy and seizures. It is thought to be related to an increase in vascular wall reactivity and hemodynamic changes resulting from increasing red cell mass. The changes in vascular reactivity may be related to endothelin release and/or changes in the balance between vasoconstricting and vasorelaxant prostanoids.[29] The clinical guidelines recommend monitoring blood pressure closely, especially during the initiation of rHuEPO therapy. Treatment may require the institution of antihypertensive therapy, intensified ultrafiltra-

tion, and/or a reduction in the dose of rHuEPO. Some studies have reported the frequency of access thrombosis to be around 12-14%.[28] In a recent Amgen study in which patients with cardiac disease were permitted to attain higher hematocrits, there was an increase in the thrombosis of native and synthetic arteriovenous grafts. However, the National Kidney Foundation panel concluded that there was no evidence that rHuEPO therapy increased the risk of native fistula thrombosis.[27] The panel also concluded that, with the exception of patients who had hypertensive encephalopathy, there was no evidence of an increased risk of seizures in patients treated with rHuEPO. Iron deficiency is the most common cause of resistance to rHuEPO. Only recently has the true magnitude of this problem become known.[30] Section III of the panel's guidelines addresses iron support.[27]

Cancer and Multiple Myeloma

Quality of life is an increasingly important issue as the regimens developed to treat cancer become more intense. The anemia associated with cancer and cancer treatment can cause symptoms such as fatigue, dyspnea, and listlessness, which decrease the quality of life. Survey instruments have been developed to assess specifically the effect of treatment regimens on symptoms caused by anemia.[31] For many years, the pathophysiology of the normochromic normocytic anemia associated with cancer was poorly understood, and transfusions were the only treatment available. Then, studies conducted among solid tumor patients demonstrated that for any given hematocrit, erythropoietin levels in these patients were lower than they were in a group of control subjects with iron deficiency anemia.[32] Two preliminary studies of rHuEPO in patients with multiple myeloma revealed a response rate of 82-85%, with complete correction of anemia in some patients.[33,34] A larger study of 30 patients (22 with solid tumors and 8 with lymphoma) demonstrated a 50% response to rHuEPO.[35] The variable response rate led to additional trials in patients with different types of cancer on a variety of chemotherapy regimens. In reviewing the results

Table 20-2. Essentials of the NKF-DOQI* Clinical Practice Guidelines for the Treatment of Anemia of Chronic Renal Failure (CRF)[27]

Section	Topic	Guide-lines	Recommendations	Rationale
I	Anemia work-up	1 - 3	1. Definition: Hct <33% (Hb <11g/dL) in premenopausal females and prepubertal patients; Hct <37% (Hb <12 g/dL) in adult males and postmenopausal females. 2. Evaluation: automated Hct/Hb with red blood cell indices and reticulocyte count, serum iron, total iron-binding capacity, percentage transferrin saturation (TSAT), serum ferritin - test for occult blood in stool. Evaluation should be completed before erythropoietin (EPO) therapy is begun. 3. EPO deficiency may develop early in CRF with serum creatinine as low as 2.0 mg/dL.	Definition of anemia is based on 80% of the mean level for healthy normal subgroups. Anemia of CRF is usually normochromic normocytic. Microcytosis may reflect iron deficiency, aluminum excess, or hemoglobinopathy. Macrocytosis may be associated with folate or B12 deficiency. Iron deficiency is present in about 25% of patients with anemia of CRF.
II	Target hematocrit (Hct)/ hemoglobin (Hb)	4	Target range for Hct/Hb is 33% (Hb 11 g/dL) to 37% (Hb 12 g/dL).	Survival of dialysis patients declines as the Hct decreases below the range of 30-33%. Left ventricular hypertrophy (LVH) is more likely in predialysis patients with Hct <33%. Partial correction of anemia results in partial regression of LVH. Quality of life and physiologic parameters improve as the Hct/Hb increases above 30-36%.
III	Iron support	5-10	Iron status should be monitored by percent TSAT and the serum ferritin. CRF patients should have sufficient iron to achieve Hct 33-36%. To achieve this, TSAT should be ≥20% and serum ferritin should be ≥100 ng/mL. If a patient has TSAT ≥20% and serum ferritin ≥100 ng/mL but has Hct <33%, a course of IV iron 50-100 mg once per week for 10 weeks should be tried. If TSAT ≥50% and serum ferritin level is ≥800 ng/mL, further increase in Hct or reduction in EPO dose unlikely. Monitoring of iron status should be monthly in patients not receiving IV iron and at least once every 3 months in patients receiving IV iron until target Hct is reached; thereafter, Hct/Hb TSAT and serum ferritin should be determined every 3 months. Supplemental iron should be administered to prevent iron deficiency and to maintain adequate iron stores. For adult predialysis, home hemodialysis, and peritoneal dialysis patients, oral iron may be adequate to maintain stores. Oral iron should be administered as 200 mg of elemental iron in adults and 2-3 mg/kg in pediatric patients. Most hemodialysis patients will require intravenous (IV) iron to maintain iron stores. In adults, 100 mg of iron may be administered IV at every hemodialysis for 10 doses. A test dose of IV iron should be given before beginning therapy.	More than 50% of end-stage renal disease patients receiving EPO are iron deficient. Absolute iron deficiency in CRF patients is defined as serum ferritin level <100 ng/mL and TSAT <20%. Many patients with TSAT >20% have functional iron deficiency. Low doses of IV iron improve Hct/Hb and can reduce EPO requirements. Immediate and delayed side effects may occur with IV iron dextran. An immediate anaphylaxis-like reaction may occur shortly after beginning an infusion. The delayed reaction consists of arthralgias and myalgias.

Table 20-2. Essentials of the NKF-DOQI* Clinical Practice Guidelines for the Treatment of Anemia of Chronic Renal Failure (CRF)[27] (continued)

Section	Topic	Guide-lines	Recommendations	Rationale
IV	Administration of erythropoietin	11-19	Predialysis and peritoneal dialysis patients should be given EPO subcutaneously. The preferred route in hemodialysis patients is also subcutaneous (SC). Injection sites should be rotated.	The dose of EPO required to maintain a given Hct is lower when EPO is administered subcutaneously compared with intravenously.
			Initial dosing subcutaneous by: Adults 80-120 U/kg/week in 2-3 doses. Children <5 years - 300 U/kg/week. Initial dosing - IV (adults) 120-180 U/kg/week in 3 divided doses.	In most countries outside the United States, EPO is administered subcutaneously. EPO requirements are 15-50% less with SC dosing than with IV dosing.
			Whenever possible, patients should be switched from IV to SC EPO.	
			Hct/Hb should be monitored every 1-2 weeks when initiating therapy. If Hct increase has been <2 percentage points over 2-4-week period, EPO dose should be increased 50%.	
			If Hct exceeds target or Hct increase exceeds 8 percentage points per month, EPO dose should be reduced 25%.	
			EPO should be given IV if patient is unable to tolerate SC dosing.	
V	Inadequate EPO response	20-22	CRF patients should be evaluated and treated for the following conditions: infection/inflammation, chronic blood loss, osteitis fibrosa, aluminum toxicity, hemoglobinopathies, folate or B12 deficiency, multiple myeloma, malnutrition, hemolysis.	Iron deficiency is the most common reason for an inadequate response to EPO. In the iron-replete patient, those are the most likely explanations.
VI	Role of red blood cell transfusions	23	Red blood cell transfusions are indicated in severely anemic symptomatic patients and EPO-resistant patients with chronic blood loss.	Transfusions are indicated only if signs or symptoms are likely to be reversed by transfusion.
VII	Possible adverse effects related to EPO therapy	24-28	Hypertension: Blood pressure should be monitored in all CRF patients, particularly with initiation of EPO therapy. Initiation of antihypertensive therapy or an increase in antihypertensive medication and reduction in EPO dose if there has been a rapid rise in Hct/Hb may be required to control blood pressure.	Twenty-three percent of patients developed hypertension or an increase in blood pressure.
			Seizures: Except in the case of hypertensive encephalopathy, there appears to be no evidence of an increased risk of seizures in CRF patients treated with EPO.	The incidence of seizures among patients receiving EPO is 3% (range 0-13%). In one controlled study of end-stage renal disease patients not on EPO, 5% of patients had seizures.
			Access thrombosis: There is no need for increased surveillance of access thrombosis in hemodialysis patients treated with EPO.	The average incidence of thrombosis of any access in patients on EPO was 7.5%.
			Heparin dose: EPO-treated hemodialysis patients do not need more heparin than patients not treated with EPO.	In North American multicenter studies, there is no evidence that increasing red cell mass increased dialyzer heparin requirements. One European study noted an increase in heparin requirements.
			Hyperkalemia: EPO-treated dialysis patients do not need more intensive potassium monitoring than patients not treated with EPO.	In two series accounting for 1000 patients, the incidence of hyperkalemia was less than 1%. When patients receiving EPO were compared with patients not receiving EPO, the incidence of hyperkalemia in EPO-treated patients was less than or equal to that in non-EPO-treated patients.

*National Kidney Foundation - Dialysis Outcomes Quality Initiative.

of rHuEPO treatment in patients with multiple myeloma, it was observed that patients with EPO levels up to 100 U/L were more likely to respond to treatment than patients with elevated EPO levels and that the kinetics of response varied with the type of treatment given for myeloma.[36] Patients receiving chemotherapy regimens containing cisplatin were of special interest because of the large percentage of patients developing anemia and the nephrotoxicity sometimes observed with cisplatin.[37,38] A randomized, double-blind, placebo-controlled trial of rHuEPO in such patients was conducted.[39] Patients received 100 U/kg rHuEPO subcutaneously three times a week. A response was defined as an increase in the hemoglobin level to no more than 10 g/dL. At the third week of treatment, 58% of patients had responded, and by the ninth week 82% had responded. Larger trials conducted in multiple myeloma and lymphoma revealed that 60% of patients responded to an 8-week course of subcutaneous administration of 5000 U or 10,000 U/day.[40,41]

Because of the expense of therapy, several studies have focused on identifying patients who are the best candidates for rHuEPO. The data from these studies were summarized in 1996.[42] Patients with a hemoglobin level of up to 11 g/dL and with a decrease in hemoglobin of at least 2 g/dL by the start of the second cycle of chemotherapy have a 98% chance of receiving a transfusion. When evaluated prior to chemotherapy, patients with a baseline EPO level up to 100 mU/mL are likely to respond to treatment with rHuEPO. In patients on chemotherapy, EPO levels have less predictive value. Once treatment with rHuEPO has been started, there are some early indicators of patient response. After 2 weeks of treatment, an EPO level of up to 100 mU/mL and an increase in hemoglobin of at least 0.5 g/dL are predictive of a response 95% of the time; a serum ferritin level of up to 400 ng/mL predicts a positive response 88% of the time. A retrospective analysis of 413 patients with cancer divided the patients into chemotherapy and nonchemotherapy groups. In the nonchemotherapy group, an increase in hemoglobin of at least 0.5 g/dL with an increase in the reticulocyte count of

at least 40,000 cells/μL after 2 weeks correlated with a positive response 91% of the time. For patients on chemotherapy, evaluation at 4 weeks was more informative. If the hemoglobin had increased at least 1 g/dL combined with a reticulocyte increase of at least 40,000/μL above baseline, there was an 84% likelihood of a positive response.

The result obtained in a well-controlled clinical trial cannot always be reproduced in a clinical setting. A Phase IV study of the impact of rHuEPO on anemia in patients with nonmyeloid malignancies was conducted in a community oncology setting,[43] and 2342 patients were enrolled through more than 500 community-based oncologists. Data were available for 2030 patients, of whom 1047 completed 4 months of therapy. The mean hematocrit/hemoglobin was 27.55%/9.2 g/dL. The mean patient age was 62.2 years, and 62% were women. Transfusions in the prestudy period were 0.57 per patient per month. The mean quality-of-life score was 45 on a scale of 100. Ninety-nine percent of patients received chemotherapy while on the study. Therapy was initiated with 150 U/kg rHuEPO administered subcutaneously three times a week; if there was no response after 8 weeks, the dose could be increased to 300 U/kg. However, physicians did not always increase the dose of rHuEPO when a patient was not responding to the initial dose. A response, defined as an increase in hemoglobin of at least 2 g without transfusion, was achieved by 53.4% of patients. Treatment was associated with a 50% decrease in the number of patients receiving transfusions and the number of transfusions per patient. In addition, there were medium to large increases in the score for the three parameters of quality-of-life—energy, activity, and overall quality of life. Overall, these studies indicate that rHuEPO has improved the hemoglobin level, decreased the need for transfusion, and improved the quality of life in cancer patients.

Anemia of Prematurity

The pathophysiology of neonatal anemia in normal and premature infants has been summarized elsewhere.[44] In normal infants, the lowest observed hemoglobin is approximately 9 g/dL, occurring at 10-12 weeks of age. In premature infants, the hemoglobin level is lower and occurs earlier. In infants weighing 1-1.5 kg, the hemoglobin nadir is approximately 8 g/dL, and in infants weighing less than 1.0 kg, the nadir is 7 g/dL. Superimposed on this naturally occurring anemia is iatrogenic blood loss related to the laboratory tests, which must be performed to manage critically ill infants. Estimates of the volume of blood removed for laboratory tests vary from 0.8 to 3.1 mL/kg per day.[45]

Current models of the anemia of prematurity are based on a deficient erythropoietic response due largely to inappropriately low EPO levels.[46] At term, erythropoietin production is primarily hepatic and it is postulated that hepatic erythropoietin production is less responsive to hypoxia than renal production. Erythroid progenitors in premature infants are normal in number and in their responsiveness to stimulation with EPO. Altered metabolism of EPO in premature infants may contribute to the inappropriately low levels of EPO observed.

In the past, allogeneic blood transfusions were routinely used to treat the anemia of prematurity and to replace blood losses related to laboratory tests. Neonatologists, concerned about transfusion-transmitted diseases and the immunosuppression associated with blood transfusion, have pursued parallel approaches in reducing the volumes of allogeneic blood transfused to neonates. They have tried to identify infants who would benefit most from treatment with rHuEPO and have worked to define the dosage and schedule for producing the optimal response. In addition, they have worked with blood banks to develop more conservative transfusion policies, allowed hematocrits to reach lower levels before transfusion, and worked to limit donor exposure.

The major clinical trials using rHuEPO to treat the anemia of prematurity were reviewed in 1997.[46] Most studies focused on infants weighing less than 1.5 kg. All studies used iron supplementation; some used protein supplementation. Use of vitamin E and multiple vitamin supplements varied. The studies were divided into those in which EPO was administered during the first week of life and those in which administration was begun about the third week of life. Seven trials initiated EPO therapy within the first week of life. The dose of EPO varied from 70 to 1400 U/kg per week. At doses below 300 U/kg per week, there was no evidence of an effect, and the results at 300 U/kg per week were equivocal. However, at doses of 750 U/kg per week, the study groups showed higher reticulocyte counts and hemoglobins and/or hematocrits. The number of patients transfused was lower in the study group, as was the number of transfusions given. A study of EPO in extremely-low-birthweight infants (<750 g) in whom therapy was started in the first 72 hours of life also shows promising results.[47] Infants were given EPO (200 U/kg/day) or placebo for 14 days and were maintained on the study for 21 days with similar transfusion guidelines. All infants received iron 1 mg/kg per day in their total parenteral nutrition solution. The number and volume of transfusions received were lower in the study group than in the placebo group (4.7±0.7 transfusions at 70±11 mL/kg per patient in the EPO group vs 7.5±1.1 transfusions at 112±17 mL/kg per patient in the control group). The reticulocyte count was higher and the ferritin concentration lower in the EPO group at day 14. Twelve trials evaluated EPO therapy initiated at week three. Doses below 300 U/kg per week produced no effect; doses between 450 and 500 U/kg per week produced higher hematocrits and reticulocyte counts but no difference in transfusions. At doses of 600-900 U/kg per week, however, reticulocyte counts and hematocrits were higher in 11 of the 12 studies. Fewer infants were transfused in the treated group and fewer transfusions were given.

Altogether, the results of these clinical trials indicate a positive effect of rHuEPO on the anemia of prematurity as manifested by decreased numbers and volumes of transfusions. Preliminary studies indicate that infants with severe hemolytic disease of the newborn and bronchopulmonary dysplasia might also benefit from rHuEPO treatment.[47-49] Although studies suggest that iron supplementation is needed, it is not yet clear that oral iron supplementation permits EPO-driven erythropoiesis without the development of iron deficiency in all patients. Some infants may require parenteral iron. Earlier concerns about reduced neutrophil counts have not been a concern in more recent trials. Measurements of PBPCs in patients receiving 300 U rHuEPO subcutaneously three times a week did not identify an effect on myeloid progenitors using colony-forming assays and flow cytometry.[50]

The recommended treatment for anemia of prematurity in a 1997 review was that rHuEPO be started early in premature infants 750-1300 g in weight at a dose of 250 U/kg subcutaneously three times a week (from week 1 to week 6 of life) with iron supplementation (elemental iron 5 mg/kg/day).[13] Although there are clearly benefits associated with rHuEPO use, however, the cost-effectiveness of this treatment relative to the cost of modifications in transfusion practices is a serious issue.

A single center review of neonatal transfusion practices for the years 1982, 1989, and 1993 indicated that the number of transfusions given to neonates gradually declined from 7±7.4 in 1982 to 2.3±2.7 in 1993.[51] While the percentage of very-low-birthweight infants never receiving transfusions increased from 17% in 1982 to 64% in 1993, more than 95% of infants weighing less than 1 kg were transfused in each year. Thus, there will be a population of infants who are so ill that transfusion will be required even with rHuEPO treatment.

Some blood banks have a practice of assigning one unit to a specific patient. When policies required that neonatal patients always be tranfused with anticoagulated (CPDA-1) blood less than 7 days old, it was difficult to reduce donor exposure. A study comparing clinical and biochemical parameters in patients receiving CPDA-1 blood up to 7 days old and receiving additive solution (AS-1) blood up to 42 days old for small replacement transfusions demonstrated no difference in the patient groups, making it possible to extend the shelf life of the assigned unit.[52] Implementation of this type of program reduced donor exposure. Patients receiving AS-1 red cells were exposed to 1.6 donors, whereas patients receiving CPDA-1 units were exposed to 3.7 donors. This benefit was confirmed in another study, which used an expiration period of 30 days for neonatal units, where 56% of neonates were exposed to one donor and 89% of neonates to one to two donors.[53]

Studies that have tried to evaluate the cost-effectiveness of standard transfusions vs rHuEPO therapy with transfusion as needed have had variable results. One of the large European trials concluded that the cost of treatment with rHuEPO was $1262 and the cost for controls was $1203, including an adjustment for hepatitis C exposure. A US study reported that the cost of transfusion and rHuEPO was $129 per patient whereas the cost of transfusions alone was $256.[46] However, another US study concluded that treatment with rHuEPO cost 3.6 times more than the standard management with transfusion.[54] Studies that provide a better understanding of the pharmacokinetics in extremely-low-birthweight and very-low-birthweight infants may provide information leading to the more effective use of rHuEPO in this very vulnerable age group.

HIV Infection

Anemia, a common hematologic abnormality in patients with HIV infection, may be related to many different factors.[55] Hematopoiesis may be depressed by direct infection with the virus, and viral infection of marrow endothelium reduces stromal production of hematopoietic growth factors. Tumor necrosis factor-α production may be increased and erythropoietin levels are low.[55,56] In untreated patients, the most common form of anemia is the normochromic normocytic anemia seen in patients with chronic disease. The reticulocyte count is low and the serum ferritin concentration is elevated. Treatment with antiretroviral drugs, especially zidovudine, causes the anemia to increase in severity and the red cells become macrocytic. In early clinical trials, 31.3% of patients had a hemoglobin level below 7.0 g/dL and 46% required red cell transfusions. In a randomized, double-blind, placebo-controlled trial of rHuEPO (100 U/kg three times a week IV bolus) in patients treated with zidovudine, both the number of patients transfused and the number of transfusions per patient appeared to be reduced by the second month of the study.[57] The response to rHuEPO was observed in patients with serum EPO levels of up to 500 U/L prior to study entry. Subsequent combined analysis of the original and three other clinical trials confirmed the ability of rHuEPO (at doses of 100-200 U/kg three times a week) to increase the hematocrit and reduce the transfusion requirement in zidovudine-treated acquired immune deficiency syndrome (AIDS) patients with EPO levels up to 500 U/L.[58] An open-label, multicenter trial of rHuEPO among 1943 patients demonstrated an increase in hematocrit from a baseline of 28% to 33.8% at week 24 of the study. Further, 40% of patients required at least one transfusion in the 6 weeks prior to study, but only 18% of patients required transfusion by week 24. Two other trials of rHuEPO in AIDS patients not treated with zidovudine also demonstrated clinical responses when the serum rHuEPO level was not more than 500 U/L.[59,60] The few trials of rHuEPO performed in pediatric patients suggest that rHuEPO is equally effective in children.[61,62]

Chronic Inflammatory Diseases

Anemia is a common problem in patients with chronic inflammatory diseases such as rheumatoid arthritis and inflammatory bowel disease. Inappropriately low serum EPO levels and increased production of proinflammatory cytokines such as IL-1 and tumor necrosis factor-α have been described in many of these disorders. However, other factors may play a substantial role in the development of anemia. For example, iron deficiency related to gastrointestinal blood loss and vitamin deficiencies caused by malabsorption should be considered in inflammatory bowel disease. In systemic-onset juvenile chronic arthritis, a severe microcytic anemia is often present, which might suggest the involvement of an erythropoietin deficiency. The elevated levels of IL-6 in this disease appear to correlate with disease activity and would tend to support the impression that this anemia is the anemia of chronic disease. However, laboratory evaluation of a group of such patients revealed that EPO levels were appropriate and that iron deficiency was playing a major role in the anemia.[63] The patients appeared to have a defect in iron absorption and problems with iron mobilization. Intravenous, but not oral, iron corrected the anemia. Thus, even when patients have a chronic inflammatory condition in which inflammatory cytokines are known to increase, other causes for anemia must be excluded.

Early clinical trials in rheumatoid arthritis demonstrated that rHuEPO corrected anemia in many patients but did not appear to improve their ability to perform activities of daily living or to decrease their pain.[64] The investigators recommended that EPO therapy be reserved for severely anemic patients and for patients scheduled for elective orthopedic surgery. A 1997 study has demonstrated that rHuEPO can be used to facilitate preoperative autologous donation in rheumatoid arthritis patients.[65] Iron supplementation may be needed.

The anemia associated with inflammatory bowel disease has also been treated with rHuEPO.[66-68] A placebo-controlled trial of rHuEPO and iron saccharate was conducted among patients with Crohn's disease. The treated group received rHuEPO 150 U/kg three times a week with IV iron saccharate; the control group received only iron. Ninety-four percent of the treated group had an increase in hemoglobin of at least 2 g compared with 66% of the placebo group. However, the increase in hemoglobin, which was associated with increased quality of life in both groups, was faster and higher in the EPO-treated group. A small study among pediatric patients with Crohn's disease had similar results.[68] In another study that included 15 patients with ulcerative colitis as well as 19 patients with Crohn's disease, anemia refractory to iron therapy was treated with either rHuEPO (150 U/kg subcutaneously twice a week) and oral iron supplementation or placebo. Hemoglobin levels in the treated group increased from 8.81±0.27 g/dL to 10.52±0.41 g/dL, whereas the hemoglobin concentration decreased in the placebo group. These studies suggest that the correction of anemia in patients with inflammatory bowel disease can lead to important improvements in their quality of life.

Myelodysplastic Syndromes and Other Stem Cell Disorders

The myelodysplastic syndromes are a group of heterogeneous stem cell disorders characterized by ineffective hematopoiesis and variable degrees of peripheral cytopenia. Symptomatic anemia requiring transfusion is one of the most common clinical problems encountered in these patients, although neutropenia and variable degrees of thrombocytopenia are also present. Patients with myelodysplastic syndromes may have elevated or normal levels of serum EPO. Both in-vivo and in-vitro erythropoiesis are ineffective and data suggest that impaired responses to erythropoietin are present. Recent studies demonstrated that receptors are present in normal numbers in marrow cells from patients with myelodysplasia and that the binding of EPO to its receptor occurs. However, signal transduction following EPO binding is abnormal.[69] In normal marrow erythroid cells, STAT5 is activated after EPO binds to its receptor. However, following stimulation with EPO in 15 samples from patients with myelodysplasia, STAT5 activation was absent in 11 and greatly depressed in 4.

Early clinical trials of rHuEPO in myelodysplastic syndromes produced variable results. A meta-analysis of 205 patients from 17 studies revealed that 16% of patients showed a significant response to treatment.[70] Patients with refractory anemia with ringed sideroblasts had a lower response rate than other groups. Patients not requiring transfusion had a better response rate than patients needing transfusion (44% vs 10%), and responders also had lower serum EPO levels. In an open-label, multicenter, compassionate treatment trial, 100 patients received rHuEPO beginning at 150 U/kg three times a week, with escalations of up to 300 U/kg three times a week.[71] Clinical responses were defined as a six-point increase in hematocrit or a 50% decrease in transfusion requirement. Ten of 100 patients achieved a clinical response using the hematocrit criterion, and 18 patients had a reduction in transfusion requirement for an overall response rate of 28%. Thirty-nine percent of patients with the refractory anemia subtype responded to

rHuEPO, and 54% of patients in this category with EPO levels below 100 mU/mL were responders.

In-vitro studies demonstrated synergy between EPO and G-CSF in normal and myelodysplastic syndrome erythropoiesis, leading clinical investigators to evaluate the combination in clinical trials.[72] Twenty-four patients received G-CSF at 1 μg/kg daily, adjusted to normalize or double the neutrophil count, and rHuEPO 100 U/kg per day with dose escalations up to 300 U/kg per day was added. Ten of 24 patients (42%) had erythroid responses, and 6 of these were able to discontinue red cell transfusions during the treatment period. In 1996, the investigators reported follow-up on the original patients and additional patients enrolled in this treatment protocol.[73] Of the 55 patients enrolled in the extended study, 44 were evaluable for an erythroid response. Twenty-one patients (48%) were erythroid responders and 17 of 21 (80%) continued to respond during the maintenance phase. Eight patients were subsequently maintained on EPO alone, and seven required G-CSF plus EPO. Responders had lower pretreatment serum EPO levels and lower transfusion requirements. The dose of EPO required to produce the response was high, generally 300 U/kg per day. The median duration of response was 11 months with 35% of maintenance-phase responders having durable responses for 15-36 months.

The anemia of aplastic anemia is not considered to be responsive to treatment with EPO.[12] However, there is a 1997 report in which rHuEOP and G-CSF produced an erythroid response in patients with nonsevere aplastic anemia, suggesting that growth factor therapy may be helpful in a small subset of patients.[74] There is also a report of pure red cell aplasia following peripheral stem cell transplantation that responded to rHuEPO.[25]

Sickle Cell Anemia and Thalassemia

Erythropoietin levels in patients with sickle cell anemia have been reported to be low for the degree of anemia and to be appropriate or elevated in thalassemia. Erythropoietin has the ability to stimulate synthesis of fetal hemoglobin (HbF). In sickle cell disease, increased HbF levels are associated with milder disease. In thalassemia, increased production of gamma chains could decrease the number of unpaired insoluble alpha globin chains. The administration of exogenous EPO to baboons increases gamma chain synthesis, resulting in an increase in HbF.[75] In preliminary clinical studies, EPO with iron supplementation transiently increased F-reticulocyte production in sickle cell anemia patients.[76] The administration of rHuEPO to thalassemic mice and the retrovirus-mediated transfer of the EPO gene in thalassemic mice improves the ratio of alpha/nonalpha chains, improving erythrocyte survival.[77] In clinical studies of patients with sickle cell anemia, administration of EPO alone did not increase HbF synthesis, but when rHuEPO with iron supplementation alternating with hydroxyurea was given, HbF and F-cell levels were higher than they were with hydroxyurea treatment alone.[78] In thalassemia intermedia, a preliminary clinical trial of rHuEPO 1,000 U/kg twice a week in three patients produced an increase in hemoglobin/hematocrit without consistent changes in total HbF, F cells, or F reticulocytes.[79] In another small trial in thalassemia intermedia, two patients experienced an increase in hemoglobin preceded by an increase in F reticulocytes and F cells, but no increase in overall HbF levels.[80] For one patient, the increase in hematocrit was associated with an increase in the level of HbF. In a larger trial, 8 of 10 patients with thalassemia intermedia treated with 500-1000 U/kg subcutaneously three times a week showed an increase in hemoglobin of at least 2 g/dL during the study, with only one patient requiring blood transfusion.[81] There was once again no change in HbF or F cells. Hemoglobin levels returned to normal over 1-2 months after rHuEPO was discontinued. In thalassemia major, a trial of rHuEPO 750 U/kg three times a week in 10 patients from four separate families produced an increase in hemoglobin in six of seven splenectomized patients and in one of three nonsplenectomized patients.[82] There was no increase in HbF, but the percentage of F cells increased in three patients and that of F reticulocytes increased in five patients. The administration of rHuEPO to a larger group of 26 patients with transfusion-dependent β-thalassemia was less successful, with only 3/26 patients demonstrating an increase in hemoglobin.[83] Further research is needed to determine which HbF-inducing agents provide optimal clinical results with the least toxicity. Preclinical studies in the β-thalassemic mouse model suggest that combination therapy with erythropoietin, hydroxyurea, and clotrimazole might be a combination to consider.[84]

Myeloid Hematopoietic Growth Factors: Granulocyte-Macrophage Colony-Stimulating Factor and Granulocyte Colony-Stimulating Factor

GM-CSF and G-CSF were purified and cloned in the mid-1980s. GM-CSF is a glycoprotein that promotes the survival, proliferation, and differentiation of myeloid precursors. In vivo, pharmacologic doses of GM-CSF lead to an increase in the number of neutrophils, eosinophils, and monocytes in the peripheral blood. G-CSF, also a glycoprotein, promotes the proliferation and differentiation of neutrophilic precursors, producing an increase in neutrophilic granulocytes in the peripheral blood. Both factors mobilize hematopoietic progenitor cells into the peripheral blood and enhance the function of mature cells.

In 1991, the FDA approved both factors for clinical use. Initially, GM-CSF [sargramostim (Leukine); Immunex, Seattle, WA] was approved to accelerate neutrophil recovery following autologous marrow transplantation for lymphoid malignancies, and G-CSF [filgrastim (Neupogen); Amgen] was approved to decrease the incidence of febrile neutropenia in patients receiving myelosuppressive chemotherapy. Over the next few years, clinical trials identified other potential applications in patients with solid tumors and hematologic malignancies and demonstrated that the neutropenia associated with myelodysplasia and other forms of acquired and congenital neutropenia might respond to treatment with G-CSF or GM-CSF.

As clinicians gained experience using these growth factors, some expressed a preference for G-CSF over GM-CSF. In the United States, more than 80% of physicians queried preferred to use G-CSF, the most common reasons being concerns about toxicity, efficacy, and the original FDA approval indication.[85] Studies exploring potential transfusion medicine applications in healthy blood donors have primarily used G-CSF because of concerns about the adverse effects of GM-CSF, as discussed below under pharmacokinetics. Currently, G-CSF is being used on an investigational basis to mobilize hematopoietic progenitor cells in related and unrelated stem cell donors and to increase the granulocyte yield in apheresis procedures.

Granulocyte-Macrophage Colony-Stimulating Factor

Biology

The biology of GM-CSF is summarized in earlier reviews.[86,87] Human GM-CSF was isolated from conditioned medium from the T-lymphoblast cell line Mo. The gene for human GM-CSF, cloned independently by two laboratories, is located on chromosome 5 (5q21-32). The gene encodes a protein of 127 amino acids. The molecular weight of the protein moiety alone is approximately 14,000 daltons. Both natural and recombinant human GM-CSF vary in molecular weight from 14,000 to 30,000 daltons because of differences in glycosylation.

GM-CSF mediates its effects by binding to a specific cell surface receptor. These receptors are located primarily on normal hematopoietic cells, which have 100-300 receptors per cell, but they have also been found on myeloid and lymphoid leukemia cells and on a variety of tumor cell lines, including melanoma, small cell carcinoma of the lung, and osteogenic sarcoma. Circulating soluble receptors have also been identified. The number of receptors on myeloid cells increases as cells mature. Early studies of GM-CSF receptors referred to high-affinity and low-affinity receptors. Cloning studies of GM-CSF receptors have demonstrated

that the receptor has two subunits, an alpha subunit involved with ligand-specific binding and a beta subunit that is shared by GM-CSF, IL-3, and IL-5.[88] Both chains appear to participate in signal transduction. Experimental data suggest that some GM-CSF receptor alpha and beta complexes are present prior to ligand binding but that binding of GM-CSF promotes subunit heterodimerization. Once GM-CSF has bound to the receptor, the receptor is rapidly internalized.

GM-CSF is produced by a large number of cell types, including T lymphocytes, macrophages, endothelial cells, and fibroblasts. Under normal circumstances, GM-CSF is not detectable in the circulation, which suggests that it is not the primary regulator of leukocyte production. GM-CSF knockout mice have normal basal hematopoiesis. However, such mice develop a syndrome similar to human pulmonary alveolar proteinosis.[89] When GM-CSF is overexpressed in marrow cells transduced with a retrovirus carrying the cDNA for murine GM-CSF, the mice develop a nonmalignant but fatal myeloproliferative disorder.[90]

In-vitro studies demonstrated that GM-CSF supports the development of murine and human multilineage colonies containing neutrophils, eosinophils, and macrophages. In the murine system, high doses of GM-CSF also support the development of multilineage colonies and megakaryocytes. GM-CSF maintains the viability of neutrophils in culture by inhibiting apoptosis.[91] In combination with erythropoietin, human GM-CSF stimulates multipotential progenitor cells and early erythroid progenitors.

In normal animals and humans, SC and IV doses of GM-CSF initially cause a transient leukopenia beginning within 5 minutes, with neutrophils, eosinophils, and monocytes disappearing from the circulation. By 2 hours, the cells begin to return to the circulation with neutrophil counts peaking at 8 hours after a single dose. Neutrophilia persists and increases with continued dosing.[92] After a single dose of GM-CSF, the peak counts for eosinophils and monocytes occur at 24 hours. The increase in neutrophils during the first 72 hours of treatment is thought to be caused by mobilization of neutrophils and neutrophil precursors from the marrow. Beyond 72 hours, increased marrow production of neutrophils is responsible for the elevated counts. GM-CSF increased neutrophil production 1.5-fold.[86,87]

GM-CSF enhances the function of mature effector cells.[86,87,92] Neutrophils have enhanced degranulation, chemotaxis, phagocytosis, superoxide generation, arachidonic acid release, and synthesis of leukotrienes and plasminogen-activating factor. There is also decreased L-selectin expression, enhanced antibody-dependent tumor killing, and inhibition of random migration. Eosinophils also demonstrate evidence of degranulation, decreased L-selectin expression, and leukotriene synthesis. Monocytes exhibit increased phagocytosis; increased intracellular killing; increased antibody-dependent cell cytotoxicity and tumor killing; increased gene expression or release of G-CSF, IL-1, IL-6, tumor necrosis factor-α and GM-CSF; increased expression of major histocompatibility comple Class II antigens; and augmented antigen presentation.

Pharmacokinetics

For GM-CSF (sargramostim), the usual adult dose is 250 μg/m² per day. The dose may be administered intravenously over 2-4 hours or subcutaneously once a day. For mobilization of PBPCs and myeloid reconstitution after marrow transplantation, a 24-hour IV infusion or SC administration is recommended. Pharmacokinetic studies in children indicate that a higher dosage is needed to obtain the same biologic effect.[93] In studies using a yeast-expressed GM-CSF, children required at least 750 μg/m² to achieve the same effect as 250-500 μg/m² in adults. The half-life of clearance for the 2-hour infusion is 1.5-2 hours. With SC administration, blood levels peak at 2 hours and the half-life is 3 hours.

Fever, myalgia, headache, bone pain, rash, local reactions at the injection site, excessive leukocytosis, edema, capillary leak syndrome, pericardial and pleural effusions, supraventricular arrhythmias, and respiratory symptoms, as well as eleva-

tion of creatinine, bilirubin, and liver enzymes, have been observed after administration. Respiratory symptoms that occur shortly after administration may be related to pulmonary sequestration of leukocytes.[94]

Some patients have also had a very severe first-time reaction characterized by flushing, hypotension, tachycardia, dyspnea, nausea, vomiting, and hypoxia. This reaction appears to be more common with IV administration and usually responds to symptomatic treatment. Although rare, eosinophilic pneumonia has also been reported.[95]

Granulocyte Colony-Stimulating Factor

Biology

The biology of G-CSF and its receptor are summarized in reviews from 1996.[96,97] G-CSF was first identified as a granulocyte-macrophage differentiation factor in serum from endotoxin-treated mice.[96] This factor could induce the differentiation of the murine myelomonocytic leukemia cell line WEHI-3B(D⁺). The scientific observations leading to the recognition of G-CSF as a unique myeloid hematopoietic growth factor are described in an earlier review.[96] The gene for G-CSF, located on chromosome 17 (17q21-22), encodes a polypeptide chain of 174 amino acids. The predicted molecular weight of the protein is 18,672 daltons; the purified natural protein has a molecular weight of 19,600 daltons. Recombinant human G-CSF produced in *Escherichia coli* and Chinese hamster ovary cells has a molecular weight of 18,700 daltons and 21,600 daltons, respectively. The protein expressed in Chinese hamster ovary cells is glycosylated.

The biologic effects of G-CSF are mediated by interaction with a specific receptor.[97] The gene of the G-CSF receptor is located on chromosome 1 (1p35-34.3). G-CSF receptors are expressed on myeloid progenitor cells, myeloid leukemia cells, mature neutrophils, monocytes, platelets, and some B- and T-lymphoid cell lines. They have also been identified on endothelial cells, placenta, and some small cell lung carcinoma cell lines. The number of receptors increases as granulocytic precursors mature, with mature neutrophils having 200-1000 receptors per cell. Molecular cloning of G-CSF receptors indicates that the human receptor is a transmembrane polypeptide of 813 amino acids with singular extracellular, transmembrane, and cytoplasmic domains. The first 200 N-terminal amino acids are important for ligand binding. Five different G-CSF receptor classes arise from alternative splicing of mRNA. One form (Class II) codes for a soluble receptor. Neutrophils express primarily high-affinity Class I receptors, as well as lower levels of Class IV and V receptors. Human placenta expresses Class II and IV receptors. HL-60 also expresses Class II receptors. Class I and IV receptors can generate mitogenic signals, but only Class I receptors can transduce maturation signals when transfected into receptor-negative myeloid cell lines. When G-CSF binds to its receptor, the receptor is internalized.

In healthy individuals, the level of G-CSF is usually below the limits of detection of the most sensitive immunoassays (≤ 30 pg/mL). During infection, stress, and neutropenia, blood levels of G-CSF may exceed 2000 pg/mL. G-CSF knockout mice appear healthy but have chronic neutropenia, with blood neutrophil levels that are 20-30% of those found in the wild-type mouse. In the marrow, neutrophilic precursors are decreased 50%. G-CSF knockout mice have impaired ability to control infections with *Listeria* monocytogenes, demonstrating a defect in infection-driven granulopoiesis and monocyte production.[98]

In-vitro studies indicate that the effects of G-CSF are primarily on cells of the neutrophilic lineage. Cultures of marrow cells enriched for CD34+, CD33- cells produce few neutrophilic colonies when stimulated by G-CSF. However, G-CSF can effectively stimulate CD34+, CD33+ cells that are committed to myeloid differentiation. G-CSF alone cannot support the growth of multilineage hematopoietic cells, but it exhibits synergistic activity with GM-CSF, IL-3, and IL-6 in supporting multilineage hematopoiesis.

The administration of G-CSF results in an immediate but transient leukopenia, caused by a decrease of neutrophils in the peripheral blood.[86,99] The nadir in leukocyte count occurs 5-15 minutes after IV administration and 30-60 minutes after SC administration. The neutropenia lasts less than an hour, and then the neutrophils increase in number with the neutrophilia being dose-dependent. The leukocytosis induced by G-CSF is associated, with a left-shifted myelopoiesis, and myelocytes, promyelocytes, and even myeloblasts may be seen. Neutrophil production is increased 9.4-fold by G-CSF. At doses greater than 10 µg/kg per day, G-CSF can also induce an increase in monocytes and lymphocytes. Most studies have not demonstrated an effect of G-CSF on eosinophils. However, a recent investigation using 7.5-10 µg/kg per day for 6 consecutive days in healthy donors reported an increase in eosinophil counts from $0.22 \pm 0.04 \times 10^9$/L to $0.6 \pm 0.098 \times 10^9$/L.[100] This increase in eosinophils, first occurring on day 2 of treatment, was accompanied by an increase in serum levels of eosinophil granule proteins. Because eosinophils do not have a G-CSF receptor, the effect must be indirect. At high doses of G-CSF (10-60 µg/kg per day), a decrease in platelets is observed. Once G-CSF is discontinued, leukocyte counts return to normal in 4-7 days.

Pharmacokinetics

The two most commonly used forms of G-CSF available are filgrastim, a nonglycosylated recombinant G-CSF produced in *E. coli*, and lenograstim, a glycosylated G-CSF. As of August 1998, only filgrastim has been approved for use in the United States, but both products are available in Europe. In some studies, lenograstim appears to be more efficacious than filgrastim for mobilization of PBPCs. When normal donors were given first one and then the other at a dose of 5 µg/kg per day for 6 days in crossover studies, the average GM-CFU count on days 5, 6, and 7 was 28% higher with lenograstim, even though higher serum concentrations were obtained with filgrastim.[101] A brief report published in 1997 emphasizes that mass units are not equivalent for recombinant products and that when bioequivalent doses are used (using the World Health

Organization international potency standard), the in-vivo effects on PBPC mobilization are the same.[102]

G-CSF can be administered subcutaneously or intravenously.[103] When G-CSF was administered intravenously at 3.5 μg/kg to healthy volunteers, the half-life was 163 ± 7.4 minutes, with G-CSF levels returning to normal within 14-18 hours. In other studies, the terminal phase elimination half-lives ranged from 1.3 to 7.2 hours. Following SC administration, absorption is variable and peak levels may be reached between 2 and 8 hours. The half-life elimination time is approximately 3 hours. Serum G-CSF levels remain above baseline levels for 10-16 hours. Adverse effects associated with G-CSF use include fatigue, arthralgias, myalgias, medullary bone pain, mild to moderate headache, skin rash, itching, excessive leukocytosis, and redness or pain at the injection site. Sweet's syndrome has also been reported.[104] The development of osteoporosis has been described in patients with congenital neutropenia.[105]

Clinical Applications of Granulocyte Colony-Stimulating Factor and Granulocyte-Macrophage Colony-Stimulating Factor

Normal Donors

G-CSF is being used (with Institutional Review Board approval in the United States) to improve the yield of granulocytes collected with apheresis procedures[106-109] and to mobilize and collect PBPCs from HLA-identical related and unrelated stem cell donors.[110-112] The doses used for granulocyte collections have varied from 3.5 to 10 μg/kg per day subcutaneously with the first dose being given 12 hours before the apheresis procedure was scheduled. With G-CSF stimulation, the yield of granulocytes is reported to be sixfold greater than that collected from historic controls. Either hydroxyethyl starch or dextran is used to accelerate sedimentation. A regimen using the combination of G-CSF (600 μg subcutaneously) and dexamethasone (8 mg orally) appears to provide better results than G-CSF alone.[109] In a Phase I/II clinical trial of

granulocyte transfusions obtained from unrelated donors stimulated with this protocol, the median granulocyte number in transfusions was 7.8×10^{10}. In addition to granulocytes, these products also contain substantial numbers of platelets. No side effects were experienced by 28% of donors but bone pain, headache, and insomnia were reported by 41%, 30%, and 30%, respectively. Data are inadequate to determine if these transfusions improve clinical outcomes.

G-CSF mobilization of progenitor cells was initially used for patients receiving autologous stem cell transplants.[110] Since 1995, a number of centers have been reporting the use of allogeneic PBPCs in patients with advanced hematologic malignancies.[111-115] In most instances, the allogeneic donor is an HLA-identical sibling or alternative family donor,[113] but the National Marrow Donor Program is collecting PBPCs for some retransplantations in which the original stem cell donation was marrow. Because of the increasing use of G-CSF to mobilize PBPCs in healthy donors, two scientific groups convened to discuss the scientific and ethical issues relating to this practice.[114,115] The European Group for Blood and Marrow Transplantation made five recommendations: 1) that donors should be mobilized with G-CSF at a dose of 10 μg/kg per day, with leukapheresis initiated on the day following the fourth dose; 2) that leukapheresis should be performed on a continuous flow blood cell separator using peripheral veins, with each procedure processing 15 L of blood; 3) that the minimum dose of $CD34^+$ cells should be $2-3 \times 10^{10}$ cells per kg of recipient weight; 4) that PBPCs should be given without cryopreservation whenever possible; and 5) that recipients should receive standard conditioning and graft-vs-host disease prophylaxis. Finally, the group suggested that follow-up on the donor and the recipient should be made to a registry.[114]

A subsequent meeting involving the International Bone Marrow Transplant Registry, the National Marrow Donor Program, and the aforementioned European group focused specifically on donor safety issues.[115] Tnis group affirmed that G-CSF treatment and stem cell collection appear to be safe and that doses up to 10 µg/kg per day show a consistent dose-response relationship for the mobilization of CD34$^+$ PBPCs and are acceptable for routine clinical use.[115] They observed that many centers were concerned about excessive leukocytosis (70 × 10^9/L) and were reducing the G-CSF dose to maintain a lower leukocyte count. They further stated that transient postdonation cytopenias of granulocytes, lymphocytes, and platelets might occur and are in part related to the apheresis procedure, are self-limiting, and require no treatment. They recommended reinfusion of autologous platelet-rich plasma if postdonation thrombocytopenia was expected (≤80-100 × 10^9). They agreed that donors should meet the same eligibility criteria that apply to the donors of apheresis platelets, except that pediatric donors are acceptable. This group also recommended the development of a registry to monitor donor and recipient outcomes.

Cancer

The American Society of Clinical Oncology has developed evidence-based clinical practice guidelines for the use of CSFs in cancer patients.[116] Initially published in 1994, these guidelines were reviewed and updated in 1996.[117] The guidelines address primary and secondary prophylaxis; the use of CSFs in afebrile and febrile neutropenia, stem cell transplantation, and myeloid leukemia; the role of CSFs in increasing chemotherapy dose intensity; concurrent chemotherapy and radiotherapy; pediatric applications; dosing and duration of therapy; and comparative activity of G-CSF and GM-CSF. These recommendations are summarized in a quick reference form in Table 20-3. CSFs are not recommended for the treatment of afebrile neutropenia, and one recently published trial provides continuing support for that recommendation.[118] Recent clinical trials using G-CSF and GM-CSF in cancer patients are summarized in Table 20-4.[118-126]

In acute leukemia, CSFs are used to limit myelotoxicity and to alter the chemoresistance of residual disease. Priming with CSFs to alter chemoresistance is considered experimental. However, for acute myeloid leukemia (AML), use of CSFs to shorten the duration of neutropenia after completion of induction chemotherapy, especially in patients at least 55 years of age, is recommended. Five major studies in patients with acute leukemia have been published since the last revision of the American Society of Clinical Oncology guidelines, two in children[119,120] and four in adults.[121-124] In children with acute lymphoblastic leukemia treated with G-CSF 10 µg/kg per day beginning one day after completion of remission induction chemotherapy, there was no difference in the rates of hospitalization for febrile neutropenia and no decrease in the number of severe infections, but there was a decrease in the number of documented infections and there were shorter hospital stays.[120] In a large, randomized, placebo-controlled trial of adult patients with de-novo AML, treatment with G-CSF 5 µg/kg per day beginning 24 hours after the last dose of induction or consolidation chemotherapy accelerated neutrophil recovery and decreased the frequency and duration of hospitalization.[123] The number of patients requiring systemic antifungal therapy was also reduced. It is noteworthy that a Phase II study of G-CSF with a consolidation cycle using aziridinyl benzoquinone and mitoxantrone also demonstrated a decrease in the frequency and duration of hospitalization.[121] A large, prospective, randomized trial of GM-CSF in AML demonstrated accelerated neutrophil recovery but not a difference in clinical outcomes.[122] For adults with acute lymphoblastic leukemia, the use of G-CSF also appears to have clinical benefit.[124] In all these studies, the use of G-CSF or GM-CSF did not affect survival or disease-free survival. Two studies published in 1997 used G-CSF after PBPC transplantation.[125,126] In addition to accelerated neutrophil recovery, both studies demonstrated a decreased hospital stay. The dose of G-CSF in one study was 50 µg/m^2, a dose that could make the use of G-CSF more cost-effective.[125]

Overall, these studies provide additional support for the use of G-CSF in adults with leukemia to shorten the duration of neutropenia and reduce infection, and they suggest that the use of CSFs is not associated with relapse or a shorter duration of re-

Table 20-3. American Society of Clinical Oncology Clinical Guidelines for the Use of Hematopoietic Colony-Stimulating Factors (CSFs)[116]

Guideline	Recommendation
1. Primary prophylactic CSF administration	
General circumstances	*CSF administration reserved for patients expected to have an incidence of neutropenia ≥40%.
Special circumstances	Additional factors that might warrant CSF administration include 1) preexisting neutropenia due to disease, or previous extensive chemotherapy or radiation to pelvis or other areas containing marrow; 2) history of recurrent febrile neutropenia on similar or lesser dose intensity; 3) other conditions enhancing the risk of infection, such as decreased immune function, open wounds, or tissue infection; 4) poor performance status and more advanced cancer.
2. Secondary prophylactic CSF administration	CSF can decrease the probability of febrile neutropenia in subsequent cycles of chemotherapy after documented occurrence.
	If prolonged neutropenia is causing excessive dose reduction or delay in chemotherapy, CSF administration may be considered.
3. CSF therapy	
Afebrile patients	Not recommended.
Febrile patients	May be useful in patients with prognostic factors that predict clinical deterioration, such as pneumonia, hypotension, multiorgan dysfunction, or fungal infection.
4. CSFs to increase chemotherapy dose intensity	Reserved for clinical research trials in which dose-intensive therapy does not require progenitor/stem cell support and incidence of febrile neutropenia is ≥40%.
5. CSFs as adjuncts to progenitor-cell transplantation	Routinely recommended as adjuncts to allogeneic and autologous progenitor cell transplantation, for mobilization, and to speed hematopoietic reconstitution following transplantation of marrow or peripheral blood progenitor cells.
6. CSFs in patients with myeloid malignancies	
Acute myeloid leukemia	Primary administration of CSF can be used after completion of induction chemotherapy in patients ≥55 to shorten duration of neutropenia.
	May be applicable to other patients, but data not available.
	CSFs given before and/or concurrent with chemotherapy for primary effects cannot be recommended outside a clinical trial.
Myelodysplastic syndromes	Data supporting routine long-term continuous use are lacking.
	Intermittent administration of CSFs may be considered in a subset of patients with severe neutropenia and recurrent infection.

(continued)

Table 20-3. American Society of Clinical Oncology Clinical Guidelines for the Use of Hematopoietic Colony-Stimulating Factors (CSFs)[116] (continued)

Guideline	Recommendation
7. CSFs in patients receiving concurrent chemotherapy and irradiation	CSFs should be avoided in patients receiving concomitant chemotherapy and radiation therapy.
8. CSFs in pediatric population	Guidelines recommended for adults are generally applicable to the pediatric age group. Optimal CSF doses need to be determined. Further clinical research in support of chemotherapy and progenitor cell transplantation is needed.

9. CSF dosing and route of administration	Adults
	  G-CSF 5 μg/kg/day
	  GM-CSF 250 μg/m^2/day
	  May be administered SC or IV as clinically indicated.

10. Initiation and duration of CSF administration	Starting G-CSF or GM-CSF between 24 and 72 hours subsequent to chemotherapy may provide optimal neutrophil recovery. Continuation of CSF until occurrence of absolute neutrophil count of 10,000/μL is safe and effective but a shorter duration of therapy that is sufficient to achieve clinically adequate neutrophil recovery is a reasonable alternative.
11. Comparative clinical activity of G-CSF and GM-CSF	Data are insufficient to make a recommendation.

*Recommendations reflect 1996 revisions. Since this manuscript was submitted for publication, the FDA has approved filgrastim to reduce the time to neutrophil recovery and the duration of fever following chemotherapy in patients with acute myelogenous leukemia.

Table 20-4. Recent Clinical Trials Using Granulocyte Colony-Stimulating Factor (G-CSF) and Granulocyte-Macrophage Colony-Stimulating Factor (GM-CSF) in Cancer Patients

Investigators	Age	Study Group	Number of Patients/Episodes	Type of Study	Growth Factor	Dosage	Results
Hartmann et al[118]	Adults	Afebrile neutropenia following chemotherapy for solid tumors or lymphoma	138 (T=71 P=67)	Randomized, double-blind placebo-controlled trial	G-CSF (filgrastim)	5 µg/kg/day subcutaneously until absolute neutrophil count (ANC) = 2000/µL or for maximum of 14 days	Median time to ANC >500/µL was 2 days in G-CSF group vs 4 days for placebo (p<0.001) No effect on rate of hospitalization, number of days in hospital, duration of treatment with parenteral antibiotics, or number of culture-positive infections.
Mitchell et al[119]	Pediatric	Febrile neutropenia following chemotherapy for acute lymphoblastic leukemia (ALL), acute myeloid leukemia (AML), lymphoma, and solid tumors	112 patients with 186 episodes of febrile neutropenia T=94 P=92	Randomized double-blind placebo-controlled trial comparing treatment with antibiotics alone vs antibiotics and G-CSF	G-CSF (filgrastim)	5 µg/kg/day intravenously commencing within 24 hours of antibiotic therapy	Shorter hospital stay (median 5 vs 7 days p-0.04), fewer days of antibiotic use (median 5 vs 6 days, p=0.02) in G-CSF group; possible cost savings
Pui et al[120]	Pediatric	ALL after induction chemotherapy	164 randomized 148 evaluable T=73 P=75	Randomized, placebo-controlled trial	G-CSF (filgrastim)	10 µg/kg/day subcutaneously commencing 1 day after the completion of remission-induction therapy and continuing until ANC≥1000/µL for 2 days	Shorter median hospital stays (6 days vs 10 days, p=0.011) and fewer documented infections (12 vs 27, p=0.009) in G-CSF-treated group. No difference in the rate of hospitalization for febrile neutropenia; no decrease in the number of severe infections; no difference in the likelihood of event-free survival at 3 years.

(continued)

Table 20-4. Recent Clinical Trials Using Granulocyte-Colony-Stimulating Factor (G-CSF) and Granulocyte-Macrophage Colony-Stimulating Factor (GM-CSF) in Cancer Patients (continued)

Investigators	Age	Study Group	Number of Patients/Episodes	Type of Study	Growth Factor	Dosage	Results
Moore et al[121]	Adults <60	AML in complete remission with daunorubicin receiving sequential high-dose consolidation therapy with high-dose cytarabine, cycloposphamide/etoposide, aziridinyl benzoquinone (AZQ), and mitoxantrone	123 62-No CSF with AZQ-mitoxantrone 61-G-CSF +AZQ-mitoxantrone 27 AZQ-24 mg/m^2 34-AZQ-28 mg/m^2	Phase II	G-CSF (filgrastim)	5 μg/kg/day commencing on day 4 of the AZQ/mitoxantrone course until ANC >500/μL for 2 successive days	Decrease in the duration of neutropenia in the groups receiving AZQ- mitoxantrone +G-CSF (p<0.001) Decrease in the frequency of hospitalization (p=0.05) and the duration of hospitalization in G-CSF-treated groups; decrease in frequency of severe infections; no effect on median survival time or duration of complete remission.
Lowenberg et al[122]	Adults >61	AML during remission induction with daunomycin-cytosine arabinoside	318 T=157 P=161	Prospective, randomized, multicenter trial	GM-CSF (molgramostim)	5 μg/kg/day continuous infusion starting 1 day before the start of chemotherapy and continuing until ANC ≥500/μL for 3 days but not beyond day 28	Median time to recovery of neutrophils shorter in GM-CSF-treated group (23 vs 25 days p=0.0002) No difference in nights spent in hospital or in infections No difference in survival and disease-free survival at 2 years

Table 20-4. Recent Clinical Trials Using Granulocyte-Colony-Stimulating Factor (G-CSF) and Granulocyte-Macrophage Colony-Stimulating Factor (GM-CSF) in Cancer Patients (continued)

Investigators	Age	Study Group	Number of Patients/Episodes	Type of Study	Growth Factor	Dosage	Results
Heil et al[123]	Adults	AML (de novo) in remission induction and consolidation	521 T=259 P=262	Randomized, blinded, placebo-controlled trial	G-CSF (filgrastim)	5 μg/kg/day subcutaneously beginning 24 hours after the last dose of chemotherapy until ANC ≥1.0 × 10⁹/L for 3 consecutive days or ANC ≥10 × 10⁹/L for 1 day	Reduction in the duration of neutropenia for induction and consolidation chemotherapy (p=0.0001 induction 1, p=0.015 induction 2, p=0.0001 consolidation 1) Reductions in the duration of fever (7 vs 8.5 days, p=0.009) Parenteral antibiotic use (15 vs 18.5 days p=0.001), and hospitalization (20 vs 25 days p=0.0001) Reduction in number of patients requiring systemic antifungal therapy No difference in median disease-free survival or overall median survival
Geissler et al[124]	Adults	ALL induction chemotherapy	53* T=25 P=26	Randomized, placebo-controlled trial	G-CSF (filgrastim)	5 μg/kg/day subcutaneously starting day 2 of chemotherapy until ANC ≥2000/uL on 2 consecutive days but not less than day 22	Reduced the median proportion of days with neutropenia less than 1000/μL (29% vs 84%, p<0.00005) Reduced the incidence of febrile neutropenia (12% vs 42%, p=0.05) and documented infections No significant difference in remission rate, remission, survival, or disease-free survival

(continued)

Table 20-4. Recent Clinical Trials Using Granulocyte-Colony-Stimulating Factor (G-CSF) and Granulocyte-Macrophage Colony-Stimulating Factor (GM-CSF) in Cancer Patients (continued)

Investigators	Age	Study Group	Number of Patients/Episodes	Type of Study	Growth Factor	Dosage	Results
McQuaker et al[125]	Adults	Lymphoma and myeloma treated with high-dose chemotherapy and autologous peripheral blood stem cell transplantation	38 T=19 P=19	Randomized placebo-controlled trial	G-CSF (filgrastim)	50 µg/m² starting the first day after transplant and continuing until ANC >0.5×10⁹/L	More rapid neutrophil engraftment (10 vs 14 days, p<0.0001) Fewer patients required amphotericin (16% vs 58%, p=0.029) Lower dose of G-CSF makes treatment cost-effective
Linch et al[126]	Adults	Lymphoma treated with high-dose chemotherapy and peripheral blood stem cell transplantation	90 62 evaluable T=34 NT=28	Prospective, randomized trial	G-CSL (lenograstim)	263 µg subcutaneously daily beginning the day after peripheral blood progenitor cell (PBPC) reinfusion and continuing until ANC ≥0.5×10⁹/L for 3 days or ≥1.0 × 10⁹/L for 1 day	Median time to neutrophil recovery shorter (9 vs 12.5 days, p=0.0001) Median duration of hospital stay decreased (13 vs 15.5 days, p=0.0002) No difference in incidence of infections or other hematologic parameters

*Two patients who were enrolled did not meet criteria and dropped out, leaving the treated and placebo group.

T = Patients on active treatment

P = Patients on placebo

NT = Not treated

Overall, these studies provide additional support for the use of G-CSF in adults with leukemia to shorten the duration of neutropenia and reduce infection, and they suggest that the use of CSFs is not associated with relapse or a shorter duration of remission. For dose intensification in protocols not requiring stem cell support, the use of CSFs is experimental. For some protocols, hematologic toxicity has been reduced, allowing patients to get higher and/or full doses of planned chemotherapeutic agents. For other protocols, hematologic toxicity has been reduced but dose intensification has not been possible because of limitations imposed by toxicity to other organ systems.

HIV Infection

Neutropenia is common in advanced HIV infection.[55] It may be caused directly by the HIV virus or by viral proteins. In addition, inhibitors of neutrophil production and decreased serum G-CSF levels in individuals with afebrile neutropenia have been reported. Accelerated neutrophil apoptosis may also play a role in neutropenia.[127] Although infection of CD34+ hematopoietic progenitors has not been proven to be a contributory factor, HIV coreceptors have been described on these cells.[128] Also, many of the drugs used to treat opportunistic infections and HIV-related malignancies are myelosuppressive. Prospective observation of 62 HIV-infected patients with polymorphonuclear leukocyte counts below $1000/mm^3$ has provided information on risk factors for infection.[129] The causes of neutropenia in this group were lymphoma (4), chemotherapy (7), zidovudine therapy (32), trimethoprim-sulphamethoxazole (28), and ganciclovir (11). Fifteen patients with neutropenia developed infectious complications. Infection occurred more often with neutropenia related to lymphoma or chemotherapy. In multivariate analysis, neutropenia in the previous 3 months, an indwelling central venous catheter, and the occurrence of a nadir in the polymorphonuclear leukocyte count were risk factors for infection.

A number of studies have documented the ability of G-CSF and GM-CSF to reverse the neutropenia observed in AIDS.[55,130-133] GM-CSF is associated with a higher frequency of adverse effects and is believed to promote viral replication, so G-CSF is the preferred growth factor. The use of growth factors has permitted HIV-infected patients to remain on essential myelosuppressive medications. In an open label, noncompetitive, multicenter study of filgrastim in 200 HIV-infected patients, therapy was initiated at 1 µg/kg per day for 28 days and adjusted to maintain an absolute neutrophil count of $2\text{-}5 \times 10^9/L$.[134] Ninety-six percent of patients achieved reversal of neutropenia with a dose of less than 300 µg per day. Ganciclovir, zidovudine, and pyrimethamine were the drugs most often considered to cause neutropenia. Filgrastim therapy allowed more than 80% of patients to maintain dose levels of their medications.

Severe Chronic Neutropenia

Severe chronic neutropenia is a heterogeneous group of hematologic disorders in which the absolute neutrophil count is decreased (usually <0.5 × $10^9/L$) and patients experience recurrent fever, oropharyngeal ulcers, and severe infections. There are three main syndromes: congenital forms of neutropenia, cyclic neutropenia, and idiopathic neutropenia. A preliminary report published in 1989 described the administration of recombinant human G-CSF to five patients with severe congenital neutropenia.[135] Within 9 days of beginning treatment, all five patients responded with an increase in their neutrophil count. The absolute neutrophil count rose from below 100 to between 1300 and 9500 cells/µL. The elevations were maintained for long periods of time. Preexisting chronic infections resolved and new infections were reduced. In 1993, the results of a Phase III randomized, controlled trial of recombinant human G-CSF in severe chronic neutropenia were published.[136] On therapy, 108/120 patients had a median absolute neutrophil count of at least 1.5 × $10^9/L$. Marrow aspirates showed increasing proportions of maturing neutrophils. The incidence and duration of infection-related events were reduced and there was a 70% reduction in the duration of antibiotic use. This trial established recombinant human G-CSF as the standard therapy for severe congenital neutropenia. Not every patient responded to G-CSF treatment, and in-vitro studies of these patients suggest that there might be a problem with signal transduction following the binding of G-CSF to the G-CSF receptor. In 1994, a nonsense mutation in the G-CSF receptor was identified in two patients with severe congenital neutropenia.[137,138] This mutation led to a truncation of the cytoplasmic domain of the receptor. The patients with the truncated receptor developed acute myelogenous leukemia.

In 1994, an international registry was established for patients with severe chronic neutropenia to improve their care and to further understanding of the disease. A 1997 review has summarized the safety and effectiveness of recombinant human G-CSF in this patient group.[139] One of the adverse events reported to the registry is the development of AML in patients with Kostmann's syndrome, a form of congenital neutropenia with autosomal recessive inheritance, normal erythroid and megakaryocytic maturation, but arrest of myeloid maturation at the promyelocytic stage of maturation. Twenty-three of 249 patients with congenital neutropenia—approximately 9%—have developed either myelodysplasia or acute myelogenous leukemia. No cases of myelodysplasia or AML have occurred in patients with cyclic or idiopathic neutropenia. There is concern that the development of AML/myelodysplasia is related to G-CSF therapy and the development of an abnormal G-CSF receptor. Molecular analysis of the G-CSF receptor in 28 patients with severe congenital neutropenia revealed that four had a point mutation in the cytoplasmic domain of the receptor.[140] All four patients had been investigated regularly, and there was no association between the development of receptor mutations and G-CSF therapy. When the parents of patients who developed AML were tested, the G-CSF receptor was nor-

mal. It was also normal in two siblings who also had congenital neutropenia. Thus, preliminary investigations suggest that the development of the receptor mutations is independent of G-CSF treatment. Further studies are needed in this area.

Secondary Neutropenias

Myelopoietic growth factors have been evaluated in secondary neutropenias associated with Felty's syndrome in rheumatoid arthritis,[141,142] neonatal alloimmune neutropenia,[143] neutropenia secondary to glycogen storage disease type 1b,[144,145] and drug-induced agranulocytosis.[146-152] Both GM-CSF and G-CSF have been used to treat the neutropenia of Felty's syndrome successfully. Flares of arthritis and the development of leukocytoclastic vasculitis with growth factor therapy seem more common in Felty's syndrome than in other disorders. The flare in arthritis seems to occur more often with GM-CSF than with G-CSF treatment. Several cases of neonatal alloimmune neutropenia have been successfully treated with G-CSF. GM-CSF and G-CSF have also both been used to treat neutropenia in glycogen storage disease type 1b. A clinical response has not always been associated with an improvement in respiratory burst activity. It is of interest that a recent report of Sweet's syndrome occurring in such a patient followed therapy with G-CSF.[145] Drug-induced agranulocytosis related to the use of clozapine,[146] sulphasalazine,[147] chlorpromazine,[148] propylthiouracil,[149] methimazole,[150] deferiprone,[151] and ticlopidine[152] has been reported to respond to treatment with G-CSF.

Nonneutropenic Infected Patients

G-CSF and GM-CSF activate mature neutrophils, enhancing normal effector functions such as phagocytosis and bacterial killing. In addition, they prime neutrophils for enhanced superoxide production after exposure to normal physiologic stimuli. This enhancement of neutrophil function has led to preliminary clinical trials of G-CSF in nonneutropenic-infected patients with normal or elevated neutrophil counts. A preliminary trial of filgrastim as an adjunct to antibiotic therapy in the treatment of community-acquired pneumonia demonstrated no effect on pneumonia-related clinical variables.[153] However, a randomized, placebo-controlled trial of filgrastim in 40 diabetic patients with foot infections under treatment with antibiotics and diabetes control therapy demonstrated earlier eradication of pathogens, quicker resolution of cellulitis, shorter duration of antibiotic therapy, and a shorter hospital stay in the treated group.[154] In addition, surgical intervention in the form of amputation or surgical debridement was needed in four patients in the placebo group but in none of the treated group. Superoxide production in the treated group was greater than in the placebo group when measured 7 days after the beginning of treatment. Previous studies had documented decreased production of reactive oxygen intermediates and bactericidal killing in animal models of diabetes and diabetic patients with poor diabetes control.[155] Further studies of this type are clearly warranted.

Thrombopoietic Growth Factors

Recombinant human growth factors and cytokines that have been investigated for the ability to stimulate megakaryocytopoiesis and thrombopoiesis include IL-1, IL-3, IL-6, IL-11, PIXY 321 (fusion cytokine of IL-3 and GM-CSF), thrombopoietin (TPO), and megakaryocyte growth and development factor (MGDF), a truncated form of TPO. At this time, only IL-11 has received FDA approval for clinical use.

Interleukin-11

Biology

Interleukin-11 is a pleiotropic cytokine that alone and in combination with other growth factors stimulates multiple stages of hematopoiesis and promotes the growth and development of a variety of nonhematopoietic tissues. The biology of IL-11 and the results of preclinical and clinical studies have been summarized elsewhere.[156-158] IL-11 was first described in 1990 as a novel growth factor in conditioned medium prepared from the immortalized marrow-derived stromal cell line PU-34.[159] When conditioned medium was screened for mitogenic activity with T1165, an IL-6-dependent murine plasmacytoma cell line, stimulatory activity remained after neutralization of IL-6. The cDNA for this stimulatory activity contained an open reading frame of 597 nucleotides, which predicted a polypeptide of 199 amino acids with a protein secretory leader of 21 amino acids. The gene for human IL-11 was subsequently cloned in 1992; it is located on chromosome 19q13.3-19q13.4.[160] The mature polypeptide is composed of 178 amino acids. The recombinant form of human IL-11 available for clinical use is a polypeptide of 177 amino acids, which lacks the aminoterminal proline residue.[161]

The receptor for human IL-11 consists of an alpha chain (IL-11Rα) coded for by genes on chromosome 9 (9p13) and a beta chain, which is the gp130 common receptor subunit shared by IL-6, oncostatin M, leukemia inhibitory factor, and ciliary neutrotrophic factor.[162] To generate a biologic signal, a cell must coexpress IL-11Rα and gp130. The IL-11/IL-11α complex induces heterodimerization, tyrosine phosphorylation, and gp130 activation. The stages of signal transduction have been reviewed.[163]

Murine studies indicate that IL-11 is expressed in a large number of normal tissues as well as in the hematopoietic microenvironment. These tissues include neurons of the hippocampus and spinal cord, lung fibroblasts and epithelial cells, osteoblasts,[164] chondrocytes, synoviocytes, uterine fibroblasts, and endometrial tissue, as well as trophoblast (summarized in reference 158). The IL-11Rα is also expressed widely in tissues. The IL-11Rα has been detected in hematopoietic tissue (including megakaryocyte precursors), liver, brain, heart, kidney, and epithelial cells from salivary glands and the gastrointestinal tract.[165]

IL-11 acts in synergy with IL-3, IL-4, IL-7, IL-12, IL-13, stem cell factor (SCF), flt3-ligand, and GM-CSF to stimulate the proliferation of primitive hematopoietic stem cells and of multipotential and committed progenitor cells.[166-169] Studies indicate that the proliferative effect is related to the entry of cells into the active cell cycle. In the presence of IL-3 or SCF, IL-11 can stimulate various stages of erythroid differentiation. In the presence of IL-3-containing cultures, IL-11 appears to promote multilineage colonies and erythroid colonies, including BFU-Es and CFU-Es. The stimulation of BFU-E colonies persists in the absence of EPO. In later erythroid maturation, IL-11 alone supports the maturation of CFU-Es from marrow cells. IL-11, in combination with SCF, stimulates myeloid colony formation and, in combination with SCF and IL-4, supports accessory-cell-dependent B-cell differentiation. IL-11 also appears to support the growth of stromal cells in the hematopoietic microenvironment and, with other cytokines, to mobilize primitive hematopoietic progenitor cells. Data concerning the role of IL-11 in early hematopoiesis are conflicting. Transplantation of hematopoietic progenitors expanded with IL-3, IL-6, IL-11, and SCF has suggested impaired engraftment of IL-11 expanded cells. Transplantation studies with IL-11 and SCF-expanded cells have been associated with sustained engraftment. To clarify the physiologic conditions under which IL-11 stimulates primitive hematopoietic stem cells and under which it promotes differentiation, investigators have performed transplantation studies in lethally irradiated mice with marrow cells transduced with a defective retrovirus carrying murine IL-11 cDNA.[170] In these studies, ectopic production of murine IL-11 accelerated the recovery of platelets and neutrophils in primary, secondary, and tertiary transplant recipients, suggesting that IL-11 expression may result in enhanced maintenance of primitive hematopoietic progenitor cells.

Megakaryocytopoiesis and thrombopoiesis in murine and human marrow cells are stimulated by IL-11 in combination with IL-3, TPO, or SCF.[171-176]T The SC administration of IL-11 to rodents, nonhuman primates, and humans stimulates megakaryocytopoiesis, increasing production, differentiation, and maturation. Marrow examination of patients treated with recombinant human IL-11 at doses of 50 µg/kg per day or higher showed an increased number of megakaryocytes with a shift toward cells of higher ploidy (64N).[175] The percentage of megakaryocytes staining with a monoclonal antibody that recognizes the proliferating cell nuclear antigen also increased. Increases in peripheral blood platelet counts were seen with doses as low as 10 µg/kg per day. A physiologic role for IL-11 in normal thrombopoiesis is supported by the elevated IL-11 and TPO levels observed in marrow transplant recipients with thrombocytopenia following myeloablative therapy. Of equal interest is the observation that in immune thrombocytopenia with decreased platelet survival but intact marrow megakaryocytopoiesis, IL-11 was elevated but TPO levels were undetectable.[177] Preclinical studies in rodents indicate that IL-11 improves the survival rate and accelerates multilineage recovery in marrow transplantation, chemotherapy, and chemoradiation models.[178-180]

Clinical Studies

Three clinical studies were paramount in establishing the ability of recombinant human (rh)IL-11 (Neumega, Genetics Institute, Inc) to ameliorate the thrombocytopenia produced by chemotherapy. The first of these, a Phase I trial of rhIL-11 in women receiving chemotherapy for breast cancer, was published in 1996.[174,181] In this study, cohorts of three to five women were given daily SC doses of rhIL-11 (10, 25, 50, 75, and 100 µg/kg per day) before and after dose-intensive chemotherapy with cyclophosphamide (1500 mg/m^2) and doxorubicin (60 mg/m^2). Patients receiving 10, 25, 40, and 75 µg/kg per day experienced mean increases in platelet counts of 76%, 93%, 108%, and 185%, respectively. Patients receiving doses of 25 µg/kg or greater had less thrombocytopenia in the first two chemotherapy cycles. Fatigue and myalgia/arthralgia were observed at doses of at least 75 µg/kg per day. Fever was not observed, but weight gain and edema were observed even at lower doses. A decrease in hematocrit believed to be related to increased plasma volume was also observed.

The second study was a multicenter, randomized, placebo-controlled trial among 93 patients with cancer (breast cancer, non-Hodgkin's lymphoma, small cell and non-small-cell lung cancer, and other solid tumors) who had developed severe thrombocytopenia requiring platelet transfusion during a previous cycle of chemotherapy.[182] While continuing chemotherapy, patients were assigned to receive placebo or rhIL-11 (25 μg or 50 μg/kg per day) subcutaneously for 14-21 days beginning 1 day after chemotherapy. Fewer patients treated with the 50 μg/kg per day dose of rhIL-11 required platelet transfusions when compared with control subjects. Although a similar trend was seen with the 25 μg/kg per day dose, the difference was not significant.

In the third study, 77 patients with advanced breast carcinoma receiving cytoxan (3200 mg/m^2) and doxorubicin (75 mg/m^2) plus G-CSF (5 μg/kg per day) were randomly assigned to receive either placebo or rhIL-11 at 50 μg/kg per day subcutaneously for 10-17 days after the first two chemotherapy cycles.[183] Using the intention-to-treat analysis, 68% of the patients receiving rhIL-11 (as compared with 41% in the control group) did not require platelet transfusions. The total number of platelet transfusions was also lower for the rhIL-11 treated group. A multicenter Phase I/II trial of rhIL-11 and G-CSF in pediatric patients with solid tumors treated with ifosfamide, etoposide, and carboplatin demonstrated an accelerated platelet recovery and a reduction in platelet transfusions compared with those given G-CSF treatment alone.[184] However, efficacy studies have not yet been performed among pediatric populations.

Based on the three studies conducted among adults, the FDA has approved rhIL-11 (Neumega) for "the prevention of severe thrombocytopenia and the reduction of the need for platelet transfusions following myelosuppressive chemotherapy in patients with nonmyeloid malignancies who are at high risk of severe thrombocytopenia."[161] The recommended dosage is 50 μg/kg per day subcutaneously beginning 6-24 hours following the completion of chemotherapy dosing. The reader should consult Neumega Professional Prescribing Information for details of dosing and precautions regarding adverse events.[161]

Thrombopoietin

Thrombopoietin (also called Mpl-ligand) is the primary humoral regulator of megakaryocytopoiesis and thrombopoiesis.[185,186] It stimulates the production of megakaryocyte precursors from marrow CD34$^+$ cells, increases megakaryocyte size and ploidy, and promotes megakaryocyte maturation. Under conditions of myelosuppression, it also has multilineage effects. The concept of a humoral regulator of platelet production was first proposed in the late 1950s, but thrombopoietin was not isolated and cloned until 1994. A chronology of the critical scientific observations leading to the discovery of thrombopoietin is presented in a 1995 review.[185] Two forms of recombinant human thrombopoietin are available for investigative studies: a full-length, 332-amino acid polypeptide chain generally referred to as TPO; and a truncated but fully functional polypeptide containing the receptor domain and consisting of the first 153 amino acids, referred to as megakaryocyte growth and development factor (MGDF). Because MGDF has a shorter half-life in the circulation than the full-length molecule, the molecule was conjugated to polyethylene glycol, and this pegylated recombinant human MGDF (Peg-MGDF) has been used in most investigative studies. Although neither form of thrombopoietin is approved by the FDA for clinical use, preclinical and early clinical studies suggest potential applications in increasing platelet yields from healthy apheresis donors, decreasing the severity of thrombocytopenia following chemotherapy, increasing the mobilization of PBPCs, and expanding megakaryocyte precursors and other hematopoietic progenitor cells ex vivo.

Biology

The discovery of the retrovirus that induces a myeloproliferative syndrome in mice and the subsequent cloning of the transforming gene, v-mpl, were critical developments in the discovery of TPO. The structure of the transforming gene suggested a polypeptide that was a cytokine receptor.[185] When c-mpl, the human homolog of v-mpl, was subsequently identified, it became clear that the gene coded for a protein that was a member of the hematopoietic growth factor receptor superfamily. The distribution of c-mpl on hematopoietic progenitor cells, megakaryocyte precursors, platelets, and cell lines with surface markers indicating a commitment to megakaryocyte development established a relationship between megakaryocytopoiesis and c-mpl. Antisense oligodeoxynucleo- tides to c-mpl were found to inhibit c-mpl RNA synthesis, and this reduced synthesis correlated with the inhibition of megakaryocyte colony formation in culture. Scientists at two companies (Genentech, San Francisco, CA, and Amgen) used soluble c-mpl to isolate mpl-ligand from plasma obtained from aplastic animals. The strategy used by a third group of scientists (Zymogenetics, Corp, Seattle, WA) involved the use of mutagens to promote gene activation of mpl-ligand in a cell line transduced to express c-mpl and grown under culture conditions where there was a survival advantage for mutants expressing c-mpl and producing c-mpl-ligand. Other laboratories used conventional protein purification and sequencing techniques to isolate cDNA clones for mpl-ligand.

The gene for thrombopoietin maps to the long arm of chromosome 3 (3q26) and is similar in structure to the gene for EPO. It has five coding exons, which can be aligned with those of EPO. The human gene codes for a polypeptide 332 amino acids in length. Thrombopoietin has a two-domain structure: a cytokine domain and a C-terminal domain. The receptor-binding moiety and the physiologic activity of the peptide are associated with the first 153 amino acids. The role of the C-terminal domain is not understood at this time but may involve stabilization of the molecule in the circulation. The TPO molecule has a half-life of 18-24 hours, but the unmodified MGDF has a half-life of 1.5 hours.

The mRNA for thrombopoietin is expressed primarily in the liver, kidney, and muscle, with lesser amounts expressed in the spleen and marrow.[187] Studies of primary cell cultures have identified thrombopoietin mRNA in endothelial cells and fibroblasts. Most cultures of marrow-derived stromal cells from CD34+ and CD34– cells also express the mRNA for thrombopoietin.[188] Most studies of thrombopoietin levels during thrombocytopenia and thrombocytosis indicate an inverse relationship between platelet levels and thrombopoietin levels.[189,190] However, the expression of mRNA for thrombopoietin does not change during periods of thrombocytopenia.[190] Human and mouse studies suggest that plasma levels of thrombopoietin are regulated through the binding of thrombopoietin to high-affinity c-mpl receptors on platelets and megakaryocytes.[191-196] The average human platelet is estimated to have 25-35 such receptors. Mpl receptors have also been identified on BFU-Es, supporting other observations of a TPO effect on erythroid progenitors. Thrombopoietin is internalized and degraded by platelets.

The details of signal transduction following the binding of TPO to the c-mpl receptor are not known. However, tyrosine phosphorylation of c-mpl itself and a number of cellular proteins (Jak-2, Tyk-2, Shc, STAT3, and STAT5) occurs following such binding.[193,194] Phosphorylation of Vav, a 95-kD protein expressed in hematopoietic cells, has also been reported following the binding of TPO to human platelets.[195]

The development of TPO and c-mpl knockout mice has provided information to substantiate further the crucial role of TPO in platelet development.[197,198] In both animal models, there is an 85-90% reduction in circulating platelets (and megakaryocytes), but other blood cells are present in normal numbers. The remaining platelets are normal and adequate for hemostasis. There is also a reduction in erythroid and myeloid progenitors, which again suggests that TPO may directly affect other hematopoietic progenitor cells. The knockout mouse for NF-E2, a transcriptional factor that is believed to have a role in erythroid cell globin gene expression, has served to remind us of the complex nature of platelet production.[199] The NF-E2 knockout mouse has severe thrombocytopenia, which routinely causes death from hemorrhage. Megakaryocytes are present but do not mature properly. Initially, there was concern because TPO levels were not elevated in this model. However, further investigations indicate that the TPO is bound to mega-karyocytes, which are increased in number.[199]

In-vitro and preclinical studies in normal and myelosuppressed animals have consistently supported a major role for thrombopoietin in megakaryocyte and platelet production but have been in conflict with regard to the efffect of thrombopoietin on other lineages.[200] Recombinant TPO alone induces proliferation of megakaryocyte progenitors and their maturation. In colony-forming assays, the effects of IL-3 and IL-6 are additive and that of SCF is synergistic.

Preclinical Studies

In normal animals, TPO seems to affect primarily platelet production and to have little or no effect on erythroid and myeloid production. In normal mice, daily administration of Peg-MGDF caused dose-related increases in the platelet count, with peak counts of five times normal by day 10.[201] In baboons, Peg-MGDF administered daily (0.05-5 µg/kg/day subcutaneously) for 28 days increased the platelet count threefold by 7 days and fivefold by day 28.[202] Platelet appearance and aggregation remained normal, but Peg-MGDF did sensitize platelets to normal aggregating reagents such as adenosine diphosphate, collagen, thrombin, and epinephrine. Platelets induced by thrombopoietin do not express surface markers of activation and do not appear to promote thrombosis.[202,203] There is some in-vitro evidence that TPO stimulates thromboxane A2 formation and serotonin secretion, but it is unclear how these observations relate to in-vivo events.[204]

Preclinical models of myelosuppression show that TPO/MGDF accelerates platelet recovery.[205-209] Peg-MGDF and murine G-CSF improved survival and neutrophil and platelet recovery compared with control and single cytokine treatment regimens.[205] Treatment with MGDF, Peg-MGDF, or Peg-MGDF and G-CSF beginning on day 1 diminished the duration and severity of thrombocytopenia in primates receiving 700 cGy of total body irradiation, and TPO produced similar results in rhesus monkeys receiving 500 cGy.[206,207] Moderate

myelosuppression (3.5 Gy) in a mouse model can be ameliorated with a single dose of Peg-MGDF given 1 hour after irradiation, with accelerated red cell, white cell, and platelet recovery.[208] In rhesus monkeys receiving 5Gy total body irradiation (TBI), a single IV dose of TPO one day after TBI counteracted the need for platelet transfusions and accelerated platelet recovery to normal levels 2 weeks earlier than it did in control subjects.[209] The combination of TPO and G-CSF provided similar platelet recovery and shortened the period of severe neutropenia.

Clinical Studies

Selected published and preliminary reports of clinical studies of recombinant forms of thrombopoietin are summarized in Table 20-5.[2,210-219] The first published report was a Phase I study of Peg-MGDF in patients with advanced cancer.[210] Peg-MGDF was given in doses of 0.03-1.0 µg/kg daily by subcutaneous injection for up to 10 days. Thirteen patients received the active drug and four received placebo. Those receiving doses of 0.3 and 1.0 µg/kg had an increase in platelet count from 51% to 584%. The platelet count began to rise on about day 6 and peaked between days 12 and 18, remaining above normal for up to 21 days. There were no adverse effects associated with drug administration. The platelets induced by treatment were normal in appearance and function and did not demonstrate spontaneous aggregation or express activation markers. However, a sensitivity to normal aggregating agents was observed, as in earlier preclinical studies.

A trial of Peg-MGDF in patients with non-small-cell lung cancer demonstrated a higher nadir and accelerated platelet recovery, but few patients had clinically significant thrombocytopenia.[211] More recently, a study of patients with advanced cancer treated with carboplatin (600 mg/m) and cytoxan (1200 mg/m) and randomly assigned to receive placebo plus G-CSF (5 µg/kg/day) or MGDF at escalating doses plus G-CSF demonstrated an earlier return to baseline platelet counts in the MGDF-treated group.[212] Overall, studies suggest a possible

Table 20-5. Selected Clinical Studies Using Human Recombinant Thrombopoietin (TPO) or Pegylated Megakaryocyte Growth and Development Factor (Peg-MGDF)

Investigator	Study Population	Product/Dosage	Results	Comments
Basser et al[210]	Patients with advanced solid tumors Randomization in study to drug or placebo	Peg-MGDF/0.03-1.0 µg/kg/day subcutaneously for up to 10 days	Increase in platelet count with 0.3 and 1.0 µg/kg dosage varying from 51% to 584% Increase in platelet count began on day 6 and peaked between day 12 and day 18, remaining above normal for 21 days Increase in marrow megakaryocytes	Platelet morphology and function normal No adverse effects from drug No antibodies to Peg-MGDF Single episode of spontaneously resolving thrombophlebitis
Fanucchi et al[211]	Patients with lung cancer treated with carboplatin and paclitaxel Randomized, double-blind, placebo-controlled trial	Peg-MGDF/0.03-5.0 µg/kg/day subcutaneously before and after chemotherapy	Median nadir platelet count higher in treated group (188,000/µL vs 111,000/µL) Platelet count recovery to base-line levels faster in treated group (14 days vs 21 days)	One episode of deep venous thrombosis and pulmonary embolism One episode of superficial thrombophlebitis Adverse events same in treated and placebo groups
Basser et al[212]	Patients with advanced cancer treated with carboplatin and cyclophosphamide Randomized, blinded, placebo-controlled trial	Peg-MGDF/0.03-5.0 µg/kg/day subcutaneously beginning the day after chemotherapy for 7-20 days G-CSF 5 µg/kg/day	Recovery to baseline platelet count earlier in treated group (17 days vs 22 days) Earlier platelet nadir in treated group but no difference in depth of nadir Enhanced mobilization of PBPC with Peg-MGDF + G-CSF vs G-CSF alone (measured at day 15)	One episode of pulmonary embolism in patient with lung cancer One self-limiting episode of thrombophlebitis Adverse events same in treated and placebo groups No antibodies to Peg-MGDF
Vadhan-Raj et al[213]	Phase I/II study of patients with sarcoma at high risk for severe thrombocytopenia	TPO/single IV dose (0.3-2.4 µg/kg) 3 weeks before chemotherapy	Increase in platelet counts of 61-213% above baseline Increase began on day 4 and peaked on median of day 12 Increase in marrow megakaryocytes 5.7 to 10-fold increase in hematopoietic progenitors in peripheral blood	Normal platelet morphology and function No significant adverse events attributable to TPO 1/12 patients developed transient nonneutralizing antibody to full-length TPO

Table 20-5. Selected Clinical Studies Using Human Recombinant Thrombopoietin (TPO) or Pegylated Megakaryocyte Growth and Development Factor (Peg-MGDF) (continued)

Investigator	Study Population	Product/Dosage	Results	Comments
Vadhan-Raj et al[214]	Phase I/II study of patients with gynecologic malignancy on high-dose carboplatin	TPO/0.6-3.6 mcg/kg/day subcutaneously prior to and for four doses following a second cycle of chemotherapy	Optimal dose of TPO determined to be 1.2 mcg/kg 71% of patients receiving optimal dose in second chemotherapy cycle were able to avoid platelet transfusion	
Nash et al[215]	Phase I study of patients with delayed platelet recovery (≥35 days) following hematopoietic stem cell transplantation	TPO/single and multiple IV doses of 0.6-2.4 mg/kg	No evidence of clinical benefit	
Beveridge et al[216]	Randomized, double-blind, placebo-controlled trial in patients with breast cancer receiving STAMP V high-dose chemotherapy followed by autologous marrow transplantation	Peg-MGDF/5 μg/kg/day or 10 μg/kg/day from day 0 until count recovered to ≥250 × 10^9/L	34% reduction in duration of thrombocytopenia 48% reduction in use of platelet transfusions	
Bolwell et al[217]	Randomized placebo-controlled study of breast cancer patients treated with STAMP I regimen and G-CSF-mobilized PBPCs	Peg-MGDF/1.0-10.0 μg/kg/day subcutaneously from day 0 to platelets >50 × 10^9/L	No effect on duration or severity of thrombocytopenia	
Glaspy et al[218]	Randomized placebo-controlled study of breast cancer patients treated with STAMP I regimen and G-CSF mobilized PBPCs	Peg-MGDF/1-30 μg/kg/day subcutaneously on day −14 to day −8 and post PBPC infusion	No impact on either platelet recovery or platelet transfusions	
Bertolini et al[219]	Phase 1 study of cancer patients (8 breast, 2 non-Hodgkins' lymphoma) undergoing PBP rescue following chemotherapy Retrospective control group	Peg-MGDF + SCF + IL-3 + IL-6 + IL-11+ Flt ligand + MIP-1 expanded megakaryocyte progenitors. Unmanipulated PBPCs and expanded PBPCs infused	No bacterial contamination of expanded product No adverse effect of infusion	
Kuter et al[2]	Normal platelet apheresis donors Randomized, placebo-controlled blinded, crossover, sequential-dose escalation study	Peg-MGDF single subcutaneous dose of 1 μg/kg or 3 μg/kg in 28-day period	Increased platelet count in donors 366 × 10^9/L for 1 μg/kg dose 599 × 10^9/L for 3 μg/kg dose	Donors with personal family history indicating predisposition to thrombosis excluded

benefit of Peg-MGDF treatment for patients with solid tumors receiving high-dose chemotherapy.[211-214] However, the results in stem cell transplantation have been disappointing so far.[215-218] These results may reflect both damage to the hematopoietic microenvironment and stem cells from previous treatment and the absence of cells able to respond to a humoral stimulus.

A preliminary report of the first use of Peg-MGDF in normal plateletpheresis donors is encouraging.[220] The platelet yield of the apheresis product was considerably increased by a single subcutaneous injection of Peg-MGDF, and (not unexpectedly) recipients had higher counts following the transfusion of a larger number of platelets. In this highly selected donor group, there were no adverse events, and most donors did not mind the inconvenience of the extra visit. There are two issues to be considered when one discusses the use of Peg-MGDF in normal donors. First, there is very little information about the long-term effects of treatment with Peg-MGDF. Most plateletpheresis donors are individuals who provide many donations over a period of years and could be exposed to MGDF with some regularity. Second, it is unclear if patients will benefit from this development. One study reported the transient occurrence of a non-neutralizing antibody to TPO.[213] Another study reported that 2 of 30 patients receiving Peg-MGDF for multiple cycles of chemotherapy developed neutralizing antibodies.[221] Several hundred patients have received Peg-MGDF, but only two have developed antibodies. The clinical significance of these antibodies is not known at this time. There have been no reports of antibodies developing in normal donors. The 1997 report of the induction of a fatal myeloproliferative syndrome in irradiated mice engrafted with marrow cells infected with a retrovirus carrying murine TPO cDNA also raises concerns about potential adverse effects in normal donors.[222]

The other issue is whether the patient or the blood center would receive the benefit from the collection of larger numbers of platelets. When the technology for apheresis improved and larger numbers of platelets were collected, blood centers began splitting a single donation into two products when feasible. This could happen with increasing frequency if Peg-MGDF is used to increase the platelet yield. For a patient to benefit from a product with a higher yield, it would be necessary to change standards so that the average number of platelets in an apheresis product is higher than that currently required.

A study published in 1997, which demonstrates another potential transfusion medicine application of Peg-MGDF, deals with ex-vivo expansion of megakaryocyte precursors and transfusion of this expanded product.[219] The ability to increase the number and maturity of megakaryocyte precursors in a stem cell product (PBPC or cord blood) could result in clinically meaningful reductions in the severity and duration of thrombocytopenia.

Other Thrombopoietic Growth Factors

IL-1, IL-3, and IL-6 are multilineage hematopoietic growth factors, and PIXY-321 is a fusion protein containing IL-3 and GM-CSF. In-vitro and preclinical studies suggested that these growth factors had the potential to reduce thrombocytopenia following myelosuppressive chemotherapy. Preliminary clinical trials of IL-1 in cancer patients receiving chemotherapy regimens, including carboplatin, demonstrated that IL-1 has the ability to reduce the severity and duration of thrombocytopenia. However, most patients had fever, chills, nausea, vomiting, myalgia, and headache, and more than 50% of patients had mild to moderate hypotension. These side effects were considered unacceptable for the degree of clinical benefit obtained. IL-3 hastened platelet recovery, but the benefits were once again considered modest, and IL-3 administration was also accompanied by some toxicity. Initially, PIXY-321 appeared to improve platelet recovery following chemotherapy in sarcoma patients, but controlled clinical trials comparing GM-CSF and PIXY-321 in patients with advanced breast cancer and with non-Hodgkin's lymphoma following autologous marrow transplantation have demonstrated that PIXY-321 is not superior to GM-CSF in ameliorating thrombocytopenia. IL-6 administration accelerated platelet recovery without affecting the platelet nadir and was associated with side effects of fever and headache, which could be managed with acetaminophen therapy. A polyethylene-glycol-modified IL-6 has been developed, which has a longer half-life and greater thrombopoietic activity than native IL-6. Preclinical studies suggest that this modified IL-6 produces a greater thrombopoietic effect than native IL-6 without side effects.

Hematopoietic Growth Factors in Transfusion Medicine: The Next Decade

The first-generation application of hematopoietic growth factors in transfusion medicine involved the administration of a lineage-dominant growth factor to an individual (patient or healthy donor) and depended on the hematopoietic microenvironment to provide defined and undefined accessory growth factors to produce clinical results. With the identification of hematopoietic growth factors that act on stem cells, and an increasing knowledge base about how these growth factors interact with CSFs and other growth factors that are synergystic, it has become possible to duplicate hematopoiesis (or at least some aspects of it) ex vivo. While initial experiments involving ex vivo expansion were successful in expanding committed hematopoietic progenitors, more recent studies suggest that it might be possible to amplify primitive hematopoietic progenitors as well.[223] There are clinical situations in which it might be desirable to expand committed progenitors while maintaining the number of stem cells, and other situations in which it may be desirable to expand both committed progenitors and stem cells. Umbilical cord blood is one hematopoietic stem cell product for which the direction of expansion might depend on the age of the recipient. For a pediatric recipient, in whom the stem cell number appears adequate but posttransplantation thrombocytopenia and neutropenia are prolonged, one might want to maintain the number of stem cells but expand committed progenitors to shorten the posttransplantation neu-

tropenia and thrombocytopenia. For an adult recipient, the goal might be to expand the number of stem cells and committed progenitor cells. For an autologous PBPC transplant for a patient with a malignancy, one might want to maintain stem cells and committed progenitor cells in culture until contaminating tumor cells have died, and then expand committed progenitors so that myelopoiesis and thrombopoiesis reconstitute more rapidly. As preliminary clinical trials are under way, new therapies with products expanded ex vivo may be less than 5 years away.

Note in proof: On August 18, 1998, Amgen announced that it had discontinued platelet donation clinical trials, including a multi-dose trial of its megakaryocyte growth and development factor (PEG-rHuMGDF), following the development of thrombocytopenia and neutralizing antibodies.

References

1. Bowden R, Price T, Boeckh M, et al. Phase I/II study of granulocyte transfusions from G-CSF-stimulated unrelated donors for treatment of infections in neutropenic blood and marrow transplant (BMT) patients (abstract). Blood 1997;90(Suppl 1):435a.
2. Kuter D, McCullough J, Romo J, et al. Treatment of platelet (PLT) donors with pegylated recombinant human megakaryocyte growth and development factor (PEG-rHuMGDF) increases circulating PLT counts (CTS) and PLT apheresis yields and increases platelet increments in recipients of PLT transfusions (abstract). Blood 1997;90(Suppl 1):579a.
3. Lieberman J, Skolnik PR, Parkerson GR III, et al. Safety of autologous, ex-vivo expanded human immunodeficiency virus (HIV)-specific cytotoxic T-lymphocyte infusion in HIV-infected patients. Blood 1997;90:2196-206.
4. To LB, Haylock DN, Simmons PJ, Juttner CA. The biology and clinical uses of blood stem cells. Blood 1997;84:2233-58.
5. Egrie JC, Dwyer E, Lykos M, et al. Novel erythropoiesis stimulating protein (NESP)

has a longer serum half-life and greater in vivo biological activity than recombinant human erythropoietin (rHuEPO) (abstract). Blood 1997;90(Suppl 1):56a.

6. Curtis BM, Williams DE, Broxmeyer HE, et al. Enhanced hematopoietic activity of a human granulocyte/macrophage colony-stimulating factor-interleukin 3 fusion protein. Proc Natl Acad Sci U S A 1991;88:5809-13.

7. Krantz SB. Erythropoietin. Blood 1991;77:419-34.

8. Winearls CG, Oliver DO, Pippard MJ, et al. Effect of human erythropoietin derived from recombinant DNA on the anaemia of patients maintained by chronic haemodialysis. Lancet 1986;2:1175-8.

9. Eschbach JW, Abdulhadi MH, Browne JK, et al. Recombinant human erythropoietin in anemic patients with end-stage renal disease. Results of a Phase III multicenter clinical trial. Ann Intern Med 1989;111:992-1000.

10. Goodnough LT, Monk TG, Andriole GL. Erythropoietin therapy. N Engl J Med 1997;336:933-8.

11. Youssoufian H, Longmore G, Neumann D, et al. Structure, function, and activation of the erythropoietin receptor. Blood 1993;81:2223-36.

12. Fisher JW. Erythropoietin: Physiologic and pharmacologic aspects. Proc Soc Exp Biol Med 1997;216:358-69.

13. Cazzola M, Mercuriali F, Brugnara C. Use of recombinant human erythropoietin outside the setting of uremia. Blood 1997;89:4248-67.

14. Shinjo K, Takeshita A, Higuchi M, et al. Erythropoietin receptor expression on human bone marrow erythroid precursor cells by a newly devised quantitative flow-cytometric assay. Br J Haematol 1997;96:551-8.

15. Li Y, Juul SE, Morris-Wiman JA, et al. Erythropoietin receptors are expressed in the central nervous system of mid-trimester human fetuses. Pediatr Res 1996;40:376-80.

16. Morishita E, Masuda S, Nagao M, et al. Erythropoietin receptor is expressed in rat hippocampal and cerebral cortical neurons and erythropoietin prevents in vitro glutamate-induced neuronal death. Neuroscience 1997;76:105-16.

17. Matthews DJ, Topping RS, Cass RT, Giebel LB. A sequential dimerization mechanism for the erythropoietin receptor. Proc Natl Acad Sci U S A 1996;93:9471-6.

18. Miura O, Nakamura N, Quelle FW, et al. Erythropoietin induces association of the JAK2 protein tyrosine kinase with the erythropoietin receptor in vivo. Blood 1994;84:1501-7.

19. Barber DL, Corless CN, Xia K, et al. Erythropoietin activates Raf1 by an Shc-independent pathway in CTLL-EPO-R cells. Blood 1997;89:55-64.

20. De la Chapelle A, Traskelin A-L, Juvonen E. Truncated erythropoietin receptor causes dominantly inherited benign human erythrocytosis. Proc Natl Acad Sci U S A 1993;90:4495-9.

21. McMahon GF, Vargas R, Ryan M, et al. Pharmacokinetics and effects of recombinant human erythropoietin after intravenous and subcutaneous injections in healthy volunteers. Blood 1990;76:1718-22.

22. Widness JA, Veng-Pederson P, Peters C, et al. Erythropoietin pharmacokinetics in premature infants: Developmental, nonlinearity, and treatment effects. J Appl Physiol 1996;80:140-8.

23. Krishnan R, Shankaran S, Krishnan M, et al. Pharmacokinetics of erythropoietin following single-dose subcutaneous administration in preterm infants. Biol Neonate 1996;70:235-40.

24. Schaller R, Sperschneider H, Thieler H, et al. Differences in intravenous and subcutaneous application of recombinant human erythropoietin: A multicenter trial. Artif Organs 1994;18:552-8.

25. Peces R, de la Torre R, Alcazar R, Urra JM. Antibodies against recombinant human

erythropoietin in a patient with erythro-
poietin-resistant anemia. N Engl J Med 1996;
335:523-4.

26. Prabhakar SS, Muhlfelder T. Antibodies to recombinant human erythropoietin causing
pure red cell aplasia. Clin Nephrol 1997;47:
331-5.

27. NKF-DOQI clinical practice guidelines for the
treatment of anemia of chronic renal failure.
Am J Kidney Dis 1997;30(Suppl 3):S194-
S237.

28. Muirhead N. Renal disease: The clinical impact of recombinant erythropoietin. J R Coll
Physicians Lond 1997;31:125-30.

29. Bode-Boger SM, Boger RH, Kuhn M, et al.
Recombinant human erythropoietin enhances vasoconstrictor tone via endothelin-1
and constrictor prostanoids. Kidney Int
1996;50:255-61.

30. Ahluwalia N, Skikne BS, Savin V, Chonko A.
Markers of masked iron deficiency and effectiveness of EPO therapy in chronic renal failure. Am J Kidney Dis 1997;30:532-41.

31. Cella D. The functional assessment of cancer
therapy anemia (FACT-An) scale: A new tool
for the assessment of outcomes in cancer
anemia and fatigue. Semin Hematol 1997;34
(Suppl 2):13-9.

32. Miller CB, Jones RJ, Piantadosi S, et al. Decreased erythropoietin response in patients
with the anemia of cancer. N Engl J Med
1990;322:1689-92.

33. Ludwig H, Fritz E, Kotzmann H, et al.
Erythropoietin treatment of anemia associated with multiple myeloma. N Engl J Med
1990;322:1693-9.

34. Oster W, Herrmann F, Gamm H, et al.
Erythropoietin for the treatment of anemia of
malignancy associated with neoplastic bone
marrow infiltration. J Clin Oncol 1990;8:
956-62.

35. Platanias LC, Miller CB, Mick R, et al. Treatment of chemotherapy-induced anemia with
recombinant human erythropoietin in cancer patients. J Clin Oncol 1991;9:2021-6.

36. Barlogie B, Beck T. Recombinant human
erythropoietin and the anemia of multiple
myeloma. Stem Cells 1993;11:88-94.

37. Henry D, Keller A, Kugler J, et al. Treatment
of anemia in cancer patients on cisplatin chemotherapy with recombinant human
erythropoietin. Proc Am Soc Clin Oncol 1990;
90:703.

38. Miller CB, Platanias LC, Mills SR, et al. Phase
I-II trial of erythropoietin in the treatment of
cisplatin-associated anemia. J Natl Cancer
Inst 1992;84:98-103.

39. Cascinu S, Fedeli A, Del Ferro E, et al. Recombinant human erythropoietin treatment
in cisplatin-associated anemia: A randomized, double-blind trial with placebo. J Clin
Oncol 1994;12:1058-62.

40. Cazzola M, Messinger D, Battistel V, et al.
Recombinant human erythropoietin in the
anemia associated with multiple myeloma or
non-Hodgkin's lymphoma: Dose finding and
identification of predictors of response.
Blood 1995;86:4446-53.

41. Osterborg A, Boogaerts MA, Cimino R, et al.
Recombinant human erythropoietin in
transfusion-dependent anemic patients with
multiple myeloma and non-Hodgkin's lymphoma—a randomized multicenter study.
Blood 1996;87:2675-82.

42. Henry DH III, Thatcher N. Patient selection
and predicting response to recombinant human erythropoietin in anemic cancer patients. Semin Hematol 1996;33(Suppl
1):2-5.

43. Glaspy J, Bukowksi R, Steinberg D, et al. Impact of therapy with epoetin-alpha on clinical
outcomes in patients with nonmyeloid malignancies during cancer chemotherapy in
community oncology practice. J Clin Oncol
1997;15:1218-34.

44. Strauss RG. Neonatal anemia: Pathophysiology and treatment. Immunol Invest 1995;
24:341-51.

45. Strauss RG. Red blood cell transfusion practices in the neonate. Clin Perinatol 1995;22:
641-55.

46. Doyle JJ. The role of erythropoietin in the anemia of prematurity. Semin Perinatol 1997;21:20-7.

47. Ohls RK, Harcum J, Schibler KR, Christensen RD. The effect of erythropoietin on the transfusion requirements of preterm infants weighing 750 grams or less: A randomized, double-blind, placebo-controlled study. J Pediatr 1997;131:661-5.

48. Scaradavou A, Inglis S, Peterson P, et al. Suppression of erythropoiesis by intrauterine transfusions in hemolytic disease of the newborn: Use of erythropoietin to treat the late anemia. J Pediatr 1993;1223:279-84.

49. Ovali F, Samanaci N, Dagoglu T. Management of late anemia in rhesus hemolytic disease: Use of recombinant human erythropoietin (a pilot study). Pediatr Res 1996;39: 831-4.

50. Meister B, Maurer H, Simma B, et al. The effect of recombinant human erythropoietin on circulating hematopoietic progenitor cells in anemic premature infants. Stem Cells 1997; 15:359-63.

51. Widness JA, Seward VJ, Kromer IJ, et al. Changing patterns of red blood cell transfusion in very low birth weight infants. J Pediatr 1996;129:680-7.

52. Strauss RG, Burmeister LF, Johnson K, et al. AS-1 red cells for neonatal transfusions: A randomized trial assessing donor exposure and safety. Transfusion 1996;36:873-8.

53. Asch J, Wedgwood JF. Optimizing the approach to anemia in preterm infants: Is there a role for erythropoietin therapy? J Perinatol 1997;17:276-82.

54. Fain J, Hilsenrath P, Widness JA, et al. A cost analysis comparing erythropoietin and red cell transfusions in the treatment of anemia of prematurity. Transfusion 1995;35:936-43.

55. Moses A, Nelson J, Bagby GC Jr. The influence of human immunodeficiency virus-1 on hematopoiesis. Blood 1998;91:1479-95.

56. Spivak JL, Barnes DC, Fuchs E, Quinn TC. Serum immunoreactive erythropoietin in HIV-infected patients. JAMA 1989;261: 3104-7.

57. Fischl M, Galpin JE, Levine JD, et al. Recombinant human erythropoietin for patients with AIDS treated with zidovudine. N Engl J Med 1990;322:1488-93.

58. Henry DH, Beall GN, Benson CA, et al. Recombinant human erythropoietin in the treatment of anemia associated with human immunodeficiency virus (HIV) infection and zidovudine therapy. Ann Intern Med 1992; 117:739-48.

59. Henry DH, Jemsek JG, Levin AS, et al. Recombinant human erythropoietin and the treatment of anemia in patients with AIDS or advanced ARC not receiving ZDV. J Acquir Immune Defic Syndr 1992;5:847-52.

60. Phair JP, Abels RI, McNeill MV, et al. Recombinant human erythropoietin treatment: Investigational new drug protocol for the anemia of the acquired immunodeficiency syndrome. Arch Intern Med 1993;153: 2669-75.

61. Caselli D, Maccabruni A, Zuccotti GV, et al. Recombinant erythropoietin for treatment of anaemia in HIV-infected children. AIDS 1996;10(8):929-31.

62. Rendo P, Freigeiro D, Braier J, et al. Double-blind multicenter randomized study of recombinant human erythropoietin in HIV+ children with anemia treated with antiretrovirals (abstract). Blood 1996;88:348a.

63. Cazzola M, Ponchio L, de Benedetti F, et al. Defective iron supply for erythropoiesis and adequate endogenous erythropoietin production in the anemia associated with systemic-onset juvenile chronic arthritis. Blood 1996;87:4824-30.

64. Pincus T, Olsen NJ, Russell IJ, et al. Multicenter study of recombinant human erythropoietin in correction of anemia in rheumatoid arthritis. Am J Med 1990;89:161-8.

65. Goodnough LT, Marcus RE. The erythropoietic response to erythropoietin in patients with rheumatoid arthritis. J Lab Clin Med 1997;130:381-6.

66. Gasche C, Dejaco C, Waldhor T, et al. Double-blind, placebo-controlled trial of erythropoietin and iron saccharate for anemia in Crohn's disease (abstract). Gastroenterology 1995;108:A821.

67. Schreiber S, Howaldt S, Schnoor M, et al. Recombinant erythropoietin for the treatment of anemia in inflammatory bowel disease. N Engl J Med 1996;334:619-23.

68. Dobil R, Hassall E, Wadsworth LD, Israel DM. Recombinant human erythropoietin for treatment of anemia of chronic disease in children with Crohn's disease. J Pediatr 1998; 132:155-9.

69. Hoefsloot LH, van Amelsvoort MP, Broeders LCAM, et al. Erythropoietin-induced activation of STAT5 is impaired in the myelodysplastic syndrome. Blood 1997;89:1690-700.

70. Hellstrom-Lindberg E. Efficacy of erythropoietin in the myelodysplastic syndrome: A meta-analysis of 205 patients from 17 studies. Br J Haematol 1995;89:67-71.

71. Rose EH, Abels RI, Nelson RA, et al. The use of rHuEPO in the treatment of anaemia related to myelodysplasia (MDS). Br J Haematol 1995;89:831-7.

72. Negrin RS, Stein R, Vardiman J, et al. Treatment of the anemia of myelodysplastic syndrome using recombinant human granulocyte colony-stimulating factor in combination with erythropoietin. Blood 1993;82:737-43.

73. Negin RS, Stein R, Doherty K, et al. Maintenance treatment of the anemia of myelodysplastic syndromes with recombinant human granulocyte colony-stimulating factor and erythropoietin: Evidence for in vivo synergy. Blood 1996;87:4076-81.

74. Bessho M, Hirashima K, Asano S, et al. Treatment of the anemia of aplastic anemia patients with recombinant human erythropoietin in combination with granulocyte colony-stimulating factor: A multicenter randomized controlled study. Eur J Haematol 1997;58:265-72.

75. Al-Khatti A, Veith RW, Papayannopoulou T, et al. Stimulation of fetal hemoglobin synthe-sis by erythropoietin in baboons. N Engl J Med 1987;317:415-20.

76. Nagel RL, Vichinsky E, Shah M, et al. F reticulocyte response in sickle cell anemia treated with recombinant human erythropoietin: A double-blind study. Blood 1993; 81:9-14.

77. Villeval J-L, Rouyer-Fessard P, Blumenfeld N, et al. Retrovirus-mediated transfer of the erythropoietin gene in hematopoietic cells improves the erythrocyte phenotype in murine β-thalassemia. Blood 1994;84:928-33.

78. Rodgers GP, Dover GJ, Uyesaka N, et al. Augmentation by erythropoietin of the fetal-hemoglobin response to hydroxyurea in sickle cell disease. N Engl J Med 1993;328: 73-80.

79. Rachmilewitz EA, Goldfarb A, Dover G. Administration of erythropoietin to patients with β-thalassemia intermedia: A preliminary trial. Blood 1991;78:1145-7.

80. Olivieri NF, Freedman MH, Perrine SP, et al. Trial of recombinant human erythropoietin: Three patients with thalassemia intermedia. Blood 1992;80:3258-60.

81. Nisli G, Kavakli K, Vergin C, et al. Recombinant human erythropoietin trial in thalassemia intermedia. J Trop Pediatr 1996;42: 330-4.

82. Rachmilewitz EA, Aker M, Perry D, Dover G. Sustained increase in haemoglobin and RBC following long-term administration of recombinant human erythropoietin to patients with homozygous beta-thalassemia. Br J Haematol 1995;90:341-5.

83. Nisli G, Kavakli K, Aydinok Y, et al. Recombinant erythropoietin trial in children with transfusion-dependent homozygous beta-thalassemia. Acta Haematol 1997;98:199-203.

84. De Franceschi L, Rouyer-Fessard P, Alper SL, et al. Combination of erythropoietin hydroxyurea, and clotrimazole in a β-thalassemic mouse: A model for human therapy. Blood 1996;87:1188-95.

85. Bennett CL, Smith TJ, Weeks JC, et al. Use of hematopoietic colony-stimulating factors: The American Society of Clinical Oncology Survey. J Clin Oncol 1996;14:2511-20.

86. Lieschke GJ, Burgess AW. Granulocyte colony-stimulating factor and granulocyte-macrophage colony-stimulating factor. N Engl J Med 1992;327:28-35 and 99-106.

87. Nemunaitis J. Granulocyte-macrophage-colony-stimulating factor: A review from preclinical development to clinical application. Transfusion 1993;33:70-83.

88. Bagley CJ, Woodcock JM, Stomski FC, Lopez AF. The structural and functional basis of cytokine receptor activation: Lessons from the common β subunit of the granulocyte-macrophage colony-stimulating factor, interleukin-3 (IL-3) and IL-5 receptors. Blood 1997;89:1471-82.

89. Dranoff G, Crawford AD, Sadelain M, et al. Involvement of granulocyte-macrophage colony-stimulating factor in pulmonary homeostasis. Science 1994;264:713-6.

90. Johnson GR, Gonda TJ, Metcalf D, et al. A lethal myeloproliferative syndrome in mice transplanted with bone marrow cells infected with a retrovirus expressing granulocyte-macrophage colony-stimulating factor. EMBO J 1989;8:441-8.

91. Brach MA, de Vos S, Gruss H-J, Herrmann F. Prolongation of survival of human polymorphonuclear neutrophils by granulocyte macrophage colony-stimulating factor is caused by inhibition of programmed cell death. Blood 1992;80:2920-4.

92. Van Pelt LJ, Huisman MV, Weening RS, et al. A single dose of granulocyte-macrophage colony-stimulating factor induces systemic interleukin-8 release and neutrophil activation in healthy volunteers. Blood 1996;87:5305-13.

93. Stute N, Furman WL, Schell M, Evans WE. Pharmacokinetics of recombinant human granulocyte-macrophage colony-stimulating factor in children after intravenous and subcutaneous administration. J Pharm Sci 1995;84:824-8.

94. Honkoop AH, Hoekman K, Wagstaff J, et al. Continuous infusion or subcutaneous injection of granulocyte-macrophage colony-stimulating factor: Increased efficacy and reduced toxicity when given subcutaneously. Br J Cancer 1996;74:1132-6.

95. Seebach J, Speich R, Fehr J, et al. GM-CSF-induced acute eosinophilic pneumonia. Br J Haematol 1995;90:963-5.

96. Welte K, Gabrilove J, Bronchud MH, et al. Filgrastim (r-metHuG-CSF): The first 10 years. Blood 1996;88:1907-29.

97. Avalos BR. Molecular analysis of the granulocyte colony-stimulating factor receptor. Blood 1996;88:761-77.

98. Lieschke GJ, Grail D, Hodgson G, et al. Mice lacking granulocyte colony-stimulating factor have chronic neutropenia, granulocyte and macrophage progenitor cell deficiency, and impaired neutrophil mobilization. Blood 1994;84:1737-46.

99. Anderlini P, Przepiorka D, Champlin R, Korbling M. Biological and clinical effects of granulocyte-colony stimulating factor in normal individuals. Blood 1996;88:2819-25.

100. Karawajczyk M, Hoglund M, Ericsson J, Venge P. Administration of G-CSF to healthy subjects: The effects on eosinophil counts and mobilization of eosinophil granule proteins. Br J Haematol 1997;96:259-65.

101. Watts MJ, Addison I, Long SG, et al. Crossover study of the haematological effects and pharmacokinetics of glycosylated and nonglycosylated G-CSF in healthy volunteers. Br J Haematol 1997;98:474-9.

102. de Arriba F, Lozano ML, Ortuno F, et al. Prospective randomized study comparing the efficacy of bioequivalent doses of glycosylated and nonglycosylated rG-CSF for mobilizing peripheral blood progenitor cells. Br J Haematol 1997;96:418-20.

103. Kuwabara T, Kobayashi S. Pharmacokinetics and pharmacodynamics of a recombinant human granulocyte colony-stimulating factor. Drug Metab Rev 1996;28:625-58.

104. Jain KK. Cutaneous vasculitis associated with granulocyte colony-stimulating factor. J Am Acad Dermatol 1994;31:213-5.

105. Bonilla MA, Dale D, Ziedler C, et al. Long-term safety of treatment with recombinant human granulocyte colony-stimulating factor (R-metHuG-CSF) in patients with severe congenital neutropenia. Br J Haematol 1994; 88:723-30.

106. Grigg A, Lusk J, Szer J. G-CSF stimulated donor granulocyte collections for neutropenic sepsis. Leuk Lymphoma 1995;18:329-34.

107. Grigg A, Vecchi L, Bardy P, Szer J. G-CSF stimulated donor granulocyte collections for prophylaxis and therapy of neutropenic sepsis. Aust N Z J Med 1996;26:813-8.

108. Adkins D, Spitzer G, Johnston M, et al. Transfusions of granulocyte-colony-stimulating factor-mobilized granulocyte components to allogeneic transplant recipients: Analysis of kinetics and factors determining post-transfusion neutrophil and platelet counts. Transfusion 1997;37:737-48.

109. Liles WC, Huang JE, Llewellyn C, et al. A comparative trial of granulocyte-colony-stimulating factor and dexamethasone, separately and in combination, for the mobilization of neutrophils in the peripheral blood of normal volunteers. Transfusion 1997;37:182-7.

110. Sheridan WP, Begley CG, Juttner CA, et al. Effect of peripheral-blood progenitor cells mobilised by filgrastim (G-CSF) on platelet recovery after high-dose chemotherapy. Lancet 1992;339:640-4.

111. Grigg AP, Roberts AW, Raunow H, et al. Optimizing dose and scheduling of filgrastim (granulocyte colony-stimulating factor) for mobilization and collection of peripheral blood progenitor cells in normal volunteers. Blood 1995;86:4437-45.

112. Anderlini P, Przepiorka D, Huh Y, et al. Duration of filgrastim mobilization and apheresis yield of CD34+ progenitor cells and lymphoid subsets in normal donors for allogeneic transplantation. Br J Haematol 1996;93:940-2.

113. Beelen DW, Ottinger HD, Elmaagacli A, et al. Transplantation of filgrastim-mobilized peripheral blood stem cells from HLA-identical sibling or alternative family donors in patients with hematologic malignancies: A prospective comparison on clinical outcome, immune reconstitution, and hematopoietic chimerism. Blood 1997;90:4725-35.

114. Russell N, Gratwohl A, Schmitz N. Annotation: The place of blood stem cells in allogeneic transplantation. Br J Haematol 1996;93:747-53.

115. Anderlini P, Korbling M, Dale D, et al. Allogeneic blood stem cell transplantation: Considerations for donors (editorial). Blood 1997;90:903-8.

116. American Society of Clinical Oncology recommendations for the use of hematopoietic colony-stimulating factors: Evidence-based clinical practice guidelines. J Clin Oncol 1994;12:2471-508.

117. Update of the recommendations for the use of hematopoietic colony-stimulating factors: Evidence-based clinical practice guidelines. J Clin Oncol 1996;14:1957-60.

118. Hartmann LC, Tschetter LK, Habermann TM, et al. Granulocyte colony-stimulating factor in severe chemotherapy-induced afebrile neutropenia. N Engl J Med 1997;336:1776-80.

119. Mitchell PLR, Morland B, Stevens MCG, et al. Granulocyte colony-stimulating factor in established febrile neutropenia: A randomized study of pediatric patients. J Clin Oncol 1997;15:1163-70.

120. Pui C-H, Boyett JM, Hughes WT, et al. Human granulocyte colony-stimulating factor after induction chemotherapy in children with acute lymphoblastic leukemia. N Engl J Med 1997;336:1781-7.

121. Moore JO, Dodge RK, Amrein PC, et al. Granulocyte-colony stimulating factor (filgrastim) accelerates granulocyte recovery after intensive postremission chemotherapy for acute myeloid leukemia with aziridinyl benzoquinone and mitoxantrone: Cancer and leukemia group B study 9022. Blood 1997;89:780-8.

122. Lowenberg B, Suciu S, Archimbaud E, et al. Use of recombinant granulocyte-macrophage colony-stimulating factor during and after remission induction chemotherapy in patients aged 61 years and older with acute myeloid leukemia (AML): Final report of AML-11, a Phase III randomized study of the leukemia cooperative group of European Organisation for the Research Treatment of Cancer (EORTC-LCG) and the Dutch Belgian Hemato-Oncology Cooperative Group (HOVON). Blood 1997;90: 2952-61.

123. Heil G, Hoelzer D, Sanz MA, et al. A randomized, double-blind, placebo-controlled, Phase III study of filgrastim in remission induction and consolidation therapy for adults with de novo acute myeloid leukemia. Blood 1997;90:4710-8.

124. Geissler K, Koller E, Hubmann E, et al. Granulocyte colony-stimulating factor as an adjunct to induction chemotherapy for adult acute lymphoblastic leukemia—a randomized Phase-III study. Blood 1997;90:590-6.

125. McQuaker IG, Hunter AE, Pacey S, et al. Low-dose filgrastim significantly enhances neutrophil recovery following autologous peripheral-blood stem-cell transplantation in patients with lymphoproliferative disorders: Evidence for clinical and economic benefit. J Clin Oncol 1997;15:451-7.

126. Linch DC, Milligan DW, Winfield DA, et al. G-CSF after peripheral blood stem cell transplantation in lymphoma patients significantly accelerated neutrophil recovery and shortened time in hospital: Results of a randomized BNLI trial. Br J Haematol 1997;99: 933-8.

127. Pitrak DL, Tsai HC, Mullane KM, et al. Accelerated neutrophil apoptosis in the acquired immunodeficiency syndrome. J Clin Invest 1996;98:2714-9.

128. Deichmann M, Kronenwett R, Haa R. Expression of the human immunodeficiency virus type I co-receptors, CXCR-4 (fusin, LESTR) and CKR-5 in CD34$^+$ hematopoietic progenitor cells. Blood 1997;89:3522-8.

129. Meynard J-L, Guiguet M, Arsac S, et al. Frequency and risk factors of infectious complications in neutropenic patients infected with HIV. AIDS 1997;11:995-8.

130. Kimura S, Matsuda J, Ikematsu S, et al. Efficacy of recombinant human granulocyte colony-stimulating factor on neutropenia in patients with AIDS. AIDS 1990;12: 1251-5.

131. Hardy WD. Combined ganciclovir and recombinant human granulocyte-macrophage colony-stimulating factor in the treatment of cytomegalovirus retinitis in AIDS patients. J Acquir Immune Defic Syndr 1991;4(Suppl 1):S22-8.

132. Kaplan LD, Kahn JO, Crowe S, et al. Clinical and virologic effects of recombinant human granulocyte-macrophage colony-stimulating factor in patients receiving chemotherapy for human immunodeficiency virus-associated non-Hodgkin's lymphoma: Results of a randomized trial. J Clin Oncol 1991;9:929-40.

133. Garavelli PL, Berti P. Efficacy of recombinant granulocyte colony-stimulating factor in the long-term treatment of AIDS-related neutropenia. AIDS 1993;7:589-90.

134. Hermans P, Rozenbaum W, Jou A, et al. Filgrastim to treat neutropenia and support myelosuppressive medication dosing in HIV infection. G-CSF 92105 study group. AIDS 1996;10:1627-33.

135. Bonilla MA, Gillio AP, Ruggeiro M, et al. Effects of recombinant human granulocyte colony-stimulating factor on neutropenia in patients with congenital agranulocytosis. N Engl J Med 1989;320:1574-80.

136. Dale DC, Bonilla MA, Davis MW, et al. A randomized controlled Phase III trial of recombinant human granulocyte colony-stimulating factor (filgrastim) for treatment of severe chronic neutropenia. Blood 1993; 81:2496-502.

137. Guba SC, Sartor CA, Hutchinson R, et al. Granulocyte colony-stimulating factor (G-

CSF) production and G-CSF receptor structure in patients with congenital neutropenia. Blood 1994;83:1486-92.

138. Dong F, Hoefsloot LH, Schelen AM, et al. Identification of a nonsense mutation in the granulocyte-colony-stimulating factor receptor in severe congenital neutropenia. Proc Natl Acad Sci U S A 1994;91:333:4480-4.

139. Welte K, Boxer LA. Severe chronic neutropenia: Pathophysiology and therapy. Semin Hematol 1997;34:267-78.

140. Tidow N, Pilz C, Teichmann B, et al. Clinical relevance of point mutations in the cytoplasmic domain of the granulocyte colony-stimulating factor receptor gene in patients with severe congenital neutropenia. Blood 1997;89:2369-75.

141. Hazenberg BPC, van Leeuwen MA, van Ryswyk MH, et al. Correction of granulocytopenia in Felty's syndrome by granulocyte-macrophage colony stimulating factor. Simultaneous induction of interleukin-6 release and flare-up of the arthritis. Blood 1989;74:2769-74.

142. Bhalla K, Ross R, Jeter E, et al. G-CSF improves granulocytopenia in Felty's syndrome without flare-up of arthritis. Am J Hematol 1993;42:230-1.

143. Rodwell RL, Gray PH, Taylor KM, Minchinton R. Granulocyte colony stimulating factor treatment for alloimmune neonatal neutropenia. Arch Dis Child Fetal Neonatal Ed 1996;75:F57-8.

144. Hurst D, Kilpatrick L, Becker J, et al. Recombinant human GM-CSF treatment of neutropenia in glycogen storage disease-Ib. Am J Pediatr Hematol Oncol 1993;15:71-6.

145. Gartz BZ, Levy I, Nitzan M, Barak Y. Sweet's syndrome associated with G-CSF treatment in a child with glycogen storage disease type Ib. Pediatrics 1996;97:401-3.

146. Lamberti JS, Bellnier TJ, Schwarzkopf SB, Schneider E. Filgrastim treatment of three patients with clozapine-induced agranulocytosis. J Clin Psychiatry 1995;56:256-9.

147. Roddie P, Dorrance H, Cook MK, Rainey JB. Treatment of sulphasalazine-induced agranulocytosis with granulocyte macrophage-colony stimulating factor. Aliment Pharmacol Ther 1995;9:711-2.

148. Kendra JR, Rugman FP, Flaherty TA, et al. First use of G-CSF in chlorpromazine-induced agranulocytosis: A report of two cases. Postgrad Med J 1993;69:885-7.

149. Balkin MS, Buchholtz M, Ortiz J, Green AJ. Propylthiouracil (PTU)-induced agranulocytosis treated with recombinant human granulocyte colony-stimulating factor (G-CSF). Thyroid 1993;3:305-9.

150. Magner JA, Snyder DK. Methimazole-induced agranulocytosis treated with recombinant human granulocyte colony-stimulating factor (G-CSF). Thyroid 1994;4:295-6.

151. Al-Refaie FN, Wonde B, Hoffbrand AV. Deferiprone-associated myelotoxicity. Eur J Haematol 1994;53:298-30.

152. Marinella MA. Agranulocytosis associated with ticlopidine: A possible benefit of filgrastim. Ann Clin Lab Sci 1997;27:418-21.

153. de Boisblana BP, Mason CM, Andersen J, et al. Phase I safety trial of filgrastim (r-metHuG-CSF) in non-neutropenic patients with severe community-acquired pneumonia. Respir Med 1997;91:387-94.

154. Gough A, Clapperton M, Rolando N, et al. Randomised placebo-controlled trial of granulocyte-colony stimulating factor in diabetic foot infection. Lancet 1997;350:855-9.

155. Sato N, Kashima K, Tanaka Y, et al. Effect of granulocyte-colony stimulating factor on generation of oxygen-derived free radicals and myeloperoxidase activity of neutrophils from poorly controlled NIDDM patients. Diabetes 1997;46:133-7.

156. Du XX, Williams DA. Interleukin-11: A multifunctional growth factor derived from the hematopoietic microenvironment. Blood 1994;82:2023-30.

157. Yang Y-C. Interleukin-11 (IL-11) and its receptor: Biology and potential applications in thrombocytopenic states. In: Kurzrock R, ed.

Cytokines: Interleukin and their receptors. Norwell, MA: Kluwer Academic Publishers, 1995;321-40.

158. Du X, Williams D. Interleukin 11: Review of molecular, cell biology, and clinical use. Blood 1997;89:3897-908.

159. Paul SR, Bennett F, Calvetti JA, et al. Molecular cloning of a cDNA encoding interleukin-11, a stromal cell derived lymphopoietic and hematopoietic cytokine. Proc Natl Acad Sci U S A;1990;87:7512-6.

160. McKinley D, Wu Q, Yang-Feng T, Yang Y. Genomic sequence and chromosomal location of human interleukin 11 (IL-11) gene. Genomics 1992;13:814-9.

161. Neumega Professional Prescribing Information, Genetics Institute, Inc., Cambridge, MA, 1998.

162. Hilton DJ, Hilton AA, Raicevic A, et al. Cloning of a murine IL-11 receptor alpha-chain;requirement for gp130 for high-affinity binding and signal transduction. EMBO J 1994;13:4765-75.

163. Kishimoto T, Akira S, Narazaki M, et al. Interleukin-6 family of cytokines and gp130. Blood 1995;86:1243-54.

164. Girasole G, Passeri G, Jilka RL, Manolagas SC. Interleukin-11: A new cytokine critical for osteoclast development. J Clin Invest 1994;93:1516-24.

165. Keith JC Jr, Albert L, Sonis ST. IL-11, a pleiotrophic cytokine: Exciting new effects of IL-11 on gastrointestinal mucosal biology. Stem Cells 1994;12:79-90.

166. Musashi M, Yang Y, Paul SR. Direct and synergistic effects of interleukin-11 on murine hematopoiesis in culture. Proc Natl Acad Sci U S A 1991;88:765-9.

167. Quesniaux VFJ, Clark SC, Turner K, Fagg B. Interleukin-11 stimulates multiple phases of erythropoiesis in vitro. Blood 1992;80:1218-23.

168. Kobayashi S, Teramura M, Sugawara I, et al. Interleukin-11 acts as an autocrine growth factor for human megakaryoblastic cell lines. Blood 1993;81:889-93.

169. Weich NS, Wang A, Fitzgerald M, et al. Recombinant human interleukin-11 directly promotes megakaryocytopoiesis in vitro. Blood 1997;90:3893-902.

170. Hawley RG, Hawley TS, Fong AZC, et al. Thrombopoietic and serial repopulating ability of murine hematopoietic stem cells constitutively expressing interleukin-11. Proc Natl Acad Sci U S A 1996;93:10297-302.

171. Cairo MS, Plunkett JM, Nguyen A, et al. Effect of interleukin-11 with and without granulocyte colony-stimulating factor on in vivo neonatal rat hematopoiesis: Induction of neonatal thrombocytosis by interleukin-11 and synergistic enhancement of neutrophilia by interleukin-11 + granulocyte colony-stimulating factor. Pediatr Res 1993;34:56-61.

172. Yonemura Y, Kawakita M, Masuda T, et al. Effect of recombinant human interleukin-11 on rat megakaryopoiesis and thrombopoiesis in vivo: Comparative study with interleukin-6. Br J Haematol 1993;84:16-23.

173. Leonard JP, Neben TY, Lozita MK, et al. Constant subcutaneous infusion of rhIL-11 in mice: Efficient delivery enhances biological activity. Exp Hematol 1996;24:270-6.

174. Gordon MS, McCaskill-Stevens WJ, Battiato LA, et al. A Phase I trial of recombinant human interleukin-11 (Neumega rhIL-11 growth factor) in women receiving breast cancer chemotherapy. Blood 1996;87:3615-24.

175. Orazi A, Cooper RJ, Tong J, et al. Effects of recombinant human interleukin-11 (Neumega™ rhIL-11 growth factor) on megakaryocytopoiesis in human bone marrow. Exp Hematol 1996;24:1289-97.

176. Anderson KC, Morimoto C, Paul SR, et al. Interleukin-11 promotes accessory cell-dependent B-cell differentiation in humans. Blood 1992;80:2797-804.

177. Chang M, Suen Y, Meng G, et al. Differential mechanisms in the regulation of endogenous levels of thrombopoietin and interleukin-11 during thrombocytopenia: Insight into the

regulation of platelet production. Blood 1996; 88:3354-62.

178. Leonard JP, Quinto CM, Kozitza MK, et al. Recombinant human interleukin-11 stimulates multilineage hematopoietic recovery in mice after a myelosuppressive regimen of sublethal irradiation and carboplatin. Blood 1994;83:1499-506.

179. Galmiche MC, Vogel CA, Delaloye AB, et al. Combined effects of interleukin-3 and interleukin-11 on hematopoiesis in irradiated mice. Exp Hematol 1996;24:1298-306.

180. Yonemura Y, Kawakita M, Miyake H, et al. Effects of interleukin-11 on carboplatin-induced thrombocytopenia in rats and in combination with stem cell factor. Int J Hematol 1997;65:397-404.

181. Ault KA, Mitchell J, Knowles C. Recombinant human interleukin-11 (Neumega rHuIL-11 growth factor) increases plasma volume and decreases urinary sodium excretion in normal human subjects (abstract). Blood 1994;84:276a.

182. Tepler I, Elias L, Smith JW, et al. A randomized placebo-controlled trial of recombinant human interleukin-11 in cancer patients with severe thrombocytopenia due to chemotherapy. Blood 1996;87:3607-14.

183. Isaacs C, Roberts NJ, Bailey FA, et al. Randomized placebo-controlled study of recombinant human interleukin-11 to prevent chemotherapy-induced thrombocytopenia in patients with breast cancer receiving dose-intensive cyclophosphamide and doxorubicin. J Clin Oncol 1997;15:3368-77.

184. Kirov I, Goldman S, Blazer B, et al. Recombinant human interleukin-11 (Neumega) is tolerated at double the adult dose and enhances hematopoietic recovery following ifosfamide, carboplatin and etoposide (ICE) chemotherapy in children. Correlation with rapid clearance, lack of induction of inflammatory cytokines and mobilization of early progenitor cells (abstract). Blood 1997;90 (Suppl 1):581a.

185. Kaushansky K. Thrombopoietin: The primary regulator of platelet production. Blood 1995;86:419-31.

186. Eaton DL, de Sauvage FJ. Thrombopoietin: the primary regulator of megakaryocytopoiesis and thrombopoiesis. Exp Hematol 1997; 25:1-7.

187. Sungaran R, Markovic B, Chong BH. Localization and regulation of thrombopoietin mRNA expression in human kidney, liver, bone marrow, and spleen using in situ hybridization. Blood 1997;89:101-7.

188. Guerriero A, Worford L, Holland HK, et al. Thrombopoietin is synthesized by bone marrow stromal cells. Blood 1997;90:3444-55.

189. Emmons RVB, Reid DM, Cohen RL, et al. Human thrombopoietin levels are high when thrombocytopenia is due to megakaryocyte deficiency and low when due to increased platelet destruction. Blood 1996;87:4068-71.

190. Nagata Y, Shozaki Y, Nagahisa H, et al. Serum thrombopoietin level is not regulated by transcription but by the total counts of both megakaryocytes and platelets during thrombocytopenia and thrombocytosis. Thromb Haemost 1997;77:808-14.

191. Debili N, Wendling F, Cosman D, et al. The Mpl receptor is expressed in the megakaryocytic lineage from late progenitors to platelets. Blood 1995;85:391-401.

192. Broudy VC, Lin NL, Sabath DF, et al. Human platelets display high-affinity receptors for thrombopoietin. Blood 1997;89:1896-904.

193. Miyakawa Y, Oda A, Druker BJ, et al. Thrombopoietin induces tyrosine phosphorylation of Stat3 and Stat5 in human blood platelets. Blood 1996;87:439-46.

194. Drachman JG, Sabath DF, Fox NE, Kaushansky K. Thrombopoietin signal transduction in purified murine megakaryocytes. Blood 1997;89:483-92.

195. Miyakawa Y, Oda A, Druker BJ, et al. Thrombopoietin and thrombin induce tyrosine phosphorylation of Vav in human blood platelets. Blood 1997;89:2789-98.

196. Fielder PJ, Hass P, Nagel M. Human platelets as a model for the binding and degradation of thrombopoietin. Blood 1997;89:2782-8.

197. de Sauvage FJ, Carver-Moore K, Luoh S-M, et al. Physiologic regulation of early and late stages of megakaryocytopoiesis by thrombopoietin. J Exp Med 1996;183:651-6.

198. Alexander WS, Roberts AW, Nicola NA, et al. Deficiencies in progenitor cells of multiple hematopoietic lineages and defective megakaryocytopoiesis in mice lacking the thrombopoietin receptor c-Mpl. Blood 1996;87:2162-70.

199. Shivadasani RA, Fielder P, Keller GA, et al. Regulation of the serum concentration of thrombopoietin in thrombocytopenic NF-E2 knockout mice. Blood 1997;90:1821-7.

200. Papayannopoulou T, Brice M, Farrer D, Kaushansky K. Insights into the cellular mechanisms of erythropoietin-thrombopoietin synergy. Exp Hematol 1996;24:660-9.

201. Arnold JT, Dau NC, Stenberg PE, et al. A single injection of pegylated murine megakaryocyte growth and development factor (MGDF) into mice is sufficient to produce a profound stimulation of megakaryocyte frequency, size, and ploidization. Blood 1997;89:823-33.

202. Harker LA, Marzec UM, Hunt P, et al. Dose-response effects of pegylated human megakaryocyte growth and development factor on platelet production and function in nonhuman primates. Blood 1996;88:511-21.

203. O'Malley CJ, Rasko JEJ, Basser RL, et al. Administration of pegylated recombinant human megakaryocyte growth and development factor to humans stimulates the production of functional platelets that show no evidence of in vivo activation. Blood 1996;88:3288-98.

204. Fontenay-Roupie M, Huret G, Loza JP, et al. Thrombopoietin activates human platelets and induces tyrosine phosphorylation of p80/85 cortactin. Thromb Haemost 1998;79:195-201.

205. Hokom MM, Lacey D, Kinsler O, et al. Megakaryocyte growth and development factor abrogates the lethal thrombocytopenia associated with carboplatin and irradiation in mice. Blood 1995;86:4486-92.

206. Farese AM, Hunt P, Grab LB, MacVittie TJ. Combined administration of recombinant human megakaryocyte growth and development factor and granulocyte colony-stimulating factor enhances multilineage hematopoietic reconstitution in nonhuman primates after radiation-induced marrow aplasia. J Clin Invest 1996;97:2145-51.

207. Neelis KJ, Dubbelman YD, Wognum AW, et al. Simultaneous administration of TPO and G-CSF after cytoreductive treatment of rhesus monkeys presents thrombocytopenia, accelerates platelet and red cell reconstitution, alleviates neutropenia, and promotes the recovery of immature bone marrow cells. Exp Hematol 1997;25:1084-93.

208. Shibuya K, Akahori H. Takahashi K, et al. Multilineage hematopoietic recovery by a single injection of pegylated recombinant human megakaryocyte growth and development factor in myelosuppressed mice. Blood 1998;91:37-45.

209. Neelis KJ, Hartong SCC, Egeland T, et al. The efficacy of single-dose administration of thrombopoietin with coadministration of either granulocyte/macrophage or granulocyte-colony stimulating factor in myelosuppressed rhesus monkeys. Blood 1997;90:2565-73.

210. Basser RL, Rasko JEJ, Clarke K, et al. Thrombopoietic effects of pegylated recombinant human megakaryocyte growth and development factor (PEG-rHuMGDF) in patients with advanced cancer. Lancet 1996;348:1279-81.

211. Fanucchi M, Glaspy J, Crawford J, et al. Effects of polyethylene glycol-conjugated recombinant human megakaryocyte growth and development factor on platelet counts after chemotherapy for lung cancer. N Engl J Med 1997;336:404-9.

212. Basser RL, Rasko JEJ, Clarke K, et al. Randomized, blinded, placebo-controlled phase

I trial of pegylated recombinant human megakaryocyte growth and development factor with filgrastim after dose-intensive chemotherapy in patients with advanced cancer. Blood 1997;89:3118-28.

213. Vadhan-Raj S, Murray LJ, Bueso-Ramos C, et al. Stimulation of megakaryocyte and platelet production by a single dose of recombinant human thrombopoietin in patients with cancer. Ann Intern Med 1997; 126:673-81.

214. Vadhan-Raj S, Verschraegen C, McGarry L, et al. Recombinant human thrombopoietin (RhTPO) attenuates high-dose carboplatin (c)-induced thrombocytopenia in patients with gynecologic malignancy (abstract). Blood 1997;9(Suppl 1):580a.

215. Nash R, Kurzrock R, Di Persio J, et al. Safety and activity of recombinant human thrombopoietin (rhTPO) in patients (pts) with delayed platelet recovery (DPR) (abstract). Blood 1997;90(Suppl 1):262a.

216. Beveridge R, Schuster M, Waller E, et al. Randomized double-blind, placebo-controlled trial of pegylated recombinant human megakaryocyte growth and development factor (PEG-rHuMGDF) in breast cancer patients (pts) following autologous bone marrow transplantation (ABMT) (abstract). Blood 1997;90(Suppl 1):580a.

217. Bolwell B, Vrendenburgh J, Overmoyer B, et al. Safety and biologic effect of pegylated recombinant human megakaryocyte growth and development factor (PEG-rHuMGDF) in breast cancer patients following autologous peripheral blood progenitor cell transplantation (PBPC) (abstract). Blood 1997;90(Suppl 1):171a.

218. Glaspy J, Vrendenburgh J, Demetri GD, et al. Effects of PEG-ylated recombinant human megakaryocyte growth and development factor (PEG-rHuMGDF) before high dose chemotherapy (HDC) with peripheral blood progenitor cell (PBPC) support (abstract). Blood 1997;90(Suppl 1):580a.

219. Bertolini F, Battaglia M, Pedrazzoli P, et al. Megakaryocytic progenitors can be generated ex vivo and safely administered to autologous peripheral blood progenitor cell transplant recipients. Blood 1997;89:2679-88.

220. McCullough J, Peterson R, Clay M, et al. Donors' willingness to participate in a trial of pegylated megakaryocyte growth and development factor (PEG-rHuMGDF) for platelet apheresis (abstract). Blood 1997;90(Suppl 1):135b.

221. Crawford J, Glaspy J, Belani et al. A randomized, placebo-controlled, dose scheduling trial of pegylated recombinant human megakaryocyte growth and development factor (PEG-rHuMGDF) with filgrastim support in non-small cell lung cancer (NSCLC) patients treated with paclitaxel and carboplatin during multiple cycles of chemotherapy (abstract). Proc ASCO 1998;17:73a.

222. Villeval J-L, Cohen-Solal K, Tulliez M, et al. High thrombopoietin production by hematopoietic cells induces a fatal myeloproliferative syndrome in mice. Blood 1997;90: 4369-83.

223. Dooley DC, Xiao M, Oppenlander BK, et al. Flt 3 ligand enhances the yield of primitive cells after ex vivo cultivation of $CD34^+$ $CD38^{dim}$ cells and $CD34^+38^{dim}$ $CD33^{dim}$ $HLA-DR^+$ cells. Blood 1997;90:3903-13.

In: Mintz PD, ed.
Transfusion Therapy: Clinical Principles and Practice
Bethesda, MD: AABB Press, 1999

21

Quality Assessment and Improvement of Blood Transfusion Practices

PAUL D. MINTZ, MD

 ASSESSING THE TRANSFUSION practices of colleagues is difficult. Factors that contribute to this difficulty include disagreement regarding when a transfusion is indicated and unavailability of the information needed to make an informed decision to transfuse. These factors affect the decision to transfuse every blood component. However, because Red Blood Cells (RBCs) are the most frequently transfused component, the following discussion uses red cell transfusion as a specific example to illustrate broader concepts.

Clinicians disagree regarding what constitutes an appropriate hemoglobin concentration for prescribing a transfusion. The role of red cell transfusion in improving peripheral red cell volume (and thereby gastrointestinal perfusion) as well as hemostasis has been raised as a reason for considering more liberal transfusion practices than have been recently deemed acceptable.[1] Furthermore, there is a continuing disagreement regarding an appropriate target hemoglobin concentration in unstable, acutely ill patients.[2,3] In this regard, the consensus statement on red cell transfusion from the Royal College of Physicians of Edinburgh concluded, "... there is no general agreement at which point transfusion should be given or on the optimum target concentration (of hemoglobin) to be achieved. There is no single critical hemoglobin or hematocrit value applicable to all patients."[4(p177)]

A refined and meaningful assessment of the appropriateness of any transfusion requires a careful consideration of the patient's unique circumstances present at the time the decision to prescribe the transfusion was made. While a single criterion such as hemoglobin concentration, platelet count,

Paul D. Mintz, MD, Associate Chair and Professor of Pathology, Professor of Internal Medicine, and Director, Clinical Laboratories and Blood Bank, University of Virginia Health Sciences Center, Charlottesville, Virginia

or activated partial thromboplastin time may serve as a means to guide practice, it does not necessarily indicate when any particular transfusion is absolutely necessary.

Physicians assessing transfusion practices must be aware that the actual information needed to define the need for any individual transfusion is not available. For example, we do not know the mitochondrial pO_2 of myocardial cells. We do not know if the delivery of oxygen to specific organs or tissues is adequate; in fact, we do not know their actual oxygen requirements. Thus, physicians must resort to using surrogate markers to inform their decisions. Unfortunately, measurement of hemoglobin concentration may not be well correlated in any patient with the amount of oxygen reaching critically important cells, owing to variability in cardiovascular and pulmonary function. Thus, those assessing transfusion practices should be careful to consider, in addition to the patient's unique circumstances, the information that was and was not available when the decision to transfuse was made.

Despite these difficulties, the assessment of transfusion practices by clinical staff is a requirement of accrediting organizations and may serve as a means of education and improved clinical care. With more than 11 million transfusions of red cells annually in the United States,[5] utilization review of blood transfusions requires significant resources.

There has been a long-standing interest in the assessment of clinical practice. The increasing role of accreditation standards and regulatory requirements, a growing appreciation by patients and the general public of the risks of medical treatment, the increasing amount of litigation related to health care, and the development of hospital health-care evaluation divisions have all contributed to increased activity in assessing the quality of care.

Industrial practices have been applied to assessment programs in clinical medicine.[6,7] In these programs, cycles of continuous improvement are created in the course of designing, measuring, assessing, and refining work processes.[6]

These activities have resulted in measurable improvements in health care.[6] The principles and practices of continuous quality improvement may be applied to organizational performance and clinical care in all patient services, including blood transfusions.

For any quality assessment program to work successfully in a hospital, the clinical staff must give a high priority to the process and the hospital administration must make available the resources necessary to ensure its development, implementation, refinement, and continuing support. Although criteria used in evaluating clinical care are ideally created from scientific data, this information is not always available, and it may be necessary to use consensus opinion.[8] In practice, clinical staff often find it appropriate to use explicit criteria to separate cases that should not require further assessment (because they are most likely to have met accepted standards of practice) from cases that need to be reviewed individually (using implicit criteria or a combination of implicit and explicit criteria).

The persons who develop the criteria may exert significant control over clinical practices and organizational procedures. As clinical staff assess transfusion practices and other processes, as further clinical information becomes available, and/or as a different level of performance is deemed necessary, the criteria may need to be modified.

History

The quality assessment of blood transfusion practices is as old as human transfusion itself. Jean Denis performed the first human transfusions in 1667 in Paris by transfusing animal blood into humans. Other physicians, many of whom preferred bloodletting, did not welcome his experiments. Eventually, a decree was issued prohibiting the practice of blood transfusion unless approved by the faculty of medicine of Paris.[9] Thus, prospective auditing of transfusion practices dates back to the 17th century.

In 1936, Bock emphasized the need to create clear indications for transfusion practice.[10] The following year, Fantus stated that too many transfusions were being done at Cook County Hospital in Chicago and discussed the development of a multidisciplinary committee to review blood transfusion practices there.[11] The Ministry of Health in England, in 1951, requested the review of blood use,[12] and an editorial in the *New England Journal of Medicine* in the same year noted that some transfusions were being given inappropriately.[13] In an early audit of transfusion practices published in 1953, Straus and Torres concluded that 49 of 290 transfusions were not indicated.[14] They recommended educational programs for clinicians to improve transfusion practices. A number of other publications in the 1950s supported these findings and emphasized the potential liability of physicians if an unnecessary transfusion were administered.[15-19] In 1960, Graham-Stewart stated that "All routine dogma concerning transfusion should be abandoned and each case should be dealt with on its merits."[20(p424)]

In 1961, the Joint Commission on Accreditation of Hospitals noted the need to review transfusion practices,[21] and MacDonald declared that a patient with a hemoglobin level of 11 g/dL preoperatively was generally safer donating blood than receiving it.[22] In 1962, Crosby recommended the establishment of a hospital transfusion board to oversee transfusion practices and noted the educational role that such a committee would serve.[23] In 1964, Walz demonstrated that a transfusion committee could conduct effective utilization review and decrease unnecessary transfusions.[24,25] Thus, utilization review of transfusion practices is not a new phenomenon.

Regulatory and Accreditation Requirements

Several accrediting and regulatory agencies in the United States have developed standards regarding the assessment and improvement of transfusion practices. Since 1961, such review has been a part of the accreditation process of the Joint Commission on Accreditation of Healthcare Organizations (JCAHO).[21] In fact, between 1985 and 1991, the JCAHO actually required the evaluation of all transfusions. Although only a minority of hospitals were ever reported as having complied with this require-

ment, this component of JCAHO accreditation was, nevertheless, the single most influential driving force behind enhanced blood utilization review in the United States. Since 1991, the JCAHO has made a series of modifications to this standard.

Currently, JCAHO standard PI.3.2.3 requires hospitals to measure "all blood use processes performed by the hospital, such as ordering; distributing, handling, and dispensing; administering; and monitoring blood and blood component effects on patients."[26(pPI-19)] Examples of measuring such processes are included in the section below on the functions of a transfusion committee. Surveyors are instructed to assess documentation of ongoing reviews. With respect to the appropriateness of transfusions, institutions are advised to evaluate at least 5% of transfusions if more than 600 transfusions are performed quarterly, or at least 30 transfusions if fewer than 600 transfusions are given quarterly, or all cases if there are fewer than 30 transfusions quarterly.[26(pPI-19)] The current scoring system regarding these measurements stipulates a score of 1 if the hospital is found to measure systematically its processes for the use of blood and blood components on an ongoing basis and a score of 5 if it does not.[24(pPI-23)]

JCAHO standard PI.4.5.3 specifies that the hospital should intensively assess all confirmed transfusion reactions.[26(pPI-29)] A score of 1 is achieved if this occurs in 100% of cases, a score of 3 if this occurs in 95-99% of cases, and a score of 5 if fewer than 95% of transfusion reactions are intensively assessed.[26(pPI-32)] Also, JCAHO standard MS.8.1.3 requires members of the medical staff to assess the use of blood components as a part of their "performance-improvement activities."[26(pMS-13)] Scoring for this standard is either 1 for compliance or 5 for noncompliance.[26(pMS-81)] The JCAHO also stipulates that each clinical department must develop its own criteria for determining the ability of an applicant to the clinical staff to provide patient care services within the scope of clinical privileges requested.[26(pMS-33)] The JCAHO *Comprehensive Accreditation Manual for Hospitals* states that for renewing or revising clinical privileges, these criteria could include a physician's blood prescribing practices.[26(pMS-34)]

The American Association of Blood Banks (AABB) *Standards for Blood Banks and Transfusion Services* requires all transfusing facilities to "use a peer-review program that documents monitoring of transfusion practices for all categories of components."[27(p2)] The AABB *Standards* also requires the facility to have a method for evaluating ordering practices, specimen collection, usage and discard of blood components, blood administration policies, and the ability of the transfusion service to meet patient needs. Such a requirement first appeared in the 14th edition of the *Standards*, published in 1991; prior to this, the AABB standards did not address blood utilization review.

The College of American Pathologists' blood bank inspection checklist (question 05.4085) calls for documentation confirming the participation of the medical director of the blood bank or transfusion service in establishing criteria for blood transfusion and in reviewing cases that do not meet these criteria.[28] Noncompliance with this requirement, however, is a Phase I deficiency and does not preclude achieving accreditation.

The Code of Federal Regulations requires that there be procedures for investigating adverse donor and recipient transfusion reactions[29] and that reports of such investigations be available.[30] Federal regulations relating to Medicare and Medicaid specify that hospitals must "make recommendations to the medical staff regarding improvements in transfusion procedures" and that there must be an investigation of transfusion reactions according to an institution's own established procedures.[31]

It is noteworthy that none of the standards or requirements of the accrediting and regulatory agencies mandates that an institution have a transfusion committee. However, such a committee facilitates the assessment of transfusion practices.

The Transfusion Committee

The clinical staff's governing body for each hospital must decide how it wishes to assess transfusion practices. A committee concerned exclusively with blood bank and transfusion practices is a logical solution. Such a committee should report either to the institution's medical policy committee directly or to the health care evaluation committee or office.

Structure

The committee members should represent those departments that are the principal prescribers of blood for transfusion. Representatives from hematology and/or oncology, surgery, obstetrics and gynecology, anesthesiology, and pediatrics should ordinarily be appointed to the committee. In addition, clinicians from surgical subspecialities (eg, cardiovascular surgery) and from services that may require frequent customization of blood products (eg, neonatology) should be considered for representation. Although the medical director of the blood bank must be a member, it may be preferable for this individual not to serve as chair. If the committee is perceived by the clinical staff as a discrete entity and not as a part of the blood bank or transfusion service, its policies may be more easily accepted. In fact, a persistent critic of transfusion service policies could be particularly effective as chair. The blood bank director should have no problem contributing significantly without serving as chair of the committee. If a prescriber of blood products serves as chair this could enhance the visibility, credibility, and effectiveness of the committee.

In addition to clinicians, it is appropriate to include other individuals in the committee's deliberations, such as the blood bank supervisor; a risk management representative; and individuals from medical records, information technology, and medical and surgical nursing services. The director of the blood center that supplies the institution may be a particularly valuable member as he or she may be able to provide comparisons of transfusion activities at other hospitals in the community as benchmarks.[32] If policies with medicolegal implications are under consideration (eg, look-back, informed consent), the hospital attorney should also attend.

A multidisciplinary transfusion committee will help to develop policies as members educate each other.[33-35] Monthly meetings of the committee will help ensure timely feedback, which may result in more effective utilization review. Both the hospital and the clinical governing bodies should implement committee recommendations promptly. Appointment to the transfusion committee should be for several years to allow for the acquisition of expertise, and such appointments should be staggered to promote continuity. The hospital administration should ensure an environment in which members of the clinical staff are recognized for committee service. In academic institutions, department chairs must support the participation of faculty on clinical staff committees. Faculty members may be able to use the committee's work as a source of clinical scholarship.

Functions

Utilization Review

The assessment of transfusion practices may have multiple beneficial effects. These include the potential to improve the quality of patient care; educate clinical staff; help ensure compliance with regulatory and accreditation standards; lower costs; reduce the risk of litigation; provide information about the clinical practices of individual physicians, divisions, and departments; conserve blood; and create, document, sustain, and demonstrate a high quality of care within the institution.

Undertransfusion. A patient is more likely to be harmed by not receiving a transfusion that is indicated than by receiving one that is not necessary. While most attention has been focused on identifying unnecessary transfusions, transfusion committees should be mindful of the opportunity to determine whether patients may not be receiving transfusions that are indicated. For example, the committee could review the medical records of patients with hemoglobin levels below 5.0 g/dL who were not transfused.

If the blood bank is not releasing units in a timely manner, undertransfusion can occur.[36] The unrelenting publicity regarding the real and potential risks of blood transfusion and the numerous ar-

ticles regarding inappropriate transfusion, in concert with strict policies, procedures, regulatory requirements, and accreditation standards, have created the possibility of a rigid adherence to procedures that may, in certain instances, prevent the flexibility required for rapid release of blood components for transfusion.

Surveys by the College of American Pathologists suggested that this may be a problem. In 1991 survey J-D, a 65-year-old man who had symptoms of intestinal obstruction and a hematocrit of 22% was found to have an ABO blood grouping discrepancy. Fifty-three percent of 3476 institutions stated that they would not release RBCs for transfusion until the discrepancy was resolved. Since there would have been no harm in releasing Group O RBCs in this situation and there could have been considerable harm in not doing so, this is a worrisome response. In 1992, survey J-A described a patient who was Group A Rh-negative and who had received four units of RBCs. In this report, more than 14% of 413 institutions that responded stated that they "would not transfuse" a crossmatch-compatible Group O Rh-positive unit even though no Group A RBCs were available for this patient. In this instance, it would even be appropriate to provide uncrossmatched Group O Rh-positive blood. In 1985 survey J-B, more than 11% of responding institutions said that they would have "refused to provide any component" to a patient who had red cell T activation and to whom a "plasma-containing product must be given." Thus, it would be reasonable for the transfusion committee to assure itself that excessive concern about exceptions to routine policies and procedures does not delay the release of urgently required components from the blood bank.

Unnecessary Transfusion: The Development of Screening Criteria. The assessment of transfusion practices has traditionally focused on evaluating the appropriateness of prescribed transfusions. Transfusion committee members should determine the scope of the review. It is almost always unnecessary and unduly burdensome to review retrospectively each transfusion in an institution. Instead, many hospitals have used predetermined screening criteria to evaluate all or a large number of transfusion episodes. Transfusions that meet these criteria are not subject to further review; those that do not meet the screening criteria undergo more complete evaluation. In addition, an intensive assessment of a particular transfusion may be initiated as a result of concerns by a third-party payer, patient, or provider.

Screening criteria do not constitute an absolute standard of practice. They are designed to select transfusion episodes for more intensive review. Each clinician who performs retrospective clinical assessments must remember that not every patient who has met a screening criterion necessarily has required a blood transfusion and that some patients who may require a transfusion may not have met the screening criteria. In this regard, the committee members may choose to review a few cases in which a transfusion has been given to a patient who has met one of the screening criteria. It is essential to distinguish between what has been used to select a clinical record for more intensive review and what constitutes appropriate clinical practice. Nevertheless, those who have developed screening criteria may, in fact, exert significant influence on an institution's transfusion practices.

Members of the clinical staff develop the screening criteria and perform the more intensive review. In most hospitals, these individuals are members of the transfusion committee, who will also evaluate and refine the auditing process. For such a program to work, physicians must devote a sufficient amount of time to this process, and the hospital administration must make appropriate resources available. Each clinical service that transfuses blood components and each type of component transfused in the institution should be evaluated in the course of assessing transfusion practices. A provocative suggestion has been made that the clinical staffs of hospitals should review each other's practices to avoid the problem of assessing one's close colleagues.[37]

When criteria are developed, they could be initially liberal to capture those transfusions in which inappropriate practices are most likely to have occurred. Once these have been addressed, the criteria can be tightened. Differences in clinical judg-

ment, prevailing practices, procedures performed in an institution, and patient populations will result in different screening criteria among institutions. Whatever criteria are selected, it is reasonable to ascertain initially that they are working in practice and provide a feasible framework for a retrospective review. Some have found it preferable to limit the criteria to a few easily identified variables and to minimize exceptions to the criteria themselves. Screening criteria can also be applied to the customization of blood products (eg, gamma irradiation, and cytomegalovirus-reduced-risk or leukocyte-reduced cellular components).

The screening criteria should be approved by the staff's governing body. Input and approval by other members of the clinical staff will lessen any conflicts about their validity. Those who develop the screening criteria should also be willing to evaluate them on a regular basis. Before any clinical practices are assessed, however, policies regarding the administrative response to identified deficiencies should be publicized. New members of the clinical staff and new housestaff should receive copies of the criteria, which should be disseminated throughout the institution. During the course of assessment of transfusion practices, it may become apparent that refinement is necessary. Specialists should feel free to approach the committee to suggest modifications in light of different patient populations, new clinical practices, or information that has become available. Any changes made to the criteria should also be publicized widely.

Goodnough et al have described an alternative approach in which admission and discharge hematocrits of patients are used to determine the appropriateness of blood transfusions.[38,39] This system has the advantage of avoiding both the process of extensive chart audits and dependence on a single hematocrit level, which can be misleading. Furthermore, the inadequate documentation that makes retrospective review particularly difficult[40] may be avoided.

Timing of Assessments. The assessment of transfusion practices can be conducted prospectively, concurrently, or retrospectively. A prospective review necessitates the verification that one or more specific criteria have been met before a blood component can be released for transfusion. This validation is presumably the most beneficial with regard to preventing unnecessary transfusions, but it is difficult to perform in emergency situations and it is very labor-intensive. In addition, the ideal time to discuss appropriate transfusion practices or to provide effective education may not be during the course of providing emergency care. This prospective auditing may be most useful prior to the provision of customized blood products such as those that have undergone gamma irradiation or leukocyte reduction.

Concurrent audits are performed shortly after a transfusion—for example, within 24 hours. Although common sense indicates that this prompt feedback should be very useful, it requires a sustained effort and is not always practical to perform. Audits performed retrospectively 1 day or more after a transfusion are easier to complete but should still be done as soon after the transfusion as possible to achieve maximal effectiveness.

One approach has been to combine prospective justification with a retrospective audit. This has been accomplished using either a computer-generated ordering form or a requisition slip. In each case, screening criteria can be used as an integral part of the blood prescription process. The ordering clinician notes the transfusion criteria met by a patient or provides a different clinical justification for transfusion. Table 21-1 contains examples of such screening criteria that could be used.[41] Various other screening criteria for adult and pediatric blood transfusion practices have been published.[42-48] Subsequently, some or all of the "other" options that have been provided as justification prospectively are reviewed more intensively. Transfusions thought to pose the most significant risk, or those deemed the most likely to be inappropriate on the basis of other laboratory values noted in the patient, could be selected for review. It is unlikely to be feasible, as a routine practice, to review retrospectively every order in which another indication has been selected. The members of the transfusion committee should rotate their review among differ-

ent clinical services or different procedures. For hospitals that have not implemented screening criteria as part of the ordering process, unusual transfusion episodes are a logical place to focus blood utilization review. Although retrospective audits are usually performed by members of a clinical staff transfusion committee, it is possible that one individual or a less formal small group could be as effective in some institutions. As noted, the clinician conducting a retrospective review must always consider both the information available to the physician as well as the patient's clinical condition at the time the transfusion was prescribed.

Consequences of Utilization Review. The JCAHO *Comprehensive Accreditation Manual for Hospitals* states that results of peer review of clinical performance must be included when physicians are being considered for renewal or revision of clinical privileges.[26(pMS-40)]

The conclusions of the individuals performing retrospective review should be presented to the transfusion committee as a whole, if this is the body performing the assessment. There should be an opportunity to discuss the reviewer's recommendation. If it is determined that a particular transfusion may have deviated from acceptable clinical practice, an appropriate course is to invite, in writing, the physician who ordered the transfusion to provide an explanation for the transfusion in question. A sample letter to the prescribing physician is presented in Fig 21-1. Once the physician's response is received, the committee can make a final determination regarding the appropriateness of the transfusion and then inform the physician. If the physician's response satisfies the members of the committee, the committee should promptly communicate this to the clinician. If the physician chooses not to respond, the judgment of the committee should be made a part of the permanent record of the committee's deliberations. A copy of all correspondence with the physician should be made available to the clinician's department chair as well as to the risk management staff. In addition, the findings from transfusion practice assessments should be summarized for department chairs and division directors. Since it is likely that transfusion

Table 21-1. Criteria That May Be Used to Preclude More Intensive Review of the Appropriateness of Blood Component Transfusion and That May Be Incorporated into Blood Ordering Procedures*

Red Blood Cells:

1. Hematocrit <25% and/or hemoglobin <8 g/dL

2. Acute blood loss greater than 20% of estimated blood volume

3. Coronary or cerebral vascular disease and hematocrit <30%

4. >10% surface burns and hematocrit <30%

5. To improve oxygen delivery in a patient with sepsis, septic shock, or acute respiratory distress syndrome, and hemoglobin <12 g/dL

6. Neonate: hematocrit <40% with respiratory distress; otherwise, hematocrit <30% or blood loss >10% of blood volume

Platelet Concentrate:

1. Bleeding or a planned invasive or surgical procedure and any one or more of the following:

    a. platelet count <80,000/μL (neonate: <100,000/μL)

    b. bleeding time >7.5 minutes

    c. documented platelet function disorder

    d. infusion of > one blood volume of red blood cells and other volume-expanding fluids in the previous 24 hours

2. Platelet count <100,000/μL in a patient who either:

    a. has retinal or cerebral hemorrhage

    b. has undergone a cardiopulmonary bypass procedure

3. Prophylactically for platelet count <10,000/μL (neonate: <40,000/μL)

4. Infusion of > one blood volume of red blood cells and other volume-expanding fluids in the previous 24 hours

Fresh Frozen Plasma:

1. Bleeding or a planned invasive or surgical procedure and any one or more of the following:

    a. prothrombin time >1.5 times the midpoint of the reference range

    b. partial thromboplastin time >1.5 times the top of the reference range

    c. documented deficiency of Factor II, V, VII, X, or XI

    d. infusion of > one blood volume of red blood cells and other volume-expanding fluids in the previous 24 hours

2. Thrombotic thrombocytopenic purpura

3. Hemolytic-uremic syndrome

Cryoprecipitate-Depleted Plasma:

1. Thrombotic thrombocytopenic purpura

2. Hemolytic-uremic syndrome

3. Deficiency of Factor II, V, VII, X, or XI

Table 21-1. Criteria That May Be Used to Preclude More Intensive Review of the Appropriateness of Blood Component Transfusion and That May Be Incorporated into Blood Ordering Procedures* (continued)

Cryoprecipitate:

Bleeding or a planned invasive or surgical procedure and any one or more of the following:

    a. documented deficiency of fibrinogen (<80 mg/dL)

    b. von Willebrand disease

    c. uremic platelet dysfunction (bleeding time >7.5 minutes)

    d. documented deficiency of Factor XIII

Granulocyte Concentrate:

Neutropenia (<1000/µL) with documented infection unresponsive to antibiotics

Rh Immune Globulin:

1.   postpartum D-negative mother with D-positive infant

2.   antepartum D-negative woman at 28 weeks' gestation or with risk of recent fetomaternal hemorrhage

3.   D-negative female after abortion, ectopic pregnancy, miscarriage, amniocentesis, percutaneous umbilical blood sampling, chorionic villus sampling, or death in utero

4.   transfusion of D-positive cellular blood components to a D-negative patient

---

*These screening criteria are not absolute indications for blood component transfusion.

Adapted with permission from Mintz PD.[41(pp222-3)]

---

practices will be audited selectively, the review should be rotated among the different clinical divisions. Committee minutes with collected information appended should also be provided to the entity to which the transfusion committee reports. If specific problems with transfusion practices are identified, the practices should be subject to repeated evaluation.

An important element of the assessment of any clinical practice is the communication of conclusions regarding good practices to clinicians, division directors, and department chairs. These communications may reinforce appropriate practices and may also lead to the willingness of practitioners to accept comments in the future that may be less supportive. The committee should see its overriding purpose as one of staff education rather than viewing its work as a punitive activity. The latter approach obviously can antagonize the individuals whom the process is designed to instruct. Utilization review can actually be an important element in documenting continuing excellence or ongoing improvement in clinical practice. If utilization review finds no opportunities for improvement, the screening criteria and methods used to perform retrospective review should be assessed to determine their validity.

Results of Utilization Review. A number of reports have documented that assessing transfusion practices and providing educational programs improve clinical practice. Toy found that the most successful programs combined individual education of the prescribing clinician with audits of clinical practice either prior to or within 1-2 days after

Dear Dr. _____:

The Transfusion Committee is charged with reviewing transfusion practices. At its meeting on _____, the members of the Committee reviewed the transfusion of _____ prescribed by you on _____ for _____ (history number _____). The members of the Committee did not find documentation in the medical record justifying the transfusion.

The members of the Committee understand that there may be reasons for prescribing the transfusion that are not apparent from reviewing the patient's medical record. Therefore, we would appreciate any additional information that you can provide regarding the reasons for ordering this transfusion. Such information will afford the Committee the opportunity to conduct a more complete review. We appreciate your responding to this request by ____*(date)*____. Thank you for your attention to this matter.

Sincerely,

_____
Chair, Transfusion Committee

Figure 21-1. Transfusion Committee communication with prescribing physician. (Adapted from *Guidelines for Blood Utilization Review.*[46(p25)])

transfusion.[49] Discussions regarding blood usage for specific patients have reportedly prompted changes in practice where lectures had not done so.[50] Shanberge demonstrated a 77% reduction in the use of Fresh Frozen Plasma (FFP) over a 2-year period after the implementation of a next-day review complemented by an educational program.[51] Simpson reported on a prospective audit of platelet transfusions that led to a significant improvement in ordering practices and a 56% reduction in platelet use.[52]

Solomon et al reported a 52% decrease in FFP use after the implementation of a retrospective audit, a revised FFP request form that required the prescribing physician to indicate the reason for the request, an educational program, and prior approval in patients lacking documentation of abnormal coagulation results.[53] McCullough et al performed an audit of platelet use, subsequently modified practice guidelines, and then applied these guidelines prospectively to requests for platelets. This program led to a 14% decrease in the number of platelet transfusions during the subsequent year.[54] Silver et al reported that a prospective review resulted in more appropriate transfusion practices, a significant reduction in donor exposures, and substantial cost savings.[55] Lepage et al reported a drop in the hematocrits of persons being transfused from 28.6% to 27.7% as well as a reduction in the number of transfusion orders requiring review after the computerized screening of blood transfusion requests was implemented.[56]

Morrison et al reported a 75% decrease in the total number of red cells transfused by an obstetrics and gynecology service after a year-long audit and educational program.[57] Rosen et al noted a significant decrease in allogeneic donor exposures and substantial cost savings after establishing transfusion guidelines based on national standards and implementing a system that required physicians to record medical indications for all nonemergency transfusions.[58] Hawkins et al reported that a mandatory pretransfusion approval program resulted in a 33% decrease in FFP transfusions.[59]

Cheng et al demonstrated a significant reduction in inappropriate platelet and FFP transfusions after they introduced a new component request form with transfusion guidelines printed on it.[60] Tuckfield et al also noted a significant decrease in inappropriate RBC, platelet, and FFP transfusions after the request form was modified to include the indications for transfusion and relevant clinical and laboratory data.[61] Joshi et al demonstrated improved transfusion practices in patients undergoing total hip arthroplasty during an ongoing quality assurance program.[62] Marconi et al implemented the practice of permitting only a limited number of physicians to submit nonurgent blood prescriptions, accompanied by a computerized prospective audit of blood requests. They demonstrated a high level of appropriateness for RBC and platelet requests and improved ordering practices for plasma.[63] Although this novel approach would not be feasible in every institution, their report illustrates the usefulness of specialists in improving transfusion practices. Toy has reviewed how systematic audits and targeted education can improve transfusion practice.[64] She noted how multi-institutional audits[65,66] can serve as useful benchmarking tools.

Other Related Activities

A transfusion committee can pursue a variety of useful activities in addition to assessing blood transfusion practices. As noted, JCAHO accreditation standards require measuring performance with regard to ordering, distributing, handling, dispensing, and administering blood components[26(pPI-19)]

and also require monitoring the effects of blood transfusion on patients. Table 21-2 is a template for a checklist that an institution could develop for complying with these requirements.

While it is obviously not possible for the committee continually to conduct reviews on every activity related to transfusion, the following list is designed to serve as a menu from which individuals charged with ensuring compliance with the JCAHO recommendations may select activities they find appropriate for their own institution.

1. Review that transfusions are appropriately documented in the medical record. The institution's policies regarding appropriate documentation should be followed. The transfusion record may be audited to ensure that it includes the information the institution requires regarding the recipient's identification, the results of compatibility testing, the transfusion volume administered, the expiration time or date of the component, the time of transfusion, the identification of the person administering the transfusion, and information about the patient's clinical status during the transfusion. A program for nurses providing information about documenting and monitoring transfusions has been reported to improve these practices.[67]

2. Review compliance with the informed consent process for blood transfusion.

3. Review that the medical record contains documentation of the indications for transfusion, the prescription for the transfusion, and the outcome of the transfusion.

4. Ensure that there are adequate policies and procedures for detecting, reporting, and evaluating transfusion reactions as well as for reviewing the timeliness and adequacy of the ensuing investigations.

5. Review the hospital's look-back activities and ensure that they comply with federal regulations and guidelines.

6. Evaluate the utilization of devices used with blood transfusions. This could include verification that adequate quality control has been performed on infusion pumps and blood

Table 21-2. Monitoring the Ordering, Dispensing, Handling, and Administration of Blood Components

1. Time request for blood component was received.
2. Was there a prescription for the transfusion?
3. Was the request submitted correctly?
4. Was the correct component selected for issue?
5. Was the component inspected?
6. Was the component outdated?
7. Was documentation prior to issue completed correctly?
8. Time transportation was notified component was available.
9. Time component was issued.
10. Was the correct filter issued?
11. Was documentation regarding transportation completed correctly?
12. Time component was delivered by transportation.
13. Was the blood component unattended after release from the blood bank? Where was it?
14. Was informed consent obtained in accord with written procedure?
15. Were patient and blood component identification properly performed in accord with written procedure before transfusion was started?
16. Was documentation on the transfusion slip accurate and complete?
17. Were pretransfusion vital signs taken and recorded?
18. Was filter attached properly?
19. Was arm/port preparation properly performed?
20. Time transfusion was started. Was this documented?
21. Were only approved solutions in contact with the component?
22. Were only approved solutions mixed with the component?
23. If utilized, was a blood warmer and/or infusion pump used in accord with written procedure?
24. Were vital signs taken and recorded during the transfusion in accord with written procedure?
25. Was any transfusion reaction reported to a physician and the blood bank in accord with written procedure?
26. Time transfusion was completed. Was this documented?
27. Were vital signs taken and recorded and was the patient observed after transfusion in accord with written procedures?
28. Were the component bag and other materials disposed of correctly?
29. Were written instructions about adverse reactions provided if the recipient was an outpatient or at home?
30. Was all documentation placed in the patient's permanent record in accord with written procedure?
31. Was the outcome of the transfusion documented in the medical record?

warmers and that appropriate personnel have reviewed the policies for using these devices.

7. Review aspects of autologous blood use and collection, if performed. Allison and Toy reported how a quality improvement team improved the availability of autologous and directed donor blood and had a far-reaching impact on quality improvement methodology throughout the medical center.[68]

    Although the risk of bacterial contamination, clerical error, and hypervolemia exist with autologous blood, and although autologous blood should not be given simply because it is available, the transfusion committee could establish a more liberal policy when reviewing autologous transfusions because they are safer than allogeneic blood. The same auditing criteria, however, may be used to determine which cases require more intensive review. The use of perioperative autologous transfusion services is also properly within the committee's purview.

8. Review the performance of the blood transfusion service regarding its timeliness of response, its productivity, and the outdating of blood products.

9. Audit the use of customized products, such as cytomegalovirus-reduced-risk blood components, gamma-irradiated components, leukocyte-reduced components, uncrossmatched blood, and "fresh" blood.

10. Audit the use and underuse of single-unit transfusions in particular circumstances. A single-unit transfusion may often represent good clinical practice. If one transfusion has provided sufficient oxygen delivery, there should be no need for additional transfusions. The committee may wish to audit carefully the last unit or units given as a series of red cell transfusions (see 11 below). It may be more likely that these are unnecessary than are single-unit transfusions.

11. Review the last unit or few units of consecutive transfusions to one patient. There may have been one determination of a low hemoglobin concentration or one episode of hemorrhage that led to the transfusion of a number of units of blood of which the last unit or few units may have been unnecessary. In many auditing strategies, these transfusions may not routinely be called to the attention of the committee because the patient may have initially met a particular screening criterion. Nevertheless, these may be among the least needed transfusions provided. Therefore, the committee members may wish to review situations in which more than a single unit of blood has been transfused on the basis of a specific criterion to determine whether each of the units was truly indicated. Gillham and Mark noted that two-unit transfusions were commonly given to patients undergoing total hip replacement when one would have sufficed.[69] Determining the patient's hematocrit prior to the transfusion of each unit of blood could reduce the number of RBC transfusions significantly.[70]

12. Audit whether the hospital's preoperative blood crossmatch ordering guidelines for elective surgery are followed.[71] Murphy et al demonstrated that effectively using crossmatch guidelines for elective surgery did not compromise patient care.[72]

13. Audit the truthfulness of physicians in choosing the criteria that are selected to justify blood transfusion. The author has periodically performed such audits in his hospital and found complete veracity in this regard.

14. Review the wastage of blood owing to the failure to return unused units to the blood bank.[73]

15. Evaluate staff adherence to the institutional policies regarding the dispensing and handling of blood and ensure that such policies are regularly reviewed (eg, every 12 months).

16. Observe the administration of transfusions to ensure that proper patient and blood component identification has been completed prior to the transfusion according to written procedure.

Monitoring the ordering, handling, dispensing, and administration of transfusions is important because fatal hemolytic transfusion reactions are most commonly due to an error in patient, specimen, or blood component identification, resulting in an ABO-incompatible transfusion.[74] When Shulman et al introduced a program that permitted direct oversight of transfusionists' practices, they noted that the percentage of transfusions at variance from institutional policy decreased from 50% to nearly zero as a result of this activity.[75] Shulman and Jones described in detail how such monitoring can be accomplished successfully,[76] suggesting that it should generally be done randomly but that some instances could be intentionally selected to review performance in specific clinical services. They emphasized that these assessments should include intraoperative transfusions and should be ongoing to monitor the effects of personnel turnover and new equipment. They noted that their programs had found system flaws and educational opportunities in both hospitals studied; variances from procedures were due to insufficient knowledge, carelessness, and system defects. They concluded that internal assessment must be accompanied by training, in-service education, and competency assessment. Boone et al demonstrated how careful monitoring can effectively identify correctable errors in blood administration.[77]

In addition to selecting the aforementioned activities to comply with JCAHO standards, the committee may focus its attention on a number of other activities:

1. Review accreditation and inspection reports and the results of proficiency testing from the blood bank and transfusion service.
2. Review the adequacy and timeliness of delivery of blood components from the hospital's blood supplier. In this regard, it may be helpful to have the director of the blood center attend those committee meetings that address this issue if he or she is not a committee member.
3. Review the crossmatch:transfusion ratio from selected services or within the whole institution. Although there is no accreditation requirement to determine this ratio and

its utility has been overstated in the past, there may be selected divisions within the institution that have a significantly elevated ratio. An appropriate ratio is typically less than 2:1.
4. Develop hospital policies related to transfusion practices. The committee may be instrumental in such areas as informed consent for blood transfusion and the development of look-back procedures for patients who have received blood from donors subsequently found to be infected with an agent that is potentially transmissible by blood transfusion.
5. Serve as an advocate for the blood bank and transfusion service to the institution's administrative and clinical staff for personnel, space, or equipment needs.

The transfusion committee will typically select areas for review that will help the institution maintain compliance with the JCAHO accreditation standards as well as monitor those areas that the members view as most in need of oversight or improvement. All written communications related to the committee's activities should be marked as part of the hospital's quality assessment program. This may make these communications less likely to be available in the discovery process for legal proceedings. The members of the committee should be familiar with state laws and regulations regarding the discoverability of these materials (eg, committee minutes, records, reports, and correspondence). Some states' statutes may prevent their routine discoverability but may, in fact, allow courts to order the disclosure of these records if extraordinary circumstances warrant it.

Conclusion

Although successful quality assessment programs create "an environment of watchful concern,"[8(p1747)] they should be conducted in a professional, nonadversarial, and educational manner. Despite the difficulties caused by disagreement regarding treatment options (such as when RBC transfusions are indicated in the acutely anemic patient) and the necessity of using surrogate markers due to unavailability of data (such as that needed to establish oxygen deficit), the assessment of transfusion practices provides many benefits. It can improve the judgment and enhance the knowledge of physicians and other health-care professionals; provide useful information about patient management; decrease the risk of litigation; reduce costs; help to ensure compliance with accreditation and regulatory requirements; conserve the blood supply; provide an opportunity to demonstrate a high level of quality and value to the public and institutional oversight boards; and help create, document, and sustain excellence in patient care.

References

1. Valeri CR, Crowley JP, Loscalzo J. The red cell transfusion trigger: Has a sin of commission now become a sin of omission? Transfusion 1998;38:602-10.

2. Weiskopf RB. Do we know when to transfuse red cells to treat acute anemia (editorial)? Transfusion 1998;38:517-21.

3. Allain J-P, Williamson LM. How can we best achieve optimal transfusion practice (editorial)? Med J Aust 1997;167:462-3.

4. Royal College of Physicians of Edinburgh. Consensus statement on red cell transfusion. Transfus Med 1994;4:177-8.

5. Wallace EL, Churchill WH, Surgenor DM, et al. Collection and transfusion of blood and blood components in the United States, 1994. Transfusion 1998;38:625-36.

6. Headrick LA, Neuhauser D. Quality healthcare. JAMA 1994;271:1711-2.

7. Kritchevsky SB, Simmons BP. Continuous quality improvement: Concepts and applications for physician care. JAMA 1991;266:1817-23.

8. Donabedian A. The quality of care: How can it be assessed? JAMA 1988;260:1743-8.

9. Brown HM. The beginnings of intravenous medication. Ann Med Hist 1917;1:177-97.

10. Bock AV. Use and abuse of blood transfusions. N Engl J Med 1936;215:421-5.

11. Fantus B. The therapy of Cook County Hospital. JAMA 1937;109:128-31.

12. Use of blood for transfusions. Lancet 1951;2:1044.

13. Garland J, Smith RM, Lanman TH, et al. Abuse of transfusion therapy (editorial). N Engl J Med 1951;245:745-6.

14. Straus B, Torres JM. Use and abuse of blood transfusion. JAMA 1953;151:699-701.

15. Crisp WE. One pint of blood. Obstet Gynecol 1956;7:216-7.

16. Cantor D. A legal look at blood transfusions. GP 1957;16:82-4.

17. Crosby WH. Misuse of blood transfusions. Blood 1958;13:1198-200.

18. Crosby WH. Misuse of blood transfusions. Med Bull U S Army, Europe 1958;15:7.

19. Friesen R. The use and abuse of blood in abortions. Can Med Assoc J 1959;80:802-5.

20. Graham-Stewart CW. A clinical survey of blood transfusion. Lancet 1960;2:421-4.

21. Bulletin of Joint Commission on Accreditation of Hospitals, publication 26, March 1961. Oakbrook Terrace, IL: Joint Commission on Accreditation of Hospitals, 1961.

22. MacDonald I. Editorial. Bull L A Co Med Assoc 1961;91:57-8.

23. Crosby WH. The hospital transfusion board. Transfusion 1962;2:1-2.

24. Walz DV. An effective hospital transfusion committee. JAMA 1964;189:660-2.

25. The transfusion of blood (editorial). JAMA 1964;189:116.

26. Comprehensive accreditation manual for hospitals. Oakbrook Terrace, IL: Joint Commission on Accreditation of Healthcare Organizations, 1998.

27. Menitove JE, ed. Standards for blood banks and transfusion services. 18th ed. Bethesda, MD: American Association of Blood Banks, 1997.

28. Inspection checklist, transfusion procedures. Northfield, IL: College of American Pathologists, 1998.

29. Code of federal regulations. 21 CFR 606.100 (9). Washington, DC: US Government Printing Office, 1998 (revised annually).

30. Code of federal regulations. 21 CFR 606.160 (b)(1)(iii), (b)(6), and 606.170. Washington, DC: US Government Printing Office, 1998 (revised annually).

31. CCH Medicare and Medicaid guide. 22,142F. 482.27(d)(6). Riverwoods, IL: Commerce Clearing House, (continuously updated).

32. Chapman RG. The role of the community blood center in improving transfusion practice. In: Wallas CH, Muller VH, eds. The hospital transfusion committee. Arlington, VA: American Association of Blood Banks, 1982:87-94.

33. Sandlow LJ, Bashook PG, Maxwell JA. Medical care evaluation: An experience in continuing education. J Med Educ 1981;56:580-6.

34. Bashook PG, Maxwell JA, Sandlow LJ. Increasing the educational value of medical care evaluation: A model program. J Med Educ 1982;57:701-7.

35. Maxwell JA, Sandlow LJ, Bashook PG. Effect of a medical care evaluation program on physician knowledge and performance. J Med Educ 1984;59:33-8.

36. Mintz PD. Undertransfusion (editorial). Am J Clin Pathol 1992;98:150-1.

37. Epstein BH, Kaufman A. Hospital peer review: A new proposal. JAMA 1994;271:1485.

38. Goodnough LT, Verbrugge D, Vizmeg K, et al. Identifying elective orthopedic surgical patients transfused with amounts of blood in excess of need: The transfusion trigger revisited. Transfusion 1992;32:648-53.

39. Goodnough LT, Vizmeg K, Riddell J IV, et al. Discharge haematocrit as clinical indicator for blood transfusion audit in surgery patients. Transfus Med 1994;4:35-44.

40. Audet AM, Goodnough LT, Parvin CA. Evaluating the appropriateness of red blood cell transfusions: The limitations of retrospective medical record reviews. Int J Qual Health Care 1996;8:41-9.

41. Mintz PD. Quality assessment and improvement of transfusion practices. Hematol/Oncol Clin North Am 1995;9:219-32.

42. Silberstein LE, Kruskall MS, Stehling LC, et al. Strategies for the review of transfusion practices. JAMA 1989;262:1993-7.

43. Blanchette VS, Hume HA, Levy GJ, et al. Guidelines for auditing pediatric blood transfusion practices. Am J Dis Child 1991;145:787-96.

44. Pediatric Hemotherapy Committee. Guidelines for conducting pediatric transfusion audits. 3rd ed. Bethesda, MD: American Association of Blood Banks, 1992.

45. Stehling L, Luban NLC, Anderson KC, et al. Guidelines for blood utilization and review. Transfusion 1994;34:438-48.

46. Transfusion Practices Quality Assurance Committee. Guidelines for blood utilization review. Bethesda, MD: American Association of Blood Banks, 1994.

47. Cummings JP. Technology assessment: Red blood cell transfusion guidelines. Oak Brook, IL: University HealthSystem Consortium Clinical Practice Advancement Center, 1997.

48. Cummings JP. Technology assessment: Platelet transfusion guidelines. Oak Brook, IL: University HealthSystem Consortium Clinical Practice Advancement Center, 1998.

49. Toy PTCY. Effectiveness of transfusion audits and practice guidelines. Arch Pathol Lab Med 1994;118:435-7.

50. Bergin JJ. The composition and function of the hospital transfusion committee: Historical perspective. In: Wallas CH, Muller VH, eds. The hospital transfusion committee. Arlington, VA: American Association of Blood Banks, 1982:7-13.

51. Shanberge JN. Reduction of fresh-frozen plasma use through a daily survey and education program. Transfusion 1987;27:226-7.

52. Simpson MB. Prospective-concurrent audits and medical consultation for platelet transfusions. Transfusion 1987;27:192-5.

53. Solomon RR, Clifford JS, Gutman SI. The use of laboratory intervention to stem the flow of fresh-frozen plasma. Am J Clin Pathol 1988;89:518-21.

54. McCullough J, Steeper TA, Connelly DP, et al. Platelet utilization in a university hospital. JAMA 1988;259:2414-8.

55. Silver H, Tahhan HR, Anderson J, Lachman M. A non-computer-dependent prospective review of blood and blood component utilization. Transfusion 1992;32:260-5.

56. Lepage EF, Gardner RM, Laub RM, Golubjatnikov OK. Improving blood transfusion practice: Role of a computerized hospital information system. Transfusion 1992;32:253-9.

57. Morrison JC, Sumrall DD, Chevalier SP, et al. The effect of provider education on blood utilization practices. Am J Obstet Gynecol 1993;169:1240-5.

58. Rosen NR, Bates LH, Herod G. Transfusion therapy: Improved patient care and resource utilization. Transfusion 1993;33:341-7.

59. Hawkins TE, Carter JM, Hunter PM. Can mandatory pretransfusion approval programmes be improved? Transfus Med 1994; 4:45-50.

60. Cheng G, Wong HF, Chan A, Chui CH. The effects of a self-educating blood component request form and enforcements of transfusion guidelines on FFP and platelet usage. Clin Lab Haematol 1996;18:83-7.

61. Tuckfield A, Haeusler MN, Grigg AP, Metz J. Reduction of inappropriate use of blood products by prospective monitoring of transfusion request forms. Med J Aust 1997;167:473-6.

62. Joshi G, McCarroll M, O'Rourke P, Coffey F. Role of quality assessment in improving red blood cell transfusion practice. Ir J Med Sci 1997;166:16-9.

63. Marconi M, Almini D, Pizzi MN, et al. Quality assurance of clinical transfusion practice by implementation of the privilege of blood prescription and computerized prospective audit of blood requests. Transfus Med 1996; 6:11-9.

64. Toy PTCY. Audit and education in transfusion medicine. Vox Sang 1996;70:1-5.

65. Toy PT, Strauss RG, Stehling LC, et al. Predeposit autologous blood for elective surgery: A national multicenter study. N Engl J Med 1987;316:517-20.

66. Goodnough LT, Soegiarso RW, Birkmeyer JD, Welch HG. Economic impact of inappropriate blood transfusions in coronary artery bypass graft surgery. Am J Med 1993;94:509-14.

67. Devine P, McClure PL. Quality assurance of hospital transfusion practices: The role of nursing staff. Qual Rev Bull 1988;14:250-3.

68. Allison MJ, Toy P. A quality improvement team on autologous and directed-donor blood availability. Joint Commission Journal on Quality Improvement 1996;22:801-10.

69. Gillham M, Mark A. A retrospective audit of blood loss in total hip joint replacement surgery at Middlemore Hospital. N Z Med J 1997;110:294-7.

70. Tartter PI, Barron DM. Unnecessary blood transfusions in elective colorectal cancer surgery. Transfusion 1985;25:113-5.

71. Mintz PD, Nordine R, Henry JB, Webb W. Expected hemotherapy in elective surgery. N Y State J Med 1976;76:532-7.

72. Murphy WG, Phillips P, Gray A, et al. Blood use for surgical patients: A study of Scottish hospital transfusion practices. J R Coll Surg Edinb 1995; 40:10-3.

73. Clark JA, Ayoub MM. Blood and component wastage report: A quality assurance function of the hospital transfusion committee. Transfusion 1989;29:139-42.

74. Sazama K. Reports of 355 transfusion-associated deaths: 1976–1985. Transfusion 1990;30:583-90.

75. Shulman IA, Lohr K, Derdiarian AK, Picukaric JM. Monitoring transfusionist practices: A strategy for improving transfusion safety. Transfusion 1994;34:11-5.

76. Shulman IA, Jones FS. Practical aspects of the self-assessment of the issue and administration of blood. Am J Clin Pathol 1997;107: S17-22.

77. Boone DJ, Steindel D, Herron R, et al. Transfusion medicine monitoring practices. A study of the College of American Pathologists/Centers for Disease Control and Prevention Outcomes Working Group. Arch Pathol Lab Med 1995;119:999-1006.

Index